W9-BCN-856

The Law

of Healthcare

Administration

EIGHTH
EDITION

The Law
of Healthcare
Administration

J. STUART SHOWALTER

AUPHA

Health Administration Press, Chicago, Illinois

Association of University Programs in Health Administration, Washington, DC

21 20 19 18   5 4 3 2

Library of Congress Cataloging-in-Publication Data

Names: Showalter, J. Stuart, author.
Title: The law of healthcare administration / J. Stuart Showalter.
Description: Eighth Edition. | Chicago, Illinois : Health Administration Press; Washington, DC : Association of University Programs in Health Administration, 2017.
Identifiers: LCCN 2016045989 (print) | LCCN 2016046145 (ebook) | ISBN 9781567938760 (print : alk. paper) | ISBN 9781567938777 (Ebook) | ISBN 9781567938784 (Xml) | ISBN 9781567938791 (Epub) | ISBN 9781567938807 (Mobi)
Subjects: LCSH: Medical care—Law and legislation—United States. | Hospitals—Law and legislation—United States. | Medical laws and legislation—United States.
Classification: LCC KF3825 .S65 2017 (print) | LCC KF3825 (ebook) | DDC 344.7303/21 dc23
LC record available at https://lccn.loc.gov/2016045989

The paper used in this publication meets the minimum requirements of American National Standard for Information Sciences—Permanence of Paper for Printed Library Materials, ANSI Z39.48-1984. ∞ ™

Acquisitions editor: Janet Davis; Project manager: Theresa L. Rothschadl; Cover designer: James Slate; Layout: Cepheus Edmondson

Found an error or a typo? We want to know! Please e-mail it to hapbooks@ache.org, mentioning the book's title and putting "Book Error" in the subject line.

For photocopying and copyright information, please contact Copyright Clearance Center at www.copyright.com or at (978) 750-8400.

Health Administration Press
A division of the Foundation of the American
  College of Healthcare Executives
One North Franklin Street, Suite 1700
Chicago, IL 60606-3529
(312) 424-2800

Association of University Programs
  in Health Administration
1730 M Street
Suite 407
Washington, DC 20036
(703) 894-0940

BRIEF CONTENTS

DETAILED CONTENTS

PREFACE

Overview

As in prior editions, this newest *The Law of Healthcare Administration* attempts to offer a thorough treatment of health law in the United States in plain language for ease of use. The eighth edition moves from broad-brush treatments of the US legal system and the history of medicine to specific issues that affect healthcare leaders on a daily basis: contracts, torts, taxation, antitrust law, regulatory compliance, and of course health insurance reform. For this latter topic, the Affordable Care Act (ACA) takes center stage.

The ACA Is Prominent

We saw important changes in the healthcare sector after the ACA became law in 2010. It has been the most significant development in healthcare since Medicare and Medicaid were passed half a century ago.

Government figures show that by early 2016 an estimated 20 million people had gained insurance coverage under the ACA—the uninsured rate declined from 16.0 percent (49 million people) in 2010 to 9.1 percent (29 million) in 2015. The reasons for these improved numbers include Medicaid expansion, creation of the health insurance exchanges, and requirements that private insurance plans cover preexisting conditions and allow young adults to stay on their parents' plans to age 26.[1]

Chapter 3, titled "Health Reform, Access to Care, and Admission and Discharge," reviews the history of reform efforts, discusses the implications of Medicaid expansion, and goes to considerable length to present *NFIB v. Sebelius* and *King v. Burwell*, the two most serious legal challenges. Taken together, those decisions seem to have settled the most significant constitutional issues; despite the ACA's landmark status, however, its future is in doubt as the Donald J. Trump administration takes over. Readers will need to stay tuned for future developments.

Other Highlights of the Eighth Edition

This edition also contains new material on the following topics:

- The history of nursing, which has been added to chapter 2
- The status of Medicare's inpatient admission standards and the "two-midnight rule"

- The "dual capacity" doctrine in worker's compensation
- End-of-life topics including the Physician Orders for Life-Sustaining Treatment (POLST) paradigm and "death with dignity" laws in some states, which allow physicians to aid terminally ill patients in ending their own lives
- Prominent antitrust cases from Ohio, Idaho, and North Carolina
- The *Whole Woman's Health* case, in which the Supreme Court again reaffirmed the essential holdings of *Roe v. Wade* and related cases
- The Supreme Court's decision on "implied certification," plus other false claims and fraud-related issues

In Addition

Throughout the book I have updated citations, added current URLs, and made editorial changes to minimize (or at least clarify) legal jargon and make the text as accessible to nonlawyers as possible.

Like the editions before it, the eighth edition of *The Law of Healthcare Administration* is a practical text for students and educators in health administration, public health, nursing, and similar programs or disciplines.

Chapter Contents

Chapter 1: The Anglo-American Legal System

This chapter discusses the history of law, its sources, the relationships among the three branches of government, the basic structure of the federal and state court systems, and some basics of legal procedure in civil cases.

Chapter 2: A Brief History of Medicine

Because "a page of history is worth a volume of logic," chapter 2 adds to the foundational concepts of chapter 1 and sets the stage for material explored in the remaining 13 chapters.

Chapter 3: Health Reform, Access to Care, and Admission and Discharge

This chapter discusses the ACA's major changes, important decisions regarding the act by the US Supreme Court, and the potential that the legislation might be undone by the Trump administration. The chapter also presents traditional rules about hospital admission and discharge, law relating to emergency services, and the conflict between managed care organizations' desire to limit healthcare expenditures and providers' moral and legal duties to give quality patient care.

Chapter 4: Contracts and Intentional Torts

This chapter addresses the essential elements of a valid contract (competent parties, "meeting of the minds," consideration, and legality of purpose) and the importance of contract law in the relationships between patients and their physicians and between patients and hospitals. The chapter also briefly discusses issues related to workers' compensation and intentional tort, pointing out that both can affect physician–patient and hospital–patient relationships.

Chapter 5: Negligence

This chapter outlines the four basic elements of proof in a tort case, the ways the standard of care can be proven, and the concept of causation. It addresses *respondeat superior* (vicarious liability), the "school rule," *res ipsa loquitur*, defenses to malpractice suits, and alternatives to the tort system.

Chapter 6: The Organization and Management of a Corporate Healthcare Institution

This chapter reviews some basic concepts of corporation law, including a corporation's "personhood," its ability to shield owners from personal liability, the foundations and limitations of corporate power, and the duties of a corporation's governing board. The concept of piercing the corporate veil and the various reasons for and methods of restructuring a healthcare corporation are also explored. Attention is also given to hospital–physician joint ventures and their potential for renewal due to the effects of the ACA and other factors in the healthcare environment.

Chapter 7: Liability of the Healthcare Institution

This chapter shows that the law has come a long way in recent years as it relates to healthcare organizations: The shift from charitable immunity to application of respondeat superior in the healthcare setting is one example. The demise of the "captain-of-the-ship" and "borrowed-servant" doctrines is another. These notions have now expanded to the point that the independent contractor defense seems no longer viable in the healthcare field. The chapter also addresses the rise of managed care in the 1980s and 1990s, the conflicts that sometimes arise between advancing patient welfare and reducing healthcare costs, and the phenomenon of Employee Retirement Income Security Act (ERISA) preemption providing immunity for some managed care organizations.

Chapter 8: Medical Staff Privileges and Peer Review

This chapter focuses on decisions about medical staff privileges. It points out that management and the medical staff are responsible for the credentialing process and may recommend physician applicants (including doctors of osteopathy, dentistry, podiatry, and chiropractic, as well as other physicians, depending on state law). The ultimate responsibility for appointing a competent medical staff lies with the hospital governing board, however. The chapter also addresses issues related to the peer review and quality assurance functions, both of which are efforts to monitor the quality of care. It concludes with some thoughts about accountable care organizations, complementary and alternative medicine practices, and "integrative healthcare."

Chapter 9: Health Information Management

The title of this chapter reflects a belief that the term *medical records* is passé because information about a person's health (or payment for health-related services) can be maintained in many types of media other than paper. Regardless of the form in which it is maintained, health information must be accurate and its confidentiality must be ensured. This chapter reviews the various ways in which health information is properly used, such as for documentation of treatment, for accurate billing, and as evidence in legal forums. It also discusses the Health Insurance Portability and Accountability Act (HIPAA) and other state and federal laws that govern the protection of health information. It outlines circumstances in which third parties may legitimately access individuals' health information with and without patient consent, and it points out the pitfalls that one can encounter when that information is improperly disclosed inadvertently or through "hacking" by cyberthieves.

Chapter 10: Emergency Care

This chapter reviews the common-law rule that individuals have no duty to provide emergency care and the rule's numerous exceptions, both judicial and statutory. It provides considerable detail on the federal Emergency Medical Treatment and Labor Act (EMTALA), which currently sets the standard for emergency department personnel's review of patients' conditions, and presents examples of liability for failure to meet those standards. The chapter concludes with a brief discussion of Good Samaritan statutes, which are probably unnecessary but have afforded some medical personnel a measure of emotional comfort.

Chapter 11: Consent for Treatment and Withholding Consent

This chapter explores the difference between consent and informed consent and outlines the minimum requirements for the latter. It also considers consent issues in emergency situations and such thorny issues as the right to die (i.e., refusal to consent to life-sustaining treatment), consent for patients who are not competent to make choices for themselves, and physicians' role in helping terminally ill patients end their lives legally. The chapter ends with discussion of various methods of documenting and enforcing patients' end-of-life preferences—including living wills and durable powers of attorney—and discusses "death with dignity" laws that allow physicians to aid certain terminal patients to end their own lives. Appendixes present examples of an advance directive form and a Physician Order for Life-Sustaining Treatment form.

Chapter 12: Taxation of Healthcare Institutions

This chapter addresses the taxation of healthcare organizations, primarily not-for-profit corporations. All tax-exempt organizations are not-for-profit, but not all not-for-profits are tax exempt. The standards for income and property tax exemption are also discussed, as are the occasions in which some income of a tax-exempt organization may be taxable. The chapter raises the question of what it means to be a charity and what implications that designation may have under federal and state law. It closes with a review of a 2010 decision that, if followed by other states, augurs rough sailing ahead for non-profit hospitals' property tax exemptions, especially if the Affordable Care Act continues to decrease the number of uninsured Americans.

Chapter 13: Competition and Antitrust Law

This chapter reviews the basic concepts of antitrust law, including laws against restraints of trade, monopolization, and price discrimination. It distinguishes among the various per se violations and shows how cases that do not fit one of those categories are decided on the basis of a "rule-of-reason analysis." Exemptions from the antitrust laws include implied repeal, state action, Noerr-Pennington, and the business of insurance doctrines. This chapter reviews the factors used in defining the appropriate market for individual cases, and it concludes with a discussion of what to expect in the coming years, especially now that the ACA is being implemented. A significant US Supreme Court decision from North Carolina has been added to The Court Decides, and other cases (from Ohio and Idaho) are also discussed.

Chapter 14: Issues of Reproduction and Birth

This chapter reviews many of the sensitive and contentious legal questions surrounding reproduction. These include sterilization, wrongful life, wrongful birth, surrogate parenting, in vitro fertilization (IVF), stem cell research, and abortion. The hospital's role in reproduction issues is discussed, including whether the hospital can be required to provide such services and whether government programs will pay for the procedures if the hospital does provide them. The chapter also points out that stem cell research will continue to be an issue, but in light of the *Whole Woman's Health* case, it may be some time before abortion again comes before the Supreme Court.

Chapter 15: Fraud Laws and Corporate Compliance

This chapter addresses one of the most salient issues in healthcare today: the prevention of fraud and abuse in governmental healthcare programs. The major fraud laws are reviewed, as are the aggressive enforcement activities of federal and state regulators, and the severe monetary and criminal penalties that can be imposed for violations of these laws are emphasized. The chapter also discusses some of the changes to the fraud laws occasioned by the passage of the ACA, and it reviews the basics of a proper corporate compliance program, an essential preventive measure and a valuable resource for a wide range of legal and ethical issues.

J. Stuart Showalter, JD, MFS
San Diego

Note

1. U.S. Dep't of Health and Human Serv., *Health Insurance Coverage and the Affordable Care Act, 2010–2016* (March 3, 2016), https://aspe.hhs.gov/pdf-report/health-insurance-coverage-and-affordable-care-act-2010-2016.

Instructor Resources

This book's Instructor Resources include a test bank; two versions of a PowerPoint presentation; and an updated instructor's manual with chapter overviews, answers to end-of-chapter discussion questions, and answers to end-of-case discussion questions.

For the most up-to-date information about this book and its Instructor Resources, go to ache.org/HAP and browse for the book's title or author name.

This book's Instructor Resources are available to instructors who adopt this book for use in their course. For access information, please e-mail hapbooks@ache.org.

THE ANGLO-AMERICAN LEGAL SYSTEM

After reading this chapter, you will

- understand that law comes from four basic sources—constitutions, statutes, administrative regulations, and judicial decisions;
- know that no one branch of government in the US legal system is meant to be more powerful than the others;
- be able to find judicial opinions in the reporter system;
- understand the importance of stare decisis and due process; and
- be familiar with basic aspects of legal procedure.

Some History

Before we discuss Anglo-American law specifically, let's discuss some of the history of "law" itself. Nearly 3,800 years ago, King Hammurabi of Babylon inscribed a set of laws on an eight-foot-tall black stone monument. Lost for centuries but rediscovered in 1901, the Code of Hammurabi is the oldest known example of written laws for the governance of a society (see exhibit 1.1).

The code is known for its "eye for an eye, tooth for a tooth" philosophy (*lex talionis* is a Latin phrase meaning "the law of retaliation"). Adultery and theft were punishable by death. A slave who disobeyed his master lost an ear, which was an ancient symbol of obedience. If a surgeon caused injury, his hand was cut off; this provision may have been the first version of malpractice law known to humankind. In addition to these harsh standards, the code contained

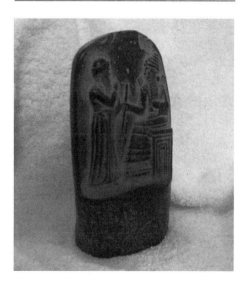

EXHIBIT 1.1
Code of Hammurabi Stele (top portion)

rules for everyday social and commercial affairs—sale and lease of property, maintenance of lands, commercial transactions (contracts, credit, debt, banking), marriage and divorce, estates and inheritance, and criminal procedure. Given Hammurabi's reputation as a lawgiver, his depiction can be found in several US government buildings, including the US Capitol and the Supreme Court.

Fast-forward to the fourth century BCE and we find Aristotle, the father of *natural law*—the idea that there exists a body of moral principles common to all persons and recognizable by reason alone. Natural law is distinguished from *positive law*—the formal legal enactments of a particular society.[1]

Centuries later, Saint Thomas Aquinas distinguished natural law from eternal, divine, and human-made law in his *Summa Theologica* (circa 1274). A few other legal philosophies (and representative adherents) over the centuries have included the following:

- Law as a social contract (Thomas Hobbes, *Leviathan*, 1651)
- Analytic jurisprudence (David Hume, *A Treatise of Human Nature*, 1739)
- Utilitarianism (Jeremy Bentham and John Stuart Mill, nineteenth century)
- Legal positivism (John Austin, nineteenth century)
- Legal realism (Oliver Wendell Holmes Jr., Roscoe Pound, and others, twentieth century)
- Libertarianism (John Nozick and Ron Paul, late twentieth century)

The point here is not to make legal philosophers out of you but to demonstrate that various systems of thought have influenced the US legal system over the centuries.

common law
the body of law based on custom and judicial precedents, as distinct from statutory law; its historical roots are the traditional laws of England that developed over many centuries and were carried over to the American colonies and thus the United States.

Anglo-American Law

In Charles Dickens's *Oliver Twist*, Mr. Bumble has been proven an accessory to his wife's attempt to deprive poor Oliver of a rightful inheritance. Bumble asserts that if the law holds him responsible, then "the law is an ass—an idiot."[2] This argument is ineffective, however. Bumble and his wife lose their jobs and become inmates of the very workhouse where Oliver's mother died while giving birth to him. Ah! The law is not so asinine after all. It has impressed and fascinated authors and scholars for millennia, and the US legal system has done the same for two and a half centuries.

One can study law simply by reading statutes and judicial decisions, but for a full understanding one must also read history, sociology, public policy, politics, economics, ethics, religion, and other relevant fields. Because the roots of Anglo-American law can be traced back to the Norman Conquest of England in 1066 and beyond, some view the richness of the US legal tradition with a respect that approaches reverence (see Legal Brief).

Stated in the simplest and arguably most important way, the purpose of a legal system is to prevent anarchy and provide an alternative to personal revenge as a method of resolving disputes. Considering the size and complexity of our nation, the litigious temperament of our people, and the wide range of possible disputes, our legal system is remarkably successful in achieving its purpose. It has its shortcomings, to be sure, but at least it stands as a bulwark against self-help and blood feuds.

The law permeates today's healthcare field. The US medical system is perhaps the most heavily regulated enterprise in the world, subject not only to the principles that affect all businesses (everything from antitrust to zoning) but also to myriad regulations peculiar to healthcare. For these reasons, students of healthcare administration need to become familiar with the law and legal system. Almost every decision made and every action taken by healthcare administrators have legal implications, and all such decisions and actions are explicitly or implicitly based on some legal standard. Furthermore, students must understand basic legal principles well enough to recognize when professional legal advice is needed. The main purpose of this book is to help you and your organization stay out of trouble.

This chapter outlines general concepts essential to any study of law. It emphasizes three areas:

Legal Brief

The **common law** is the result of centuries of judicial decisions, decrees, customs, and ordeals in the pursuit of justice. People from many backgrounds have influenced its development over the years.

More than a millennium ago, the Anglo-Saxon inhabitants of what was to become England began to centralize their various kingships to ward off enemies and maintain peace. In the process, they created a legal system that came to include concepts still familiar today, such as writs (court orders); the offices of sheriff, bailiff, and mayor; taxation; complex legal record keeping; the use of sworn testimony; and stare decisis (respect for legal precedent).

The common law grew along with the further cohesion of the country following the conquest of England by Duke William of Normandy ("William the Conqueror"; 1028–1087) in 1066. Under King Henry II (1133–1189), tribunals such as the King's Court and circuit courts were added to the legal system, and the decisions of those bodies became part of the law common to the whole of England. Henry is sometimes described as the father of English common law. Also part of the common law are the Magna Carta (1215), the Habeas Corpus Act (1679), the Petition of Right (1628), and the English Bill of Rights (1689). These instruments describe certain basic concepts—the authority of the sovereign (king or state), freedom of speech, limitations on the use of martial law, the separation of judicial and legislative powers, and recognition that statutes are not the sole basis of law—that applied to colonial America and remain woven through the fabric of US law to this day.

1. Sources of law
2. Workings of the court system
3. Basic legal procedure

The Definition of *Law*

law
a system of standards to govern the conduct of people in an organization, a community, a society, or a nation

In its broadest sense, **law** is a system of principles and rules devised by organized society or groups in society to set norms for human conduct. Societies and groups must have standards of behavior and means to enforce those standards; otherwise, they devolve into vigilantism. The purpose of law, therefore, is to prevent conflict among individuals and between government and its subjects. When conflicts occur, legal institutions and doctrines supply the means of resolving the disputes.

Because law is concerned with human behavior, it is not an exact science. Indeed, "it depends" is a law instructor's most frequent answer to students' questions. This response is frustrating for both the students and the instructor, but it is honest. The law provides only general guidance; it is not an exact blueprint for living. Its application varies according to the circumstances of the case. However, this inherent ambiguity is a great strength; its adaptability fosters creativity. Legal rigidity would inhibit initiative, stunt the growth of social institutions, and ultimately result in decay.

Viewed in proper light, law is a landscape painting that captures the beliefs of society in a given location at a certain point in time. But it is not static; law is a work in progress, a constantly changing piece of art—a hologram, perhaps—that moves with society. Most often it moves at a glacial pace—slowly and quietly, the land shifting beneath it. At other times, it moves seismically, as was the case in 2010 with the passage of a legislative temblor known as the **Affordable Care Act (ACA)**, or "Obamacare."[3] Despite outcries from some segments of the political spectrum, the US Supreme Court in June 2012 held the ACA to be constitutional. Most of the ACA's reforms took effect in 2014, and the aftershocks will be felt for years. Until the dust settles completely, we will not know how much the act has altered the legal topography.

Affordable Care Act (ACA)
the health reform law enacted by Congress in 2010; full name: Patient Protection and Affordable Care Act, Pub. L. No. 111-148

Types and Sources of Law

Law can be classified in various ways. One of the most common ways is to distinguish between public law and private law. *Public law* concerns the government and its relations with individuals and businesses. *Private law* refers to the rules and principles that define and regulate rights and duties among persons. These categories overlap, but they are useful in illustrating Anglo-American legal doctrine.

Private law comprises the law of contracts, property, and tort, all of which usually concern relationships between private parties. It also includes, for example, such social contracts as canon law in the Catholic Church and the regulations of a homeowners' association. Public law, on the other hand, regulates and enforces rights in which the government has an interest (e.g., labor relations, taxation, antitrust, environmental regulation, criminal prosecution). The principal sources of public law are as follows:

- Written constitutions (both state and federal)
- Statutes enacted by a legislative body (federal, state, local)
- Administrative law
- Judicial decisions

Constitutions

The US Constitution is aptly called the "supreme law of the land" because it sets standards against which all other laws are judged. Other sources of law must be consistent with the Constitution.

The Constitution is a grant of power from the states to the federal government (see Legal Brief). All powers not granted to the federal government in the Constitution are reserved by the individual states. This grant of power to the federal government is both express and implied. For example, the Constitution expressly authorizes the US Congress to levy and collect taxes, borrow and coin money, declare war, raise and support armies, and regulate interstate commerce. Congress may also enact laws that are "necessary and proper" to carry out these express powers. For example, the power to coin money includes the implied power to design US currency, and the power to regulate interstate commerce embraces the power to pass antidiscrimination legislation, such as the Civil Rights Act of 1964.

The main body of the Constitution establishes, defines, and limits the power of the three branches of the federal government:

1. The legislature (Congress) has the power to enact statutes.
2. The executive branch has the power to enforce the laws.
3. The judiciary has the power to interpret the laws.

Each branch plays a different role, and the branches' interaction is governed

Legal Brief

The United States is not a union; it is a federation (from the Latin word *foedus*, meaning "covenant") of 50 self-governing states that have ceded some of their sovereignty to the central (federal) government to promote the welfare of all.

by a system of checks and balances (see exhibit 1.2). The president can nominate federal judges, but the Senate must confirm those nominations; Congress can remove high-ranking federal personnel (including judges and the president) through the impeachment and trial process; and the judiciary can declare laws unconstitutional. The president can veto a congressional bill, but Congress can override a veto by a two-thirds vote of each chamber.

Twenty-seven amendments follow the main body of the Constitution. The first ten—ratified in 1791—are known as the Bill of Rights, which includes the rights to

due process of law
a fundamental principle of fairness in legal matters, both civil and criminal; the requirement that all legal procedures set by statute and court practice be followed so that no unjust treatment results

- exercise freedom of speech,
- practice religion,
- bear arms,
- be secure from unreasonable searches and seizures,
- demand a jury trial,
- be protected against self-incrimination, and
- be accorded substantive and procedural **due process of law**.

Of the remaining amendments, two cancelled each other: the Eighteenth, which established Prohibition, and the Twenty-First, which repealed the Eighteenth. As of this writing, only 15 substantive changes have been made to the basic structure of US government since 1791. The first ten

---

EXHIBIT 1.2
Checks and
Balances

1. Impeach/convict
2. Appoint
3. Veto
4. Override or not confirm

5. Interpret or rule unconstitutional
6. Amend law
7. Change regulation

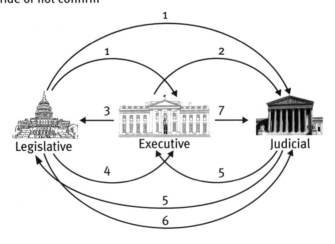

---

amendments apply only to the federal government. However, the Fourteenth Amendment—ratified in 1870—declares that no state may "deprive any person of life, liberty, or property, without due process of law." The US Supreme Court has held that most of the rights set forth in the Bill of Rights apply to the states because of the Fourteenth Amendment's Due Process Clause. (An example of a due process case is *Simkins v. Moses H. Cone Mem. Hosp.*, presented in The Court Decides at the end of this chapter.) Consequently, neither the states nor the federal government may infringe on the rights mentioned earlier.

In addition to the US Constitution, each state has its own constitution. A state's constitution is the supreme law of the particular state, but it is subordinate to the federal constitution. State and federal constitutions are similar, although state constitutions are more detailed and cover such matters as the financing of public works and the organization of local governments.

Statutes

Statutes are positive law enacted by a legislative body. Because our federal system is imbricate with national, state, and local jurisdictions, the legislative body may be Congress, a state legislature, or a deliberative assembly of local government (e.g., county council, city council). Statutes enacted by any of these bodies may apply to healthcare organizations. For example, hospitals must comply with federal statutes such as the Civil Rights Act of 1964 and the Hill-Burton Act, which prohibit discrimination at patient admission. Most states and a number of large cities have also enacted antidiscrimination statutes.

Judges face the task of interpreting statutes. Interpretation is especially difficult when the wording of a statute is ambiguous, as it usually is. To clarify statutes, the courts have developed several *rules of construction*, which in some states are themselves the subject of a separate statute. Regardless of their source, the rules are designed to help judges ascertain the intent of the legislature. Common rules of construction include the following:

- Interpretation of a statute's meaning must be consistent with the intent of the legislature.
- Interpretation of a statute's meaning must give effect to all of its provisions.
- If a statute's meaning is unclear, its purpose, the result to be attained, legislative history, and the consequences of one interpretation over another must all be considered.

Whether of constitutions or statutes, judicial interpretation is the pulse of the law. A prominent example appears later in this chapter in the discussion of *Erie R. R. Co. v. Tompkins*, a case in which the meaning of a venerable federal statute was at issue. And in chapter 12, the section on taxation of real estate discusses numerous cases concerning the meaning of "exclusive use" of a piece of property for charitable purposes. These cases are just a few of the many examples of judicial interpretation that permeate this text. Be alert for others, and try to discern the different philosophies of judicial interpretation that the cases' outcomes represent.

Administrative Law

Administrative law is the type of public law that deals with the rules of government agencies. According to one scholar, "Administrative law . . . determines the organization, powers, and duties of administrative authorities."[4] Administrative law has greater scope and significance than is sometimes realized. In fact, administrative law is the source of much of the substantive law that directly affects the rights and duties of individuals and businesses and their relation to governmental authority (see the discussion of federal healthcare privacy regulations in chapter 9).

The executive branch of government carries out (administers) the law as enacted by the legislature and interpreted by the courts. However, the executive branch also makes law (through administrative regulations) and exercises a considerable amount of quasi-judicial (court-like) power. The term *administrative government* means all departments of the executive branch and all governmental agencies created for specific public purposes.

Administrative agencies exist at all levels of government: local, state, and federal. Well-known federal agencies that affect healthcare are the National Labor Relations Board, Federal Trade Commission, Centers for Medicare & Medicaid Services, and Food and Drug Administration. At the state level, there are boards of professional licensure, Medicaid agencies, workers' compensation commissions, zoning boards, and numerous other agencies whose rules affect healthcare organizations.

Legislative bodies delegate lawmaking and judicial powers to administrative government as necessary to implement statutory requirements; the resulting rules and regulations have the force of law, subject to the provisions of the Constitution and statutes. The Food and Drug Administration, for example, has the power to make rules controlling the manufacturing, marketing, and advertising of foods, drugs, cosmetics, and medical devices. Similarly, state Medicaid agencies make rules governing eligibility for Medicaid benefits and receipt of funds by participating providers.

The amount of delegated legislation increased tremendously during the twentieth century, especially after World War II. The reason for this increase is clear: Economic and social conditions inevitably change as societies become more complicated. Legislatures cannot directly provide the detailed rules necessary to govern every particular subject. Delegation of rulemaking authority puts this responsibility in the hands of experts, but the enabling legislation will stipulate the standards to be followed by an administrative agency when it writes the regulations. Such rules must be consistent with their underlying legislation and the Constitution.

Judicial Decisions

The third major source of law is the judicial decision. All legislation, whether federal or state, must be consistent with the US Constitution. The power to legislate is, therefore, limited by constitutional doctrines, and the federal courts have the power to declare an act of Congress or of a state legislature unconstitutional.[5] Judicial decisions are subordinate to the Constitution and to statutes as long as the statutes are constitutional. Despite this subordinate role, however, judicial decisions are the primary domain of private law, and private law—especially the law of contracts and torts—traditionally has had the most influence on healthcare and thus is of particular interest to healthcare administrators.

Common law—judicial decisions based on tradition, custom, and precedent—was developed after the Norman Conquest in 1066 and produced at least two important concepts that endure today: writ and stare decisis. A *writ* is a court-issued order directing the recipient to appear before the court or to perform, or cease performing, a certain act.

The doctrine of **stare decisis** (Latin for "to stand by a decision")—the concept of precedent—requires that courts look to past disputes involving similar facts and principles and determine the outcome of the current case on the basis of the earlier precedents as much as possible. This practice engenders a general stability in the Anglo-American legal system (see Legal Brief).

stare decisis
the principle that a court must respect decisions of higher courts (precedents) on a settled legal issue applicable to the instant case

Consider, for example, the opening sentence of the 1992 abortion decision, *Planned Parenthood of S.E. Pennsylvania v. Casey*. The case involved the question of whether to uphold or overturn the precedent set in *Roe v. Wade*, the landmark abortion decision of 1973. Justice Sandra Day O'Connor's opinion in the *Casey* case sums up stare decisis in nine words: "Liberty finds no refuge in a jurisprudence of doubt" (see The Court Decides at the end of this chapter).

Stare decisis applies downward, but not horizontally. An Ohio trial court, for example, is bound by the decisions of Ohio's Supreme Court and the US Supreme Court but not by the decisions

Legal Brief

Use of precedent to determine the substance of law distinguishes common-law jurisdictions from code-based civil law systems, which traditionally rely on a comprehensive collection of rules. The civil law system is the basis for the law in Europe, Central and South America, Japan, Quebec, and (because of its French heritage) the state of Louisiana.

of other Ohio trial courts or out-of-state courts. Courts in one state may, but are not required to, examine judicial decisions of other states for guidance, especially if the issue is new to the state. Similarly, a federal trial court is bound by the decisions of the Supreme Court and the appellate court of its circuit but not by the decisions of other appellate or district courts.

The doctrine of stare decisis should not be confused with a related concept—*res judicata*, which literally means "a thing or issue settled by judgment." (In Latin, the word *res* means "thing.") In practical terms, once a legal dispute has been resolved in court and all appeals have been exhausted, res judicata prohibits the same parties from later bringing suit regarding the same matters.

The Court System

In a perfect world, we would not need courts and lawyers. This idea may have inspired Shakespeare's famous line in *Henry VI*, "The first thing we do, let's kill all the lawyers."[6] At the time—the sixteenth century—resentment against lawyers ran high in England. Shakespeare was perhaps engaged in a little lawyer bashing, and his intention may have been to express his indictment of a corrupt system. On the other hand, the remark may have been a compliment; the character who utters the famous words was an insurgent who would not want skillful lawyers around to uphold law and order. Or maybe the Bard was just trying to get a laugh out of the audience. Regardless of one's interpretation of the play, we do not live in a utopia, so we need courts and lawyers, and we always will.

There are more than 50 court systems in the United States. In addition to the state and federal courts, the District of Columbia, the Virgin Islands, Guam, the Northern Mariana Islands, and Puerto Rico have their own systems. The large number of court systems makes the study of US law complicated, but the decentralized nature of federalism adds strength and vitality. As various courts adopt different approaches to a novel issue, the states become a testing ground on which a preferred solution eventually becomes apparent.

State Courts
The federal courts and the court systems of most states use a three-tier structure comprising the trial courts, the intermediate courts of appeal, and a supreme court (see exhibit 1.3). In a state court system, the lowest tier—the trial courts—is often divided into *courts of limited jurisdiction* and *courts of general jurisdiction*. Typically, the courts of limited jurisdiction hear only specific types of cases, such as criminal trials involving lesser crimes (e.g.,

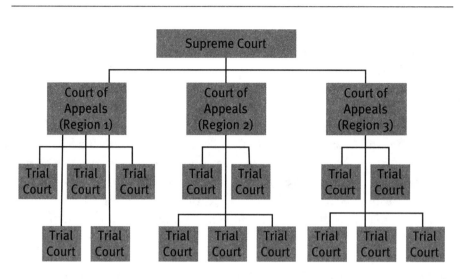

EXHIBIT 1.3
Model of a
Typical Three-
Tier Court
Structure

misdemeanors, traffic violations) or civil cases involving disputes of a certain amount (e.g., in small claims court, lawyers are not allowed and complex legal procedures are relaxed). State courts of general jurisdiction hear more serious criminal cases involving felonies and civil cases involving larger sums of money.

The next tier in most states is the intermediate appellate courts. They hear appeals from the trial courts. In exercising their jurisdiction, appellate courts are usually limited to the evidence from the trial court and to interpreting questions of law, not questions of fact.

The highest tier in the state court system is a state supreme court. This court hears appeals from the intermediate appellate courts—or from trial courts if the state does not have intermediate courts—and, like the trial courts, the supreme court has limited jurisdiction and hears only certain types of cases. (Texas and Oklahoma are a little different: each has two separate highest courts, one for civil and the other for criminal cases.) The high court is also charged with administrative duties, such as adopting rules of procedure and disciplining attorneys.

The states are not uniform in naming the various courts. A trial court of general jurisdiction, for example, may be called a circuit, superior, common pleas, or county court. New York is unique in that its trial court is known as the "supreme court"; its intermediate appellate court is the "Supreme Court Appellate Division." In most states, the highest court is named the supreme court, but in Maine and Massachusetts the high court is styled the "Supreme Judicial Court," and in New York, Maryland, and the District of Columbia, the highest court is called the "Court of Appeals." In West Virginia the highest court is the Supreme Court of Appeals.

Federal Courts
US District Courts

The federal court system is similar to the state court system. At its bottom tier, federal district (trial) courts hear nearly all categories of cases, including criminal matters arising under federal statutes and civil cases between parties from different states or based on federal law. There are now 94 district courts—at least one in each state and in the District of Columbia, Puerto Rico, the Virgin Islands, Guam, and the Northern Mariana Islands. Each district also has a US bankruptcy court, which is a unit of the district court. The federal courts (beginning with the district courts) have exclusive jurisdiction over certain kinds of cases, such as violations of federal antitrust or securities laws, **admiralty**, bankruptcy, and issues related to the Employee Retirement Income Security Act.

Federal and state courts have *concurrent* jurisdiction in cases arising under the US Constitution or under any federal statute that does not confer exclusive jurisdiction to the federal court system. A federal district court may hear suits based on state law in which a citizen of one state sues a citizen of another state if the amount in dispute is more than $75,000.[7] These suits are called *diversity of citizenship* cases. A prime example is *Erie R. R. Co. v. Tompkins*.[8] In this famous case, Tompkins, a citizen of Pennsylvania, was injured by a passing train while walking along the Erie Railroad's right-of-way in that state. He sued the railroad for negligence in a New York federal court, asserting diversity jurisdiction. The railroad was a New York corporation, but the accident occurred in Pennsylvania, and the railroad pointed out that Tompkins was trespassing on its property. Under Pennsylvania's court decisions, trespassers could not recover for their injuries. Tompkins countered that because there was no state statute on the subject, only judicial decisions, the railroad could be held liable in federal court as a matter of "general law."

At issue in this case was the interpretation of a section of the Federal Judiciary Act, which reads as follows:

> The laws of the several States, except where the Constitution, treaties, or statutes of the United States otherwise require or provide, shall be regarded as rules of decision in trials at common law, in the courts of the United States, in cases where they apply.[9]

Swift v. Tyson,[10] an 1842 case, had concluded that this language applied only to a state's statutes, not its common law. On the basis of *Swift*, the lower courts held for Tompkins. The Supreme Court disagreed, however, citing various plaintiffs' use of diversity jurisdiction and the *Swift* doctrine to circumvent an unfavorable state law. Thus, the court reversed the judgment in favor of Tompkins and overturned the precedent set by *Swift*, stating that

> experience in applying the doctrine of *Swift v. Tyson*, had revealed its defects, political and social; and the benefits expected to flow from the rule did not accrue.

admiralty
the system of law that applies to accidents and injuries at sea, maritime commerce, alleged violations of rules of the sea over shipping lanes and rights of way, and crimes aboard a ship

Persistence of state courts in their own opinions on questions of common law prevented uniformity; and the impossibility of discovering a satisfactory line of demarcation between the province of general law and that of local law developed a new well of uncertainties.

. . . The mischievous results of the doctrine had become apparent. Diversity of citizenship jurisdiction was conferred [by the Constitution] in order to prevent apprehended discrimination in state courts against those not citizens of the state. *Swift v. Tyson* introduced grave discrimination by noncitizens against citizens. It made rights enjoyed under the unwritten "general law" vary according to whether enforcement was sought in the state or in the federal court; and the privilege of selecting the court in which the right should be determined was conferred upon the noncitizen. Thus the doctrine rendered impossible equal protection of the law. In attempting to promote uniformity of law throughout the United States, the doctrine had prevented uniformity in the administration of the law of the state.

The Court concluded:

Except in matters governed by the Federal Constitution or by acts of Congress, the law to be applied in any case is the law of the state. And whether the law of the state shall be declared by its Legislature in a statute or by its highest court in a decision is not a matter of federal concern. There is no federal general common law. Congress has no power to declare substantive rules of common law applicable in a state whether they be local in their nature or "general," be they commercial law or a part of the law of torts. And no clause in the Constitution purports to confer such a power upon the federal courts.

Claims involving federal statutes and the US Constitution may also be tried in state court, depending on the situation.

US Courts of Appeals

There are 13 US Courts of Appeals. The 94 judicial districts (trial courts) are organized geographically into 11 numbered circuits plus one for the District of Columbia. These courts hear appeals from the district courts located in their respective geographical regions and, in the case of the DC Circuit, from decisions of federal agencies. In addition, the thirteenth court of appeals, the "US Court of Appeals for the Federal Circuit," has subject matter responsibilities rather than oversight of a given region. This court hears appeals in specialized cases, such as those involving patent laws or specific statues assigned to it by Congress (see exhibit 1.4).[11]

US Supreme Court

At the highest level of the federal court system is the US Supreme Court. The Supreme Court hears appeals of cases involving federal statutes, treaties, or the US Constitution from the US courts of appeals and from the highest state

EXHIBIT 1.4
Map of US
Courts of
Appeals

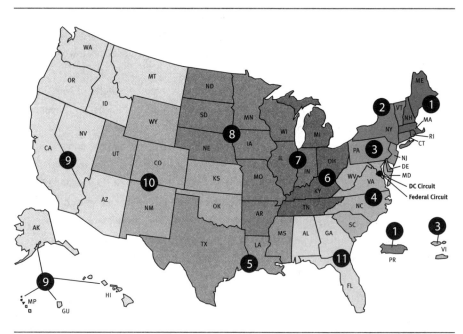

writ of certiorari
an order from a
higher court to
a lower court,
requesting that the
record of a case be
sent up for review

courts. In most cases litigants have no absolute right to have their case heard by the Supreme Court. Instead, they must petition for a **writ of certiorari**— an order to the lower court requiring that the case be sent up for the high court's review—and must persuade at least four of the nine justices that the issue merits their attention. The Supreme Court normally decides only about 150 cases per year from the eight to ten thousand "cert petitions" it receives.

In the words of Chief Justice William H. Taft, the justices see their function being "for the purpose of expounding and stabilizing principles of law for the benefit of the country, passing upon constitutional questions, [and] to preserve uniformity of decision among the intermediate courts of appeal."[12] As a result, the Supreme Court grants certiorari only in cases that present questions of extraordinary legal or social significance or when the federal courts of appeals have differed in deciding cases involving the same legal issue. Because the court has considerable discretion in which cases it chooses to hear, lower courts decide most of the important legal issues.

The Constitution vests the judicial power of the United States "in one supreme Court, and in such inferior Courts as the Congress may from time to time ordain and establish" (Article III, Section 1). Unlike state judges, federal judges are given lifetime appointments and can be removed only by impeachment and conviction. Congress may create additional courts and may redefine the jurisdiction of all tribunals below the Supreme Court level. Over the years, it has complemented the district courts and the courts of appeals with several federal courts that have specialized functions—for example, the US Federal Claims Court (which hears certain contract claims brought against the government), the US Court of International Trade, the US Tax Court, and the US Court of Appeals for the Armed Forces.

Alternative Dispute Resolution

There are two popular alternatives to the court system for resolving disputes. The first is resort to the quasi-judicial power of an administrative agency or tribunal. (Workers' compensation commissions are a familiar example.) Administrative bodies settle far more disputes today than do the judicial courts, and administrative agencies usually have the statutory responsibility and power to enforce their own decisions (which courts do not have). Thus, the agency that wrote the regulations often brings the initial proceeding, hears the case, and decides the dispute as well. The Federal Trade Commission, for example, is empowered to compel an alleged offender to cease and desist from practicing unfair methods of competition under the commission's regulations.

Statutes prescribe the powers of administrative bodies. The role of ordinary courts is generally limited to preventing administrative authorities from exceeding their powers and to granting remedies to individuals who have been injured by wrongful administrative action. Sometimes statutes grant the right of appeal of an adverse administrative decision to a judicial court.

The second alternative method for dispute resolution is **arbitration**, which is often faster, less complicated, more confidential, and less costly than a lawsuit. Arbitration involves submission of a dispute for decision by a third person or a panel of experts outside the judicial process. When the parties to a dispute voluntarily agree to have their differences resolved by an arbitrator or by a panel and to be bound by the decision, arbitration becomes a viable alternative to the court system. Statutory law in most states favors voluntary, binding arbitration and frequently provides that an agreement to arbitrate is enforceable by the courts.[13] Arbitration is different from *mediation*, in which a third party—the mediator—simply attempts to persuade adverse parties to agree to settle their differences. The mediator has no power to require a settlement.

arbitration
an extrajudicial hearing sometimes used in medical liability cases to avoid a court trial and conducted by a person or a panel of people who are not necessarily judges

Legal Procedure

Substantive law is the type of law that creates and defines rights and duties. Most of this book is devoted to substantive law as it relates to healthcare providers. *Procedural law*, as the term implies, provides the specific processes for enforcing and protecting rights granted by substantive law. The branch of procedural law discussed in this section is law relating to trial of a case.

Commencement of Legal Action: The Complaint

To begin a lawsuit (an *action*), a claimant (the *plaintiff*) files a complaint against another party (the *defendant*). The complaint states the nature of the plaintiff's injury or claim and the amount of damages or other remedy sought from the defendant. (The complaint and other papers subsequently filed in court are *pleadings*.) A copy of the complaint, along with a summons, is then served on the defendant. The summons advises the defendant that he must answer the complaint or take other action within a limited time (e.g., 30 days) and that the plaintiff will be granted judgment by default if the defendant fails to act.

The Defendant's Response: The Answer

In response to the summons, the defendant files an answer to the complaint, admitting to, denying, or pleading ignorance to each allegation. The defendant may also file a complaint against the plaintiff (a *countersuit* or *counterclaim*) or against a third-party defendant whom the original defendant believes is wholly or partially responsible for the plaintiff's alleged injuries.

At this stage in the proceeding, the defendant may ask the court to dismiss the plaintiff's complaint if the court lacks jurisdiction, a judgment has already been made on the same matter, or the plaintiff's complaint failed to state a legal claim. Although the terminology differs from state to state, the motion to dismiss is usually called a *motion for summary judgment* or a *demurrer*. If the court grants the motion to dismiss, the judgment is final and the plaintiff can appeal the decision immediately.

Discovery

In rare cases, the court's decision quickly follows the complaint and answer stages (see Law in Action). Usually, however, especially in urban areas, several months elapse between commencement of the action and trial. During this time, each party engages in *litigation*, or *discovery*, in an attempt to determine the facts and strength of the other party's case.

Discovery is a valuable device that can be used, for example, to identify prospective defendants or witnesses or to uncover other important evidence. For example, in one hospital case, a patient had fallen on the way to the washroom and fractured a hip.[14] During discovery, the hospital was required to disclose the identity of the nurse who had directed the patient to the washroom instead of giving bedside attention.

Law in Action

In one instance of procedural law, a wife and mother of young children had lost two-thirds of her blood supply because of a ruptured ulcer, but her husband refused to approve blood transfusions because they were Jehovah's Witnesses. The hospital petitioned the district court for permission to administer blood; the district court denied permission; and the case was taken to a court of appeals, where an order was signed allowing the transfusion—all in a matter of hours.[15]

During the discovery phase, parties may use any or all of the following five methods to discover the strength of the other party's case:

1. Deposition
2. Written interrogatories
3. Inspection and copying of documents
4. Physical or mental examination of a party
5. Request for admission of facts

Only relevant facts and matters that are not privileged or confidential may be solicited through these methods.

Deposition

The most common and effective discovery device is the *deposition*, whereby a party subpoenas a witness to testify under oath before a court reporter, who transcribes the testimony. The opposing attorney is also present during the deposition to make objections and, if appropriate, to cross-examine the witness. The transcript of the deposition may be read into evidence at the trial itself if the witness is unable to testify in person and can be used to impeach the witness's testimony if her "story" has changed.

Written Interrogatories

A second method of discovery, written interrogatories, are similar to depositions except the questions are written. The procedure for using written interrogatories sometimes varies, depending on whether they are directed toward an adverse party or other witnesses. Interrogatories are somewhat less effective than oral depositions because there is little opportunity to ask follow-up questions.

Inspection and Copying of Documents

A party using the third method of discovery (a method especially relevant to healthcare cases) may request to inspect and copy documents, inspect tangible items in the possession of the opposing party, enter and inspect land under the control of the other party, or inspect and copy items produced by a witness served with a **subpoena duces tecum**—a subpoena requiring the witness to produce certain books and documents, such as medical records. There are special rules governing subpoenas to produce hospital records because of the sensitivity of these records.

subpoena duces tecum
a court order, issued at the request of one of the parties to a suit, that asks a witness to bring to court or to a deposition any relevant documents under the witness's control

Physical or Mental Examination of a Party

A physical or mental examination, the fourth discovery device, may be used when the physical or mental condition of a party to the lawsuit is in dispute and good cause for the examination is shown.

Request for Admission of Facts

A party using this final discovery method requests that the opposing party admit certain facts. By making and fulfilling these requests, the parties may save the time and expense involved in proving facts in court and may substantially limit the factual issues to be decided by the court.

The Trial

A trial begins with the selection of a jury if either party has requested a jury trial. After jury selection, each attorney makes an opening statement that explains matters to be proven during the trial. The plaintiff then calls witnesses and presents other evidence, and the defense attorney is given an opportunity to cross-examine each of the witnesses. After the plaintiff has rested the case, in many cases the defendant's attorney asks the court to direct a verdict for the defense. Courts will grant the directed verdict if the jury, viewing the facts most favorably to the plaintiff, could not reasonably return a verdict in the claimant's favor that would be in accord with the law. If the motion is denied, the defendant proceeds with evidence and witnesses supporting the defense's case, subject to cross-examination by the plaintiff.

judgment NOV (non obstante veredicto) a verdict "notwithstanding the verdict" entered by the court when a jury's verdict is clearly unsupported by the evidence

When all the evidence has been presented, either party may move for a directed verdict. If the judge denies the motion, she gives instructions to the jury concerning applicable law and the jury retires to deliberate until it reaches a verdict. Many times, after the jury has reached its decision, the losing party asks the court for a "judgment notwithstanding the verdict"—also known as **judgment NOV**, an abbreviation for the Latin term *non obstante veredicto*—and a new trial. The motion is granted if the judge decides that the verdict is clearly not supported by the evidence.

The judge and the jury play key roles in the trial. The judge has the dominant role, deciding whether evidence is admissible and instructing the jury on the law before deliberation begins. The judge also has the power to take the case away from the jury by means of a directed verdict or a judgment notwithstanding the verdict. The role of the jury is thus limited to deciding the facts and determining whether the plaintiff has proven the allegations by a preponderance of the evidence.

Because the jury's role is to decide the facts, the impartiality of the jury is of utmost importance. If there is evidence that a jury member might have been biased, many courts overturn the verdict. In cases tried without a jury, the judge assumes the jury's fact-finding role. (Because either a judge or jury can assume this role, it is often referred to as the role of "trier of fact.")

Appeal and Collection

The next stage in litigation is often an appeal. For various reasons (e.g., satisfaction with the verdict, a party's unwillingness to incur additional expenses), not all cases go to an appellate court.

The party who appeals the case (the losing party in the trial court) is usually the *appellant,* and the other party is the *appellee.* When reading appellate court decisions, one must not assume that the first name in the case heading is the plaintiff's because many appellate courts reverse the order of the names when the case is appealed (see exhibit 1.5). The appellate court's function is limited to a review of the law applied in the case; it accepts the facts as determined by the trier of fact. In its review, the appellate court may affirm the trial court decision, modify or reverse the decision, or reverse it and remand the case for a new trial.

The final stage of the litigation process is collection of the judgment. The most common methods of collection are execution and garnishment. A *writ of execution* entitles the plaintiff to have a local official seize the defendant's property and to have that property sold to satisfy the judgment. A *garnishment* is an order to a third person who is indebted to the defendant to pay the debt directly to the plaintiff to satisfy the judgment. Often, the third party is the defendant's employer, who, depending on local laws, may be ordered to pay a certain percentage of the defendant's wages directly to the plaintiff.

Summary

This chapter discusses the history of law, its sources, the relationships among the three branches of government, the basic structure of the federal and state court systems, and some basics of legal procedure in civil cases. (The procedures followed in criminal cases are somewhat different and are beyond the scope of this text.)

Discussion Questions

1. Why is some knowledge of the history of law important to understanding the law more fully?
2. What are the four sources of law in the United States?
3. Describe the three branches of government and the role of each, including the system of checks and balances.
4. What is the hierarchy among the sources of law in the federal government?
5. What is the system for citing judicial opinions?
6. What are due process and stare decisis, and why are they important?
7. Describe the structure of the federal judicial system.
8. What is the Affordable Care Act?

EXHIBIT 1.5
Legal Citation
System

The legal system uses a unique citation method.* The citation in the *Simkins v. Moses H. Cone Mem. Hosp.* case is a good example. Its heading efficiently conveys a sizable amount of information, as follows:

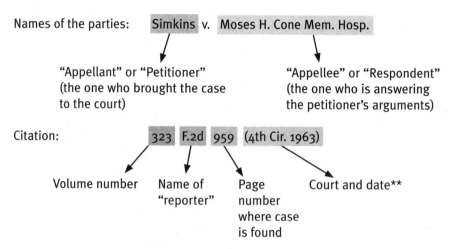

Names of the parties: Simkins v. Moses H. Cone Mem. Hosp.

"Appellant" or "Petitioner"   "Appellee" or "Respondent"
(the one who brought the case   (the one who is answering
to the court)   the petitioner's arguments)

Citation: 323 F.2d 959 (4th Cir. 1963)

Volume number   Name of   Page   Court and date**
                 "reporter"   number
                              where case
                              is found

The *reporter* is the publication in which the decision is documented. Supreme Court decisions are published in the *U.S. Reports* (abbreviated *U.S.*). Federal appellate decisions, such as the *Simkins* case decision, are published in the *Federal Reporter* (abbreviated as *F., F.2d,* or *F.3d*).

Many federal district court and most state trial court decisions are not published formally; however, the captions of the cases retain the same style—the name given first is that of the person who initiated the action. Thus, for example, in *Smith v. Jones*, Smith would be the plaintiff and Jones, the defendant. If Jones loses at the trial court, the appellate decision might read *Jones v. Smith*. A caption that reads something like *State v. Jones* is most likely a criminal prosecution. If a federal trial court decision is published, it will appear in the *Federal Supplement* (F. Supp. or F. Supp. 2d).

State appellate decisions can be found in publications of the West Publishing Company and in official reporters published by some states. The West reporters are grouped regionally and contain the decisions of the courts of nearby states—for example:

Northeast Reporter (N.E., N.E.2d)
Southern Reporter (So., So. 2d)
Pacific Reporter (P., P. 2d)

A designation of *2d* or *3d* indicates that a publisher began a new numbering sequence at a certain point, beginning with volume 1 of the later series.

* These conventions vary slightly in some states' official reports, but they generally hold throughout the country.
** Court designation is not necessary if implicit in the name of the reporter.

The Court Decides

Simkins v. Moses H. Cone Mem. Hosp.
323 F.2d 959 (4th Cir. 1963)

Sobeloff, Chief Judge

The threshold question in this appeal is whether the activities of the two defendants, Moses H. Cone Memorial Hospital and Wesley Long Community Hospital, of Greensboro, North Carolina, which participated in the Hill-Burton program, are sufficiently imbued with "state action" to bring them within the Fifth and Fourteenth Amendment prohibitions against racial discrimination. . . .

The plaintiffs are Negro physicians, dentists and patients suing on behalf of themselves and other Negro citizens similarly situated. . . . The basis of their complaint is that the defendants have discriminated, and continue to discriminate, against them because of their race in violation of the Fifth and Fourteenth Amendments to the United States Constitution. The plaintiffs seek an injunction restraining the defendants from continuing to deny Negro physicians and dentists the use of staff facilities on the ground of race; an injunction restraining the defendants from continuing to deny and abridge admission of patients on the basis of race . . .; and a judgment declaring unconstitutional [the statute and regulations], which authorize the construction of hospital facilities . . . on a "separate-but-equal" basis. . . .

Factual Background
Six of the plaintiffs are physicians and three are dentists, and all of them are duly licensed and practice their professions in Greensboro. Before filing the complaint they sought staff privileges at the defendant hospitals, which were denied them because of racial exclusionary policies. Two of the plaintiffs are

persons in need of medical treatment who desire to enter either of the defendant hospitals which, they contend, possess the most complete medical equipment and the best facilities available in the Greensboro area. They also desire to be treated by their personal physicians who are Negroes. . . .

The claims of racial discrimination were . . . clearly established. In fact the hospitals' applications for federal grants for construction projects openly stated, as was permitted by statute and regulation, that "certain persons in the area will be denied admission to the proposed facilities as patients because of race, creed or color." These applications were approved by [a state agency], and [by] the Surgeon General of the United States under his statutory authorization.

Both Cone and Long are nonprofit hospitals owned and governed by boards of trustees, and under state law they are duly constituted charitable corporations. The Long Hospital is governed by a self-perpetuating board of twelve trustees. The Cone Hospital, however, is governed by fifteen trustees, five of whom are selected by various state agencies, and one is appointed by a "public agency." . . . Neither hospital's charter contains any explicit or implicit authorization or requirement for the exclusion of Negro professionals or patients.

By far the most significant governmental contact of these two hospitals is their participation in the federally assisted Hill-Burton [program]. As a result . . . both hospitals have received large amounts of public funds, paid by the United States to the State of North

(continued)

(continued from previous page)

Carolina and in turn by North Carolina . . . to the hospitals. They received these funds as part of a "state plan" for hospital construction, which allocates available resources for hospitals within the state and contemplates and authorizes the defendants to exclude Negroes. . . .

A state, to participate in the Hill-Burton program, is required to submit for approval by the Surgeon General a state plan setting forth a "hospital construction program" which, among other things, "meets the requirements as to lack of discrimination on account of race, creed, or color, and for furnishing needed hospital services to persons unable to pay therefor, required by regulations. . . ."

Both state plans and project applications are subject to this general nondiscrimination requirement. However, the Act authorizes the Surgeon General . . . to provide an exception to the general racial nondiscrimination rule by making "equitable provision" for separate hospitals for separate population groups. Thus, by statute and regulation, the states may [discriminate in any area where separate but equal facilities exist]. Where a "separate-but-equal" plan is in operation, the individual applicant for aid need not give any assurance that it will not discriminate and, in fact, may expressly indicate on its application form, as did each of the defendant hospitals, that "certain persons in this area will be denied admission to the proposed facilities as patients because of race, creed, or color. . . ."

The Legal Issue

Upon this factual foundation the District Court formulated the question for determination as follows: "Whether the defendants have been shown to be so impressed with a public interest as to render them instrumentalities of government, and thus within the reach of the Fifth and Fourteenth Amendments to the Constitution of the United States." After first examining separately [the various] points of governmental contact [which included $3.25 million in construction funds, state agency supervision, and federal operational standards,] the [trial] court concluded that none was sufficient to impress the hospitals with the necessary "public interest. . . ." Having found no "state action" the court declined to pass upon the constitutionality of [the Hill-Burton Act and its regulations]. . . .

[I]t is our conclusion that the case was wrongly decided. In the first place we would formulate the initial question differently. . . . In our view the initial question is . . . whether the state or the federal government, or both, have become so involved in the conduct of these otherwise private bodies that their activities are also the activities of these governments. . . .

[Justifying its conclusion, the court cites "massive use of public funds and extensive state-federal sharing in the common plan." The opinion then continues as follows.] But we emphasize that this is not merely a controversy over a sum of money. Viewed from the plaintiffs' standpoint it is an effort by a group of citizens to escape the consequences of discrimination in a concern touching health and life itself. As the case affects the defendants it raises the question of whether they may escape constitutional responsibilities for the equal treatment of citizens, arising from participation in a joint federal and state program allocating aid to hospital facilities throughout the state. . . .

[T]he defendant hospitals operate as integral parts of comprehensive joint or intermeshing state and federal plans or programs designed to effect a proper allocation of available medical and hospital resources for the best possible promotion and maintenance of public health. Such involvement in discriminatory action "it was the design of the Fourteenth Amendment to condemn." *[Quoting a 1961 Supreme Court case.]* . . .

[T]he challenged discrimination has been affirmatively sanctioned by both the state and the federal government pursuant to federal law and regulation. It is settled that governmental sanction need not reach the level of compulsion to clothe what is otherwise private discrimination with "state action." . . .

These federal provisions undertaking to authorize segregation by state-connected institutions are unconstitutional. . . .

Unconstitutional as well under the Due Process Clause of the Fifth Amendment and the Equal Protection Clause of the Fourteenth are the relevant regulations implementing this passage in the statute. . . .

Giving recognition to its responsibilities for public health, the state elected not to build publicly owned hospitals, which concededly could not have avoided a legal requirement against discrimination. Instead it adopted and the defendants participated in a plan for meeting those responsibilities by permitting its share of Hill-Burton funds to go to existing private institutions. The appropriation of such funds to the Cone and Long Hospitals effectively limits Hill-Burton funds available in the future to create non-segregated facilities in the Greensboro area. In these circumstances, the plaintiffs can have no effective remedy unless the constitutional discrimination complained of is forbidden.

The order of the District Court is reversed. . . . ■

Discussion Questions

Other cases, notably *Jackson v. Metropolitan Edison Co.*, 419 U.S. 345 (1974), have seemingly come to the opposite conclusion. In *Jackson*, a public utility company—privately owned but highly regulated and "affected with the public interest"—summarily turned off the plaintiff's electric service for nonpayment. She filed suit, claiming violation of her due process rights. The US Supreme Court found in favor of the utility company. (You can read the opinion online by entering the case name in any search engine.)

1. What arguments can be made to distinguish *Jackson* from *Simkins*? In what ways are the two cases similar?
2. If *Jackson* had been decided differently—that is, if the court had held that extensive government regulation turns the corporation's activities into "state action"—what would the implications have been for healthcare organizations?
3. In *Simkins*, Judge Sobeloff said the issue was "whether the state or the federal government, or both, have become so involved in the conduct of these otherwise private bodies that their activities are also the activities of these governments." Given that Medicare and Medicaid regulation of hospitals is much more extensive than the regulation under the Hill-Burton Act, why are all actions of a hospital today not considered state actions under the due process clause? Should they be?

~ ◍ ~

The Court Decides

Planned Parenthood of S.E. Pennsylvania v. Casey
505 U.S. 833 (1992)

O'Connor, Justice

Liberty finds no refuge in a jurisprudence of doubt. Yet 19 years after our holding that the Constitution protects a woman's right to terminate her pregnancy in its early stages, that definition of liberty is still questioned. . . . . . .

[T]he Court's legitimacy depends on making legally principled decisions under circumstances in which their principled character is sufficiently plausible to be accepted by the Nation. . . .

The Court is not asked to [overrule prior decisions] very often. . . . But when the Court does [so], its decision requires an equally rare precedential force to counter the inevitable efforts to overturn it and to thwart its implementation. Some of those efforts may be mere unprincipled emotional reactions; others may proceed from principles worthy of profound respect. But whatever the premises of opposition may be, only the most convincing justification under accepted standards of precedent could suffice to demonstrate that a later decision overruling the first was anything but a surrender to political pressure, and an unjustified repudiation of the principle on which the Court staked its authority in the first instance. So to overrule under fire in the absence of the most compelling reason to reexamine a watershed decision would subvert the Court's legitimacy beyond any serious question. . . .

The promise of constancy, once given, binds its maker for as long as the power to stand by the decision survives and the understanding of the issue has not changed so fundamentally as to render the commitment obsolete. From the obligation of this promise this Court cannot and should not assume any exemption when duty requires it to decide a case in conformance with the Constitution. A willing breach of it would be nothing less than a breach of faith, and no Court that broke its faith with the people could sensibly expect credit for principle in the decision by which it did that. . . .

The Court's duty in the present case is clear. In 1973, it confronted the already divisive issue of governmental power to limit personal choice to undergo abortion, for which it provided a new resolution based on the due process guaranteed by the Fourteenth Amendment. Whether or not a new social consensus is developing on that issue, its divisiveness is no less today than it was in 1973, and pressure to overrule the decision, like pressure to retain it, has grown only more intense. A decision to overrule *Roe*'s essential holding under the existing circumstances would address error, if error there was, at the cost of both profound and unnecessary damage to the Court's legitimacy, and to the Nation's commitment to the rule of law. It is therefore imperative to adhere to the essence of *Roe*'s original decision, and we do so today. ∎

Discussion Questions

1. What is the significance of the first sentence in this excerpt?
2. In your opinion, is this defense of the principle of stare decisis persuasive?
3. If you were attempting to get this case overruled, what arguments might you make to counter this position?

~ ~

Notes

1. *See, e.g.*, J. Dolhenty, *An Overview of Natural Law* (published January 29, 2012), at www.themoralliberal.com/2012/01/29/an-overview-of-natural-law.

2. CHARLES DICKENS, OLIVER TWIST 279 (2nd ed., vol. 3, Richard Bentley 1839).

3. Pub. L. No. 111-148, 124 Stat. 119, codified as amended at various titles and sections of the United States Code.

4. W. IVOR JENNINGS, THE LAW AND THE CONSTITUTION (5th ed., University of London Press 1959).

5. Marbury v. Madison, 5 U.S. (1 Cranch) 137 (1803), established the court's power to declare federal legislation unconstitutional.

6. WILLIAM SHAKESPEARE, 2 HENRY VI (act 4, scene 2).

7. 28 U.S.C. § 1332.

8. 304 U.S. 64 (1938).

9. 28 U.S.C. § 725.

10. 41 U.S. (16 Pet.) 1 (1842). Before the current system took hold, early Supreme Court reports were published by the court clerk, and the name of the reporter was an abbreviation of that official's name. For example, this citation for *Swift v. Tyson* was first published when the clerk was a man named Peters.

11. United States Courts, *Court Role and Structure* (accessed July 13, 2016), at http://www.uscourts.gov/FederalCourts/Understandingthe FederalCourts/CourtofAppeals.aspx.

12. Hearings before the Committee on the Judiciary of the House of Representatives on H.R. 10479, 67th Cong., 2d Sess., at 2 (1925).

13. *See, e.g.*, Ohio Rev. Code Ann. § 2711.03 at http://codes.ohio.gov/orc/2711.03.

14. *Cidilko v. Palestine*, 24 Misc.2d 19, 207 N.Y.S.2d 727 (1960).

15. Application of President and Directors of Georgetown College, Inc., 331 F.2d 1000 (D.C. Cir. 1964), *cert. denied*, 377 U.S. 398 (1964).

A BRIEF HISTORY OF MEDICINE

2

After reading this chapter, you will

- have a greater appreciation for the evolution of medicine over the centuries,
- understand that "modern medicine" is a recent phenomenon, and
- recognize that the structure of today's US health system is the result of political compromises made over the course of decades.

Supreme Court Justice Oliver Wendell Holmes Jr. (1840–1835) famously wrote: "The life of the law has not been logic; it has been experience."[1] In other words, as you learned in chapter 1, to understand the US legal system well, you must know some history. The same can be said about the healthcare system. Without some background, we may be in danger of concluding that our health system is timeless and ineluctable; it is neither. It was not predestined, and surely no creator would have designed it thusly on a tabula rasa. We must, therefore, understand how our health system came to be the peculiar creature it is.[2]

Answers to these and similar questions help broaden our perspective on the state of the US health system and the law's place in it:

- What did healthcare look like 50 or 100 years ago—or earlier?
- Why do doctors no longer make house calls?
- Why have families stopped providing as much care in the home as they used to?
- What can "scientific medicine" learn from the arts of shamanism, acupuncture, Chinese medicine, and other alternative modalities?
- Why do most of us receive health insurance through our employers?
- Why do we not have a system of national health insurance as do most other developed countries?

Some milestones in the history of medicine are shown in exhibit 2.1, and appendix 2.1 contains a more extensive timeline.

A page of history is worth a volume of logic.

—Oliver Wendell Holmes Jr.[44]

EXHIBIT 2.1
Milestones in the History of Medicine

• **ca. 2600 BCE**
Imhotep, an Egyptian polymath and the first physician known by name

• **ca. 1790 BCE**
The Code of Hammurabi includes the first known medical malpractice standards, mostly criminal punishments

• **ca. 1000 BCE**
The "four humors" are the dominant medical theory

• **ca. 460–370 BCE**
Hippocrates, the "father of Western medicine"

• **384–322 BCE**
Aristotle

• **129–ca. 200**
Galen, Greek-born philosopher and physician to the court of Roman Emperor Marcus Aurelius

• **ca. 450–900**
The early Middle Ages; widespread ignorance in Europe; Islamic physicians make scientific progress that goes unnoticed elsewhere

• **ca. 1250–1475**
The Bubonic Plague in Europe; humoral theory persists

• **ca. 1850**
"Modern medicine" begins

2500 BCE   2000 BCE   1500 BCE   1000 BCE   500 BCE   0   500 CE   1000 CE   1500 CE   2000 CE

"Modern medicine" spans only a small fraction of that history, but in a little more than a century and a half, we moved from mysticism and bloodletting to germ theory, antiseptic surgical technique, antibiotics and vaccines, X-ray and other noninvasive imaging techniques, insulin therapy, organ transplantation, renal dialysis, chemotherapy, coronary bypass surgery, and stem cell research. HIV was identified as the cause of AIDS in 1983, and smallpox and polio were declared eradicated (although prematurely in the case of polio) in 1980 and 1994, respectively. By 2003, the human genome was fully deciphered, thus leading to better treatments for various inherited and acquired diseases. Just since 2006, we have seen facial transplants; bionic limbs; new vaccines for human papilloma virus, pneumonia, and shingles; and other wonders.

We should be gratified by such progress, but not smug. If the learning curve continues at this exponential rate, unimaginable medical advances are in store in the next few decades.

Early History
The Pharaohs and Babylonians

The state of medicine before the nineteenth century can be summarized in two words: mysticism and superstition. Various ancient cultures had beliefs concerning the benefits of ingrained dietary habits and the pharmacological effects of certain plants, such as tobacco and peyote. They had little knowledge of natural disease processes, however, so they usually relied on shamans to invoke what they believed to be the healing powers of the spirit world. Forms of shamanism persist in various indigenous cultures today, including, among others, those of some Native Americans, the Hmong of Southeast Asia, certain African tribes, and a few mestizo (mixed-race) peoples in Central and South America.[3]

Medicine in ancient Egypt was perhaps not as rudimentary as we might think.[4] Homer writes in *The Odyssey*, "Everyone in the whole country is a skilled physician."[5] They were familiar with anatomy (perhaps because of their embalming practices), were aware of the connection between pulse and the heart, could diagnose and treat numerous diseases, and were adept at simple surgery and orthopedics. The Edwin Smith Papyrus, sometimes credited to the court physician Imhotep, is one of the first examples of medical literature. It contains descriptions of medical techniques still in use today: simple suturing, immobilization of spinal injuries, and use of splints for fractures.

Magic and superstition remained prevalent throughout Egyptian culture, however, and some of their medical practices were ineffective—even harmful.[6] In any event, what useful knowledge they amassed was not communicated widely, perhaps because of their use of hieroglyphic writing, which was not deciphered in the Western world until the nineteenth century.

Around the same time, Babylonian physicians introduced the concepts of diagnosis and prognosis, wrote prescriptions, and used logic and observation to advance medical knowledge. A diagnostic handbook appeared around 1050 BCE. Like their Egyptian counterparts, however, Babylonian physicians did not spread their science widely, and when patients were not cured by the basic medicine of the day, exorcism and similar techniques were the only remaining options.

Hippocrates and Galen Yield to Modern Medicine

Western medicine was generally uninformed by the concepts and practices developed in Egypt and the Middle East, so the Greek physicians Hippocrates (circa 460–370 BCE) and Galen (circa 131–201 CE) were essentially working from a clean slate. *Humoralism*—the belief that the body consisted of four basic substances ("humors")—was the prevailing school of thought. Under this theory, the balance of the four humors determined one's state of health; an imbalance was said to be the cause of disease and disability. The four humors and their corresponding attributes are summarized in exhibit 2.2.

Humoralism (also known as "humorism") was challenged by certain Islamic physicians in the Middle Ages, but it dominated Western medical practice for more than 2,000 years. Given persistent ignorance of etiology, pathology, bacteriology, pharmacology, and similar disciplines, physicians were severely limited in their treatment choices. Even human anatomy was not well known. Not until the early 1600s, for instance, did William Harvey (1578–1657) become the first to describe in detail the circulatory system, and practices such as bloodletting, administration of emetics, purging, and application of poultices continued for at least two more centuries thereafter. These treatments were usually ineffective and often did more harm than good.

For example, several twentieth-century scholars surmise that President George Washington, who died in December 1799 at 84, succumbed to acute

EXHIBIT 2.2 The Four Humors			
Humor	**Organ**	**Personal Characteristic**	**Disposition**
Blood	Liver	Sanguine	Courage, amorousness
Yellow bile	Gallbladder	Choleric	Anger, bad temper
Black bile	Spleen	Melancholic	Depression, irritability, sleeplessness
Phlegm	Brain/lungs	Phlegmatic	Peacefulness and calm

inflammatory edema of the larynx (and resultant suffocation) secondary to a septic sore throat. His condition was probably aggravated by the removal of up to half his blood volume in the hours before his death.[7]

Although the picture of early medicine began to change slowly in the mid-1800s, throughout most of that century physicians still had little else to offer than comfort, compassion, and concern, as illustrated in the famous Victorian era painting *The Doctor*, shown in exhibit 2.3. In the span of about a quarter century, however, a few major developments started the process that gradually led to what we now call "modern medicine."

One of these occurred in 1846 when John C. Warren, MD (1778–1856), and dentist William T. G. Morton (1819–1868) performed the first significant public demonstration of anesthesia at Massachusetts General Hospital. Using diethyl ether, and with Morton as his anesthetist, Dr. Warren removed a tumor from a patient's jaw. After the patient, Gilbert Abbott, awoke and reported that he had felt no pain, Warren proudly announced to the audience of physicians and medical students, "Gentlemen, this is no humbug."[8] The era of painless surgery and dentistry had officially begun in the Western world (see "Anesthesia: A Brief History").

As most high school science students know, another development was the discovery by Frenchman Louis Pasteur (1822–1895) of the cause and prevention of disease. Considered the father of germ theory (1860s)

EXHIBIT 2.3
The Doctor,
Sir Luke Fildes
(1891)

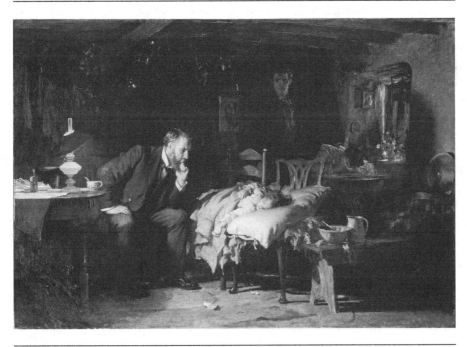

Source: Tate, London 209. Used with permission.

Anesthesia: A Brief History

Hanaoka Seishu (1760–1835), a Japanese surgeon, is said to have been the first person to perform surgery using general anesthesia when he treated a patient's breast cancer in 1804.[45] Because of the country's isolation, however, this development was unknown outside of Japan for many years.

The American surgeon C. W. Long (1815–1878) performed successful surgery using diethyl ether as an anesthetic in 1842, but he did not publish his results until 1849.[46] Morton and Warren were unaware of Long's success when they performed their operation in 1846.

The term *anesthesia* (also the prefix *anaes-*) was coined by Oliver Wendell Holmes Sr. (1819–1894), a physician, poet, and philosopher and the father of the famous US Supreme Court justice.[47]

and one of the founders of microbiology, he disproved the myth of spontaneous generation; developed vaccines for rabies, cholera, and anthrax; and created a process (now known as *pasteurization*) to slow the growth of microbes in food. An earlier pioneer, the Hungarian physician Ignaz Philipp Semmelweis (1818–1865), showed that the incidence of puerperal (childbirth) fever could be reduced drastically with antiseptic technique and hand washing in obstetrical clinics, but he was roundly ridiculed until Pasteur provided scientific proof of his theories.[9]

Next was the promotion by Joseph Lister (1827–1912) of antiseptic surgery at the University of Glasgow, Scotland. Building on Pasteur's discoveries, and consistent with Semmelweis's beliefs, Lister treated instruments with a carbolic acid solution and required surgeons to wear clean gloves and wash their hands before and after operations. As a result of these new practices, he noted a profound drop in the number of wound infections. The results were published in a widely respected British medical journal, and Lister was later elected to the Royal Society.[10] Listerine mouthwash is named in his honor, as is the bacterial genus *Listeria*.

And last, coincident with medical advances came improvements in the practice of nursing. The primary meaning of *to nurse* is to feed at the breast or to suckle,[11] thus it is no coincidence that nursing was long considered solely "women's work." And for centuries much of nursing care was provided by women religious: Catholic nuns and women of other faiths. This gender bias was reinforced during wartime—men went off to do battle, and women were left to care for the wounded. Even today, the nursing field is 90 percent female.[12]

The first inklings that nursing is a profession with standards of its own arose during the Crimean War in the early 1850s, when Florence Nightingale (1820–1910) led a group of women to serve as nurses for English troops and began to bring true order to nursing services for the first time. In addition to dressing wounds and comforting casualties, she organized supplies, improved sanitation, attended to dietary needs, and addressed similar aspects of patient care of the time. In 1860, with generous public donations, Nightingale established the first official nurses' training program, and her legacy lives on at the Florence Nightingale School of Nursing and Midwifery, a subdivision of King's College London.[13] Because of her fame and her influential books *Notes on Hospitals* (1858) and *Notes on Nursing* (1859), Nightingale (often called "the lady with the lamp") is generally regarded as the founder of modern nursing.

In this country the US Civil War brought similar pressures for nursing services, and the first US nursing schools opened during that conflict. Prominent among these institutions were nurse training programs at the New England Hospital for Women and Children (1860) and the Philadelphia Women's Hospital (1861). These were followed by similar programs at Bellevue Hospital in New York, Connecticut's New Haven Hospital, and Massachusetts General Hospital in Boston (all in 1873). According to one source, by the end of the nineteenth century, "somewhere between 400 to 800 schools of nursing were in operation in the country."[14]

With the need for nurses and nursing schools growing, and as nursing began to consider itself a profession, not merely a trade, it was inevitable that the field would seek to organize (see "What Is a Profession?"). The late 1890s saw the creation of the American Society of Superintendents of Hospital Training Schools (now the National League for Nursing), and the Nurses Associated Alumnae of the United States (the forerunner of today's American Nurses Association).

These national organizations were soon followed by state societies and associations, annual conventions, elections of officers, publication of professional materials and educational standards, and similar activities typical of most trade groups today. The groups even developed the modern title "registered nurse" and lobbied successfully for enactment of nurse licensure statutes, a "significant legislative accomplishment at a time when women held little political power."[15]

The demand for nurses increased dramatically, of course, during each of the two world wars in the twentieth century, and after World War II, a debate arose about the best method of nurse training. Hospital-based nurse training programs ("diploma programs") emphasized the practicalities of bedside care, while college-level "degree programs" were focused on more advanced types of nursing. A third avenue, community college–based "associate degree programs," tried to split the difference. The debate continues, and the modern practice of nursing now includes nurse training at various levels:

- CNA: certified nursing assistant (high school diploma)
- LPN: licensed practical nurse (high school diploma)
- LVN: licensed vocational nurse (high school diploma)
- RN: registered nurse (associate or bachelor's degree)
- APRN: advanced practice registered nurse (master's degree; not to be confused with an advanced registered nurse practitioner [ARNP], who

According to an April 2016 report from the Henry J. Kaiser Family Foundation, there are more than 3.9 million professionally active nurses in the United States today.[48] When compared to the approximately 908,000 active physicians,[49] that makes nursing the largest healthcare profession in the country by a factor of more than four to one.

has advanced clinical training beyond RN and is licensed to practice independently)

- DNP: doctor of nursing practice
- DNS or PhD: doctor of nursing science or doctor of philosophy in nursing

Given the progress made in the mid-nineteenth century, nursing and medical care were of better quality during the US Civil War than one might think. In particular, antiseptic techniques and anesthesia were not uncommon. According to one source:

> Exactly how often anesthesia was employed during the war is not known, but Union Army surgeons at the [Army Medical] Museum believed that a good estimate was 80,000 cases. . . . Supporting these statistics were the individual testimonies of field surgeons who noted that they "invariably," "universally," "always," "in every painful operation," used chloroform. . . . The experience with chloroform in the Civil War, along with other anesthetic agents, might help put to rest apocryphal stories of the purported widespread practice of soldiers biting on bullets, or being overdosed with whisky during surgery. But such stories linger on.[16]

These conditions notwithstanding, healthcare at the time was still rudimentary by today's standards. Military personnel had a much greater chance of dying from infection and disease than from direct combat injuries.[17]

> For the unfortunate Civil War soldier, whether he came from the North or from the South, [he] not only got into the army just when the killing power of weapons was being brought to a brand-new peak of efficiency; he enlisted in the closing years of an era when the science of medicine was woefully, incredibly imperfect, so that he got the worst of it in two ways. When he fought, he was likely to be hurt pretty badly; when he stayed in camp, he lived under conditions that were very likely to make him sick; and in either case he had almost no chance to get the kind of medical treatment which a generation or so later would be routine.[18]

Not until the next generation would medicine and nursing begin to be recognized as professions, not mere trades.

Post–Civil War Era Through Early 1900s

Establishments that provide medical care date back to the almshouses of the Middle Ages. The primary purpose of these pits of misery and horror for the poor and the insane was to sequester unfortunate souls from respectable society. After all, treatment as we know it today was impossible, and recovery was more a matter of God's will than of human intervention.

This picture began to change in the middle of the nineteenth century, and after the Civil War the transformation was sensational. Professor Paul Starr characterized it thus in his Pulitzer Prize–winning book, *The Social Transformation of American Medicine:*

What Is a Profession?

The accepted definition of *profession* is "an occupation, such as law, medicine, or engineering, that requires considerable training and specialized study."[50] But it could be said, whimsically, that a field is not truly a profession until it has one or more membership associations to represent it.

> Few institutions have undergone as radical a metamorphosis as have hospitals in their modern history. In developing from places of dreaded impurity and exiled human wreckage into awesome citadels of science and bureaucratic order, they acquired a new moral identity, as well as new purposes and patients of higher status. The hospital is perhaps distinctive among social organizations in having first been built primarily for the poor and only later entered in significant numbers and an entirely different state of mind by the more respectable classes. As its functions were transformed, it emerged, in a sense, from the underlife of society to become a regular part of accepted experience, still an occasion for anxiety but not horror.[19]

One might dispute whether hospitals are, even today, citadels of "bureaucratic order," but the overall thrust of Starr's argument is correct: Once a place to segregate the contagious and dying "dregs of society," the hospital as an institution rapidly gained prestige and honor when the medical profession as a whole emerged from its "dark ages" and moved into the twentieth century. As Starr put it, "No longer [was a hospital] a well of sorrow and charity but a workplace for the production of health."[20]

As scientific knowledge grew, the need for improvements in medical education and hospital care became self-evident. For centuries, physicians had received a medieval education in the classics that placed little or no emphasis on science and research. Medical training began to change after the Civil War, but it remained "highly variable and frequently inadequate."[21]

> [It] was administered through 1 of 3 basic systems: an apprenticeship system, in which students received hands-on instruction from a local practitioner; a proprietary school system, in which groups of students attended a course of lectures from physicians who owned the medical college; or a university system, in which students received some combination of didactic and clinical training at university-affiliated lecture halls and hospitals. These medical schools taught diverse types of medicine, such as scientific, osteopathic, homeopathic, chiropractic, eclectic,

Legal Brief

Licensing laws, which had been disfavored for a generation or more as being elitist and monopolistic, reappeared in the late nineteenth century. In one of the first healthcare-related cases to reach the US Supreme Court—*Dent v. West Virginia* (1889)—a state licensing law was upheld against a challenge that it unconstitutionally deprived the unlicensed appellant of the right to practice his trade. The court had little sympathy for the purported doctor's claim:

The power of the state to provide for the general welfare of its people authorizes it to prescribe all such regulations as in its judgment will secure or tend to secure them against the consequences of ignorance and incapacity, as well as of deception and fraud. . . .

Few professions require more careful preparation by one who seeks to enter it than that of medicine. . . . Due consideration, therefore, for the protection of society may well induce the state to exclude from practice those who have not such a license, or who are found upon examination not to be fully qualified. . . . No one has a right to practice medicine without having the necessary qualifications of learning and skill; and the statute only requires that whoever assumes, by offering to the community his services as a physician, that he possesses such learning and skill, shall present evidence of it by a certificate or license from a body designated by the state as competent to judge of his qualifications.[51]

physiomedical, botanical, and Thomsonian [a belief that application of either heat or cold could cure any disease]. In addition, wealthy and industrious medical students supplemented their education with clinical and laboratory training in the hospitals and universities of Europe, primarily in England, Scotland, France, and Germany. Because of the heterogeneity of educational experiences and the paucity of licensing examinations [see Legal Brief], physicians in America at the turn of the 20th century varied tremendously in their medical knowledge, therapeutic philosophies, and aptitudes for healing the sick.[22]

Reform of this system began with influential college presidents such as Charles Eliot (1834–1909) at Harvard University and Daniel Coit Gilman (1831–1908) at Johns Hopkins University. The number of commercial medical schools dropped, training requirements for physicians increased from a few months after high school to three or more years, and programs placed more emphasis on science and research (see "Exclusion and Education Reform").

Education reform continued in 1904 when the American Medical Association (AMA) (established in 1847) created the Council on Medical Education and thereafter supported the Carnegie Foundation's *Bulletin Number Four* (the famous "Flexner Report"). This document, issued in 1910,[23] proposed new standards for medical schools and helped increase physicians' professional stature.

In 1914, the AMA council set the first "standards for hospital internship programs" and identified the few hospitals that met them. Concurrent with these types of efforts, the Catholic Hospital Association (now the Catholic Health Association of the United States [CHA]) was established the following year. The number of Catholic hospitals was growing, and the new association said it wanted to respond to technological advances while ensuring that its hospitals' Catholic mission, identity, and values "would not be derailed by this new movement [for healthcare standardization]."[24] In 1920, CHA began publishing an official journal, *Hospital Progress* (now *Health Progress*), to further promote quality in inpatient healthcare.

Around the same time, the newly established American College of Surgeons (ACS) developed a set of minimum standards for hospitals and began on-site inspections of facilities. It found that fewer than 15 percent of hospitals met the standards. ACS would later join the AMA, the American Hospital Association (AHA; established in 1899), and other groups to form The Joint Commission on Accreditation of Hospitals. Now known as The Joint Commission, this organization has published *Standards for Hospital Accreditation* since 1953 (see Legal Brief).[25]

Exclusion and Education Reform

According to Starr, "The new [medical education] system greatly increased the homogeneity and cohesiveness of the profession."[52] In fact, "The profession grew more uniform in its social composition. The high costs of medical education and more stringent requirements limited the entry of students from the lower and working classes. And deliberate policies of discrimination against Jews, women, and blacks promoted still greater social homogeneity. The opening of medicine to immigrants and women, which the competitive system of medical education allowed in the 1890s, was now reversed."[53]

These effects undoubtedly contributed to the elite status with which US physicians have been viewed for most of the past century.

The 1920s and Beyond
Early Twentieth Century: The Birth of Health Policy and Politics

To this point in our historical narrative, legal principles have taken a back seat. People simply did not sue their "simple country doctors," hospitals were charitable organizations and thus were immune from liability, and adopting a national health policy was unthinkable. Aside from a few lawsuits about licensure and a smattering of public health statutes (discussed briefly later in this chapter), the law had little effect on the evolution of the US healthcare system until hospitals became more complex organizations, medical science advanced, and the needs of society changed.

But by the early twentieth century, hospitals were becoming high-quality organizations with state-of-the-art diagnostic and treatment methodologies. Use of X-rays (discovered in 1895) was common, as was administration of penicillin (discovered accidentally by Sir Alexander Fleming in 1928). Laboratory and other equipment became more sophisticated, not to mention more expensive. As hospitals became operationally more complex, they needed trained staff to handle personnel issues, billing, purchasing, medical records maintenance, fundraising, and similar corporate functions.

Legal Brief

The Joint Commission's standards are frequently cited to establish the standard of care in negligence cases. See the discussion of the *Darling* case in chapter 7.

Thus, a division of labor occurred: Patient care was left to physicians, nurses, and other clinicians, whereas business activities were carried out by salaried administrative personnel.

Some hospital administrators were physicians, but many were nurses by training. Their quaint titles ("superintendent" or "nurse matron") reflected the old paradigm of hospital qua asylum. These titles eventually changed as hospital administration became a recognized profession. Like any good profession, it needed an association, so the American College of Hospital Administrators (now the American College of Healthcare Executives) was established in 1933. At that time, there were more than 6,000 hospitals in the country—there had been fewer than 200 after the Civil War—and they needed professionals to run them.

What developed was a "peculiar bureaucracy" (Starr's expression)[26] with two lines of operational authority—one clinical and the other administrative. The former often considered hospitals merely to be "doctors' workshops," created for their benefit; the latter tended to see them as dedicated to serving the broader needs of the community. Adding to the anomalous situation was the fact that most hospitals were ultimately governed by a board of trustees representing local religious, business, professional, philanthropic, or other community interests. The trustees were charged with making major policy and strategic decisions that management and (presumably) physicians were expected to implement.

This peculiar governance and operating structure led to hospitals being described as resting on a "three-legged stool" of physicians, administrators, and governing board members. Few self-respecting sociologists or management consultants would recommend such a confounding arrangement, but it is what it is: a product of the political environment and historical coincidence (see "A Wry Definition").

If hospitals are a peculiar animal, similarly perplexing to many is the way government is structured in this country—an uncommon arrangement in which sovereign powers are divided between a national authority and its constituent units (the states). Given the American psyche after the Revolution, the founders chose a system that granted limited power to the federal government. From the beginning to the present day, most of our great national debates have revolved around finding a correct balance between central control and local autonomy. Loaded terms such as *states' rights* and *federal takeover* have inflamed policy

A Wry Definition

One of my colleagues at Washington University School of Medicine used to describe a hospital as "a collection of individual fiefdoms connected by a common heating, ventilating, and air conditioning system." Although most hospitals are no longer single buildings with a common HVAC system, consider to what extent the professor's point about individual fiefdoms remains valid.

discussions from the Whiskey Rebellion (1794) to the Civil War, the civil rights movement, healthcare reform, and the Tea Party movement.

For about 150 years, most responsibility for social programs resided with the states, and the federal government exerted little influence. Despite the language of the Preamble to the Constitution, the United States lagged behind other countries in ensuring the "general welfare" of the citizenry, at least with regard to health issues. Beginning with Germany in 1883, European countries were rapidly adopting broad plans of social insurance for sickness, old age, industrial accidents, and the like. But on this side of the Atlantic, these programs were slow to develop.

In 1906, the book *The Jungle* by Upton Sinclair (1878–1968) exposed horrendous working conditions in the slaughterhouses of Chicago and prompted a few pieces of social reform legislation at the federal level. Most notable were the Meat Inspection Act of 1906 and the Pure Food and Drug Act of the same year. But other topics such as workers' compensation were left to the states' discretion. President Theodore Roosevelt (1858–1919) and other Progressives supported the concept of health insurance for all Americans, but this idea essentially died with Roosevelt's defeat in the 1912 presidential election. The onset of World War I, the red scare that followed the Bolshevik Revolution in 1917, and opposition from employers and physicians prevented its revival for decades. Not until the Great Depression and implementation of the New Deal did public policy begin to consider the healthcare system, and then only tangentially.

When Franklin D. Roosevelt (1882–1945; often called "FDR") was elected president in 1932, the nation was in economic shambles (see "A Definition of Shambles") and social reform was in the air. A few states had passed old age pension laws by then, and 34 foreign countries were operating some form of social insurance program for their citizens.[27] FDR made Social Security a hallmark of his New Deal, proposing it to Congress in June 1934 (see "President Franklin D. Roosevelt to Congress, June 8, 1934"). His proposal included unemployment insurance, old age assistance, aid to dependent children, and grants to the states to provide various forms of medical care. But a proposal for the federal government even to study the concept of national health insurance was considered too politically controversial and was ultimately left out of the bill.

After some hearings and minor changes, the Social Security Act (SSA) passed both the Senate and the House of Representatives overwhelmingly, and it became law on August 14, 1935. Its passage just 14 months after FDR's message

A Definition of *Shambles*

Given the subject of Upton Sinclair's *The Jungle*, it is interesting to note that the word *shambles* derives from a Middle English usage meaning a place where meat is butchered and sold. It has come to carry the colloquial sense of "a scene of disorder or devastation; a muddle, a mess."[54]

President Franklin D. Roosevelt to Congress, June 8, 1934

Security was attained in the earlier days through the interdependence of members of families upon each other and of the families within a small community upon each other. The complexities of great communities and of organized industry make less real these simple means of security. Therefore, we are compelled to employ the active interest of the Nation as a whole through government in order to encourage a greater security for each individual who composes it. . . . This seeking for a greater measure of welfare and happiness does not indicate a change in values. It is rather a return to values lost in the course of our economic development and expansion.

to Congress is testament to the severity of the economic crisis then facing the country. National health insurance was not part of the SSA, and reform of our fragmented health system has been a contentious issue ever since.[28]

World War II to the Eisenhower Years

During World War II, when wage and price controls were in effect, employers added health coverage as a benefit in lieu of salary increases, and in 1954 their contributions to health plans were determined not to be taxable income to their employees. For this basic reason, even today—three generations later—most Americans' health insurance is tied to their place of employment.

Having insurance coverage tied to employment created what Professor Starr has called "a policy trap—a costly, extraordinarily complicated system which nonetheless protected enough of the public to make the system resistant to change."[29] This "trap" has bedeviled every attempt to reform the system from the 1940s to the present day.

In 1948, President Harry S. Truman (1884–1972) campaigned for reelection on a platform that included a plan for national health insurance. Truman defeated Governor Thomas E. Dewey (1902–1971) and Democrats regained control of Congress, but he never actually submitted a legislative proposal and his party was not successful in any attempts to pass a healthcare bill. According to Starr, "Southern Democrats in key leadership positions blocked [the Democrats'] initiatives, partly in fear that federal involvement in health care might lead to federal action against segregation at a time when hospitals were still separating patients by race."[30]

This fear was not entirely unreasonable. At Truman's urging, in 1946 Congress had passed the Hospital Survey and Construction Act (the "Hill-Burton Act"), a program of federal grants and loans designed to modernize existing hospitals and construct new ones in underserved areas. But to the consternation of some southern senators, Truman's original proposal prohibited racial discrimination in federally subsidized facilities. To ensure the Hill-Burton Act's passage, Senator Lister Hill (1894–1984) added a provision that allowed segregation of hospital facilities and services according to the concept of "separate but equal" (see "Segregation and the Hill-Burton Act"). The Hill-Burton Act thus has the dubious distinction of being the only federal law of the twentieth century to codify racial segregation.

The Hill-Burton Act is distinctive in another way, this one laudable. Hospitals that received federal money were required to provide a reasonable amount of free or reduced-cost services to persons who were unable to pay. The act was arguably the first federal law to address the problem of the healthcare uninsured, and it would be the last until President Lyndon B. Johnson (1908–1973) took office.

Segregation and the Hill-Burton Act

"Separate but equal" was struck down in the context of education in the famous 1954 US Supreme Court case *Brown v. Board of Education*, but not until 1963 was the Hill-Burton Act segregation provision declared unconstitutional.

Public policy issues aside, healthcare made significant advances in the 1930s, 1940s, and 1950s. Especially because of World War II, the federal government became more directly involved in supporting medicine. The medical programs of the military services were strengthened. Agencies such as the National Institutes of Health and the National Science Foundation were created or expanded. And the Public Health Service (created in 1798 to provide for merchant seamen) administered Social Security Administration (SSA) grants; ran the Indian Health Service; became more involved in medical research; and provided healthcare for certain populations, such as inmates, lepers, and narcotics addicts.

Outside of government, private groups such as the American Cancer Society and the March of Dimes spurred public support for scientific research on particular diseases. Polio, the most frightening disease of the time, was targeted for a cure by the National Foundation for Infantile Paralysis. When the Salk vaccine (named after its principal developer, Dr. Jonas Salk [1914–1995]) was declared effective and made available in 1955, "pandemonium swept the country,"[31] according to Starr. Today, except for a few cases in a handful of underdeveloped countries, polio has been virtually eradicated from the earth. (Suspicion of foreign health agencies has, at times, hindered vaccination efforts.)

Finally, the Depression era spawned some new concepts in hospital and physician insurance coverage. In *Blue Beginnings*, the history of the Blue Cross Blue Shield Association, the genesis of the Blue Cross and Blue Shield plans is summarized:

Born out of necessity in the Great Depression, the Blue Cross concept was created in 1929 by a pioneering businessman, Justin Ford Kimball. He offered a way for 1,300 school teachers in Dallas to finance 21 days of hospital care by making small monthly payments [$6 per person] to the Baylor University Hospital.

Around the same time, the Blue Shield concept was growing out of the lumber and mining camps of the Pacific Northwest. Serious injuries and chronic illness were common among workers in these hazardous jobs. Employers who wanted to

provide medical care for their workers made arrangements with physicians who
were paid a monthly fee for their services.

These pioneer programs provided the basis for what would become the
"modern" Blue Shield Plans.[32]

Although a "contract doctor" system had served workers on the Los Angeles
Aqueduct project from 1908 to 1912, the Blue Cross and Blue Shield plans
were more significant. They were soon followed by what is now known as
Kaiser Permanente, a consortium established to provide health coverage to
workers on the Grand Coulee Dam project and later to benefit shipbuilders
on the West Coast.[33]

These and similar private initiatives evolved into the concept we now
generally refer to as *managed care* plans—that is, insurance programs that
are "intended to reduce unnecessary health care costs through a variety of
mechanisms, including: economic incentives for physicians and patients to
select less costly forms of care; programs for reviewing the medical necessity
of specific services; increased beneficiary cost sharing; controls on inpatient
admissions and lengths of stay; the establishment of cost-sharing incentives
for outpatient surgery; selective contracting with health care providers; and
the intensive management of high-cost health care cases. The programs may
be provided in a variety of settings, such as health maintenance organizations
and preferred provider organizations."[34]

With various insurance options in place, the nation recovering from
the effects of World War II, and medical research proving effective against
polio and other diseases, a generation passed before we reached the next
milestone in our health policy journey.

The Great Society: Medicare and Medicaid

President Johnson was elected to a full term in 1964, giving Democrats an
overwhelming (more than two-thirds) majority in Congress. They dove right
in to consider the new president's legislative proposals on civil rights, poverty,
education, arts and culture, public broadcasting, consumer protection, the
environment, transportation, and healthcare.

Health insurance reform was one of Johnson's first priorities. It would
require scores of pages to describe the proposals and the political maneuver-
ings that allowed Medicare and Medicaid to pass, so a brief summary here
will have to do. (A detailed history can be found on the SSA website at
http://www.ssa.gov.)

We begin with a fundamental proposition: All legislation involves compromise and deal making. In the case of Medicare, if reforms were to be realized, the interests of hospitals, physicians, and insurance companies would need
to be addressed. These groups were represented by the AHA, the AMA, and

companies such as "the Blues"—all of which had a vested interest in maintaining the status quo and had traditionally opposed any effort to effect change.[35] President John F. Kennedy did not have enough votes or time in office to proceed, but with a huge majority in the Eighty-Ninth Congress, President Johnson did.

Needless to say, Johnson—a former Senate majority leader and wily political professional—was aware of the stiff opposition he would face as his Great Society proposals went forward. Cooperation from doctors, hospitals, and the insurance industry was therefore essential. Rather than advocate a comprehensive system of national health insurance for all Americans (an idea that never would have passed), the Johnson administration and Congressman Wilbur Mills, then chair of the House Ways and Means Committee, came up with an ingenious proposal—what one observer described as a "three-layered cake." It had something all sides could like:

1. The Democrats' plan for hospital insurance for the elderly and individuals with disabilities under Social Security (now called "Medicare Part A")
2. A Republican-backed plan for government-subsidized insurance to cover physicians' services ("Medicare Part B")
3. Assistance to the states for care of the poor (see "Medicaid")

In addition, the plan allowed healthcare providers (e.g., hospitals, physicians, long-term care facilities) to nominate private companies as go-betweens in dealing with the SSA. These Medicare Administrative Contractors (MACs)—originally known as Part A Fiscal Intermediaries and Part B Carriers—would receive the federal money and pay the providers' claims. They would also render consulting, auditing, and similar services. The arrangement seemed to assuage providers' and insurance companies' concerns enough to ensure passage of the bill, and it would ultimately prove financially rewarding for the MACs, who provide their services for a fee.

Blue Cross and Blue Shield, in particular, stood to benefit from this compromise because, not surprisingly, the overwhelming majority of providers chose its organizations to be their Medicare contractors. Thus it can be said that provider and insurance company support for Medicare was obtained by giving them more control over the funds that paid for the new system. As Starr put it, "As a result, the administration of Medicare was lodged in the private insurance systems [that were]

Medicaid

Although it is subsidized by federal funds, Medicaid is a state-run program, so its administrative structure, reimbursement rates, and coverage levels vary by jurisdiction. Physician participation is far from universal, and because the program is stigmatized as being public assistance (welfare), Medicaid has never attained Medicare's level of societal acceptance.

originally established to suit provider interests. And the federal government surrendered direct control of the program and its costs."[36]

As noted earlier, all legislation involves deals and compromises. Medicare and Medicaid were no exceptions. For a generation or more, organized medicine and conservative naysayers had predicted that rocks and shoals would lie ahead for the healthcare ship if something like Medicare were to pass. But in the end, the medical establishment reluctantly accepted the inevitable and made the best of it. In fact, in the first few years, Medicare was a bonanza because it paid hospitals on the basis of their costs and included a generous formula to cover depreciation of assets. For a time, hospitals sailed with fair winds and following seas, but there were storms on the horizon, and the concessions made to ensure Medicare's enactment have haunted policymakers for decades.

Nixon to Reagan

President Richard Nixon (1913–1994) began his first term in office in 1969, a time of great social unrest: John F. Kennedy (1917–1963), Robert F. Kennedy (1925–1968), and Martin Luther King Jr. (1929–1968) had been assassinated, huge riots took place in the Watts neighborhood of Los Angeles and later throughout the country after King's death, the Vietnam War was at its height, student protests against the military draft were common, and National Guard troops shot and killed four people at Kent State University in Ohio.

The situation in healthcare was also tumultuous. Even Nixon declared that a crisis was at hand because of increased costs and an unequal distribution of healthcare professionals. Costs were rising sharply and inflation was making healthcare unaffordable for millions of Americans, especially the poor. The rhetoric of the time eerily foreshadowed language used during the Clinton and Obama reform efforts.

The healthcare system was out of whack: there was too much emphasis on hospital treatment, not enough on primary care, and virtually none on wellness and prevention. The incentives, too, were all wrong. Accommodations made to the medical and insurance industries during the Medicare debate in Congress resulted in cost-based reimbursement, a formula under which Medicare paid doctors and hospitals whatever "usual, customary, and reasonable" fees prevailed in their service area. This arrangement practically gave providers a free hand to charge whatever they wanted, and not surprisingly, they did.

Starr describes the situation clearly:

> The dynamics of the system in everyday life are simple to follow. Patients want the best medical services available. Providers know that the more services they give

and the more complex the services are, the more they earn and the more they are likely to please their clients. Besides, physicians are trained to practice medicine at the highest level of technical quality without regard to cost. Hospitals want to retain their patients, physicians, and community support by offering the maximum range of services and the most modern technology, often regardless of whether they are duplicating services offered by other institutions nearby. Though insurance companies would prefer to avoid the uncertainty that rising prices create, they have generally been able to pass along the costs to their subscribers, and their profits increase with the total volume of expenditures. No one in the system stands to lose from its expansion. Only the population over whom the insurance costs and taxes are spread has to pay, and it is too poorly organized to offer resistance.

The obvious defect is the absence of any effective restraint. Yet this is not accidental oversight. It is . . . the outcome of a long history of accommodation to private physicians, as well as to hospitals and insurance companies.[37]

These ramifications are some of the "contradictions of accommodation," to use Starr's expression. Other unintended consequences included the disincentive to provide preventive and health promotion services (because they were not reimbursable costs) and Medicaid's burden on state and local governments, which left them with limited resources to care for people who were uninsured but not poor enough to qualify for the Medicaid program. The only option for the uninsured "near poor" was to seek treatment from community hospital emergency departments, the most expensive setting imaginable.

To address these financial challenges, the Nixon administration proposed developing prepaid health plans along the lines of the Kaiser Permanente model (discussed earlier). These *health maintenance organizations* (HMOs), as they are now called, would be paid a capitated amount (per member per month) and would be responsible, through a network of participating physicians, to care for their enrollees with the total funds provided. In theory, this model would rearrange the incentives, contain costs, and make wellness and prevention services profitable.

The HMO Act was passed in 1973. Results were mixed. The theory behind HMOs is sound, but keeping people well is only one way for insurance companies to prosper; another way is to collect premiums but provide less care, thereby keeping the medical loss ratio low and profits high (see the discussion of managed care in chapter 3). When mild economic recessions hit the country in the mid-1970s and early 1980s, HMOs began to see less income from the reserve funds they had invested, so they tightened their treatment criteria. Authorizations for hospital admission were harder to come by, and patients approved for treatment found themselves discharged "sicker and quicker" in many cases.

Other cost-control measures implemented during this period were certificate of need (CON) programs (to control hospitals' capital expenditures), health planning agencies (to review proposed projects and make recommendations on CONs and federal funding), and peer review organizations (to give advice on whether a physician's services were necessary in a given case).

None of these measures worked well. The avalanche of laws and regulations did not control costs and seemed to deepen the public's skepticism. Treatment was becoming more expensive with no noticeable improvement in the health of the population. The situation is similar today. As one report stated in 2007, "Despite having the most costly health system in the world, the United States consistently underperforms on most dimensions of performance, relative to other countries. . . . Compared with five other nations—Australia, Canada, Germany, New Zealand, the United Kingdom—the U.S. health care system ranks last or next-to-last on five dimensions of a high performance health system: quality, access, efficiency, equity, and healthy lives. The U.S. is the only country in the study without universal health insurance coverage, [which partly accounts] for its poor performance on access, equity, and health outcomes."[38]

A Difficult Decade

The 1970s were a difficult time. Healthcare costs were rising, and a crisis of confidence emerged among patients' rights advocates. Although there had never been a formal right to healthcare in American law, various groups pushed for healthcare rights (discussed in more depth throughout this book), including the right to

- receive respectful care,
- expect privacy and confidentiality,
- give or refuse informed consent,
- prepare advance directives about end-of-life treatment,
- receive psychiatric care if admitted involuntarily,
- view one's own medical records,
- obtain information about conflicts of interest among caregivers, and
- be informed about hospital policies.

The AHA even adopted a formal patient's bill of rights during this period in an apparent attempt to counter the public mistrust and skepticism that years of medical paternalism had engendered.

Apparently fed up with the lack of progress in controlling costs—and perhaps wanting to distract attention from the growing Watergate scandal—President Nixon proposed a national health insurance plan that would have provided comprehensive benefits for all Americans. In doing so, he became the first president to actually submit healthcare reform legislation to Congress. The timing was unfortunate, however. As Starr says, "If the name on the administration's plan had not been Nixon and had the time not been the year of Watergate, the United States might have had national health insurance in 1974" (see "A Difficult Decade"). As it was, another generation would pass before the time was right to try again.

Carter to Today

Few developments in healthcare occured during the four-year term of President Jimmy Carter (1924–). But the next decade brought a new emphasis on privatization, free competition, less regulation, and reduction of the government's role in virtually everything. The door was open to "an entirely new system of corporate medical enterprise,"[39] and some significant legislative developments followed in the next few years:

- The Tax Equity and Fiscal Responsibility Act of 1982 signaled the end of cost-based reimbursement and the beginning of Medicare's prospective payment system (PPS).
- The Social Security Amendments of 1983 phased in the use of diagnosis-related groups for hospital inpatient services under PPS.
- The Consolidated Omnibus Budget Reconciliation Act of 1985 enabled many employees to keep their health coverage after job loss, albeit for a short time and at their own expense.
- The Emergency Medical Treatment and Active Labor Act was passed in 1986 to prevent *patient dumping*, in which doctors passed low-income patients off to other providers, or simply turned poor people away, in favor of more profitable patients.

There is irony in the fact that these developments—especially the first two—occurred during Ronald Reagan's (1911–2004) presidency (from 1981 to 1989). Reagan was an outspoken opponent of "socialized medicine," and in the early 1960s he had warned that Medicare would mean government control of healthcare. Yet Medicare's pre-1983 "cost-based reimbursement" system contained virtually no control over the prices hospitals could charge. Only through the PPS system that Reagan signed into law did the government begin to set prices for healthcare services.

There were some medical developments during these years, as shown in the timeline in appendix 2.1. And, in tune with the zeitgeist, American medicine turned to an emphasis on corporatization. For-profit companies—notably, Hospital Corporation of America, Columbia, AMI, and Humana—began to acquire or manage healthcare facilities. Hospitals of all kinds (for-profit and not-for-profit) merged, diversified, consolidated, restructured, acquired one another, and divested one another. Simple hospital corporations became multi-institutional systems and tried to provide a spectrum of services, including preventive, primary, acute, long term, home health, and hospice. Although hospital leaders wanted the public to believe otherwise, it seemed to some observers that the goal was more to maximize reimbursement and increase market share than to serve communities' needs.

Healthcare even began to sound like corporate America. "Trustees" became "directors." "Hospital administrators" became "presidents" and "chief executive officers." "Medical records departments" became "health information management." "Nursing homes" turned into "skilled nursing facilities." Expressions such as *vertical and horizontal integration, industry concentration*, and *return on investment* seemed to displace the quaint concepts of mission, values, and service.

Starr was prescient when he wrote in the conclusion to his landmark book:

> This turn of events [corporatization] is the fruit of a history of accommodating professional and institutional interests, failing to exercise public control over public programs, then adopting piecemeal regulation to control the inflationary consequences, and, as a final resort, cutting back programs and turning them back to the private sector.
>
> But a trend is not necessarily fate. Images of the future are usually only caricatures of the present. Perhaps this picture of the future of medical care will also prove to be a caricature. Whether it does depends on choices that Americans have still to make.[40]

As it turns out, many of those choices have yet to be made, and despite the beginnings of reform during the Obama administration, there are ongoing calls for reform.

Soon after President Bill Clinton (1946–) took office in 1993, there was a serious effort to reform our healthcare system. The plan would have provided universal coverage by mandating insurance for everyone and setting up insurance cooperatives to help the poor obtain coverage. The effort barely got off the ground, however, because of the complexity of its provisions; the press of other important business; and heavy opposition from conservatives, libertarians, and the health insurance industry (see "Politics in Action").

Politics in Action

Insurance interests produced a famous (or infamous, depending on one's point of view) television ad campaign to oppose President Bill Clinton's proposal. The ads showed a fictional couple, Harry and Louise, complaining about the plan and urging viewers to contact their members of Congress. Ironically, the Harry and Louise characters returned during the 2008 presidential campaign and the first year of President Obama's term to *support* the concept of healthcare reform. This time the ads were sponsored by different organizations, not the health insurance industry.

While Clinton's plan was being considered, Republicans were looking ahead to the midterm elections and had little incentive to deal with healthcare reform. In the November 1994 election, the GOP regained control of Congress, effectively dismissing Clinton's reform plans. One year after his health reform ship set sail, it was dead in the water. Writing in the winter of 1995, Starr provided this epitaph:

The collapse of health care reform in the first two years of the Clinton administration will go down as one of the great lost political opportunities in American history. It is a story of compromises that never happened, of deals that were never closed, of Republicans, moderate Democrats, and key interest groups that backpedaled from proposals they themselves had earlier co-sponsored or endorsed.

It is also a story of strategic miscalculation on the part of the president and those of us who advised him."[41] [Starr had been on the policy team that advised the president during the process.]

President George W. Bush (1946–; in office from 2001 to 2009) devoted little attention to health policy. He and the country were preoccupied with the aftermath of the September 11, 2001, terrorist attacks; the war in Iraq; and major corporate financial scandals. But after the election of Barack Obama (1961–) in 2008, another opportunity presented itself.

Health Reform Arrives at Last (Apparently)

After a century of fits and starts and a year of intense political wrangling, in early 2010 Congress finally passed a health reform initiative—this one proposed by President Obama. Although it falls short of providing universal coverage, in some respects the policy is not unlike the Clinton proposal and in any event is the most sweeping, most significant, and most anticipated health legislation in US history. (The reforms are discussed in greater detail in chapter 3.)

Along with its accompanying technical amendments,[42] the Affordable Care Act (ACA) was intended to expand US citizens' and legal residents' access to health insurance coverage, control future costs, and improve the functioning of the healthcare delivery system.[43] Among other means, the ACA proposed to accomplish these changes through the following:

- Creating a new patient's bill of rights
- Allowing coverage of dependents up to age 26 on a parent's insurance plan
- Requiring individuals to obtain coverage or pay a penalty
- Providing premium and cost-sharing subsidies to needy individuals
- Making coverage available to persons who have been denied insurance because of a preexisting condition
- Requiring most employers to offer insurance coverage
- Creating insurance exchanges through which individuals and small businesses can purchase coverage
- Providing coverage for prevention and wellness services

- Expanding public programs such as Medicaid and the Children's Health Insurance Program
- Extending the life of the Medicare Trust Fund
- Creating other programs to improve, for example, quality, medical education, public health, and disaster preparedness

In addition, the reforms expanded various fraud and abuse statutes; increased the penalties for healthcare offenses; strengthened antikickback laws; made compliance programs mandatory; limited physician ownership of hospitals; and generally called for greater integrity of Medicare, Medicaid, and other governmental health programs. (Many of these topics are discussed in chapter 15.)

The ACA's reforms were to be phased in over a number of years (see timeline in chapter 3), while at the same time congressional Republicans have voted several dozen times to repeal all or part of it. Full repeal was impossible while President Obama remained in office, but major changes are likely under a Donald J. Trump (1946–) administration. A few more years will pass before a firm judgment can be made. Furthermore, some observers feel the law falls short of providing the public with *value* for its healthcare dollars spent and, therefore, that still other reforms are needed. Whether these additional changes result from legislation or market forces remains to be seen.

Given the political climate in Washington and the country's deep divisions on many issues at the time of this writing, the future of the ACA is anyone's guess.

From the Past to the Future

Review of a few thousand years of medical progress underscores the sagacity of Starr's comment that few institutions have changed as much in their recent history as have hospitals. Barely 200 years ago, they were horrid cesspools of suffering, infected by ignorance and medieval—even ancient—superstitions. Even as recently as the 1920s—before the discovery of penicillin, before the development of better diagnostic and surgical techniques, and before the establishment of uniform accreditation standards— hospitals were generally to be avoided. Today, just four generations later, the prospect of a sojourn in a hospital may cause some anxiety but is far less likely to inspire dread. In fact, hospital care is much more likely to be a cause for hope, recovery, and celebration of life.

As institutional healthcare changed dramatically, so did the practice of medicine by physicians, dentists, nurses, and other clinicians. As one of the baby boom generation (1946–1964), I witnessed a good deal of that change. But my father—who was born in 1916 and decided at age 5 to become a physician—saw almost all of it in his 94 years. If the country doctor who treated him at age 5 could be brought to the present à la Rip Van Winkle, he would be dazzled by today's modern medical centers and dumbfounded by what has happened to his simple trade.

As significant as those changes have been, consider what may happen in the next few decades. Universal insurance coverage, improved disease prevention, better wellness programs, genetic and stem cell therapies, better information systems, high-tech tools, online doctor visits, a team approach to care, concierge medicine for all, greater use of complementary and alternative medicine, and competition among providers on the basis of value rather than cost—these developments and others not yet imagined will make the medicine my father practiced seem as cumbersome to future generations as Civil War medicine appears to us.

Summary

Because an understanding of history helps to place almost any subject in context, this chapter traces the practice of medicine from ancient times to the present. Among the more important revelations is the fact that what we know as modern medicine is a recent development. Only in the past 100 years or so have we seen the discovery of penicillin, widespread use of vaccines, eradication of smallpox, invention of kidney dialysis, and other innovations become commonplace. If medical knowledge continues to increase geometrically, wondrous progress will occur in the coming decades.

Discussion Questions

1. In your opinion, what was the most important development in the history of medicine? Be prepared to defend your position.
2. Define when "modern medicine" began, and explain why you chose that moment in history.
3. List and describe the various attempts at health reform in the twentieth century. What factors led to the success or failure of each?
4. How many of the reforms set forth in the Affordable Care Act have been implemented, how successful were they, and which ones (if any) have been undone following the November 2016 election?

Notes

1. OLIVER WENDELL HOLMES JR., THE COMMON LAW 1 (1881).
2. These pages are synthetic historiography culled from many sources. Primary among them are CHARLES SINGER & E. ASHWORTH UNDERWOOD, A SHORT HISTORY OF MEDICINE (Oxford University

Press 1962); PAUL STARR, THE SOCIAL TRANSFORMATION OF AMERICAN MEDICINE (Basic Books 1982); and AMERICAN COLLEGE OF HEALTHCARE EXECUTIVES, COMING OF AGE: THE 75-YEAR HISTORY OF THE AMERICAN COLLEGE OF HEALTHCARE EXECUTIVES (Health Administration Press 2008).

3. A particularly striking example of the contrast between scientific medicine and traditional beliefs is found in ANNE FADIMAN, THE SPIRIT CATCHES YOU AND YOU FALL DOWN: A HMONG CHILD, HER AMERICAN DOCTORS, AND THE COLLISION OF TWO CULTURES (Farrar, Straus and Giroux 1997). The book tells the story of an epileptic Hmong child in California whose parents' strong belief in shamanistic animism led to "the collision of two cultures," as the book's subtitle puts it. Even though it covers events that occurred in the late twentieth century, *The Spirit Catches You* hints at what medicine in ancient times must have been like.

4. *See generally,* JOHN F. NUNN, ANCIENT EGYPTIAN MEDICINE (Red River Books 2002).

5. HOMER, THE ODYSSEY 40 (Samuel Butler, trans., Race Point Publishing 2015).

6. *See, e.g.,* Michael D. Parkins, *Pharmacological Practices of Ancient Egypt, in* THE PROCEEDINGS OF THE 10TH ANNUAL HISTORY OF MEDICINE DAYS (W. A. Whitelaw ed., published March 23, 2001), http://www.ucalgary.ca/uofc/Others/HOM/Dayspapers2001.pdf.

7. *See* Fielding O. Lewis, *Washington's Last Illness,* 4 ANNALS MED. HIST. 245–48 (1932); Creighton Barker, *A Case Report,* 9 YALE J. BIOLOGY & MED. 185–87 (1936); S. L. Shapiro, *Clinic-of-the-Month: General Washington's Last Illness,* 54 EYE EAR NOSE & THROAT MONTHLY 164–66 (1975).

8. Cristin O'Keefe Aptowicz, *The Dawn of Modern Anesthesia,* THE ATLANTIC (published September 4, 2014), http://www.theatlantic.com/health/archive/2014/09/dr-mutters-marvels/378688/.

9. *See* Semmelweis Society International, *Dr. Semmelweis's Biography* (accessed July 14, 2016), http://semmelweis.org/about/dr-semmelweis-biography and O. Hanninen, M. Farago, & E. Monos, *Ignaz Philipp Semmelweis, the Prophet of Bacteriology,* 4 INFECTION CONTROL 367 (1983).

10. Joseph Lister, *On the Antiseptic Principle in the Practice of Surgery,* 90 BRIT. MED. J. (1867).

11. *See* THE AMERICAN HERITAGE DICTIONARY OF THE ENGLISH LANGUAGE (5th ed. 2011).

12. US Census Bureau, *Men in Nursing Occupations* (issued February 2013), https://www.census.gov/people/io/files/Men_in_Nursing_Occupations.pdf.

13. *See* King's College London, *Florence Nightingale Faculty of Nursing and Midwifery* (accessed July 14, 2016), at www.kcl.ac.uk/schools/nursing.

14. University of Pennsylvania School of Nursing, *Nursing, History and Health Care: Introduction* (accessed August 5, 2016), http://www.nursing.upenn.edu/nhhc/Pages/Welcome.aspx.

15. U. Penn., *supra* note 14.

16. J. T. H. Connor, *Chloroform, Ether, and the Civil War*, Mil. Med. Feb. 2004, http://www.civilwarmedicalbooks.com/chloroform_Civil_War.html.

17. Michael R. Gilchrist, *Disease & Infection in the American Civil War*, 60 Am. Biology Tchr. 258 (1998), www.jstor.org/pss/4450468.

18. Shotgun's Home of the American Civil War, *Civil War Medicine* (updated November 24, 2006), at www.civilwarhome.com/civilwar medicineintro.htm.

19. Paul Starr, The Social Transformation of American Medicine 145 (1982) [hereinafter STAM].

20. *Id.* at 146.

21. Andrew H. Beck, *The Flexner Report and the Standardization of American Medical Education*, 291 J. Am. Med. Ass'n. 2139 (2004), http://jama.jamanetwork.com/article.aspx?articleid=198677.

22. *Id.*

23. American Medical Association, *Historical Timeline* (accessed July 14, 2016), at http://www.ama-assn.org/ama/pub/about-ama/our-people/ama-councils/council-medical-education/historical-timeline.page?.

24. Catholic Health Association of the United States, *Our History* (accessed July 14, 2016), at https://www.chausa.org/about/about/our-history.

25. The Joint Commission, *The Joint Commission: Over a Century of Quality and Safety* (accessed July 14, 2016), at https://www.joint commission.org/assets/1/6/TJC_history_timeline_through_2015.pdf.

26. STAM at 177.

27. *Historical Background and Development of Social Security*, https://www.ssa.gov/history/briefhistory3.html.

28. *See generally* Kaiser Family Foundation, *National Health Insurance—A Brief History of Reform Efforts in the U.S.*, Issue Brief 7871 (published March 18, 2009), www.kff.org/healthreform/upload/7871.pdf.

29. PAUL STARR, REMEDY AND REACTION 41 (rev. ed. 2013).

30. Kaiser Family Foundation, *supra* note 28.

31. STAM at 147.

32. *See, e.g.*, Consumers Union, *Blue Cross and Blue Shield: A Historical Compilation* (accessed July 14, 2016), at https://consumersunion. org/wp-content/uploads/2013/03/yourhealthdollar.org_blue-cross-history-compilation.pdf. *See also* STAM at 295.

33. STAM at 322.

34. National Center for Biotechnology Information, *Managed Care Programs* (accessed July 14, 2016), at www.ncbi.nlm.nih.gov/mesh?term= managed%20care.

35. The AMA described a Medicare proposal in the Kennedy administration as "the most deadly challenge ever faced by the medical profession" and launched an all-out effort to defeat it. *See* Social Security Administration, *Social Security History* (accessed July 14, 2016), at https://www.ssa.gov/history/corningchap4.html.

36. STAM at 375, 378.

37. STAM at 387.

38. Karen Davis, Cathy Schoen, Stephen C. Schoenbaum, Michelle M. Doty, Alyssa L. Holmgren, Jennifer L. Kriss, & Katherine K. Shea, *Mirror, Mirror on the Wall: An International Update on the Comparative Performance of American Health Care* at p. i (May 2007). Available at www.commonwealthfund.org.

39. STAM at 418.

40. *Id.* at 448–449.

41. Paul Starr, *What Happened to Health Care Reform?*, 20 AM. PROSPECT 20–31 (1995).

42. The Health Care and Education Reconciliation Act, HR 4872; Pub. L. No. 111-152 (2010).

43. *Id.*

44. New York Trust Co. v. Eisner, 256 U.S. 345, 349 (1921).

45. Masuru Izuo, *Medical History: Seishu Hanaoka and His Success in Breast Cancer Surgery Under General Anesthesia Two Hundred Years Ago*, 11 BREAST CANCER 319 (2004).

46. C. SINGER & E. A. UNDERWOOD, A SHORT HISTORY OF MEDICINE at 343 (Oxford University Press 1962).

47. *See* AM. HERITAGE DICTIONARY, *supra* note 11.

48. Henry J. Kaiser Family Foundation, *Total Number of Professionally Active Nurses* (published April 2016), http://kff.org/other/state-indicator/total-registered-nurses/.

49. Henry J. Kaiser Family Foundation, *Total Number of Professionally Active Physicians* (published April 2016), http://kff.org/other/state-indicator/total-active-physicians/.
50. AM. HERITAGE DICTIONARY, *supra* note 11.
51. Dent v. West Virginia, 129 U.S. 114 (1889).
52. STAM at 123.
53. *Id.* at 124.
54. See SHORTER OXFORD ENGLISH DICTIONARY, 6th ed., 2007.

Appendix 2.1: A Select Timeline of the History of Medicine

Date	Key Events
Third millennium BCE	• Trepanation surgery is used for purposes unknown (beginning at least 6500 BCE). • Egyptian physician Imhotep describes the diagnosis and treatment of 200 diseases (circa 2600 BCE). • Spirits and supernatural forces are thought to be the cause of disease.
Second millennium BCE	• Code of Hammurabi is inscribed (circa 1790 BCE).
Fifth century BCE	• Hippocrates, the "father of Western medicine," uses observation of the body as a basis for medical knowledge. He recommends changes in diet, rudimentary drugs, and keeping the body "in balance" (humoralism) rather than prayer and sacrifice to divinities.
Fourth century BCE	• Aristotle codifies known science. • First known anatomy book appears (circa 300 BCE), but religion still dominates medicine. • Hippocratic Oath appears.
Second century BCE	• Galen becomes physician to Roman Emperor Marcus Aurelius and builds on Hippocrates's theories of the humors but supports observation and reasoning in medical science.
Fifth to tenth century CE	• Western Europe experiences decreasing population and trade; a flood of migrants and invaders; and a paucity of literary, cultural, and scientific output. Culture continues to flourish in the Byzantine (Eastern Roman) Empire.
Eighth century CE	• Baghdad becomes "a veritable seedbed of medical learning, cross-fertilized by Persian-Mesopotamian, Byzantine-Greek, and Indian traditions" (NLM and NIH 2006). The recent introduction of paper enables knowledge to be more easily recorded and published.
Tenth century CE	• Rhazes—considered the greatest physician and practitioner of Islamic medicine during the Middle Ages—revolutionizes Islamic medicine by using careful clinical observation and notation, writes scientific treatise on infectious disease, identifies smallpox, and publishes *The Comprehensive Book on Medicine* (the *Hawi*).
Eleventh century CE	• Persian polymath Avicenna (Ibn Sina) builds on Rhazes's work and publishes *The Canon of Medicine*, an encyclopedic book dealing with pharmacology, the nature of contagious diseases, experimental and evidence-based medicine, and many other topics. It is consulted for centuries thereafter in some parts of the world.
1249	• Roger Bacon invents spectacles.

Date	Key Events
Fourteenth century	• Bubonic plague, believed by many to be a punishment from God, kills millions in Europe.
Fifteenth century	• Leonardo da Vinci and others study anatomy by dissecting corpses, much to the displeasure of the Catholic Church. • Printing press is invented (1454), enabling knowledge to be recorded and transmitted more freely.
Sixteenth century	• New drugs such as quinine and laudanum (an opiate) are discovered in North and South America. • Royal College of Physicians is formed in London (1518). • Paracelsus (1493–1541) rejects ancient texts, emphasizes natural sciences, and founds the fields of toxicology and psychology. • Zacharias Janssen invents the microscope (1590).
Seventeenth century	• William Harvey publishes *An Anatomical Study of the Motion of the Heart and of the Blood in Animals* (1628). The book forms the basis for future research on blood vessels, arteries, and the heart. • Sir Christopher Wren experiments with canine blood transfusions (1656). • Anton van Leeuwenhoek improves the microscope, discovers blood cells, and later observes bacteria (1670).
Eighteenth century	• First smallpox inoculations are developed. • James Lind discovers that citrus fruit prevents scurvy. • First successful appendectomy is performed. • Edward Jenner develops the first effective smallpox vaccine.
Early nineteenth century	• Royal College of Surgeons is formed (1800). • René Laennec invents the stethoscope. • First successful human blood transfusion is performed. • Ether and nitrous oxide are used as general anesthetics. • Benjamin Rush (1746–1813)—signatory of the Declaration of Independence, founder of Dickinson College, professor of medicine at the University of Pennsylvania, and a proponent of bloodletting and similar therapies—is considered the "father of American psychiatry." • Syringe is invented.
Mid- to late nineteenth century	• American Medical Association is founded (1847). • Louis Pasteur identifies germs as cause of disease. • Florence Nightingale lays the foundations for professional nursing and modernization of hospitals. • Joseph Lister develops antiseptic surgical techniques. • Vaccines developed for cholera, anthrax, rabies, tetanus, diphtheria, typhoid fever, and bubonic plague. • Sir William Osler (1849–1919), the "father of modern medicine" and cofounder of Johns Hopkins Hospital, establishes the first medical residency program.

(continued)

Date	Key Events
Mid- to late nineteenth century *(continued)*	• Clara Barton promotes public support for a national society to work with the International Red Cross. The American Red Cross is founded 1881. • American Public Health Association is formed (1872). • X-rays are discovered, rather accidentally, by Wilhelm Roentgen (1895). • Association of Hospital Superintendents, forerunner of the American Hospital Association, is founded (1899).
Early twentieth century	• Karl Landsteiner introduces blood classification system (types A, B, AB, and O). • X-ray technology becomes available. • US Pure Food and Drug Act is enacted (1906). • Tuberculosis skin test is introduced (1907). • The Flexner Report on medical education is published (1910). • American College of Surgeons, first of the American medical specialty colleges, is founded (1913). • Catholic Hospital Association (now Catholic Health Association of the United States) is founded (1915). • Paul Dudley White develops the electrocardiogram. • Polio epidemics break out in New York and Boston (1916) and continue elsewhere for years. • Influenza pandemic kills 15 million worldwide (1918–1919). • Edward Mellanby discovers that lack of vitamin D causes rickets (1921). • Insulin is first used to treat diabetes (1922). • Vaccines are developed for whooping cough, tuberculosis, and yellow fever. • Medical Group Management Association is founded (1926). • American Health Information Management Association is founded (1928). • Penicillin is discovered (1928). • American College of Hospital Administrators (now American College of Healthcare Executives) is founded (1933). • Vitamins A, B_1, B_2, and B_3 are identified. • First blood bank opens in Chicago (1937). • National Cancer Institute is founded (1937).
Mid-twentieth century	• Ultrasound is developed (1942). • Chemotherapy is developed for cancer treatment (1942). • Healthcare Financial Management Association is founded (1946). • Association of University Programs in Health Administration is founded (1948). • Influenza vaccines and streptomycin are developed. • First cardiac pacemaker is invented (1950). • Joint Commission on Accreditation of Hospitals (now The Joint Commission) is established (1951). • Polio vaccine is used widely (1950s).

Date	Key Events
Mid-twentieth century *(continued)*	• James Watson and Francis Crick describe the structure of the DNA molecule (1953). • First kidney transplant is performed (1954). • Vaccines for measles, mumps, rubella, chicken pox, pneumonia, and meningitis are developed. • Health Information and Management Systems Society (founded as Hospital Management Systems Society) is established (1961). • Nursing home administrators form an association (now American College of Health Care Administrators) (1962). • Medicare and Medicaid are enacted (1965). • Federation of American Hospitals (for-profit hospitals) is established (1966). • American Organization of Nurse Executives is founded (1967). • First heart transplant and coronary bypass operations are performed (1967). • Health Maintenance Organization Act is passed (1973). • American College of Physician Executives is founded (1975), previously called American Academy of Medical Directors.
Late twentieth century	• World Health Organization declares smallpox eradicated (1980). • HIV, the virus that causes AIDS, is identified (1983). • Artificial kidney dialysis machine is invented (1985). • Consolidated Omnibus Budget Reconciliation Act is passed to allow for the continuation of group health coverage after a job loss (1985). • Emergency Medical Treatment and Active Labor Act is passed to prohibit patient dumping (1986). • Hepatitis A vaccine is developed (1992). • Dolly the sheep is the first cloned mammal (1996). • Health Insurance Portability and Accountability Act is passed to provide insurance portability and new privacy standards (1996). • State Children's Health Insurance Program and Medicare+Choice (later Medicare Advantage) are established (1997). • Balanced Budget Act is enacted to cut Medicare spending and provide beneficiaries with additional choices through private health plans (1997).
Early twenty-first century	• Healthcare costs continue to rise in the United States; total healthcare spending makes up more than 17.3 percent of gross domestic product ($2.7 trillion). • The Human Genome Project is completed (2003), and the entire sequence of nearly 40,000 human genes is documented. • Medicare Part D (drug benefit) begins (2006). • Affordable Care Act (ACA) is signed into law (2010) and upheld by the US Supreme Court (2012), but Medicaid expansion is optional. • 32 states and District of Columbia expand Medicaid per ACA (by 2016). • Election of President Donald J. Trump (2016) clouds the ACA's future.

Sources

Altman and Frist, *Medicare and Medicaid at 50 Years*, 314 J. Amer. Med. Assn. 384 (2015).

AMERICAN COLLEGE OF HEALTHCARE EXECUTIVES, COMING OF AGE: THE 75-YEAR HISTORY OF THE AMERICAN COLLEGE OF HEALTHCARE EXECUTIVES (Health Administration Press 2008).

History-Timelines.org.uk, *History of Medicine Timeline* (2011), http://www.datesandevents.org/events-timelines/10-history-of-medicine-timeline.htm.

National Library of Medicine and National Institutes of Health, *Greek Medicine: Galen* (2009), www.nlm.nih.gov/hmd/greek/greek_galen.html.

———, *Medieval Manuscripts: Arabic Legacies* (2006), http://www.nlm.nih.gov/hmd/medieval/arabic.html.

———, *MEDLINEplus Goes Local with "NC Health Info"* (2003), http://www.nlm.nih.gov/pubs/nlmnews/janmar03/58n1newsline.pdf.

Terry, K. *Health Spending Hits 17.3 Percent of GDP in Largest Annual Jump* (2010), http://www.bnet.com/blog/healthcare-business/health-spending-hits-173-percent-of-gdp-in-largest-annual-jump/1117.

HEALTH REFORM, ACCESS TO CARE, AND ADMISSION AND DISCHARGE

> **After reading this chapter, you will**
>
> - understand the basic provisions of the Affordable Care Act (ACA) and the Supreme Court's decisions upholding it,
> - have additional background on the "right" to healthcare,
> - understand the hospital's duty to admit and care for patients under routine and emergency circumstances,
> - recognize that not-for-profit status carries certain obligations to provide benefits to the community,
> - understand the issues that apply to the admission and discharge of psychiatric patients, and
> - be familiar with basic issues in managed care.

The "Right" to Healthcare

We often hear the claim that the United States has "the best healthcare system in the world." But can a country that does not guarantee access to care support that claim? Even the National Academy of Sciences disputes such an assertion: "Although the United States ranks highest in per capita spending (in total and as a percentage of GDP [gross domestic product]) and ranks high in the availability of medical technology, this spending has not produced comparably high measures of health status. The health of Americans consistently ranks poorly relative to that of residents of other industrialized nations."[1] In other words, for those who are covered by some form of insurance or who can afford to pay out of pocket, the highest-quality healthcare on the planet is available in the United States, but because not everyone can access the care they need, whether we have the best healthcare *system* is arguable.

So a fundamental question arises: Do we have a legal right to healthcare? The answer is multifaceted. First, there is no *constitutional* right to healthcare. Given the level of medical knowledge in the eighteenth century (see chapter 2), healthcare is not mentioned in the Constitution and is not one of the "unalienable rights" referred to in the Declaration of Independence. Although the Constitution provides that Congress may collect taxes "to provide for the ... general Welfare,"[2] the general welfare does not perforce include the provision of healthcare.

But if there is no constitutional right, where else might a right to healthcare might be guaranteed? The answer here is twofold: (1) various statutes and common-law principles provide for legal rights relating to the healthcare field; and (2) whether one has a right to healthcare services depends on the circumstances. Here are some examples:

- In emergencies, individuals who come or are brought to a hospital have a statutory right to be seen and perhaps have their conditions stabilized.
- Persons with health insurance have a contractual right to their covered benefits.
- Persons with limited English proficiency have a statutory right to effective communication with their care providers.
- The doctor–patient relationship implies a contractual right to treatment without abandonment.
- There are common-law and statutory rights to informed consent and patient self-determination.
- Certain poor, disabled, and elderly persons have a statutory right to governmental financial assistance for healthcare services.

As one sees from this discussion, the United States does not guarantee universal access to healthcare either constitutionally or by statute. Given the contentious history of this issue (see chapter 2 and appendix 3.1) and the toxicity of today's political climate, Congress is unlikely to push for a truly universal healthcare system anytime soon. President Barack Obama's reforms in 2010 are the closest we have come thus far.

The Affordable Care Act

Congress passed the Patient Protection and Affordable Care Act and various technical amendments in March 2010.[3] Upheld by the US Supreme Court in June 2012 and again in June 2015,[4] this landmark legislation does not create a system of universal insurance, but it is the most significant attempt at health reform since the enactment of Medicare and Medicaid in the mid-1960s, and it has begun to decrease significantly the number of people who do not have health insurance (see Legal Brief).

Although generally referred to as "*the* law" or "*the* ACA" (or sometimes, derisively, as "Obamacare"), the legislation was not a single statute but was a combination of the following:

- Patient Protection and Affordable Care Act of 2010, enacted on March 21, 2010
- Health Care and Education Reconciliation Act of 2010 (HCERA), enacted on March 25, 2010
- Indian Health Care Improvement Reauthorization and Extension Act of 2009, made part of the ACA bill before final passage
- Student Aid and Fiscal Responsibility Act, a rider to HCERA

Legal Brief

The number of uninsured declined steadily after the ACA went into effect. As of October 2016, the number was under 29 million—less than 11 percent of the nonelderly population—down from more than 41 million in 2013. Coverage gains were particularly large among low-income people living in states that expanded Medicaid.[72]

The fact that the ACA was this jumble of statutes is due largely to political realities and the interplay of various affected interests. When all the amendments are counted, the ACA ran to more than 900 pages and comprised ten "titles" (major divisions) with about 400 individual sections. In general terms, it was intended to slow the rate of healthcare cost increases, improve the quality of care, and provide greater access to affordable insurance. Its most salient provisions aimed to

- expand coverage to as many as 32 million previously uninsured persons;
- require everyone to obtain insurance by 2014 or pay a penalty (the "individual mandate" and "shared responsibility payment" provisions);
- create health insurance exchanges (marketplaces) to make coverage more affordable;
- provide tax credits to low-income persons;
- prohibit denial of coverage based on preexisting conditions;
- prohibit insurance plans from placing lifetime limits on the dollar value of coverage;
- prohibit insurers from rescinding coverage except in cases of fraud;
- preserve the Children's Health Insurance Program (CHIP);
- require parents' insurance policies to cover dependent children to age 26;
- create a voluntary long-term care insurance program for the elderly (this provision was later repealed);
- strengthen fraud and abuse laws (such as the federal antikickback, false claims, and physician self-referral statutes);
- require disclosure of financial arrangements between providers and manufacturers of drugs, devices, and supplies ("sunshine" or "transparency" provisions);

- encourage physician–hospital collaboration (accountable care organizations, or ACOs) to share in Medicare cost savings;
- improve prevention and wellness programs and medical research and education; and
- improve the cost-effectiveness of the Medicare and Medicaid payment systems.

Appendix 3.2 lists select ACA reforms arranged by the segments of the sector they affect.

The Effect

The ACA was scheduled for implementation in phases throughout the 2010s (see exhibit 3.1 for a summary of the implementation timeline), and the result has been a significant decrease in the number of uninsured persons. In addition, and notwithstanding anticipated premium increases, the law has made insurance more affordable for many Americans. At least 16 states have created their own health insurance exchanges, and the rest have relied on the federal exchange, healthcare.gov. The well-publicized glitches that plagued the federal exchange at its outset have been resolved for the most part.

Governments in as many as two dozen states, most of them led by Republicans, initially refused to expand Medicaid, believing that the cost would be a significant burden. Proponents countered that under the ACA the federal share of the increased cost would be at least 90 percent, and eventually a few recalcitrant states reversed their positions after electing new governors. By the fall of 2016, 32 jurisdictions (including the District of Columbia) had expanded Medicaid by either statute or executive action.

It should be noted that Republicans in Congress have introduced more than 60 bills to repeal the ACA in its entirety, even though it was modeled in large part on reforms adopted by Massachusetts in 2006 under Republican governor and eventual presidential candidate Mitt Romney. Each of the repeal attempts failed, but the law is now in serious jeopardy with President Donald J. Trump in office and Republican majorities in both houses of Congress.

Assuming some provisions of the ACA will continue to be implemented, readers may wish to follow some of these indicators:

- Number of states that expand their Medicaid programs and accept federal funding to do so
- Number of states that reverse their previous positions on expansion, and the effect of gubernatorial elections on those decisions
- Number (total and percentage) of nonelderly uninsured, and how many of those signed up for the first time following the November 2016 election

- Number (total and percentage) of people under age 65 in the United States who report they did not have health insurance during the previous year
- How well the health insurance exchanges continue to operate as more individuals seek better deals or seek coverage for the first time
- The rate of healthcare inflation compared with all inflation
- Total US healthcare spending as a percentage of gross domestic product
- Whether health outcomes—perhaps the hardest goal of all to measure—have improved

An Uncertain Future

The ACA's implementation was planned to occur in phases through 2018. However, the future of the ACA is in serious doubt given the election in 2016 of a Republican president and Republican majorities in both houses of the 115th Congress (which is in office through the 2018 election). Repeal efforts will accelerate on Capitol Hill, and thus the major impetus for change will shift from the courts to the political arena.

Readers will wish to track how many of the implementation steps listed in exhibit 3.1 were completed, delayed, or rescinded by the new Congress, and what effect any changes have on the number of persons under the age of 65 who do not have insurance.

2010	• Various fraud/abuse provisions • Dependent coverage to age 26 • No limiting coverage for preexisting conditions in dependents under age 19 • National high-risk pool for others with preexisting conditions • Minimum coverage required for preventive services • Prohibition of rescission and lifetime limits • $250 rebate for those in the "donut hole" • Tax credits to small employers (fewer than 25 employees) • Requirement that health plans report medical-loss ratio • Reductions in Medicare market basket • Additional residency and medical education provisions • Process for reviewing insurance premiums and justifying increases • Expansion of CHIP • Various programs to study quality of care and effectiveness	**EXHIBIT 3.1** Affordable Care Act Implementation Timeline
2011	• Voluntary long-term care program for elderly • Medical malpractice demonstration project	

(continued)

EXHIBIT 3.1
Affordable
Care Act
Implementation
Timeline
(continued)

2011 *(continued)*	• Ban on physician ownership of hospitals • Medicare Advantage payment cuts • Adjustments to payments for hospital-acquired conditions • Medicaid alternative care delivery for certain chronic conditions • Expanded Medicare coverage for environmental hazards • Care coordination for dual-eligibles • Changes regarding FDA approval of generic drugs • Various prevention, wellness, and quality studies and grants • Tax changes
2012	• Accountable care organizations begin to share in cost savings • Hospital value-based purchasing • Increase in physician-quality reporting requirements • Various Medicaid demonstration projects • Increased requirements for not-for-profit status • Additional data collection on quality issues • Excess readmissions provisions go into effect • Pharmaceutical manufacturers to report information on drug samples
2013	• Disclosure of financial relationships among providers, suppliers, and manufacturers (transparency reporting) • Consumer-owned co-ops begin • Expanded coverage of preventive services (Medicaid) • Physician comparison database made available to public • Claims simplification improvements • Reductions in payments for hospital readmission • Increased reimbursement for primary care (Medicare) • Various tax provisions take effect
2014	• Individual and employer mandates take effect • Penalties for employers who do not offer benefits • Coverage expansions • Expanded Medicaid eligibility (optional, per Supreme Court ruling) • State health insurance exchanges begin • 100% federal match for new Medicaid enrollees • Employers may offer rewards for employees participating in wellness programs • Medicare and Medicaid disproportionate share payments reduced • Medicare commission to report to Congress
Through 2018	• Multistate insurance ("health choice") compacts • Further reductions of payments for hospital-acquired conditions • Independent Payment Advisory Board to propose changes to Medicare payments • Excise tax on "Cadillac" health plans

Sources: See generally, Kaiser Family Foundation, Health Reform Implementation Timeline (accessed November 3, 2016), http://www.kff.org/interactive/implementation-timeline; *and* Venson Wallin Jr. et al., *Blunting the Negative Impact of Healthcare Reform*, 64 HEALTHCARE FIN. MGMT., 62–66 (2010).

National Federation of Independent Business v. Sebelius

Literally minutes after President Obama signed the ACA into law, Florida and 12 other states filed suit in federal district court to challenge it. They were later joined by 13 other states, numerous individual plaintiffs, and the National Federation of Independent Business (NFIB) in a case that made its way to the US Supreme Court as *NFIB v. Sebelius*, 567 U.S. 1, 132 S. Ct. 2566 (2012).

The case focused on two main questions: (1) whether the requirement that individuals purchase health insurance or pay a "shared responsibility payment" (the "individual mandate") exceeds Congress's constitutional authority, and (2) whether the federal government can force states to expand their Medicaid programs.

In a rather remarkable bit of diplomacy and judicial craftsmanship, in June 2012 Chief Justice John Roberts cobbled together a 5–4 majority that held:

1. The individual mandate cannot be supported by the commerce clause of the US Constitution, *but*
2. It is a valid exercise of Congress's taxing power (see Law in Action);
3. Medicaid expansion cannot be coerced, but it is optional at each state's discretion; and
4. The rest of the reform law remains intact.

The practical effect of *NFIB v. Sebelius* was that the most salient provisions of the ACA survived: elimination of annual and lifetime benefits limitations, prevention of policy rescission because of illness, coverage of children up to 26 on

Law in Action

The first question was whether the individual mandate ("shared responsibility payment") is a tax. This issue was important because under a law known as the Anti-Injunction Act (AIA), taxes can be challenged only after they have been paid. If the payment were considered a tax, the case would have to be dismissed. In fact, that is what the Fourth Circuit had ruled.

But the chief justice and his colleagues disagreed. They found it significant that Congress used the word "penalty" to describe this payment but called other payments in the reform law "taxes." Accordingly, they held the shared responsibility payment is *not* a tax within the meaning of the AIA and the case could not be dismissed on that basis.

On the other hand, the AIA does not determine whether the penalty is a "tax" within the meaning of the Constitution's grant of authority to Congress to "lay and collect taxes."[73] That a concept can be classified as one thing for a certain purpose and as something else for another boggled the minds of some people and provided talking points for disingenuous politicians and doctrinaire commentators who opposed the ACA.

Chief Justice Roberts's distinction is not logically inconsistent, however. A concept—such as the ACA's penalty for not having insurance—can be judged by different standards depending on context and function.

A simple example may help to clarify. To a botanist, a tomato is a fruit—the fleshy, seed-bearing part of a flowering plant. To a cook, however, a tomato is a vegetable because it has less sugar than most fruits and is served as part of a salad or entrée rather than at dessert. As British journalist Miles Kington once wrote, "Knowledge is knowing that a tomato is a fruit; wisdom is not putting it in a fruit salad."[74]

To hold that it is a fruit in one context (botany) and not in another (cooking) is eminently defensible. This distinction was precisely the finding the US Supreme Court made more than a century

(continued)

(continued from previous page)

ago. In the late 1800s, US tariff laws imposed a tax on imported vegetables but not on fruits, so classification of the tomato was a matter of some legal and financial importance. In *Nix v. Hedden*, 149 U.S. 304 (1893), the Supreme Court decided that, regardless of what botanists say, the tomato is a vegetable *for purposes of customs regulations* because of how the tomato is used and the popular perception that it is more vegetable-like than fruit-like.

Like a tomato, the shared responsibility payment is one thing by one set of standards—but something else by another. It is a tax *for purposes of constitutional analysis*, but it does not qualify as a tax under the narrower definition of the AIA.

their parents' plans, guaranteed coverage for preexisting conditions, preventive services at no cost to Medicare beneficiaries, encouragement of ACOs, reforms of underwriting practices (e.g., the medical loss ratio), increased antifraud enforcement, the ban on physician-owned hospitals, and the "individual mandate." In addition, although states could not be forced to expand their Medicaid programs, federal funds are still available to cover much of the incremental cost for those states that choose to avail themselves of the opportunity.

The troublesome question left undecided by *NFIB v. Sebelius* was whether federal money could subsidize premiums for low-income individuals whose states did not establish their own health insurance exchange. This issue was the focus of the Supreme Court's second landmark healthcare decision.

King v. Burwell

Undaunted by their defeat in *NFIB v. Sebelius*, the ACA's opponents next tried to sabotage the law by arguing in *King v. Burwell* that it allows subsidies only for individuals who gain coverage through a state-run exchange, not through the federal exchange. But in a 6–3 decision Chief Justice Roberts noted that without subsidies the statute would not work as Congress intended; instead, low-income people in states relying on the federal exchange would not be able to afford coverage, and those states' insurance markets would be pushed into a "death spiral."

The court's majority was not about to let the ACA fail because of a few examples of what Roberts called "inartful drafting." Justices Antonin Scalia, Clarence Thomas, and Samuel Alito dissented vociferously, of course. (A lengthy excerpt of the case is provided in The Court Decides: *King v. Burwell* at the end of this chapter.)

Additional Observations

Despite the Supreme Court decisions in *NFIB v. Sebelius* and *King v. Burwell*, which upheld the ACA, the law's clear benefits—more insured individuals with greater access to care and drugs—are in jeopardy following the 2016 election. What comes next is uncertain and will warrant close attention. Following are a few reflections.

First, after years of emotional, rancorous, and often disingenuous political discourse (see Law in Action), the ACA was a giant step toward improving Americans' access to healthcare and controlling the costs of health services. Tumid political rhetoric to the contrary notwithstanding, the ACA was not socialized medicine or a "massive power grab" by the federal government, as opponents often claimed. Many commentators seem to feel that it was a reasonable compromise.

Second, much of the reason for the long implementation timeline had to do with Congress's desire to defer to the states and to "start small" with various demonstration projects and pilot programs. At least 40 sections of the law refer in some significant way to state initiatives that constitute a kind of public policy laboratory for experimenting with new ideas. Some of these provisions for state-based innovations include flexibility relating to insurance exchanges, flexibility to establish

Law in Action

An example of politicized discourse is the false rumor that the bill would include "death panels" that could "pull the plug on Granny" if her care cost too much.

This phony issue and the resulting outcry led legislators to eliminate a provision for Medicare to cover voluntary physician consultations about living wills, healthcare powers of attorney, hospice benefits, and similar matters. Instead, the ACA merely set up demonstration projects to study further the effectiveness of hospice care versus other treatments for the terminally ill.

Still, months after ACA's enactment, a Kaiser Family Foundation survey showed that more than a third of seniors incorrectly believed the law would "allow a government panel to make decisions about end-of-life care for people on Medicare."[75]

Despite the risk of more demagoguery on the issue, in 2015 the Obama administration revived a proposal to reimburse physicians for discussing end-of-life care with their patients.

alternative programs, an eligibility option for family planning services, new options for states to provide long-term care services, and demonstration programs to evaluate alternatives to current systems of medical tort litigation. These options and projects are, of course, subject to change by Congress and to various approaches in the several states.

Third, the ACA strengthened the government's primary fraud laws—the false claims, antikickback, and Stark self-referral statutes—and enforcement agencies will use them more aggressively. As discussed in chapter 15, regulatory agencies' increased zeal for recovering money spent unnecessarily as a result of fraud, waste, and abuse should help recoup some of the costs of new programs.

Fourth, considering all of the implementation challenges, the biggest hurdles were perhaps those the states had to face. They needed to set up insurance exchanges (or allow the federal government to operate one for them), amend their insurance codes, expand their Medicaid programs (if they chose to do so), and test alternatives to medical malpractice litigation, all while facing significant budget deficits and keeping an eye on the constantly changing political landscape. For this reason, implementation may seem to be taking forever. In the words of one health policy analyst written in 2010 but still valid today,

Implementation [often seems to be] adaptive and somewhat unpredictable; a function of real world developments, politics, the number of players and decision points and the time period involved in implementing a law. In the case of health reform, implementation [will] depend not only on what is written in the law, but also on how the political and economic landscape shifts, how governors and states respond to health reform, how the private sector responds, how health care institutions and health professionals filter the intent of the legislation on the front lines, what the media [do], and most of all, what the public's reaction to health reform is over the next several years.[5]

Some Final Thoughts

Change always brings unintended consequences, often in unrelated areas. For example, following the Supreme Court's ruling on same-sex marriage, many gay and lesbian couples found that health insurance coverage was suddenly available through a spouse's employer. But what will be the long-term cost implications for the businesses that employ same-sex couples? Will they drop "domestic partner" benefits and require employees to marry if they want coverage for the nonemployee spouse? If so, what will be the effect on unmarried opposite-sex couples? Will employers cover them even if they do not marry? Will that be legal? And if same-sex couples choose not to get married—for fear of outing themselves in a state that does not have antidiscrimation laws, for example—will the nonemployee partner be left uninsured? These and similar questions will take time to sort out.

The other major change, of course, came with the 2016 election. That seismic event cast the entire health reform effort into doubt. Only history will be able to judge accurately whether the ACA was successful, how much of it survived the 115th Congress, and what the unintended consequences of well-meaning (or even disingenuous) attempts to change it were. One thing is certain: no matter what happens, the repercussions will be felt for decades to come.

Traditional Principles on Access to Healthcare

The ACA was intended to increase access to care by making health insurance more affordable. This section discusses more traditional issues such as:

- The right to be admitted
- Admissions and discharge processes
- Nondiscrimination in health services
- Admission and treatment of mentally ill patients (including involuntary commitment and the standard of care for administering medications)
- Utilization review, peer review, and managed care

The emphasis in what follows is on hospitals, and though the criteria for service eligibility at other types of providers may differ somewhat, two basic principles pertain: Only physicians can admit and discharge patients, and only physicians (or certain other licensed personnel) can make clinical decisions and issue orders for patient care.

The Right to Care

Under common law, it was a general rule (*black-letter law*) that hospitals had no duty to treat any specific individual (see The Court Decides: *Hill v. Ohio County* at the end of this chapter). Furthermore, they accepted persons for admission and treatment only on a physician's order. Thus, even today most institutions can accept or refuse nonemergency cases with impunity as long as admission policies are not illegally discriminatory and the relevant government regulations are followed.

Clear written policies on the admission of patients are essential and must address the following kinds of factors:

- Whether the patient's condition is an emergency (see chapter 10)
- The conditions the hospital is equipped to treat (specialty hospitals, such as those established to treat only women or children, are not set up for all diagnoses)
- Whether the individual's physician has medical staff privileges (see chapter 8)
- The hospital's ownership (a government hospital is often subject to different admission standards from those imposed on private hospitals)
- Whether the facility has received federal funding under the Hill-Burton Act
- Whether civil rights or nondiscrimination laws apply
- Whether contractual arrangements (such as managed care contracts) obligate the hospital to treat members of a certain group
- Procedures and processes that differ depending on the payer type (e.g., private insurance vs. government program)

Although an individual usually has no basis for claiming a legal right to be treated at a particular hospital, many factors affect whether the patient will be admitted. Rather than focus on whether a patient has such a right, the hospital should be attentive to its mission and purpose in the community. If it adheres to its mission, the narrow legal question of a patient's right to admission usually becomes a nonissue.

Patient Registration and Admission

Hospitals must be prepared to register any patient who meets the facility's admission criteria and for whom a physician has written an order for treatment. Patients may be registered as either *inpatient* or *outpatient*. Outpatient status comprises various subcategories, such as observation, ambulatory surgery, emergency, clinic, rehabilitation, laboratory, and nonpatient (i.e., the patient is not present but the patient's specimens are in the laboratory for analysis). The registration process varies by category, and detailed policies and procedures must be in place to handle every eventuality. For example, once an order has been written to admit an individual as an inpatient, the hospital typically collects the following information:

- Demographics, such as patient name, address, telephone number, marital status, personal representative (if other than a spouse), gender, race, and Social Security number
- Religious affiliation, if the patient cares to disclose it
- Emergency contacts
- Identity and demographics of the financially responsible party (e.g., patient, parent, guardian)
- Insurance coverage
- Patient's language preferences and English proficiency
- Special needs (e.g., sign language interpretation)
- Special requests regarding release of patient information
- Generalized consent for routine care and diagnostic procedures (which must be signed and placed in the medical record and does not substitute for a detailed informed consent for significant medical procedures)

Registration personnel must review the collected information for any "red flags" of *medical identity theft*, the phenomenon of registering with another individual's insurance information, name, Social Security number, or other identifier (see Legal Brief). The Federal Trade Commission (which enforces the so-called red flag rules) has identified warning signs such as suspicious documents, inconsistent identifying information, discrepancies between mailing addresses, a reluctance to provide needed information, an inability to provide one's phone number or address, and other questionable activity.[6]

During registration, the hospital gives the patient and family a wide range of information out of both general courtesy and legal need. This information includes the following:

Legal Brief

Medical identity theft is insidious in a number of ways. Beyond the potential financial loss suffered by the healthcare provider and the possible damage done to the victim's credit, the victim has to amend his medical records lest the files contain the history, diagnosis, and treatment of the identity thief. If the victim does not strike this erroneous information from his files, it may surface years later and may be difficult to extract from the mare's nest of electronic medical and billing records. For general information on medical identity theft, see https://www.worldprivacyforum.org.

- General hospital information (maps, telephone numbers, parking restrictions, visiting hours, cafeteria location, gift shop hours)
- Instructions for storing personal belongings and valuables
- Smoking regulations
- Notice of privacy practices
- Written notice of rights under the Patient Self-Determination Act (e.g., decision-making rights, advance directives, healthcare power of attorney)

The preceding lists are not inclusive, and the requirements vary from state to state; thus, each hospital's legal counsel and other experts should advise on the full range of issues to be addressed at registration. The main point is that these matters must be covered by detailed hospital policies and procedures, and registration staff must be trained appropriately.

Medicare Inpatient Admission Standards

Merely because a patient is in a hospital bed and stays overnight does not always mean he is an "inpatient" for Medicare's purposes. (The standards may be different for Medicaid or private insurance.) Even if one is being actively observed and treated, receiving diagnostic tests, or even undergoing surgery, one becomes a Medicare inpatient only when formally admitted as such. Furthermore, inpatient status must meet certain regulatory guidelines to be eligible for Medicare inpatient coverage.

For many years the Medicare program only required that a patient be receiving care that was "medically reasonable and necessary" and which, in the physician's judgment, would require at least an overnight stay. But this standard was vague and involved a complicated medical judgement. Its application varied widely, and *Medicare auditors*—independent firms charged with identifying improper payments and paid on a contingent fee basis—were wont to deny inpatient coverage retrospectively, thus leaving patients with a higher out-of-pocket cost under the outpatient payment system.

For these reasons, the Centers for Medicare & Medicaid Services (CMS) introduced a so-called two-midnight rule (2MN) beginning in 2014. The 2MN rule states that an inpatient admission would normally be considered appropriate if the physician "expects the beneficiary to require care that crosses 2 midnights and admits the beneficiary based upon that expectation. . . . Conversely, [if] the physician expects the patient to require care less than 2 midnights, payment under Medicare Part A is generally inappropriate."[7] These requirements, codified as shown in exhibit 3.2, were controversial and were challenged by the provider community.[8] As of this writing (October 2015) the case is still pending in federal court in Washington, DC, and efforts are under way to persuade Congress and CMS to change the standard. In the meantime, whether one is or is not an "inpatient" may not always be clear, at least in Medicare's eyes.

EXHIBIT 3.2
Title 42: Public
Health

**Part 412–PROSPECTIVE PAYMENT SYSTEMS FOR INPATIENT HOSPITAL
  SERVICES**
Subpart A–General Provisions

§412.3 Admissions.

(a) For purposes of payment under Medicare Part A, an individual is considered an inpatient of a hospital, including a critical access hospital, if
formally admitted as an inpatient pursuant to an order for inpatient admission by a physician or other qualified practitioner in accordance with this
section and §§482.24(c), 482.12(c), and 485.638(a)(4)(iii) of this chapter
for a critical access hospital. This physician order must be present in the
medical record and be supported by the physician admission and progress
notes, in order for the hospital to be paid for hospital inpatient services
under Medicare Part A. In addition to these physician orders, inpatient
rehabilitation facilities also must adhere to the admission requirements
specified in §412.622 of this chapter.

(b) The order must be furnished by a qualified and licensed practitioner
who has admitting privileges at the hospital as permitted by State law,
and who is knowledgeable about the patient's hospital course, medical
plan of care, and current condition. The practitioner may not delegate the
decision (order) to another individual who is not authorized by the State
to admit patients, or has not been granted admitting privileges applicable
to that patient by the hospital's medical staff.

(c) The physician order must be furnished at or before the time of the
inpatient admission.

(d)(1) Except as specified in paragraph (d)(2) of this section, when a
patient enters a hospital for a surgical procedure not specified by Medicare
as inpatient only under §419.22(n) of this chapter, a diagnostic test, or any
other treatment, and the physician expects to keep the patient in the hospital for only a limited period of time that does not cross 2 midnights, the services are generally inappropriate for inpatient admission and inpatient payment under Medicare Part A, regardless of the hour that the patient came
to the hospital or whether the patient used a bed. Surgical procedures,
diagnostic tests, and other treatment are generally appropriate for inpatient
admission and inpatient hospital payment under Medicare Part A when the
physician expects the patient to require a stay that crosses at least 2 midnights. The expectation of the physician should be based on such complex
medical factors as patient history and comorbidities, the severity of signs
and symptoms, current medical needs, and the risk of an adverse event. The
factors that lead to a particular clinical expectation must be documented in
the medical record in order to be granted consideration.

(2) If an unforeseen circumstance, such as a beneficiary's death or
transfer, results in a shorter beneficiary stay than the physician's expectation of at least 2 midnights, the patient may be considered to be appropriately treated on an inpatient basis, and hospital inpatient payment may be
made under Medicare Part A.

Government Hospitals' Duty to Provide Services

Medicare—the federal program that pays for healthcare services provided to seniors and certain other beneficiaries—is but one of many government-supported healthcare programs at the state and federal levels. For example, some states and localities actually own and manage hospitals, and those organizations carry some special obligations not present at private hospitals.

Government hospitals are creatures of statute and are established for specific purposes. Many of the statutes regulating government hospitals sort the intended beneficiaries according to their particular disease, financial status, or place of residence. Under these statutes, a patient included in the intended class of beneficiaries has a *right* to be treated, with certain exceptions. For example, the right to treatment is subject to the hospital's ability (e.g., staffing levels, available space and equipment) to provide the care needed. The right to treatment also depends on the rules and regulations of the hospital's governing board. For example, the board might require proof of inability to pay when the hospital's statutory purpose is to serve the indigent. (However, even if the hospital's mandate is to care for the indigent, the law typically does not prevent the hospital from admitting patients who are able to pay if facilities are available and indigent patients are not disenfranchised as a result.)

Government hospitals owe the same duty of care to emergency patients that other hospitals do: to stabilize the patient's condition. Refusal to provide emergency care is not justified just because an individual is outside the class of persons the government hospital serves (see the discussion on emergency care in chapter 10).

Local Government's Duty to Pay for Care

Most states have statutes providing for payment from public funds for certain medical services furnished to indigent persons. Legislation differs significantly from state to state on the services covered, which patients are entitled to care, the process for payment, and the facilities that can render services. Typically, the statutes require municipal or county governments to pay for emergency medical care given to indigent persons wherever the care is rendered. These laws have withstood constitutional challenges.[9] Healthcare administrators must be aware of local statutes and judicial decisions that determine an institution's right to reimbursement. In addition, the health reform laws of 2010 will expand coverage under the states' Medicaid programs, and the increased number of "Medicaid eligibles" will need to be factored into the admission and registration processes.

In many states, counties are required to reimburse for emergency medical care given to indigent residents. In Arizona, for example, if an indigent patient who needed emergency care were admitted to a private hospital, the county's obligation to pay for the services would continue throughout the period of hospitalization, even after the emergency ended. In *St. Joseph's Hospital and Medical Center v. Maricopa County*, an indigent patient was admitted to a private hospital for emergency treatment. At some point thereafter, the agency responsible for paying the medical expenses could have ended its obligation to reimburse the private hospital by arranging the patient's transfer to a county-owned facility. It did not do so, and the government had to pay for the entire hospitalization.[10] Similarly, Nevada counties have a duty to pay for emergency care whether rendered at a county hospital or elsewhere, and prior governmental consent is not required if the patient's condition threatens her life or might cause permanent impairment.[11]

The duty to pay for the care of indigents is becoming a major policy issue given the increase in the number of illegal immigrants and other uninsured persons in many states. Also of concern is reimbursement for healthcare furnished to persons who (a) have been found guilty of a crime, (b) are in custody or under arrest awaiting trial, or (c) have been injured during apprehension. The duty to pay may differ depending on the status of the patient, and there is a distinction between the duty to provide or summon care and the government's duty to pay for that care.

A Prisoner's Right to Care

Failure to obtain medical assistance for a prisoner or person in custody can lead to tort liability. For example, in a 1965 Indiana case, a police officer was summoned to a man's home "for the purpose of taking [him] to the hospital for medical care." According to the court, the man was "very ill and running a high temperature," but after departing with him, the officer arrested and jailed him for being drunk and disorderly. The man died in his cell, and an autopsy showed no alcohol in his body. The cause of death was lobar pneumonia and severe congestion of both lungs. The City of Indianapolis was held liable on the grounds that the police knew or ought to have known that the person needed medical treatment.[12]

The Eighth Amendment to the US Constitution prohibits cruel and unusual punishment. It has been interpreted as requiring governments to provide convicted prisoners with adequate medical treatment.[13] The due process clauses of the Fifth and Fourteenth Amendments require that persons who have not been convicted but who have been detained or are under arrest be given essential food, shelter, clothing, and medical care.[14] On the other hand, a person not dependent on the government has no constitutional right to medical care,[15] and the right to receive care is not necessarily accompanied by the right to have the government pay for that care.

Some laws clearly state that the government must pay for care given to prisoners[16] or persons in police custody.[17] The duty to pay might be limited to cases in which the government's institutional facilities are inadequate[18] or in which the prisoner or the prisoner's family is unable to pay.[19] However, most states' laws simply uphold a prisoner's right to receive treatment and are silent on the question of the government's financial obligations.[20] Although the police generally have a duty to seek medical care for injured persons, especially those whose injuries are the result of police actions during apprehension, the government may not be obligated to pay the care provider if the patient has not been arrested. This precedent may be the reason some law enforcement agencies do not officially arrest injured suspects until after emergency treatment has been completed.

For example, in *City of Revere v. Massachusetts General Hospital*, Patrick M. Kivlin attempted to flee from the scene of a crime and was shot by a police officer.[21] The police summoned an ambulance, and the ambulance took Kivlin to Massachusetts General Hospital, where he remained for nine days. Although he was in police custody and a warrant had been issued, he was not officially arrested until the date of his discharge from the hospital. A month later, he was again hospitalized, but the city of Revere refused to pay for either hospitalization.

The Supreme Judicial Court held that Massachusetts contract law provided no basis for ordering the city to pay, but it found that the Eighth Amendment's prohibition against cruel and unusual punishment required it to do so. After granting certiorari, the US Supreme Court overruled the state court's finding on the Eighth Amendment issue, stating that the amendment did not apply because there had not yet been a formal finding of guilty at the time Kivlin needed medical care.[22] Although the Supreme Court noted that due process requires persons in Kivlin's situation be given care, local government had no duty to pay for that care in the absence of state legislation. Thus, just as the state may deny payment for an elective abortion[23] and the federal government may restrict Medicaid payments for abortions,[24] the city of Revere was not required to pay Massachusetts General Hospital.[25]

Hill-Burton Act and Mandated Free Care

The Hospital Survey and Construction Act (the Hill-Burton Act) was passed in 1946 to provide federal financing for the construction and modernization of publicly owned and not-for-profit hospital facilities.[26] For political reasons, and despite President Harry S. Truman's attempts to create a national health system, the legislation did not contain provisions requiring the government to pay for services rendered in facilities that received Hill-Burton money. Two decades passed before Congress enacted Medicare.

The Hill-Burton Act enabled the nation's hospitals to upgrade their physical plants, and in an accommodation to President Truman, it required recipients of construction grants and loans to furnish a "reasonable volume" of services to persons unable to pay. Recipient hospitals had to comply with

Law in Action

Because the ACA has reduced the number of uninsured, either the community service and uncompensated care obligations will need to be revised or hospitals will have to find innovative ways to meet them.

this requirement, known as the *uncompensated care obligation*, for 20 years after completion of construction. The statute also required that facilities financed with federal funds be available to all persons in the community, a duty commonly referred to as the *community service obligation* (see Law in Action).[27] Thus, the Hill-Burton Act was an early attempt at providing healthcare to the poor and stands as a harbinger of Medicaid and similar programs.

The Hill-Burton Act was implemented through the states, which were responsible for determining the need for facilities and for ensuring that grant recipients were complying with the uncompensated care and community service obligations. For many years, these requirements were not implemented effectively. The regulations failed to define a "reasonable volume" of services, and they did not specify patient eligibility criteria. Proper regulations were issued only after several lawsuits resulted in court orders.[28] The eventual regulations provided that an institution that received Hill-Burton financing could meet its uncompensated care obligation by budgeting a certain minimum amount for free care or simply by certifying that it did not refuse admission solely because of inability to pay. (The latter option was sometimes referred to as the "open-door policy."[29])

The community service obligation was interpreted as requiring all Hill-Burton hospitals to serve Medicaid patients and to extend emergency care to any person residing or employed in the hospital's service area regardless of ability to pay, and all services had to be nondiscriminatory with regard to race, color, creed, and national origin.[30]

In 1974, the National Health Planning and Resource Development Act (Public Law 93-641) essentially terminated the original Hill-Burton program and substituted a more restrictive scheme of providing federal funds to modernize healthcare institutions. This legislation recognized the continuing obligation of hospitals to provide uncompensated care and community service and mandated new regulations. Congress acknowledged that the Hill-Burton Act had never been effectively implemented, and thus the new law placed greater responsibility on the Department of Health, Education, and Welfare (now the Department of Health and Human Services) to enforce the provisions for care of the indigent. The statute also provided that project funding would obligate the recipients to furnish uncompensated care and community service indefinitely. However, because P. L. 93-641 was not retroactive, institutions that received funds before 1975 could still claim the 20-year limit on their uncompensated care obligation.

Over the years, restraints on the federal budget have restricted appropriations of new funds for hospital construction, so remnants of the Hill-Burton Act are hard to find. The issues of uncompensated care and service to the community have not gone away, however; for tax-exempt hospitals they live on in various ways. (These issues are discussed in chapter 12.)

Admission and Treatment of Mentally Ill Patients

The legal rights of mentally ill and incompetent patients are determined by constitutional law and state statutes. Because both of these sources of law are continually evolving, hospital management needs competent, current advice concerning emergency treatment, temporary detention, and formal admission of these persons. Hospitals must give emergency care to a mentally ill individual just as they would to any other person, but denial of admission may be justified if the hospital is not staffed or equipped for psychiatric patients. Nevertheless, hospitals must be prepared to deal with such patients for their own safety or for the protection of others. Unless statutory requirements are followed carefully, the hospital risks liability for false imprisonment, assault and battery, and other tort claims. On the other hand, when healthcare professionals act in good faith, in the patient's best interests, and according to constitutional and statutory requirements, the risks of liability are minimized.[31]

Involuntary Detention or Commitment

Because institutionalization is a significant deprivation of personal liberty, state statutes governing the civil commitment of mentally ill persons must ensure that the patient is granted both substantive and procedural due process of law.[32] A person may not be committed involuntarily unless mental illness presents a danger to the patient or to third parties.[33] Danger to self can be found if patients cannot provide the basic necessities of life or if they exhibit indications that they may harm themselves. Unless persons are adjudged dangerous to themselves or others, indefinite confinement without treatment violates their right to due process, and the officials responsible for such confinement can be personally liable under civil rights laws.[34]

When mentally ill patients present a danger to themselves, the state has a legitimate interest—under its **parens patriae** powers (Latin for *father of his country*)—to provide needed care.[35] If mentally ill patients present a danger to the community or to third parties, a psychiatric evaluation and possible civil commitment are justified by the state's inherent power to regulate matters of health, safety, and welfare. For patients to meet these criteria, psychiatrists and other professionals have to predict their behavior, a task that

parens patriae
the doctrine that the government is the ultimate guardian of all people who have a legal disability, such as minors and the mentally ill

Legal Brief

The American Psychiatric Association (APA) . . . informs us that '[the] unreliability of psychiatric predictions of long-term future dangerousness is by now an established fact within the profession.' The APA's best estimate is that two out of three [such] predictions are wrong. The Court does not dispute this proposition, and indeed it could not do so; the evidence is overwhelming.

—*Barefoot v. Estelle*, 463 U.S. 800, 920 (1983)

may be nearly impossible from a medical standpoint (see Legal Brief). Many states require evidence of a timely overt act or threat of violence to show that the patient presents a danger.

The balance between the legitimate rights of patients and the recognized interests of society depends on the answers to difficult questions of social policy and medicolegal judgment. Setting this balance involves three main risks: (1) Some patients might be detained unnecessarily, (2) some who are not dangerous might be released but not receive needed outpatient care, and (3) patients who are thought to pose no risk might be released and proceed to harm others.[36] Poor definition of *dangerousness* in both medicine and law increases the potential for error in setting the balance, and in many commitment hearings the matter is left for the jury to decide on the basis of testimony from expert witnesses. Misdiagnosis alone does not constitute negligence or malpractice; causation must also be proven. Proof may be difficult to furnish because dangerousness is difficult to predict.

Involuntary Examination of Mentally Ill and Dangerous Persons

State statutes typically allow for involuntary detention of psychiatric patients for a limited period, ranging from 48 to 72 hours. The Florida Mental Health Act (also called the Baker Act) is typical of the process.[37] Under the Florida law, if (1) there is reason to believe that a person has a mental illness, (2) the person does not agree to a voluntary examination, and (3) without care the person may suffer harm or be a danger to himself or others, the involuntary examination process can be initiated in one of three ways:

1. By court order
2. By a law enforcement officer
3. By a physician or a mental health professional

The person is taken into custody and delivered to a receiving facility (a facility designated by the state for such purposes) and must be examined within 72 hours. If she is first seen in a hospital emergency department, as is often the case, the 72-hour period begins at that time. The patient may not be held involuntarily for longer than 72 hours, at which time the facility must take one of four actions on the basis of the patient's best interests:

1. The patient shall be released, unless she is charged with a crime, in which case the patient shall be returned to the custody of a law enforcement officer;

2. The patient shall be released, subject to the provisions of subparagraph 1, for voluntary outpatient treatment;

3. The patient, unless she is charged with a crime, shall be asked to give express and informed consent to placement as a voluntary patient, and, if such consent is given, the patient shall be admitted as a voluntary patient; or

4. A petition for involuntary placement shall be filed in the circuit court when outpatient or inpatient treatment is deemed necessary. [*Involuntary placement* is Florida's term for civil commitment proceedings.] When inpatient treatment is deemed necessary, the least restrictive treatment consistent with the optimum improvement of the patient's condition shall be made available.[38]

Because civil commitment takes away a person's freedom, the patient in a civil commitment proceeding receives full due process rights. Again, the Florida statute is typical. Under Florida's process, the administrator of the receiving facility must petition for a court order, and the petition must immediately be served on the patient and the patient's guardian. The court will appoint a public defender if the patient is not already represented by counsel. An attorney representing the patient's interest must have complete access to his client. The patient is entitled to a full hearing on the petition for involuntary placement within five days. At the hearing, the court considers testimony and evidence regarding the patient's competence and mental illness. If the court concludes that the patient meets the criteria for involuntary inpatient placement, an order to that effect is entered for a period not to exceed six months (renewable for additional periods as necessary). Any such order is subject to judicial review by an appellate court.[39]

The due process protections inherent in Florida's statute reflect a nationwide emphasis on the rights of mental health patients, but as anyone who has seen the film *One Flew over the Cuckoo's Nest* knows, those rights have not always been protected; the US Supreme Court first addressed the issue in 1975. Ironically, the case *O'Connor v. Donaldson* arose in Florida, before the Florida Mental Health Act took effect. The US Supreme Court considered the plight of a man who had been confined against his will in a state mental hospital for 15 years. He was not thought to be dangerous to himself or others and was receiving no treatment. According to Justice Potter Stewart, his confinement amounted to nothing more than "a simple regime of enforced custodial care, not a program designed to alleviate or cure his supposed illness."[40] On the basis of these findings and without dissent, the Supreme Court held,

> A finding of 'mental illness' alone cannot justify a State's locking a person up against his will and keeping him indefinitely in simple custodial confinement. Assuming that that term can be given a reasonably precise content and that the 'mentally ill' can be identified with reasonable accuracy, there is still no constitutional basis for confining such persons involuntarily if they are dangerous to no one and can live safely in freedom.
>
> . . .
>
> In short, a State cannot constitutionally confine . . . a nondangerous individual who is capable of surviving safely in freedom by himself or with the help of willing and responsible family members or friends. Since the jury found, upon ample evidence, that O'Connor [the hospital superintendent], as an agent of the State, knowingly did so confine Donaldson, it properly concluded that O'Connor violated Donaldson's constitutional right to freedom.[41]

This landmark decision and others like it gave impetus to the patients' rights movement and led to the due process protections in most states' laws.

Due process does not require that civil commitment proceedings use the "beyond a reasonable doubt" standard of proof necessary for a criminal conviction.[42] However, due process also does not require the states to use a uniform standard of proof in civil commitment proceedings, so some states have adopted the criminal law standard by statute or judicial decision. Using a standard higher than that constitutionally required is permissible.

On the other hand, the "preponderance of evidence" standard applicable to most civil litigation is not considered strong enough to protect patients' rights. After all, involuntary hospitalization deprives the patient of liberty, and the risks of an erroneous decision are grave. An intermediate standard of proof is more likely to balance the rights of the mentally ill with the legitimate concerns of society. This modified standard, endorsed by the US Supreme Court, is often expressed as "clear, convincing, and unequivocal" evidence of danger to self or others.[43]

Courts distinguish between civil commitment of a mentally ill person who has not been charged with a crime and commitment of one who has been charged. In *Jones v. United States*, the defendant was acquitted in a criminal trial by reason of insanity and placed in an institution for the mentally ill. The insanity finding was based on a preponderance of evidence rather than clear and convincing proof. The majority ruling held that the less demanding standard was consistent with due process even if the period of hospital confinement would exceed the prison term for the criminal charge.[44]

Standard of Care and Administration of Medication

Once committed, psychiatric patients retain substantive constitutional rights to adequate food, shelter, clothing, medical care,[45] safe physical conditions, reasonable freedom from physical restraints, and rehabilitation or training appropriate to their diagnoses.[46] Hospital officials who fail to observe these rights can be held personally liable.[47] One federal court defined *minimally adequate medical* care as follows:

> In order to render effective care and treatment, a hospital for the mentally ill must not only hire qualified individuals, but must ensure the continuation of their training and education during their employment. . . . The court finds there are four standards generally advanced by mental health professionals as essential for minimally adequate treatment: a humane and therapeutic environment; qualified staff in sufficient numbers; an individualized treatment plan for each patient; and planned therapeutic programs and activities. It is against these standards that the conditions at a psychiatric facility must be measured in order to determine whether those operating the facility have failed to provide treatment for those mentally ill individuals involuntarily confined for such purpose in violation of the Fourteenth Amendment of the United States Constitution.[48]

With respect to conditions of confinement and the patient's right to rehabilitation and training, the US Supreme Court has held that the Constitution "only requires that the courts make certain that professional judgment in fact was exercised. . . . The appropriate standard [is] whether the defendants' conduct [is] . . . such a substantial departure from accepted professional judgment, practice, or standards in the care and treatment of this plaintiff, as to demonstrate that the defendants did not base their conduct on a professional judgment."[49] In the Supreme Court's view, this standard "affords the necessary guidance and reflects the proper balance between the legitimate interests of the State and the rights of the involuntarily committed to reasonable conditions of safety and freedom from unreasonable restraints."[50]

In several contexts, courts have developed the principle that mentally ill persons should not be presumed incompetent to make treatment decisions. The decision to commit someone involuntarily is not the same as a finding of incompetence. Thus, a competent patient has the right to consent (or refuse to consent) to care unless her or others' safety requires it. For example, competent psychiatric patients who are not a danger to themselves or others may not be given antipsychotic medications (which may have serious side effects) against their will and may not be forced to become subjects of medical research. The foundation for this rule has been described as part of a "right of privacy" or, more simply, as a principle of common law.[51]

The right to give informed consent (see chapter 11) can be overcome, and medications, restraints, and other measures can be forcibly administered, only when there are compelling reasons for doing so. In all jurisdictions, unless an immediate danger or threat of harm exists, the patient is entitled to

(1) professional determination that medication or restraint is necessary, (2) evaluation of alternatives, and (3) regular review of the recommended course of treatment. A formal hearing is not required, but a judicial determination of incompetence and the appointment of a guardian might be required.

Discharge from the Hospital

Issues relating to the mentally ill aside, hospital discharge presents few significant legal issues in most cases. As soon as they are able, most patients want to go home or to an institution that better suits their needs, and the only significant risk is liability for abandonment (i.e., discharging a patient who needs further care).

Discharge requires a physician's order (unless the patient elopes or leaves against medical advice), so the test of an abandonment claim is whether the physician's discharge order was reasonable under the circumstances.[52] For example, if the patient's condition was likely to be aggravated by the discharge and the decision was therefore deemed unreasonable, the reason the physician and hospital discharged the patient is irrelevant. (For instance, the patient's failure or inability to pay the bill is no justification.) When contemplating a patient's transfer to a less costly institution (e.g., when required by a managed care plan), attending physicians and hospital staff must be assured that the receiving institution is adequately equipped and staffed to care for the patient's condition. Most states have standards for proper patient transfers, and federal standards apply in the emergency setting.

Several cases illustrate the prospect of liability for abandonment. In *Meiselman v. Crown Heights Hospital,* the defendant was liable for discharging a minor while his legs were in casts and open wounds were draining. Further professional care at home was necessary and was to be arranged and supervised by the chief of the hospital's surgical staff. The home care proved to be inadequate, however, and the patient had to be sent to another hospital. Because the need for further care was foreseeable and there was evidence that the motive for discharging the patient was financial, the discharge was considered unreasonable.[53]

Patients can be discharged or given temporary leaves of absence only on the written order of a physician, but the hospital itself owes the patient a duty to have proper discharge policies. In one case, a physician mistakenly diagnosed a diabetic patient who was near death; he thought the patient was suffering from delirium tremens and called for the sheriff to remove him from the facility. When the patient's estate claimed that premature release was the proximate cause of death, the court held that the plaintiff was entitled to a trial on questions relating to the hospital's possible negligence.[54] "We cannot agree that the hospital operates as a slavish handmaiden to the physicians on its staff. . . . Under Alabama law a hospital [has] a duty of care to its patients."[55] Had there been hospital policies requiring trained staff to be involved in discharge planning, the death might have been prevented. (See chapter 8 for a discussion of staff physicians as independent contractors.)

If a patient is a known threat to third persons, the hospital and attending physician can be liable to persons injured by the patient after discharge. In *Semler v. Psychiatric Institute of Washington, D.C.*, a man who pleaded guilty to abducting a young girl received a suspended prison sentence contingent on continued inpatient treatment at a psychiatric institution.[56] On later recommendations of his physician and probation officer, the court approved his transfer to day care, permitting him to live at home and commute daily to the hospital with his parents. Soon, however, he began living alone and working as a bricklayer's helper, all to the knowledge of his attending physician and the court probation officer but without court approval. He then murdered a girl. The psychiatric facility, the physician, and the probation officer were all held liable for allowing the patient full outpatient status without obtaining the court's approval. Because the court had not given the probation officer authority to approve the transfer, the probation officer's approval did not shield the institution from liability, and the officer's unauthorized act made him personally liable.

When a readily identifiable potential victim suffers foreseeable harm, a person who knew of the potential for harm but failed to warn the victim may also be held liable. Depending on the circumstances, some courts have drawn a distinction between breach of duty to the community at large (negligent discharge) and breach of duty to warn a third party who is at particular risk (see Law in Action).[57]

Home care programs for any patient must be carefully planned and monitored to ensure that they meet the individual's needs. On discharge of a patient to home care, attending physicians and hospital personnel must carefully instruct the patient and family and relay medical information to professional persons responsible for the home care program.[58] Failure to do so constitutes a breach of the hospital's duty. The hospital also remains vicariously liable for the negligence of those responsible for continuing care of the patient if they are hospital employees or apparent employees. If the patient's care and treatment are rendered under the jurisdiction of the court, the orders of the court must be strictly followed.

Law in Action

The *Tarasoff* case in California is perhaps the most notorious and tragic of cases involving a duty to warn third parties of a patient's dangerous propensities. The decision is discussed in chapter 9 under the heading "Release of Information Without Patient Consent."

A problem arises when patients of sound mind insist on leaving the hospital though they still need care. Such patients may allege false imprisonment if the hospital holds them against their will,[59] but they should not be allowed simply to walk away. Attending physicians should advise these patients that remaining in the hospital is recommended, explain why they are making this recommendation, and inform the patients of the consequences of leaving early.

The hospital must have a detailed policy to cover these situations. It should include documentation of the advice given and the patient's signature on a form releasing the hospital from liability. This form should state that the patient was fully aware of the medical reasons for recommending continued stay and had been advised not to leave the hospital, that the discharge was solely on the patient's own initiative, and that the refusal to stay was a matter of the patient's free will and volition. Some patients who insist on leaving against medical advice refuse to sign the release. Patients cannot be forced to sign, but hospital policy should require that the substance of the form be explained and that the patient's refusal to sign be documented.

Hospitals are permitted to restrain patients of unsound mind from leaving the hospital if their departure would endanger their health or life or the lives or property of others.[60] On the same grounds, patients of sound mind who are suffering from a contagious disease may be detained to protect themselves and others. (The hospital may have an affirmative duty to the community to refuse to discharge such patients.) Restraint must be reasonable according to the circumstances of each case. Gathering and documenting in the medical record competent evidence of the contagious disease or the mental instability of patients detained on either of these grounds is essential.[61] Hospital policies should address this possibility.

A patient should never be held in the hospital for failure to pay a bill or until arrangements for settlement are complete. Such detainment is false imprisonment, especially if force is used or threats are made.[62] Proper policies should ensure that the payment question is addressed at the time of admission, not discharge.

Unemancipated minors under the age of discretion should be discharged only to their parents or to persons legally entitled to custody. If the whereabouts of the parents are unknown and the minor does not have a court-appointed guardian, the hospital must appoint a guardian. Social welfare agencies help hospitals in these situations. If the parents can be located but for some reason cannot come to the hospital, the patient should be discharged only to someone who has written permission from the parents.

Emancipated minors—those old enough to consent for themselves under state law—can be discharged from the hospital in the same manner as adults. Emancipation is usually a matter of agreement between the parent and child; it is a question of fact in each case and does not depend on whether the youth is living at home. In some states, minors are emancipated when they marry. Emancipation can also be decreed by a court in some cases.

Generally, discharge of an infant child to the custody of the infant's minor mother is legally sound. The hospital cannot prevent the mother from claiming her child, especially when she intends to retain custody and responsibility for raising the infant. Even if she intends to place the child for private adoption, most states recognize her legal right to claim her child, subject to local limitations and restrictions. If the mother does not claim the child but requests discharge to a third party, the child should not be discharged except on the recommendation of an approved social service agency that handles adoptions. Legal counsel should be consulted for advice consistent with law.

Most states now have safe haven ("Baby Moses") laws that allow mothers to leave unwanted children in the hands of care providers anonymously and free of interrogation. These laws were adopted to prevent infanticides and baby abandonment. They were not passed with in-hospital births in mind, but their premise is consistent with the idea that at the time of the mother's discharge from the hospital, the party to whom the baby is discharged depends on the mother's wishes (see Legal Decision Point).

In at least one state (Nebraska), the safe haven law was so broadly written that parents misused it to abandon older children. After as many as 35 children, some as old as 17, were left at various Nebraska hospitals in 2008, the law was amended to apply only to children 30 days old or younger.[63]

Utilization Review: Controls on Admission and Discharge

Thus far this chapter has discussed the health reform laws and the traditional principles concerning hospital admission and discharge. Both topics pose questions about the use—actually, the potential for overuse—of health services: questions relating to cost, quality, and value; questions relating to what is medically

Legal Decision Point

A new mother is about to be discharged but does not want custody of the baby. She has not made arrangements for private adoption, does not want to take the baby home with her, and has not named another person to take custody. If she were to leave the hospital with the baby, she could walk across the street to a fire or police station and abandon the child anonymously. She could also return to the hospital and leave the baby outside the emergency department anonymously. But if she simply leaves the baby behind when she is discharged, the abandonment is not anonymous; hospital personnel have a record of the baby's birth, the mother's name, and other information.

How should the hospital deal with privacy issues in such cases? What happens if the supposed father learns of the situation and arrives to claim the child? What happens if he or someone else alerts the media or state child protection agencies? Can hospital authorities confirm anything about the case? Why or why not? What can be said to whom, and (especially) what can be said in public?

necessary; questions about who should pay and how much. This section—indeed an entire chapter—cannot do justice to the myriad issues involved; issues of public policy and ethics are beyond the scope of this book. The ensuing paragraphs briefly discuss a few of the legal implications of utilization review (UR) not covered in chapter 7.

Most hospitals have a type of internal UR process known as *case* (or *care*) *management*. Case management departments provide ongoing concurrent reviews of patient care to determine whether treatments are medically necessary and, if not, to assist in placing patients in more appropriate (usually less costly) care settings. The departments are closely aligned with or part of the quality improvement function, and they typically track average length of stay and similar indicators. Internal case management serves an advisory purpose and does not have the authority to order a patient's discharge or transfer; for this reason, it does not present a significant legal risk.

third-party payers managed care organizations, government programs, employee benefit plans, private insurance plans, and similar entities responsible for paying for health services

As discussed in chapter 7, legal risks can arise when the financial pressures of **third-party payers** conflict with the perceived best interests of the patient. The UR decisions of third-party payers are made in a number of ways:

- Prospectively (whether to authorize payment for treatment before the treatment has begun)
- Concurrently (whether to permit treatment to continue beyond a certain point)
- Retrospectively (whether to deny payment for treatment that has been completed)

UR decisions are almost always based on physicians' recommendations and sound professional judgment related to the patient's medical needs. However, to keep their costs (medical loss ratio) as low as possible, third-party payers (managed care plans) sometimes approve payment for only a certain number of days in the hospital (see Legal Brief). In such cases, hospitals have an incentive to discharge patients "sicker and quicker."

A physician who believes the patient is not ready for discharge should carefully document the reasons for not signing a discharge order. If the physician bows to pressure and orders a discharge that is contrary to professional standards and her better judgment, she may invoke significant liability consequences (see discussion of the *Wickline* case in chapter 7). The physician and hospital usually can appeal the coverage decision, but a physician who believes treatment is necessary must ensure that the treatment is provided at whatever expense.

Conversely, if the physician sees no need for continued hospitalization and recommends discharge or transfer to a less expensive facility, patients often bear the cost of care if they choose to stay in the hospital. Attending physicians and case management staff must carefully explain coverage limitations and transfer options to patients and their family members, and together they must decide on the future course and site of care.

Hospitals and physicians should be patients' advocates if insurance coverage is threatened. The Joint Commission alludes to this responsibility in its hospital accreditation standards. In the leadership chapter, a section on ethical issues in operations states the following:

> The hospital is professionally and ethically responsible for providing care, treatment, and services within its capability and law and regulation. At times, such care, treatment, and services are denied because of payment limitations. In these situations, the decision to continue providing care, treatment, and services or to discharge the patient is based *solely on the patient's identified needs.*[64] [Emphasis added.]

Legal Brief

In insurance vernacular, *loss ratio* (LR) essentially means claims per premium dollar:

$$LR = \frac{\text{Losses} + \text{loss-related expense}}{\text{Earned premiums}}$$

In health insurance, the *medical loss ratio* (MLR) represents the percentage of premium dollars paid for medical care and related quality improvement efforts. Fewer claims paid results in a lower MLR, which in turn means higher retained earnings (profits) for the insurer. The average MLR for private insurance plans is typically 80–85 percent, and the ACA sets that range as a minimum depending on market size. If an insurer's MLR falls below the applicable level, it must provide a premium rebate to its insureds. A government program's MLR is much higher (in the 95+ percent range) because government programs are not motivated to earn a profit.

Patients whose medical conditions justify discharge or transfer have no common-law or constitutional right to remain in the hospital. A patient who remains is a trespasser, and the hospital may ask a court to issue an injunction to remove the person from the premises.[65] The courts have reasoned that hospitals have a duty to reserve their beds and facilities for patients who genuinely need them and should not permit a patient to remain when adequate care can be provided elsewhere.

On the other hand, the hospital and physician may not abandon or discharge a patient who needs further care without making appropriate arrangements for that care. Thus, someone who needs continuing care—in a nursing home, for example—presents a dilemma for all the parties involved if no appropriate facility is available, especially if the patient is unable to pay the ongoing hospital charges.

Monmouth Medical Center v. State illustrates the conflict between economic and human values in these circumstances.[66] At issue were New Jersey's administrative regulations prohibiting Medicaid reimbursement for indigent patients who no longer need hospitalization and are awaiting transfer to a nursing home. Because there was a shortage of nursing home beds, the state regulations required the hospital to absorb the cost; the hospital was unwilling to do so, and it filed suit.

The New Jersey Supreme Court pointed out that the purpose of the Medicaid program is to provide financial assistance for "medically necessary" services, and the regulations require states to furnish services "sufficient in amount, duration, and scope to reasonably achieve [their purpose]."[67] The court held that the state regulations conflicted with the federal rules; as long as the hospital exercised good faith and reasonable diligence in attempting to place patients in nursing homes, it was legally entitled to reimbursement from Medicaid. In essence, the court said that fairness required society—not the hospital—to absorb the costs even if the patient no longer needed the services of an acute care facility.

Putting the issue in sharper focus, a later case—*Monmouth Medical Center v. Harris*—upheld the government's right to deny Medicare reimbursement to a hospital for a patient who no longer required hospital or skilled nursing care.[68] The patient needed custodial care, but beds in a nursing home that provided such care were not available. The court said the unavailability of beds was irrelevant because Medicare does not reimburse for custodial care.

Federal law requires organizations that contract with Medicare to conduct utilization and quality control reviews to evaluate the services they provide to Medicare beneficiaries.[69] Through retrospective reviews of data, peer-review organizations (PROs)—also known as *quality improvement organizations*—are responsible for determining whether

- hospital services are reasonable and medically necessary,
- the quality of those services meets professional standards, and
- the services could be provided more economically elsewhere.

Each PRO is expected to conduct reviews of admission patterns and identify groups of patients whose diagnoses or contemplated treatments indicate that they could be safely cared for elsewhere than in an acute care hospital. Each PRO is empowered to set objectives for reducing inappropriate admissions in its geographic region and to identify unacceptable admission patterns in use by particular institutions and medical practitioners.

To measure the quality of care furnished to Medicare patients, the review organization has the following responsibilities:

- To ensure that patients with certain diagnoses receive adequate medical services, especially when appropriate facilities are available but are underused
- To review hospital readmissions caused by previous substandard care

- To identify instances of unnecessary surgery
- To reduce the number of preventable deaths

To achieve these objectives, PROs develop treatment protocols for particular diagnoses and set specific statistical goals. In addition to performing these functions on behalf of the federal government, PROs have the power to deny reimbursement to a Medicare provider for unnecessary or inappropriate care.[70] In certain circumstances, the review organization may also recommend penalties—ranging from monetary fines to exclusion from the Medicare program—for providers that render unnecessary or inappropriate care.

The ACA contains many provisions related to quality improvement, such as technical assistance and research, support for patient-centered medical homes, better treatment of chronic disease, regionalized emergency care systems and trauma centers, demonstration programs on quality and patient safety training, improvements to women's health, a "patient navigator" program, and studies and reports on new tort claims or causes of action generated by quality initiatives.

It remains to be seen what effects the reforms will have on quality programs generally and PROs specifically. In any event, these provisions will affect Americans' access to healthcare. (Peer review and quality issues are discussed more fully in chapter 8.)

Summary

This chapter reviews the changes wrought by the ACA and provides the anticipated timeline for those changes. Briefly stated, the ACA will affect all aspects of the US healthcare system for many years. If successfully implemented, it will extend coverage to millions of previously uninsured persons, change payment systems significantly, strengthen fraud and abuse laws, improve prevention and wellness programs, and improve quality and cost-effectiveness. The chapter also discusses the various constitutional challenges to the ACA, the issues those lawsuits raised, and the ultimate decisions of the US Supreme Court.

The chapter then turns to traditional rules about hospital admission and discharge—the black-letter law that there is no common-law right for a person to be admitted to a hospital—and discusses a number of exceptions to that principle. The discussion of the law relating to emergency services introduces a more thorough treatment of the topic in chapter 10. In addition, the chapter presents special circumstances attending the admission and discharge of psychiatric patients and the uncompensated care and community service obligations of many not-for-profit organizations.

Finally, the chapter foreshadows a section of chapter 7 by discussing the conflict between managed care organizations' desire to limit healthcare expenditures and providers' moral and legal duties to give quality patient care.

Discussion Questions

1. What are the most significant aspects of the ACA passed by Congress in 2010? Which of these have been implemented? Which have not been, and why not?

2. Which of the arguments made in the legal challenges to the ACA strike you as most persuasive?

3. Referring to Article I, Section 8 of the US Constitution, how would you define "commerce among the several states"? For example, does it include local telephone service? Your family physician? The corner drugstore? Why or why not?

4. You own and live on a commercial farm and grow wheat for sale, but you also set aside a fairly large amount for your family's personal consumption. Are you affecting interstate commerce in such a way that Congress should be able to regulate it?

5. Who has the authority to admit patients to hospitals, and in most cases why do patients not have a right to be admitted?

6. What is the current status of the "two-midnight rule," and how does it affect Medicare beneficiaries' out-of-pocket costs?

7. What is a hospital's responsibility to provide care to the indigent, and how does it differ depending on the type of care (emergency vs. nonemergency) and the type of hospital (public, private, for-profit, not-for-profit, tax exempt)?

8. What are the Hill-Burton "uncompensated care" and "community service" obligations?

9. What are the standards and processes for involuntary admission of persons who are mentally ill?

10. What kinds of issues may a hospital and physician confront when discharging a patient?

11. What are the tensions between managed care's objectives and medical judgment?

The Court Decides

King v. Burwell
135 S. Ct. 2480 (2015)

Roberts, Chief Justice

The Patient Protection and Affordable Care Act adopts a series of interlocking reforms designed to expand coverage in the individual health insurance market. First, the Act bars insurers from taking a person's health into account when deciding whether to sell health insurance or how much to charge. Second, the Act generally requires each person to maintain insurance coverage or make a payment to the Internal Revenue Service. And third, the Act gives tax credits to certain people to make insurance more affordable.

In addition to those reforms, the Act requires the creation of an "Exchange" in each State—basically, a marketplace that allows people to compare and purchase insurance plans. The Act gives each State the opportunity to establish its own Exchange, but provides that the Federal Government will establish the Exchange if the State does not.

This case is about whether the Act's interlocking reforms apply equally in each State no matter who establishes the State's Exchange. Specifically, the question presented is whether the Act's tax credits are available in States that have a Federal Exchange.

I
A
[Here the Chief Justice summarizes what he calls a "long history of failed health insurance reform" including two related concepts that several states adopted in the 1990s: a "guaranteed issue" requirement and a "community rating" requirement. Together these reforms meant that anyone who wanted

health insurance in those states could buy it, and insurers could not deny coverage or charge a higher premium because of preexisting conditions. The opinion continues.]

The guaranteed issue and community rating requirements achieved [the goal of making insurance available to all], but they had an unintended consequence: They encouraged people to wait until they got sick to buy insurance. Why buy insurance coverage when you are healthy, if you can buy the same coverage for the same price when you become ill? This consequence—known as "adverse selection"—led to a second: Insurers were forced to increase premiums to account for the fact that, more and more, it was the sick rather than the healthy who were buying insurance. And that consequence fed back into the first: As the cost of insurance rose, even more people waited until they became ill to buy it.

This led to an economic "death spiral." As premiums rose higher and higher, and the number of people buying insurance sank lower and lower, insurers began to leave the market entirely. As a result, the number of people without insurance increased dramatically.

. . . In 1996, Massachusetts adopted the guaranteed issue and community rating requirements and experienced similar results. But in 2006, Massachusetts added two more reforms: The Commonwealth required individuals to buy insurance or pay a penalty, and it gave tax credits to certain individuals to ensure that they could afford the insurance they were required to buy. The combination

(continued)

(continued from previous page)

of these three reforms—insurance market regulations, a coverage mandate, and tax credits—reduced the uninsured rate in Massachusetts to 2.6 percent, by far the lowest in the Nation.

B

[The opinion next describes the ACA's reform provisions: (1) adoption of the guaranteed issue and community rating requirements; (2) a requirement for individuals to have insurance or make a tax payment to the IRS—the "individual mandate" upheld in NFIB v. Sebelius, *see p. 67 of the textbook—and (3) the giving of tax credits to low-income persons to help make insurance more affordable.]*

These three reforms are closely intertwined. . . . Congress found that the guaranteed issue and community rating requirements would not work without the coverage requirement. And the coverage requirement would not work without the tax credits. The reason is that, without the tax credits, the cost of buying insurance would exceed eight percent of income for a large number of individuals, which would exempt them from the coverage requirement. *[The ACA exempts from the individual mandate anyone who would have to spend more than 8 percent of his income on health insurance.]*

C

In addition to those three reforms, the Act requires the creation of an "Exchange" in each State where people can shop for insurance, usually online. An Exchange may be created in one of two ways. First, the Act provides that "[e]ach State shall . . . establish an American Health Benefit Exchange . . . for the State." Second, if a State nonetheless chooses not to establish its own Exchange, the Act provides that the Secretary of Health and Human Services "shall . . . establish and operate such Exchange within the State."

The issue in this case is whether the Act's tax credits are available in States that have a Federal Exchange rather than a State Exchange. The Act initially provides that tax credits "shall be allowed" for any "applicable taxpayer." 26 U. S. C. §36B(a). The Act then provides that the amount of the tax credit depends in part on whether the taxpayer has enrolled in an insurance plan through "an Exchange *established by the State* [under § 18031 of the ACA].

[To implement these provisions, the IRS promulgated a rule that made tax credits available to applicable taxpayers who enrolled in an insurance plan through an Exchange regardless of whether the Exchange was established by the state or by HHS. At the time the opinion was written, 34 states had opted to let HHS set up their particular Exchanges. The petitioners in this case were four residents of Virginia who do not want to buy health insurance. They argue that (a) Virginia's exchange, which was set up by HHS, does not qualify as "an Exchange established by the State" under § 18031, (b) they should not receive tax credits, (c) without the credits the cost of insurance would be more than 8 percent of their income, and (d) therefore they are exempt from the individual mandate. These arguments failed at both the trial court and Court of Appeals (4th Circuit) levels; however, in a similar case the Court of Appeals for the D.C. Circuit held that the tax credits are available only for state exchanges. This split of opinion between the two appellate circuits led to the Supreme Court deciding to grant certiorari.]

II

The Affordable Care Act addresses tax credits in what is now Section 36B of the Internal Revenue Code. . . . *[Refer to the table titled "Statutory Provisions Referred to in* King v. Burwell*" on p. 100 for the text of this and other provisions referred to in the opinion. That table is provided to enable the student to follow Chief Justice Roberts's rather complex analysis.]*

The parties dispute whether Section 36B authorizes tax credits for individuals who enroll in an insurance plan through a Federal Exchange. Petitioners argue that a Federal Exchange is not "an Exchange established by the State under [42 U.S.C. §18031]," and that the IRS Rule therefore contradicts Section 36B. The Government responds that the IRS Rule *[referred to earlier]* is lawful because the phrase "an Exchange established by the State under [42 U.S.C. §18031]" should be read to include Federal Exchanges.

. . . It is . . . our task to determine the correct reading of Section 36B. If the statutory language is plain, we must enforce it according to its terms. But oftentimes the "meaning—or ambiguity—of certain words or phrases may only become evident when placed in context." *[Quoting an earlier Supreme Court case.]* So when deciding whether the language is plain, we must read the words "in their context and with a view to their place in the overall statutory scheme." Our duty, after all, is "to construe statutes, not isolated provisions."

A

We begin with the text of Section 36B. As relevant here, Section 36B allows an individual to receive tax credits only if the individual enrolls in an insurance plan through "an Exchange established by the State under [42 U.S.C. §18031]." In other words, three things must be true: First, the individual must enroll in an insurance plan through "an Exchange." Second, that Exchange must be "established by the State." And third, that Exchange must be established "under [42 U. S. C. §18031]." We address each requirement in turn.

First, all parties agree that a Federal Exchange qualifies as "an Exchange" for purposes of Section 36B. Section 18031 provides that "[e]ach State shall . . . establish an American Health Benefit Exchange . . . for the State." . . . [But] if the State chooses not to

do so, Section 18041 provides that the Secretary "shall . . . establish and operate *such Exchange* within the State."

By using the phrase "such Exchange," Section 18041 instructs the Secretary to establish and operate the *same* Exchange that the State was directed to establish under Section 18031. . . . In other words, State Exchanges and Federal Exchanges are equivalent—they must meet the same requirements, perform the same functions, and serve the same purposes. Although State and Federal Exchanges are established by different sovereigns, Sections 18031 and 18041 do not suggest that they differ in any meaningful way. A Federal Exchange therefore counts as "an Exchange" under Section 36B.

Second, we must determine whether a Federal Exchange is "established by the State" for purposes of Section 36B. At the outset, it might seem that a Federal Exchange cannot fulfill this requirement. After all, the Act defines "State" to mean "each of the 50 States and the District of Columbia"—a definition that does not include the Federal Government. But when read in context, "with a view to [its] place in the overall statutory scheme," the meaning of the phrase "established by the State" is not so clear.

. . . These provisions suggest that the Act may not always use the phrase "established by the State" in its most natural sense. Thus, the meaning of that phrase may not be as clear as it appears when read out of context.

Third, we must determine whether a Federal Exchange is established "under [42 U. S. C. §18031]." This too might seem a requirement that a Federal Exchange cannot fulfill, because it is Section 18041 that tells the Secretary when to "establish and operate such Exchange." But here again, the way different provisions in the statute interact suggests otherwise.

The Act defines the term "Exchange" to mean "an American Health Benefit Exchange

(continued)

(continued from previous page)

established under section 18031." If we import that definition into Section 18041, the Act tells the Secretary to "establish and operate such 'American Health Benefit Exchange established under section 18031.'" That suggests that Section 18041 authorizes the Secretary to establish an Exchange under Section 18031, not (or not only) under Section 18041. Otherwise, the Federal Exchange, by definition, would not be an "Exchange" at all.

This interpretation of "under [42 U. S. C. §18031]" fits best with the statutory context. All of the requirements that an Exchange must meet are in Section 18031, so it is sensible to regard all Exchanges as established under that provision. In addition, every time the Act uses the word "Exchange," the definitional provision requires that we substitute the phrase "Exchange established under section 18031." If Federal Exchanges were not established under Section 18031, therefore, literally none of the Act's requirements would apply to them. Finally, the Act repeatedly uses the phrase "established under [42 U.S.C. §18031]" in situations where it would make no sense to distinguish between State and Federal Exchanges. A Federal Exchange may therefore be considered one established "under [42 U. S. C. §18031]."

. . . The Affordable Care Act contains more than a few examples of inartful drafting. (To cite just one, the Act creates three separate Section 1563s. See 124 Stat. 270, 911, 912.) . . . Anyway, we "must do our best, bearing in mind the fundamental canon of statutory construction that the words of a statute must be read in their context and with a view to their place in the overall statutory scheme."

B
Given that the text is ambiguous, we must turn to the broader structure of the Act to determine the meaning of Section 36B. "A provision that may seem ambiguous in isolation is often clarified by the remainder of the statutory scheme . . . because only one of the permissible meanings produces a substantive effect that is

compatible with the rest of the law." [Citing a 1988 Supreme Court decision.] Here, the statutory scheme compels us to reject petitioners' interpretation because it would destabilize the individual insurance market in any State with a Federal Exchange, and likely create the very "death spirals" that Congress designed the Act to avoid. See New York State Dept. of Social Servs. v. Dublino, 413 U.S. 405, 419–420 (1973) ("We cannot interpret federal statutes to negate their own stated purposes.").

As discussed earlier, Congress based the Affordable Care Act on three major reforms: first, the guaranteed issue and community rating requirements; second, a requirement that individuals maintain health insurance coverage or make a payment to the IRS; and third, the tax credits for individuals with household incomes between 100 per cent and 400 percent of the federal poverty line. In a State that establishes its own Exchange, these three reforms work together to expand insurance coverage. The guaranteed issue and community rating requirements ensure that anyone can buy insurance; the coverage requirement creates an incentive for people to do so before they get sick; and the tax credits—it is hoped—make insurance more affordable. Together, those reforms "minimize . . . adverse selection and broaden the health insurance risk pool to include healthy individuals, which will lower health insurance premiums."

Under petitioners' reading, however, the Act would operate quite differently in a State with a Federal Exchange. As they see it, one of the Act's three major reforms—the tax credits—would not apply. And a second major reform—the coverage requirement—would not apply in a meaningful way. . . . The combination of no tax credits and an ineffective coverage requirement could well push a State's individual insurance market into a death spiral. . . .

It is implausible that Congress meant the Act to operate in this manner. See National Federation of Independent Business v. Sebelius, 567 U. S.____ (2012) (SCALIA, KENNEDY, THOMAS, and

ALITO, JJ. dissenting) ("Without the federal subsidies . . . the exchanges would not operate as Congress intended and may not operate at all."). Congress made the guaranteed issue and community rating requirements applicable in every State in the Nation. But those requirements only work when combined with the coverage requirement and the tax credits. So it stands to reason that Congress meant for those provisions to apply in every State as well. . . .

[Subpart II.C of the opinion is omitted.]

D

Petitioners' arguments about the plain meaning of Section 36B are strong. But while the meaning of the phrase "an Exchange established by the State under [42 U.S.C. §18031]" may seem plain "when viewed in isolation," such a reading turns out to be "untenable in light of [the statute] as a whole." In this instance, the context and structure of the Act compel us to depart from what would otherwise be the most natural reading of the pertinent statutory phrase.

Reliance on context and structure in statutory interpretation is a "subtle business, calling for great wariness lest what professes to be mere rendering becomes creation and attempted interpretation of legislation becomes legislation itself." *Palmer* v. *Massachusetts*, 308 U. S. 79, 83 (1939). For the reasons we have given, however, such reliance is appropriate in this case, and leads us to conclude that Section 36B allows tax credits for insurance purchased on any Exchange created under the Act. Those credits are necessary for the Federal Exchanges to function like their State Exchange counterparts, and to avoid the type of calamitous result that Congress plainly meant to avoid.

* * *

In a democracy, the power to make the law rests with those chosen by the people. Our role is more confined—"to say what the law is." *Marbury* v. *Madison*, 1 Cranch 137,

177 (1803). That is easier in some cases than in others. But in every case we must respect the role of the Legislature, and take care not to undo what it has done. A fair reading of legislation demands a fair understanding of the legislative plan.

Congress passed the Affordable Care Act to improve health insurance markets, not to destroy them. If at all possible, we must interpret the Act in a way that is consistent with the former, and avoids the latter. Section 36B can fairly be read consistent with what we see as Congress's plan, and that is the reading we adopt.

The judgment of the United States Court of Appeals for the Fourth Circuit is *Affirmed.*

JUSTICE SCALIA, with whom JUSTICE THOMAS and JUSTICE ALITO join, dissenting.

The Court holds that when the Patient Protection and Affordable Care Act says "Exchange established by the State" it means "Exchange established by the State or the Federal Government." That is of course quite absurd, and the Court's 21 pages of explanation make it no less so.

. . . This case requires us to decide whether someone who buys insurance on an Exchange established by the Secretary gets tax credits. You would think the answer would be obvious—so obvious there would hardly be a need for the Supreme Court to hear a case about it. In order to receive any money under §36B, an individual must enroll in an insurance plan through an "Exchange established by the State." The Secretary of Health and Human Services is not a State. So an Exchange established by the Secretary is not an Exchange established by the State—which means people who buy health insurance through such an Exchange get no money under §36B.

Words no longer have meaning if an Exchange that is *not* established by a State

(continued)

(continued from previous page)

is "established by the State." . . . Under all the usual rules of interpretation, in short, the Government should lose this case. But normal rules of interpretation seem always to yield to the overriding principle of the present Court: The Affordable Care Act must be saved.
. . .

I wholeheartedly agree with the Court that sound interpretation requires paying attention to the whole law, not homing in on isolated words or even isolated sections. Context always matters. Let us not forget, however, *why* context matters: It is a tool for understanding the terms of the law, not an excuse for rewriting them.

. . . Ordinary connotation does not always prevail, but the more unnatural the proposed interpretation of a law, the more compelling the contextual evidence must be to show that it is correct. Today's interpretation is not merely unnatural; it is unheard of. Who would ever have dreamt that "Exchange established by the State" means "Exchange established by the State *or the Federal Government*"?
. . .

Faced with overwhelming confirmation that "Exchange established by the State" means what it looks like it means, the Court comes up with argument after feeble argument to support its contrary interpretation. None of its tries comes close to establishing the implausible conclusion that Congress used "by the State" to mean "by the State or not by the State."

[For the next twelve pages the pugnacious and irascible Justice Scalia excoriates the majority opinion and impeaches its reasoning. He accuses his six colleagues of "jiggery-pokery" (underhanded scheming), calls a portion of the opinion "pure applesauce," and says it engages in "defense of the indefensible." He writes that the majority's logic "suffers from no shortage of flaws," and he calls it a "dismal failure." He concludes with the following peroration.]

The Court's decision reflects the philosophy that judges should endure whatever interpretive distortions it takes in order to correct a supposed flaw in the statutory machinery. That philosophy ignores the American people's decision to give *Congress* "[a]ll legislative Powers" enumerated in the Constitution. Art. I, §1. They made Congress, not this Court, responsible for both making laws and mending them. This Court holds only the judicial power—the power to pronounce the law as Congress has enacted it. We lack the prerogative to repair laws that do not work out in practice, just as the people lack the ability to throw us out of office if they dislike the solutions we concoct. We must always remember, therefore, that "[o]ur task is to apply the text, not to improve upon it." *[Quoting a 1989 case.]* . . .

. . . It is not our place to judge the quality of the care and deliberation that went into this or any other law. A law enacted by voice vote with no deliberation whatever is fully as binding upon us as one enacted after years of study, months of committee hearings, and weeks of de bate. Much less is it our place to make everything come out right when Congress does not do its job properly. It is up to Congress to design its laws with care, and it is up to the people to hold them to account if they fail to carry out that responsibility.

Rather than rewriting the law under the pretense of interpreting it, the Court should have left it to Congress to decide what to do about the Act's limitation of tax credits to state Exchanges. If Congress values above everything else the Act's applicability across the country, it could make tax credits available in every Exchange. If it prizes state involvement in the Act's implementation, it could continue to limit tax credits to state Exchanges while taking other steps to mitigate the economic consequences predicted by the Court. If Congress wants to accommodate both goals, it could make tax credits available everywhere while offering new incentives for

States to set up their own Exchanges. And if Congress thinks that the present design of the Act works well enough, it could do nothing. Congress could also do something else altogether, entirely abandoning the structure of the Affordable Care Act. The Court's insistence on making a choice that should be made by Congress both aggrandizes judicial power and encourages congressional lassitude.

. . . Today's opinion changes the usual rules of statutory interpretation for the sake of the Affordable Care Act. That, alas, is not a novelty. In *National Federation of Independent Business* v. *Sebelius*, 567 U.S. ___, this Court revised major components of the statute in order to save them from unconstitutionality. The Act that Congress passed provides that every individual "shall" maintain insurance or else pay a "penalty." This Court, however, saw that the Commerce Clause does not authorize a federal mandate to buy health insurance. So it rewrote the mandate-cum-penalty as a tax.

The Act that Congress passed also requires every State to accept an expansion of its Medicaid program, or else risk losing *all* Medicaid funding. This Court, however, saw that the Spending Clause does not authorize this coercive condition. So it rewrote the law to withhold only the *incremental*

funds associated with the Medicaid expansion. Having transformed two major parts of the law, the Court today has turned its attention to a third. The Act that Congress passed makes tax credits available only on an "Exchange established by the State." This Court, however, concludes that this limitation would prevent the rest of the Act from working as well as hoped. So it rewrites the law to make tax credits available everywhere. We should start calling this law SCOTUScare.

Perhaps the Patient Protection and Affordable Care Act will attain the enduring status of the Social Security Act or the Taft-Hartley Act; perhaps not. But this Court's two decisions on the Act will surely be remembered through the years. The somersaults of statutory interpretation they have performed ("penalty" means tax, "further [Medicaid] payments to the State" means only incremental Medicaid payments to the State, "established by the State" means not established by the State) will be cited by litigants endlessly, to the confusion of honest jurisprudence. And the cases will publish forever the discouraging truth that the Supreme Court of the United States favors some laws over others, and is prepared to do whatever it takes to uphold and assist its favorites.

I dissent. ◼

Discussion Questions

1. In his recent book, *The Court and the World: American Law and the New Global Realities* (2015), Justice Stephen Breyer writes, "Ordinarily, when deciding difficult textual questions, courts look to text, history, tradition, precedent, purpose, and consequences."[71] In your opinion, which opinion—the majority's or that of the dissent—addresses those factors more satisfactorily?
2. Can you explain the logic behind the chief justice's holding, and is it persuasive to you?
3. What are the "death spirals" he refers to?
4. What effect has the ACA had on the percentage of the population without health insurance since the individual and employer mandates began to take effect in 2014?
5. What is the current status of Medicaid expansion in your state and nationwide?

~ ⛪ ~

Statutory Provisions Referred to in *King v. Burwell*

26 U.S.C. § 36B (Internal Revenue Code)	**Refundable credit for coverage under a qualified health plan** **(a) In general** In the case of an applicable taxpayer, there shall be allowed as a credit against the tax imposed by this subtitle for any taxable year an amount equal to the premium assistance credit amount of the taxpayer for the taxable year. **(b) Premium assistance credit amount** For purposes of this section— **(1) In general** The term "premium assistance credit amount" means, with respect to any taxable year, the sum of the premium assistance amounts determined under paragraph (2) with respect to all coverage months of the taxpayer occurring during the taxable year. **(2) Premium assistance amount** The premium assistance amount determined under this subsection with respect to any coverage month is the amount equal to the lesser of— **(A)** the monthly premiums for such month for 1 or more qualified health plans offered in the individual market within a State which cover the taxpayer, the taxpayer's spouse, or any dependent (as defined in section 152) of the taxpayer and which were enrolled in through an *Exchange established by the State* under [42 U.S.C. § 18031], or **(B)** the excess (if any) of— (i) the adjusted monthly premium for such month for the applicable second lowest cost silver plan with respect to the taxpayer, over (ii) an amount equal to 1/12 of the product of the applicable percentage and the taxpayer's household income for the taxable year.
42 U.S.C. § 18031	**(b) American Health Benefit Exchanges** **(1) In general** Each State shall, not later than January 1, 2014, establish an American Health Benefit Exchange (referred to in this title as an "Exchange") for the State that— **(A)** facilitates the purchase of qualified health plans; **(B)** provides for the establishment of a Small Business Health Options Program (in this title referred to as a "SHOP Exchange") that is designed to assist qualified employers in the State who are small employers in facilitating the enrollment of their employees in qualified health plans offered in the small group market in the State; and **(C)** meets the requirements of subsection (d). [Subsection (d) relates to the Exchange being a government agency or a non-for-profit entity and other details regarding coverage, benefits, operational functions, funding, etc.]
42 U.S.C. § 18041	**(c) Failure to establish Exchange or implement requirements** **(1) In general** If [a state does not establish an Exchange as required by § 18031] . . . the Secretary shall (directly or through agreement with a not-for-profit entity) establish and operate *such Exchange* within the State and . . . take such actions as are necessary.

Note: Italics added; not in original.

The Court Decides

Hill v. Ohio County
468 S.W.2d 306 (Ky. 1971)

Smith, Special Commissioner

[This wrongful death case was filed against Ohio County, Kentucky, the owner of Ohio County Hospital. The trial court granted a motion for summary judgment in favor of the defendant without giving reasons for its decision. The "uncontradicted material facts" follow.]

Decedent approached Nurse Hartley *[who was "in charge of the floor," according to the court]* at her desk in the hospital before 9 am on May 12, 1967, said that her name was Juanita Monroe, her doctor was in Illinois, she had come to Ohio County to attend a funeral and she was afraid she would not be able to get back to Illinois before she had her baby. Nurse Hartley assumed she wanted to be admitted for obstetrical (herein OB) care.

There were only four doctors admitted to practice in the hospital. Nurse Hartley consulted her list and found that Dr. Beard (according to the doctors' informal agreement among themselves) was on call that week. He was at the time in the operating room. Upon Nurse Hartley's inquiry whether to admit decedent, Dr. Beard [replied] that he did not handle OB cases. Upon advice from the hospital administrator that another of the four doctors, Dr. Johnson, was making rounds, Nurse Hartley asked him the same question and Dr. Johnson replied that he did not handle "walk-in OBs."

Decedent did not advise that she had been delivered of a child at the Ohio County Hospital in June 1964, admitted by Dr. Charles Price of Hartford (one of the four doctors practicing in the Hospital) and had again consulted Dr. Price within the past year.

Decedent was advised that she could get OB service in Owensboro and Louisville, with doctors on call, and replied she did not want to go to Owensboro or Louisville, but would call a taxi to go home. Nurse Hartley assisted her in making the call. Being advised that decedent was still there more than an hour later, Nurse Hartley consulted with the hospital administrator and was told to call Bill Danks, ambulance driver, who promptly appeared and offered to take decedent wherever she wanted to go. She declined, and a taxi finally took her away.

Her baby was born at home (apparently unattended) during the night. Decedent called Bill Danks who came immediately, and about 6 am called Dr. Johnson, who asked some questions concerning the state of mother and child and advised Danks to take them to Owensboro. Decedent was dead on arrival at the Owensboro Hospital, some 25 miles from Hartford.

Ohio County Hospital is a public hospital, constructed (at least in part) with Hill-Burton funds which are for construction only. It is a one-floor building and the county pays the cost of operation, including an administrator (not a doctor) and at least two registered nurses. There are no salaried doctors, no residents or interns, and only four local doctors are admitted to practice. The hospital rules properly provide that no patient may be admitted without an order from a doctor to do so [and Kentucky law] provides that no one may practice medicine without being licensed to do so.

. . .

(continued)

(continued from previous page)

[The court quotes favorably from American Jurisprudence, *second edition:]*

With respect to a public hospital, it has been said that since all persons cannot participate in its benefits, no one has, individually, a right to demand admission. The trustees or governing board of a public hospital alone determine the right of admission to the benefits of the institution, and their discretion in this regard will not be reviewed by the courts at the suit of an individual applicant.
. . .

In the instant case, the decedent was not admitted to the hospital nor was the element of critical emergency apparent. The hospital nurse acted in accordance with valid rules for admission to the facility. The uncontradicted facts demonstrate that no breach of duty by the hospital occurred. The nurse could not force the private physicians to accept decedent as a patient. The nurse did all she could do for the decedent on the occasion in question. Therefore, the hospital and the nurse were entitled to a dismissal as a matter of law. The judgment is affirmed. ■

Discussion Questions

1. What other facts would you like to know about this situation to judge whether the case was decided correctly?
2. This decision is now more than 40 years old; would the case be decided differently today? If so, why?
3. In a separate portion of the opinion, the court uses the expression "plaintiff's intestate" in referring to the plaintiff, Mr. Hill. What does that expression mean? Why is Mr. Hill the plaintiff in a case involving an OB patient?
4. What is the significance, if any, of the fact that the hospital is a public hospital that received Hill-Burton funds?

Notes

1. Institute of Medicine, *Insuring America's Health: Principles and Recommendations* (2004) at 24–25, http://www.nap.edu/read/10874/chapter/3#24. *See generally* Organization for Economic Co-operation and Development (OECD), *Private Health Insurance in OECD Countries: The Benefits and Costs for Individuals and Health Systems* (2004), http://healthcare.procon.org/sourcefiles/OECDPrivateHealthInsurance.pdf.
2. U.S. Const. art. I, § 8, cl. 1.
3. Pub. L. No. 111-148, as immediately amended by the Health Care and Education Reconciliation Act of 2010, Pub. L. No. 111-152. When codified, these laws will be spread throughout various portions of the US Code, but mostly in Title 42 (The Public Health and Welfare), Chapter 7, Subchapters XVIII and XIX (The Medicare and Medicaid

Programs). A detailed summary can be found at http://www.kff.org/healthreform/upload/8061.pdf (June 18, 2010).

4. Nat'l Fed'n of Indep. Bus. v. Sebelius, 132 S.Ct. 2566 (2012) *and* King v. Burwell, 135 S.Ct. 2480 (2015).

5. Drew Altman, *Pulling It Together: Implementation Is Forever* (2010), httwww.kff.org/pullingittogether/040610_altman.cfm.

6. 16 C.F.R. Part 681.

7. 78 Fed. Reg. 50506, August 19, 2013.

8. Shands Jacksonville Medical Center v. Burwell, Nos. 14-263, 14-503, 14-536, 14-607, 14-976, and 14-1477, D.D.C.

9. Idaho Falls Consol. Hosps., Inc. v. Bingham County Bd. of County Comm'rs, 102 Idaho 838, 642 P.2d 553 (1982).

10. St. Joseph's Hosp. and Medical Center v. Maricopa County, 142 Ariz. 94, 688 P.2d 986 (1984). The county's indigent care requirement is found in Ariz. Stat. § 11-292.

11. Washoe County, Nev. v. Wittenberg & St. Mary's Hosp., 676 P.2d 808 (1984).

12. Brinkman v. City of Indianapolis, 141 Ind. App. 662, 231 N.E.2d 169 (1967). *See also* Hart v. County of Orange, 254 Cal. App. 2d 302 (1967); Porter v. County of Cook, 42 Ill. App. 3d 287, 355 N.E.2d 561 (1976).

13. Estelle v. Gamble, 429 U.S. 97, *reh'g denied*, 429 U.S. 1066 (1977) (Eighth Amendment is violated by "deliberate indifference to serious medical needs"). *See also* Bivens v. Six Unknown Federal Narcotics Agents, 403 U.S. 388 (1971) (persons subjected to constitutional violations by a federal official have a right to recover damages against the official).

14. Youngberg v. Romero, 457 U.S. 307 (1982) (an involuntarily committed mental patient was entitled to medical care).

15. Maher v. Roe, 432 U.S. 464 (1977); Harris v. McRae, 448 U.S. 297 (1980).

16. *For example*, Conn. Gen. Stat. § 18-7 (Supp. 1985); *see also* Hillcrest Medical Center v. State of Okla., ex rel. Dep't of Corrections, 675 P.2d 432 (Okla. 1983) (the county was liable for the medical expenses of a convicted murderer injured in an automobile accident while in the county's custody).

17. Idaho Code § 20-209 (1979); *but see* Sisters of Third Order of St. Francis v. County of Tazewell, 122 Ill. App. 3d 605, 461 N.E.2d 1064 (1984) (the county was not liable for care furnished an arrestee in the custody of municipal police).

18. Alaska Stat. § 33.30.050 (1982).

19. Md. Ann. Code art. 27, § 698 (Supp. 1985). *See also* Fla. Stat. § 901.35, which establishes a hierarchy of responsibility for medical expenses provided to "any person ill, wounded, or otherwise injured during or at the time of arrest." The first tier of responsibility includes (1) insurance, (2) the patient, and (3) a financial settlement relating to the cause of the injury or illness; only when those sources are not available may the provider seek reimbursement from governmental authority. On the basis of the "during or at the time of arrest" language, some law enforcement officials attempt to avoid governmental responsibility by not formally arresting the suspect until after treatment is rendered.

20. *See* William Contente, *Note and Comment, City of Revere v. Massachusetts General Hospital: Government Responsibility for an Arrestee's Medical Care*, 9 Am. J. L. & Med., 361, 369–70 (1983–84).

21. 463 U.S. 239 (1983).

22. Massachusetts Gen. Hosp. v. City of Revere, 385 Mass. 772, 484 N.E.2d 185 (1982). *Rev'd on other grounds*, City of Revere v. Massachusetts Gen. Hosp., 463 U.S. 239 (1983).

23. Maher, *supra* note 15.

24. Harris, *supra* note 15.

25. City of Revere, *supra* note 20.

26. Pub. L. No. 79-725; 42 U.S.C. §§ 291 to 291o-1.

27. Regulations regarding the uncompensated care and community service obligations may be found at 42 C.F.R. § 124. The former begin at § 124.501 and the latter at § 124.601.

28. *See, e.g.*, Cook v. Ochsner Found. Hosp., 61 F.R.D. 354 (E.D. La. 1972).

29. 42 C.F.R. § 53.111(d)(2).

30. *See* Cook v. Ochner, *supra* note 28. *See also* 42 C.F.R. § 124.603(b)(1).

31. *See, e.g.*, Jackson v. Indiana, 406 U.S. 715 (1972); Humphrey v. Cady, 405 U.S. 504 (1972).

32. Lewis v. Donahue, 437 F. Supp. 112 (W.D. Okla. 1977) (a patient released from state hospital and transferred to outpatient status may not be recommitted without due process protections). *See also* In re Anderson, 73 Cal. App. 3d 38, 140 Cal. Rptr. 546 (1977).

33. People in Interest of Paiz, 43 Colo. App. 352, 603 P.2d 976 (1979).

34. O'Connor v. Donaldson, 422 U.S. 563 (1975); 42 U.S.C. § 1983.

35. Addington v. Texas, 441 U.S. 418 (1979).

36. *See* Tobias v. Manhattan Eye and Ear Hosp., 283 N.Y.S.2d 398, 28 A.D.2d 972 (1967), *aff'd*, 23 N.Y.2d 724, 296 N.Y.S.2d 368 (1968).

37. Fla. Stat. §§ 394.451 to 394.4789.

38. Fla. Stat. § 394.463(2)(i).

39. Fla. Stat. § 394.467.

40. O'Connor v. Donaldson, 422 U.S. 563 (1975).

41. *Id.* at 576.

42. Addington, *supra* note 35.

43. *Id.*

44. 463 U.S. 354 (1983).

45. Wyatt v. Stickney, 344 F. Supp. 387 (M.D. Ala. 1972), 344 F. Supp. 373 (M.D. Ala. 1972), *aff'd in part, remanded in part*, 503 F.2d 1305 (5th Cir. 1974), *enforcing* 325 F. Supp. 781 (M.D. Ala. 1971).

46. Youngberg v. Romero, 457 U.S. 307 (an individual with an intellectual disability was not provided treatment appropriate for his diagnosis).

47. *Id.*

48. Rone v. Fireman, 473 F. Supp. 92, 104, 119 (N.D. Ohio 1979); *see also* Ohlinger v. Watson, 652 F.2d 775 (9th Cir. 1980).

49. Youngberg, *supra* note 14 at 314, quoting and adopting the view of concurring Chief Judge Seitz, Court of Appeals, Third Circuit, 644 F.2d 147, 178 (1980).

50. Youngberg, *supra* note 14 at 321.

51. Rennie v. Klein, 653 F.2d 836 (3d Cir. 1981), *vacated*, 458 U.S. 1119, *on remand*, 720 F.2d 266 (1983); Davis v. Hubbard, 506 F. Supp. 915 (N.D. Ohio 1980); Rogers v. Okin, 634 F.2d 650 (1st Cir. 1980), *vacated*, 457 U.S. 291; Goedecke v. State, 198 Colo. 407, 603 P.2d 123 (1979) (common law recognizes a mental patient's right to refuse medication).

52. *See, e.g.*, Parvi v. City of Kingston, 394 N.Y.S.2d 161, 41 N.Y.2d 553, 362 N.E.2d 960 (1977) (the city was potentially liable in negligence when intoxicated persons attempting to cross New York Thruway were struck by a car after being abandoned by the police in a rural area). *But see* Modla v. Parker, 17 Ariz. App. 54, 495 P.2d 494, *cert. denied*, 409 U.S. 1038 (1972) (the hospital was entitled to summary judgment in a suit alleging wrongful discharge when there was no evidence that the release impeded treatment or worsened the patient's condition).

53. 285 N.Y. 389, 34 N.E.2d 367 (1941); *see also* Anderson v. Moore, 202 Neb. 452, 275 N.W.2d 842 (1979).

54. Morrison v. Washington County, Ala., 700 F.2d 678 (11th Cir. 1983), *cert. denied*, 464 U.S. 864 (1983).

55. *Id.*, 700 F.2d at 683.

56. 538 F.2d 121 (4th Cir. 1976), *cert. denied*, 429 U.S. 827 (1976).

57. Chrite v. United States, 564 F. Supp. 341 (E.D. Mich. 1983) (Veterans Administration could be liable for failure to warn a patient's mother-in-law of threats of violence). *Cf.* Leedy v. Hartnett, 510 F. Supp. 1125 (M.D. Penn. 1981), *aff'd mem.*, 676 F.2d 686 (3d Cir. 1982) (Veterans Administration owed no duty to warn the plaintiff's family when a discharged mental patient posed no greater danger to the plaintiff than to the community at large).

58. Kyslinger v. United States, 406 F. Supp. 800 (W.D. Pa. 1975), *aff'd*, 547 F.2d 1161 (3d Cir. 1977) (there was no evidence to support allegations that a patient with polycystic kidney disease and his spouse were given inadequate information and training in use of home hemodialysis unit at time of discharge from hospital).

59. *See, e.g.*, Cook v. Highland Hosp., 168 N.C. 250, 84 S.E. 352 (1915); *see generally* False Imprisonment in Nursing Home, 4 A.L.R.2d 449.

60. *See, e.g.*, Marcus v. Liebman, 59 Ill. App. 3d 337, 375 N.E.2d 486 (1978) (a psychologically disturbed patient was entitled to a jury trial on the issue of whether her suspicion that force was threatened was "reasonable," thereby constituting tort of false imprisonment). *See also* Rice v. Mercy Hosp. Corp., 275 So. 2d 566 (Fla. App. 1973) *and* Paradies v. Benedictine Hosp., 431 N.Y.S.2d 175 (1980), *appeal dismissed*, 435 N.Y.S.2d 982 (1980).

61. For standards of The Joint Commission regarding use of restraint and seclusion of patients for behavioral health purposes, *see generally* "Introduction to the Standards PC.03.03.01 through PC.03.03.31," 2011 Hospital Accreditation Standards at PC-37 to PC-39; *see also* Standards PC.03.03.01 through PC.03.05.19 at PC-39 to PC-62. The medical record documentation standard is PC.03.05.15 at PC-60 to PC-61.

62. Gadsden v. Hamilton, 212 Ala. 531, 103 So. 553 (1925); Bedard v. Notre Dame, 89 R.I. 195, 151 A.2d 690 (1959). *Cf.* Bailie v. Miami Valley Hosp., 8 Ohio Misc. 193, 221 N.E.2d 217 (1966) (there was no false imprisonment when no threat of force against a mother of an infant patient existed and the patient was unaware of detention).

63. Neb. Rev. Stat. § 29-121(2008).

64. The Joint Commission, 2013 Hospital Accreditation Standards at LD-26. The entire standard reads as follows:

Standard LD.04.02.05
When internal or external review results in the denial of care, treatment, and services, or payment, the hospital makes decisions regarding the ongoing provision of care, treatment, and services, and discharge or transfer, based on the assessed needs of the patient.

Rationale for LD.04.02.05

The hospital is professionally and ethically responsible for providing care, treatment, and services within its capability and law and regulations. At times, such care, treatment, and services are denied because of payment limitations. In these situations, the decision to continue providing care, treatment, and services or to discharge the patient is based solely on the patient's identified needs.

Element of Performance for LD.04.02.05

1. Decisions regarding the provision of ongoing care, treatment, and services, discharge, or transfer are based on the assessed needs of the patient, regardless of the recommendations of any internal or external review.

2. The safety and quality of care, treatment, and services do not depend on the patient's ability to pay.

65. Jersey City Medical Center v. Halstead, 169 N.J. Super. 22, 404 A.2d 44 (1979); Lucy Webb Hayes Nat'l School v. Geoghegan, 281 F. Supp. 116 (D.C.D.C. 1967).

66. 80 N.J. 299, 403 A.2d 487 (1979), *cert. denied*, 444 U.S. 942 (1979).

67. 42 C.F.R. § 440.230(b) (1984).

68. Monmouth Medical Center v. Harris, 646 F.2d 74 (3d Cir. 1981).

69. 42 U.S.C. §§ 1320c to 1320c-13 (1983 and Supp. 1987).

70. 42 U.S.C. § 1320c-3.

71. STEPHEN BREYER, THE COURT AND THE WORLD: AMERICAN LAW AND NEW GLOBAL REALITIES 127 (Knopf 2015).

72. See, e.g., Kaiser Family Foundation, Key Facts about the Uninsured Population (published September 29, 2016), http://kff.org/uninsured/fact-sheet/key-facts-about-the-uninsured-population.

73. US Const. art. I, § 8.

74. Miles Kingston, *Heading for a Sticky End*, INDEPENDENT, March 28, 2003, http://www.independent.co.uk/voices/columnists/miles-kington/heading-for-a-sticky-end-112674.html.

75. Kaiser Family Foundation Public Opinion and Survey Research Foundation, *Kaiser Health Tracking Poll*, Publication Number 8084 (July 2010), http://kff.org/health-reform/perspective/overall-public-support-for-the-health-reform-law-is-steady-from-june.

Appendix 3.1: History of Health Reform Efforts

The tortuous history of healthcare reform in the United States runs for more than a century and a half and involves at least a dozen presidents.

Year	Event
1854	A bill that would have established asylums for the "indigent insane" as well as for the blind and deaf passes both houses of Congress but is vetoed by President Franklin Pierce. Pierce argues that the federal government should not commit itself to social welfare, which he stated was the responsibility of the states.
1865	After the Civil War, the federal government establishes the first system of national medical care in the South. Through an agency known as the Freedmen's Bureau, the government constructs 40 hospitals, employs more than 120 physicians, and treats well more than a million sick and dying former slaves. The hospitals last only from 1865 to 1870 because continuation of the bureau is opposed by President Andrew Johnson, a southerner.
1912	Former President Theodore Roosevelt champions national health insurance in his unsuccessful third-party bid for election as the "Bull Moose" candidate.
1935	President Franklin D. Roosevelt (FDR) favors creating national health insurance amid the Great Depression but decides to push for Social Security first.
1942	FDR establishes wage and price controls during World War II. Businesses cannot attract workers with higher pay, so they compete by adding benefits, including health insurance. Employer-paid health insurance grows into a workplace perk and becomes the usual source of coverage for most Americans.
1945	President Harry S. Truman calls on Congress to create a national insurance program. The American Medical Association denounces the idea as "socialized medicine" and it goes nowhere.
1960	John F. Kennedy makes healthcare a major campaign issue. Later, as president, he cannot get a plan for the elderly through Congress.
1965	President Lyndon B. Johnson's legendary arm-twisting and a Congress dominated by his fellow Democrats leads to creation of two landmark government health programs: Medicare for the elderly and Medicaid for the poor.
1974	President Richard Nixon proposes an employer mandate to offer private health insurance and reforms to Medicaid. The Watergate scandal intervenes, causing Nixon's resignation.
1976	President Jimmy Carter promotes a mandatory national health plan, but economic recession helps push it aside.
1986	President Ronald Reagan signs the Consolidated Omnibus Budget Reconciliation Act (COBRA), a requirement that employers let former workers stay on the company health plan for 18 months after leaving a job, with the workers bearing the cost.

Year	Event
1988	Congress expands Medicare by adding a prescription drug benefit and "catastrophic care" coverage. Barraged by protests from older Americans upset about paying a tax to finance the additional coverage, Congress repeals the catastrophic care law the next year.
1993	President Bill Clinton puts First Lady Hillary Rodham Clinton in charge of developing what becomes a 1,300-page plan for universal coverage. "Hillarycare" would require businesses to cover their workers and require everyone to have health insurance. The plan meets Republican opposition, divides Democrats, and comes under a firestorm of lobbying from businesses and the healthcare field. It dies in the Senate.
1997	Bill Clinton signs bipartisan legislation—the Children's Health Insurance Program (CHIP)—creating a state-federal program to provide coverage for millions of children in families of modest means whose incomes are too high to qualify for Medicaid.
2003	In a major expansion of the program for older people, President George W. Bush persuades Congress to add prescription drug coverage to Medicare.
2009	President Barack Obama and the Democratic-controlled Congress spend an intense year ironing out legislation to require most companies to cover their workers, mandate that everyone have coverage or pay a penalty to the IRS, require insurance companies to accept all comers regardless of preexisting conditions, assist people who cannot afford insurance, create state and federal health benefit exchanges, and encourage states to expand Medicaid coverage. This effort becomes the ACA, which passed in 2010 with no Republicans voting in favor.
2012	In *NFIB v. Sebelius*, the US Supreme Court upholds the "individual mandate" portion of the ACA (the penalty for individuals who do not have insurance) but strikes down the provision requiring states to expand Medicaid.
2015	In *King v. Burwell*, the court holds that the ACA's tax credits are available to applicable taxpayers in states that have a federal Exchange rather than a state Exchange.

Note: This table does not mention the many other federal health-related programs and services such as the military medical systems; the Indian Health Service; the Public Health Service; the Federal Employee Health Benefit Plan; and health plans for veterans, Peace Corps volunteers, and federal prisoners.

Appendix 3.2: Select ACA Reform Provisions

Healthcare Field Segment	Provisions
Insurers	• Report medical loss ratios and provide rebates to enrollees if the ratios are less than the prescribed percentages • Institute rate review process and consumer coverage reforms • Limit the deductibility of insurer executive or employee compensation to $500,000 per individual* ("Cadillac plans")
Non-Medicare individuals	• Free basic preventive care • No lifetime limits • Dependent coverage for adult children up to age 26 in all individual and group policies • No preexisting conditions for children • The "individual mandate"— a requirement to purchase minimum coverage or pay a penalty • Tax subsidies for low-income persons
Employers	• Tax credits to small employers that offer coverage; temporary reinsurance program for employers that offer coverage to retirees not eligible for Medicare • Requirement that certain large employers offer health insurance to employees
Hospitals and other providers	• Reduce annual market basket updates for inpatient hospital, home health, skilled nursing facility, hospice, and other providers; adjust for productivity* • Ban new physician-owned hospitals in Medicare, and require hospitals to have a provider agreement in effect by December 31, 2010; limit the growth of certain grandfathered physician-owned hospitals*; establish new rules for nonprofit hospitals • Establish a committee to develop a national workforce strategy, health professional scholarships and loans, and teaching health centers to provide Medicare payments to primary care residency programs in federally qualified health centers*
Pharmaceutical industry	Authorize the Food and Drug Administration to approve generic versions of biologic drugs, and grant to biologics manufacturers 12 years of exclusive use before generics of their products can be marketed

Healthcare Field Segment	Provisions
Medicare and Medicaid	• Free annual wellness visits for Medicare beneficiaries • Expanded options at end of life (demonstration program for hospice and curative care concurrently) • $250 rebate to beneficiaries who reach the Medicare Part D coverage gap in 2010 • Improved care coordination for dual-eligibles (persons entitled to both Medicare and Medicaid) through the Centers for Medicare & Medicaid's (CMS) new Federal Coordinated Health Care Office • Increase Medicaid drug rebates (brand-name drugs to 23.1 percent) • Funding for Medicaid and Children's Health Insurance Program (CHIP) Payment and Access Commission to include assessments of adult services
Notable new entities	• State-operated health insurance exchanges (and a federal exchange for states that choose not to develop their own) to serve as marketplaces where individuals and small businesses can enroll in plans after comparing price and coverage • Patient-Centered Outcomes Research Institute, a private, nonprofit corporation that develops and funds comparative effectiveness research • Independent Payment Advisory Board for proposals to slow the growth of Medicare and private healthcare spending and improve quality • Center for Medicare & Medicaid Innovation, a CMS entity that tests and evaluates payment structures and methods to foster patient-centered care, improve quality, and reduce the cost of care under Medicare and Medicaid

Sources: *See generally*, Kaiser Family Foundation, *Health Reform Implementation Timeline* (accessed November 3, 2016), http://www.kff.org/interactive/implementation-timeline *and* Venson Wallin Jr. et al., *Blunting the Negative Impact of Healthcare Reform*, 64 HEALTHCARE FIN. MGMT., 62–66 (2010).

*Reprinted from sources.

CONTRACTS AND INTENTIONAL TORTS

> **After reading this chapter, you will**
>
> - know the essential elements of a valid and enforceable contract,
> - understand why contract law is important to physician–patient and hospital–patient relationships,
> - appreciate how the contract principle of breach of warranty can apply to the healthcare setting, and
> - grasp the basics of intentional torts and how they apply to healthcare professionals.

Think Like a Lawyer

In the 1973 movie *The Paper Chase*, the Shakespearean actor John Houseman won an Academy Award for portraying Charles W. Kingsfield, a stern, intimidating contracts law professor. A highlight of the film is Kingsfield's description of the Socratic method—a type of philosophical inquiry commonly used in law schools. To a room filled with first-year students he explains that this technique comprises a series of questions followed by the students' answers, and that it is intended to stimulate critical thinking rather than simply convey information. The Socratic method is, essentially, *teaching by asking*.

Kingsfield struts slowly across the dais; glares at the timorous tyros before him; and announces that in his classroom there are no absolute answers, only an endless string of questions. The students are his patients on an operating table, and he is a neurosurgeon whose questions are instruments that probe their brains.

He stops. He stares. After a dramatic pause, and with a stentorian voice worthy of King Lear, he concludes: "You teach *yourselves* the law, but *I train your mind*. You come in here with a *skull full of mush*, and you leave thinking like a lawyer!" Yes, contracts law can teach you how to think like a lawyer—or at least teach you enough to know when to call on a lawyer for solid advice.

In chapter 1, you learned that law is either public or private. But law can be categorized in other ways as well—for example, there is criminal law and civil law, and civil law has subdivisions; exhibit 4.1 shows this taxonomy.

EXHIBIT 4.1
A Taxonomy
of Law

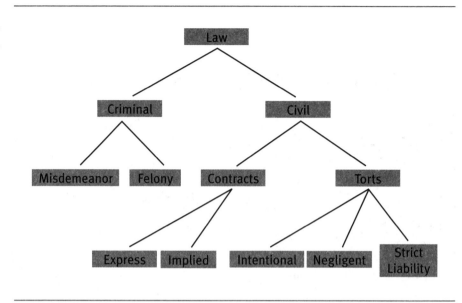

Contracts and Intentional Torts as Bases of Liability

liability
legal responsibility
for one's acts or
omissions

cause of action
the basis of a
lawsuit; sufficient
legal grounds and
alleged facts that,
if proven, would
constitute all the
requirements for
the plaintiff to
prevail

When people think of **liability** in healthcare, they usually think of medical malpractice, a form of negligence. Negligence is the most common type of malpractice,
but medical malpractice can also be based on breach of contract or the commission
of intentional torts. In fact, many malpractice suits allege more than one **cause of
action**. (The reasons for multiple allegations are discussed later in the chapter.[1])

The existence of a legal duty is essential to any liability case, and the
concept of duty tends to change as our society and values change. The legal
duty may be imposed by constitution, legislation, common law (including
negligent or intentional torts), or even contract. In healthcare, special legal
duties arise from the contractual aspects of the physician–patient relationship.[2]

This chapter does not address the law of contracts as it relates to operational issues such as employment, materials management, facilities maintenance, and procurement. Although many of the basic principles discussed
here apply to those areas, too, a full discussion of the breadth of contracts law
is beyond the scope of this text; indeed, the subject of contracts occupies an
entire semester course in the typical law school curriculum.

Elements of a Contract

In simple terms, four conditions must exist for a contract to be valid:

1. *Both parties must be legally competent to enter into the contract.*
   Contracts entered into by mentally incompetent persons are not
   valid—and neither are most contracts entered into by minors.

2. *There must be a meeting of the minds.* One party must make an offer—to buy or sell, for example—and the other party must accept that offer. The terms of the offer and acceptance must be identical.

3. *Consideration must be given.* **Consideration** is the price paid for the contract, but it need not be in the form of money. It may also be a promise (a) to do something you otherwise would not be required to do or (b) to refrain from doing something you otherwise would be able to do.

4. *The purpose of the contract must be legal.* A contract with a hit man to assassinate another person is void because its purpose is illegal. Likewise, many **exculpatory** (taken from the Latin words *ex* "from" and *culpa* "guilt") contracts—those in which a party excuses the other from liability in advance—are invalid because they are against public policy.

> **consideration**
> essentially, payment; something of value (not necessarily money) that is given (or promised) in return for what is received (or promised)

> **exculpatory**
> absolving or clearing of blame

Contracts may be *express* (written, spoken) or *implied*. Many of our day-to-day human interchanges are implied contracts. For example, consider a patron ordering lunch in a restaurant. Implicit in the situation is this message (the offer): If you serve me what I order, I will pay the bill. By taking the order and serving the food, the restaurant accepts the patron's offer and a contract exists. The offer and acceptance are rarely expressed as such in words, but the contract is valid nonetheless. Similarly, the doctor–patient relationship includes an offer (if you treat me, my insurance or I will pay you) and an acceptance (we've scheduled your appointment for next Tuesday).

The Physician–Patient Relationship

The physician–patient relationship is based on contract principles because the physician agrees to provide treatment in return for payment. Professional liability can arise if this contract is breached. In the absence of a contract between physician and patient, the law usually imposes no duty on the physician to treat the patient, although it may impose other duties on the physician. For example, like other passersby, physicians have no legal obligation to help accident victims and although **Good Samaritan statutes** provide protection if they do, with some exceptions the statutes typically do not *require* anyone to act.[3]

This principle was illustrated in *Childs v. Weis*, a Texas case decided back in 1969, before better standards for emergency care were enacted.[4] Childs, a Dallas woman who was seven months pregnant, was out of town when she began to hemorrhage and suffer labor pains. At two o'clock in the morning, Childs presented herself to a small rural hospital's emergency department where a nurse examined her; called a staff physician (presumably at home); and, on the basis of what the doctor said, told her to go to her doctor in

> **Good Samaritan statutes**
> provisions of law that provide immunity from liability for persons who provide emergency care at the scene of an accident

Legal Decision Point

You are at a beach in Florida having a picnic with your significant other. You notice a man struggling in the surf. You run to his rescue, but a minute or so later, while struggling through the waves, you notice that your companion is about to finish the last of the wine, so you abandon your effort and return to the picnic blanket before the wine is gone.

What were your legal and moral responsibilities before you began to assist the victim? Were they the same after you began? Do the answers change depending on whether you were trained in ocean rescue or CPR? What if you were an off-duty emergency medical technician? What other facts might you want to know before you answer?

Dallas. Childs left the hospital and about an hour later gave birth in her car. Twelve hours later, the infant died. The court held that the physician had no duty to Childs because no physician–patient relationship had been established.

The hospital's and nurse's duties are a different matter, of course. As noted in chapter 10, federal law now requires emergency department personnel to stabilize emergency conditions irrespective of whether a provider–patient relationship exists (see Legal Decision Point).

Creation of the Relationship

The contract necessary to form a physician–patient relationship can be *express* (e.g., when you fill out financial responsibility forms at the doctor's office), *implied* (e.g., when you make a follow-up appointment and are seen by the doctor), or even *inferred* from the circumstances. Consider this situation: A patient is unconscious or unable to consent to treatment, but an emergency exists and the physician proceeds. The law will presume (infer) that a contract exists. Although this presumption is a legal fiction, it prevents unjust enrichment by requiring the patient to pay for services he presumably would have contracted for had he been competent. Whether express, implied, or inferred, the physician–patient contract is *bilateral*; that is, it imposes duties on both parties.

Although clear enough in the abstract, these black-letter principles are often difficult to apply in practice. For example, physicians commonly and informally consult one another regarding their patients' diagnosis and treatment, and the consulted physician may not see the patient or know her name. Do these informal hallway consults create a physician–patient relationship? Generally, the answer is no.

For example, in *Oliver v. Brock*,[5] Dr. Whitfield was treating Anita Oliver in rural Demopolis, Alabama, for injuries sustained in an automobile accident. During a telephone conversation with Dr. Brock about another patient, Dr. Whitfield casually mentioned Oliver's treatment and asked for Dr. Brock's opinion. According to Dr. Whitfield's affidavit (see Legal Decision Point), Dr. Brock told him the treatment seemed to be correct under the circumstances. The conversation was apparently informal and gratuitous, and one can almost imagine Dr. Whitfield saying, "Oh, by the way, what do you think about this other situation I have?"

Dr. Brock practiced in Tuscaloosa, which is about 60 miles from Demopolis; according to his own affidavit, he never saw the patient, talked to her or her family, or even learned her name. He admitted that he occasionally talked to Dr. Whitfield by phone (apparently to discuss patients), but he continually emphasized that he did not know Oliver and had "not been employed or requested to advise anyone with regard to her medical problems." Oliver ended up suffering further injury as a result of Dr. Whitfield's course of treatment.

In her own affidavit as plaintiff, Cathy Oliver (the patient's mother) stated that he did not know Anita Oliver and had not been employed or specifically asked by anyone to consult on her medical condition.

After reviewing the evidence, such as it was, the Supreme Court of Alabama unanimously decided that there was no doctor–patient relationship between Dr. Brock and Anita Oliver, so the physician could not be held liable for the injuries

Legal Decision Point

An affidavit is a written document in which the *affiant*—the one who signs the document—swears under penalty of perjury that the facts asserted in the statement are true. Affidavits generally cannot substitute for in-court testimony because they are not subject to cross-examination. But affidavits are sometimes used to support arguments on collateral matters, especially if the opposing attorney does not object. In *Oliver v. Brock*, affidavits were used to support Dr. Brock's position that he did not have a doctor–patient relationship with Oliver, and the plaintiffs also used affidavits to support their own position.

Who do you suppose wrote the affidavits in this case? Are any of their assertions not, strictly speaking, facts? If you were opposing counsel, would you object to the use of such affidavits? If you were the judge, what weight would you give them? If you could cross-examine Dr. Whitfield (the treating physician who consulted with Dr. Brock), what questions would you ask him about his assertions?

the patient sustained as a result of the treatment. One of the justices summarized this position clearly in a concurring opinion: "The mere discussion between professional people of hypothetical situations cannot be viewed as a basis for liability. To hold otherwise would tend to adversely affect the quality of the services they offer to members of the public. Physicians, lawyers, dentists, engineers, and other professionals, by comparing problem-solving approaches with other members of their disciplines, have the opportunity to learn from one another. Possessing this freedom, they are better positioned to bring theory into practice for the benefit of those whom they serve. Our decision in this case preserves these essential learning situations for all professional people."[6]

The general rule is stated in the legal encyclopedia *American Jurisprudence* as follows:

> A physician is under no obligation to engage in practice or to accept professional employment. . . . The relation is a consensual one wherein the patient knowingly seeks the assistance of a physician and the physician knowingly accepts him as

a patient. The relationship between a physician and patient may result from an express or implied contract . . . and the rights and liabilities of the parties thereto are governed by the general law of contract. . . . A physician may accept a patient and thereby incur the consequent duties [even if] his services are performed gratuitously or at the solicitation and on the guaranty of a third person.[7]

On the other hand, a physician need not come into direct contact with a patient for a doctor–patient relationship to exist. A pathologist, for example, has a relationship with patients even though he probably never sees the people whose specimens he examines, and the patients do not know who the pathologist is or even that a pathologist is involved in their treatment.[8]

Another issue involves the duty of a physician who provides services to someone who is not a party to the contract. For example, a physician conducts a preemployment examination, examines an applicant for life insurance, or examines a plaintiff for a personal injuries case. In these situations, the general rule is that a typical physician–patient (i.e., treatment) relationship is not established and the physician owes no duty to the individual being examined—only to the party who contracted for the examination.

Some courts, however, have found at least a limited duty toward the plaintiff, even in the absence of a contractual relationship. In *James v. United States*, the plaintiff applied for a position at a shipyard and, as a condition of employment, was required to take a physical examination. A chest X-ray revealed an abnormality, but through a clerical error the physician never saw the X-ray or the radiologist's report. Almost two years later, the plaintiff was diagnosed with an inoperable cancer. The defense argued that the absence of a physician–patient relationship precluded any duty of care. The court awarded damages anyway because "having made a chest X-ray an essential part of the preemployment examination to determine an applicant's physical fitness, however, defendant failed to use due care when . . . the report on the X-ray was not brought to the attention of the examining physician."[9]

In addition, other statutes, such as the Americans with Disabilities Act and various civil rights acts, both state and federal, may limit a physician's or even a hospital's ability to decline to see a patient in certain circumstances.

Employees' Remedies and Workers' Compensation Laws

Injuries or conditions incurred on the job usually lead to physician–patient relationships for treatment. Can the employee successfully bring a lawsuit against the employer or fellow employees for the workplace injury? If treatment of the condition was rendered negligently, can the employee successfully sue the healthcare provider?

The general rule is that workers' compensation is an employee's *exclusive* legal remedy for a workplace injury or illness. Under that rule, employees are precluded from recovering from their employer or coworkers for negligence or other claims.[10] However, when an employer operates in two capacities—both as an employer and as a healthcare provider, for example—some courts have found that the second role imposes obligations outside the employment relationship and a second cause of action is possible. This exception, known as the *dual capacity doctrine*, is seen in a pair of cases.

In a 1978 case from Ohio, the plaintiff had been a laboratory technician at the defendant hospital, where she operated a blood-gas apparatus that used mercury. In her complaint against the hospital, the plaintiff alleged that she contracted mercury poisoning from the apparatus, that the hospital's clinical staff failed to diagnose her condition as mercury poisoning, and that her injuries were aggravated as a result of this alleged medical negligence.

The Ohio Supreme Court held that the hospital, as an employer, was liable for workers' compensation benefits, but in its second capacity as a hospital it was also liable for the medical negligence. "Appellant's need for protection from malpractice was neither more nor less than that of another's employee. The . . . hospital, with respect to its treatment of the appellant, did so as a hospital, not as an employer, and its relationship with the appellant was that of hospital–patient with all the concomitant traditional obligations."[11]

By way of contrast, the 2000 Maryland case *Suburban Hospital v. Kirson* illustrates the approach taken by the majority of courts.[12] Phyllis Kirson, an operating room nurse, broke her right femur on August 6, 1993, when she slipped and fell while on the job at Suburban Hospital. The injury required surgical repair, and on August 13, while still recuperating in the hospital, she fell again and reinjured the same leg. The second fall occurred because of the negligence of a hospital employee, and it led to many complications and four additional surgeries over a 15-month period.

For this string of injuries and lost wages, Kirson received total disability compensation from August of 1993 to May of 1995 and an additional 275 weeks' worth of permanent partial disability payments. The hospital was also ordered to pay all of her medical expenses.

Then, in July 1996, Kirson filed a negligence suit against the hospital, the employee who caused her second fall, and a few other individuals. The hospital raised the "exclusive remedy" defense, and Kirson countered with dual capacity. After reviewing the legal literature and cases from numerous other jurisdictions—including the *Guy* case from Ohio—the Maryland high court held that "dual capacity is not compatible with Maryland law."[13]

The court noted that it was "firmly established" in Maryland that worker's compensation applies not only to the initial workplace injury but also to any aggravation of that injury because of medical malpractice. Although the aggravation here was not the result of medical malpractice per se, it clearly resulted from the negligence of a hospital employee in causing the second fall while treating the first injury. The court disposed of Kirson's arguments as follows.

> In order for the subsequent injury to be compensable, it is necessary only to show that the injury directly resulted from improper treatment of the original compensable injury. . . . It is not necessary, as Kirson contends, to split causation hairs. . . .
>
> Fundamentally, Kirson's argument attacks the social contract on which workers' compensation is based. Suburban is obliged to pay compensation by way of disability benefits and medical expenses for the injuries sustained on August 6 and for the injuries resulting from malpractice in the treatment of the August 6 injuries. Having received compensation, Kirson wants the right to sue Suburban to recover damages which, hopefully from [her] standpoint, would exceed the amount of compensation paid. We hold, however, that, in exchange for the imposition of no fault limited liability for workplace accidents, Suburban bought peace from being considered as a third party when rendering hospital services to Kirson in fulfillment of its obligation [to provide medical care].[14]

This result, refusing to apply the dual capacity doctrine, puts Maryland in line with the majority of jurisdictions that have considered the argument. According to the *Kirson* opinion, Ohio and California are the only states in which dual capacity has "flourished," and since the *Guy* decision in 1978, even the Ohio court "has declined to apply dual capacity in other contexts."[15]

Scope of the Duty Arising from the Relationship

In the typical physician–patient relationship, the physician agrees to diagnose and treat the patient in accordance with the standards of acceptable medical practice and to continue to do so until the natural termination of the relationship. (The standards of practice and termination of the relationship are discussed later in this chapter.) For her part, the patient agrees to pay—or have her insurance pay—for the services rendered.

On the other hand, the patient does not contractually agree to follow the doctor's orders, and failure to do so may excuse the physician from liability for untoward results. Similarly, the physician does not contractually promise to cure the patient. However, in some cases, express promises made by the physician may be deemed a guarantee of a cure. If no cure results in such cases, the physician will be liable for breach of warranty. (This topic is discussed further later in this chapter.)

The physician may limit the scope of the contract to a designated geographic area or medical specialty. In *McNamara v. Emmons*, a woman sustained a bad cut and was treated by an associate of her physician.[16] The next morning the patient left for a vacation in a town 20 miles away. While there, she felt she needed further treatment and asked the physician to come to the town. He refused but gave her instructions and named a local physician whom she might call. The court held that in these circumstances the defendant physician was justified in limiting his practice to his own town. In other cases, the courts have decided that, at least when no emergency exists, the physician has no obligation to make house calls but instead may require the patient to come to the office for treatment.

Duties to Persons Other Than the Patient

In many states, the contractual relationship between the patient and the physician not only allows the physician to warn certain persons that a patient has an infectious disease but also obliges the physician to do so. For example, state law may require the healthcare provider to notify the sexual partners of persons infected with HIV or diagnosed with AIDS.

Similarly, a physician might be subject to liability when a patient injures a third party. In *Freese v. Lemmon*, a pedestrian was injured by an automobile when its driver suffered a seizure.[17] Both the driver and his physician were sued by the injured person—the physician on the theory that he was negligent in diagnosing an earlier seizure and in advising the driver that he could operate an automobile. The trial court dismissed the case against the physician, but the Supreme Court of Iowa reversed that outcome on the theory that an unreasonable risk of harm to a third party or a class of persons (i.e., other drivers) was foreseeable. The case was remanded for a trial on the merits of the evidence.

In the famous case *Tarasoff v. Regents of the University of California* (also discussed in chapter 9), the California Supreme Court ruled that despite a confidential relationship with patients, a doctor has a duty to use reasonable care to warn persons threatened by a patient's condition.[18] The patient had told his psychotherapist that he intended to kill Tarasoff, and he later made good on his threat. On these facts the court determined that the victim's parents had a valid cause of action for failure to warn.

Whether the injury to the third party is foreseeable is an important consideration in such cases. In *Brady v. Hopper*, a suit by persons injured in the assassination attempt on President Ronald Reagan in 1981, the court held that John Hinckley Jr.'s psychiatrist owed no duty to the plaintiffs because there was no evidence that Hinckley had made specific threats suggesting his intentions.[19]

Termination of the Relationship and Abandonment

Like all contracts, the one between the physician and the patient is terminated at certain points:

- When the patient is cured or dies
- When the physician and the patient mutually consent to termination

- When the patient dismisses the physician
- When the physician withdraws from the contract

Withdrawal by a physician before the patient is cured may prompt the patient to claim abandonment. Whether abandonment is a breach of contract, an intentional tort, or negligence has been a matter of some dispute, and there might be valid claims for all three, especially when the physician thought the patient had been cured and prematurely discharged her from the hospital.[20]

Abandonment may be express or implied. Express abandonment occurs when a physician notifies a patient that he is withdrawing from the case but fails to give the patient enough time to secure the services of another physician. In *Norton v. Hamilton*, the plaintiff reported that she had begun labor several weeks before her baby was due.[21] According to the plaintiff's allegations, the physician examined her and concluded that she was not in labor. When the pains continued, the plaintiff's husband called the physician twice to say that his wife was still in pain. At that point, the physician said he was withdrawing from the case. While the husband was looking for a substitute physician, the plaintiff delivered her child alone and suffered unnecessary pain and distress. The court held that the physician's acts would be abandonment, *if proven*. (The decision only concerned the legal principle that would apply; it was not a final judgment based on evidentiary findings.)

Sometimes abandonment is inferred from the circumstances, as in the 1963 Kentucky case *Johnson v. Vaughn*.[22] The facts involved "a 46-year-old colored man" who had suffered a gunshot wound to the neck in the wee hours of a Saturday morning. When the patient arrived at the hospital, a nurse phoned Dr. Vaughn, who arrived a short time later; admitted the patient; treated him somewhat (although the opinion is not clear on the extent of that treatment); and then went home, leaving word that he was to be called if the patient's condition grew worse. There is some testimony in the record that the doctor was under the influence of alcohol at the time.

Because the patient seemed dangerously injured, his son had a nurse call another doctor, Dr. Kissinger, who arrived and "gave such attention as appeared to be most urgent" but who felt he could not proceed further without a release from Dr. Vaughn. He called Dr. Vaughn, advising him that the patient was dying and needed immediate attention. At this news, Dr. Vaughn became "irate and vulgar," called Dr. Kissinger "a louse" for trying to steal his patient, and hung up. A call from the patient's son produced more verbal abuse. Finally, Dr. Vaughn said he would release the patient if he was paid $50 by nine o'clock the next morning. Meanwhile, 30 or 40 minutes had passed before Dr. Kissinger could operate, and the patient later died.

The court held that these facts were sufficient to state a claim of abandonment against Dr. Vaughn. The opinion states, in part, "It is a rule of general acceptance that a physician is under the duty to give his patient all necessary and continued attention as long as the case requires it, and that he should not leave his patient at a critical stage without giving reasonable notice or making suitable arrangements for the attendance of another physician, unless the relationship is terminated by dismissal or assent. Failure to observe that professional obligation is a culpable dereliction."[23]

As this quote from the *Johnson* case implies, physicians can raise various defenses to claims of abandonment. If the patient dismisses the physician or agrees to the latter's departure, or if the physician gives notice of withdrawal early enough for the patient to find another physician of equal ability, the claim will fail. Physicians have the right to limit their practice to a certain specialty or geographic area. A physician who is too ill to treat a patient or to find a substitute also has a valid defense to an abandonment claim. If a physician obtains a substitute physician, she has a valid defense so long as the substitute is qualified and the patient has enough time to find another if the substitute is unacceptable.

Two California cases exemplify purposeful termination of the doctor–patient relationship when a patient is uncooperative or disagreeable. In *Payton v. Weaver*, the patient was Payton, a 35-year-old indigent woman with end-stage renal disease and a history of drug and alcohol abuse. Her physician, Dr. Weaver, informed her that he would no longer continue to treat her because of her intensely uncooperative behavior, antisocial conduct, and refusal to follow instructions.[24] Payton tried without success to find alternative treatment and petitioned the court to compel the doctor to continue treating her. The parties agreed that the physician would continue if she met reasonable conditions of cooperation. When she did not keep her part of the bargain, Dr. Weaver again notified her that he was withdrawing, and she again sought a court order. This time, the trial court found that she had violated the previous conditions and in the process had adversely affected other dialysis patients. The court also found that there was no emergency requiring treatment under a California statute,[25] that the physician's notice was sufficient to end the relationship, and that the doctor was not responsible for the fact that no other dialysis unit would accept her (see Legal Decision Point). The appellate court sustained the trial court decision, and Payton died pending appeal.[26]

In another case, the court decided that a medical group and hospital must provide nonemergency care to a husband and wife. In *Leach v. Drummond Medical Group, Inc.*, the plaintiffs, who were regular patients of the group practice, had written to a state agency commenting adversely on the performance of the group's physicians.[27] The practice told the couple that, because they complained to the medical board, "a proper physician–patient relationship" could not be maintained and they would receive only 30 days

Legal Decision Point

End-stage renal disease (ESRD) is chronic kidney failure that has progressed to the point of requiring kidney dialysis or transplant. An ESRD patient needs to undergo dialysis every three or four days but lives a somewhat normal existence between treatments (subject to contributing conditions, such as high blood pressure and diabetes).

The *Payton* court stated that "there was no emergency" in Payton's case. Do you agree? Was she a patient with a chronic disease, or was she a patient who was bound to have serial emergencies? Instead of seeing Dr. Weaver as scheduled (which she did not), what if she had been taken to the emergency department every few days in extremis and in need of dialysis? If you were a hospital administrator, how would you advise the emergency department to deal with a patient such as Payton?

of care, after which they would be treated only for emergencies. The couple sued to compel continued treatment of their many health problems. (The practice was the only medical group available within 100 miles.) The trial court denied relief, but the appellate court reversed the decision and allowed the suit to continue. The court decided that although one physician may not be required to treat a patient she does not like, the group as a whole can be ordered to do so.[28] Because the patients had not publicly criticized the doctor but only discreetly contacted the appropriate state agency, the court held that denying services to them was not justified.

Some cases have extended the physician's duty to the patient even after the doctor–patient relationship has ended. In *Tresemer v. Barke*, the physician had implanted an intrauterine device (IUD) in the plaintiff in 1972.[29] The physician had seen the patient only on that one occasion. The plaintiff later suffered injury from the device (a Dalkon Shield) and filed suit against the physician. She alleged that he knew the risks of using the IUD but failed to warn her. The court held that the defendant had a duty to warn the plaintiff, noting that a physician is in the best position to alert a patient and that death or great bodily harm might be prevented as a result.[30]

Liability for Breach of Contract

In the typical physician–patient contract, the physician agrees (or implies agreement) to perform a service. Failure to perform the service with reasonable skill and care may give the patient a basis for filing a claim, not only for negligence but also for breach of contract. The previous paragraphs illustrate breach-of-contract cases based on abandonment; *Alexandridis v. Jewett* offers an example of a different kind of contractual breach.[31]

In *Alexandridis*, two obstetricians agreed that one of them would personally deliver the patient's second child. When the time came, however, the patient's labor progressed rapidly and the obstetrician whose night it was to take call could not arrive at the hospital in time. The baby was delivered by a first-year resident, who performed an episiotomy during the process and damaged the patient's anal sphincter as a result. Because the partners had contractually agreed to deliver the patient's child and were more skilled than the resident in training who delivered the child, the court found that the partners would be liable for breach of contract if their greater skill would have protected the patient from injury.

A physician who uses a procedure that is different from the one he promised to use may also be liable for breach of contract. In *Stewart v. Rudner*, the physician promised to arrange for an obstetrician to deliver a child by cesarean section.[32] The patient, a 37-year-old woman who had suffered two stillbirths, was extremely eager to have a "sound, healthy baby." While the patient was in labor, the physician told another obstetrician to "take care of this case" but did not tell him about the promise to perform a cesarean section. At the end of a lengthy labor, the baby was stillborn. The appellate court upheld a jury verdict for the patient on the ground that the physician breached his promise that a cesarean operation would be used to deliver the baby.

Liability for Breach of Warranty

Physicians are susceptible to liability not only if they promise but fail to perform a certain *service* but also especially if they promise that their treatment will yield a specific *result* but does not. A physician who guarantees a result gives the patient a contractual basis for a lawsuit if the treatment is not successful, even if it was performed skillfully. In *Sullivan v. O'Conner*, a professional entertainer thought her nose was too long.[33] She contracted with a physician to have cosmetic surgery. The physician promised that the surgery would "enhance her beauty and improve her appearance." The surgery was unsuccessful, however, and after two more operations the nose looked worse than before.

Physicians do not guarantee results simply by agreeing to perform an operation, and drawing the line between an opinion and a guarantee is often difficult. The jury decided in this case, however, that there was a guarantee, and the appellate court affirmed the jury's verdict for the plaintiff (see Legal Brief).

Guilmet v. Campbell is well known in health law circles. The plaintiff had a bleeding ulcer and talked with a surgeon about a possible operation. He testified that the surgeon said:

> Once you have an operation it takes care of all your troubles. You can eat as you want to, you can drink as you want to, you can go as you

Legal Brief

Sullivan v. O'Conner is a good example of the roles juries and appellate courts play in our legal system. The jury decides what the facts are, and the appellate court must accept those facts as true unless they are indisputably wrong.

In some respects, this rule is analogous to the instant replay rule in football. Unless the review clearly shows the decision was wrong, the call "on the field" stands.

tort
a civil offense not founded on contract; a failure to conduct oneself in a manner considered proper under the given circumstances

intentional tort
a category of torts that describes a civil wrong resulting from an intentional act on the part of the **tortfeasor**

tortfeasor
a wrongdoer; a person who commits a tort

negligence
failure to comply with established standards for the protection of others; departure from the conduct expected of a reasonably prudent person acting under the same or similar circumstances

strict liability
automatic responsibility (without having to prove negligence) for damages as a result of possession or use of inherently dangerous equipment, such as explosives, wild and poisonous animals, or assault weapons

please. Dr. Arena and I are specialists; there is nothing to it at all—it's a very simple operation. You'll be out of work three to four weeks at the most. There is no danger at all in this operation. After the operation you can throw away your pill box. In twenty years if you figure out what you spent for Maalox pills and doctor calls, you could buy an awful lot. Weigh [that cost] against an operation.[34]

With this assurance, the plaintiff underwent the operation, during which his esophagus ruptured. As a result, his weight dropped from 170 to 88 pounds, and he developed hepatitis and numerous other complications. He sued the physician on both a negligence theory and a warranty (guarantee) theory. The jury decided that the physicians were not negligent but had breached their promise to cure. The Michigan Supreme Court affirmed the decision. In response to *Guilmet*, and presumably after some heavy lobbying by the medical profession, the state legislature later passed a statute requiring that any alleged promise or guarantee of a cure will be void unless it is in writing and signed by the physician alleged to have made it.[35]

Intentional Torts

Another basis for professional liability is intentional tort. A **tort** (Latin for "wrong") is a civil wrong, not based on contract, that results in injury to another person or another person's property or reputation.[36] Torts are usually divided into three categories, each of which involves a different type of proof (see again exhibit 4.1):

- **Intentional tort**, as the name implies, is a wrongful, premeditated action that causes injury.
- **Negligence** is unintentional failure to do what a reasonably careful person would do under the circumstances.
- **Strict liability** is incurred when a person commits a wrongful act that poses high risk of harm to others, but did not do so intentionally or out of negligence.

As noted earlier, most malpractice cases are based on negligence. Strict liability is uncommon in healthcare administration, but it surfaces in relation to defective drugs and medical devices.

In healthcare, lawsuits based on intentional tort are less common than negligence cases, but they are important because they give plaintiffs some flexibility they would not have otherwise. There may also be multiple consequences for the healthcare provider who commits an intentional tort. Because intent is usually an essential element in proving both an intentional tort and a crime, many intentional torts, such as assault and battery, entail both criminal and civil liability. This point is significant because commission of a criminal act could result in revocation of one's license to practice.

Assault and Battery

"Assault and battery" is actually two intentional torts. An *assault* is conduct that places a person in apprehension of being touched in a way that is insulting, provoking, or physically harmful. *Battery* is the actual touching (see Legal Brief). Both assault and battery are acts done without legal authority or permission. A move to kiss someone without consent is an assault, and the act of kissing without consent is both assault and battery. If the person were asleep when kissed, the perpetrator would not be committing assault because the person was not apprehensive. He would, however, be committing battery. (Obviously, kissing someone with permission is neither assault nor battery but is normally an enjoyable experience.)

The question of consent to medical or surgical treatment is complex; chapter 11 features a detailed discussion of the topic. For present purposes, assault and battery cases can be grouped into three categories:

1. Those in which no consent for the touching was obtained
2. Those in which the physician exceeded the scope of the consent given
3. Those in which the consent was "uninformed"

First are the intentional acts committed by a healthcare provider with no patient consent whatsoever. In *Burton v. Leftwich*, for example, a physician who was having trouble removing sutures from the toe of a four-year-old child (whose parents were apparently not much help) smacked the tot's thigh several times with his open hand, leaving bruises that were visible for three weeks.[37] An appellate court upheld a jury verdict for the plaintiffs on the grounds that the physician had committed battery.

Compare that case with *Mattocks v. Bell*, in which a 23-month-old girl—whom a medical student was treating for a lacerated tongue—clamped her teeth on the student's finger and would not let go.[38] After a failed attempt to free his finger by forcing a tongue depressor into the child's mouth, the student slapped her on the cheek. The parents lost the battery suit. The force the student used was judged to be proper under the circumstances.

In the often-cited case *Schloendorff v. Society of New York Hospital* (discussed in more detail in chapter 11), a doctor was liable for battery after he operated on a patient who had consented only to an

Legal Brief

We accept the incidental touching that accompanies everyday life, but there are certain boundaries. For example, jostling others on a crowded subway train is not battery, but groping others is.

Battery is sometimes characterized by the aphorism, "Your right to swing your arm ends where my nose begins." (But the swing might be an assault if you see it coming.)

examination under anesthesia but not to an operation.[39] In another case, a patient signed a consent form to have his kidney stones removed by a certain urologist. After the surgery, the patient discovered that the operation had been performed not by the urologist he requested but by two other members of the urologist's medical group. He sued all three physicians for malpractice

informed consent
agreement to permit a medical procedure after disclosure of all relevant facts needed to make an intelligent decision

and failure to obtain **informed consent**. After the jury found for the defendants, the Supreme Court of New Jersey reversed the decision. It held that the plaintiff had claims for battery and malpractice and that even if no physical injury occurred, the defendants could be liable for mental anguish and perhaps even punitive damages.[40] The court stated: "Even more private than the decision who may touch one's body is the decision who may cut it open and invade it with hands and instruments. Absent an emergency, patients have the right to determine not only whether surgery is to be performed on them, but who shall perform it."[41]

The second and third categories of assault and battery cases will be discussed in more detail in chapter 11. For now it is sufficient to note that a case fitting either the second or third category can support a negligence theory in addition to the intentional tort of assault and battery. Negligence is the more common allegation, but liability on assault and battery is also possible.

Mohr v. Williams is illustrative of this point.[42] The plaintiff consented to an operation on her right ear. After she was anesthetized, the surgeon discovered that her left ear needed surgery more than the right one, so he operated on the left ear instead. On the ground, among others, that the surgeon's conduct amounted to assault and battery, the appellate court upheld a trial court's decision to let the case proceed.

Although the surgeon in *Mohr* should have consulted the patient before operating on the other ear and probably should have discussed that possibility before beginning the surgery, a surgeon may be justified in operating beyond the scope of the original consent when an emergency makes obtaining the patient's further consent impossible or dangerous. In *Barnett v. Bachrach*, a surgeon operating on a patient for an ectopic pregnancy (a pregnancy outside the uterus) discovered that the pregnancy was normal but that the patient had acute appendicitis.[43] He removed the appendix and later sued the patient for not paying the medical bill. The patient defended the collection suit by alleging that the appendix was removed without her consent. In holding for the surgeon, the court noted that if he had not taken out the appendix, both the patient and child might have been endangered.

These cases of extending the scope of surgery can be extremely complicated, and the outcome can depend on small factual differences. Generalizing about the proper course of action to take is difficult. For this reason, most hospital risk management departments have detailed surgical consent forms that anticipate all possible intraoperative complications and document the patient's permission for the medical team to make prudential judgments should those complications arise during the surgery.

Defamation

Defamation is wrongful injury to another person's reputation. Written defamation is *libel*, and oral defamation is *slander*.[44] To be actionable, the defamatory statement must be "published"—that is, the defendant must have made the statement to a third party, not just to the plaintiff. In *Shoemaker v. Friedberg*,[45] a physician wrote a letter to a patient, stating that she had a venereal disease. The patient showed the letter to two or three other women and later, in the presence of a friend, discussed the diagnosis with the physician. In suing him she alleged a breach of confidentiality, but the court held that no recovery should be allowed because the patient had published the diagnosis herself. (This result is an example of what could be called the "it's your own dumb fault" rule.)

Physicians have several defenses available to them in defamation suits:

- *The truth of a statement is an absolute defense.* Even a true statement, however, can lead to liability for invasion of privacy or breach of confidentiality. (See further discussion on this point later in the chapter and in the discussion of the Health Insurance Portability and Accountability Act [HIPAA] in chapter 9.)
- *Statements made in good faith to protect a private interest of the physician, the patient, or a third party are usually entitled to a qualified privilege.* An example is a false but good-faith report of a sexually transmitted disease diagnosis to a state health department, as required by law.
- *Some statements, such as those made during a judicial proceeding or by one physician to another in discussing a patient's treatment, are privileged and provide a defense.* In *Thornburg v. Long*, for example, a specialist advised a patient's family physician on the basis of an erroneous lab report that the patient had syphilis.[46] When the patient sued the specialist for libel, the court held that the statement was privileged because the specialist had a duty to communicate the information to the other physician and had done so with reasonable skill even though it turned out that the information was incorrect.

False Imprisonment

False imprisonment arises from unlawful restriction of a person's freedom. Many false imprisonment cases involve patients who have been involuntarily committed to a mental hospital. In *Stowers v. Wolodzko*, a psychiatrist was held liable for his treatment of a patient who had been forcibly committed against

defamation
the act of making untrue statements about another that damage the person's reputation

her will.[47] Although this type of commitment was allowed under state law, for many days the psychiatrist held the woman incommunicado and prevented her from calling an attorney or a relative. His actions amounted to false imprisonment because her freedom was unlawfully restrained. (The unusual facts of this case are laid out in The Court Decides at the end of this chapter.)

Invasion of Privacy and Breach of Confidentiality

Although truth is a defense in defamation cases, there are two other bases for possible liability: (1) invasion of privacy and (2) wrongful disclosure of confidential information. Invasion of privacy occurs when a patient is subjected to unwanted publicity. For example, in *Vassiliades v. Garfinckel's, Brooks Bros.*, the defendants (a physician and the famous department store) used "before" and "after" photographs of the plaintiff's cosmetic surgery without her permission. This action was sufficient to support a verdict for invasion of privacy and breach of **fiduciary** duty.[48] Similarly, a Michigan physician was held liable for invasion of privacy when he allowed a lay friend to observe the delivery of a baby in his patient's home. Clearly, a patient's expectation of privacy should be respected.

fiduciary
an individual or entity (e.g., a bank or a trust company) that has the power and duty to act for another (the beneficiary) under circumstances that require trust, good faith, and honesty

A suit for wrongful disclosure of confidential information was brought on behalf of a man who had been a patient at the Holyoke Geriatric and Convalescent Center.[49] His family had sought the court's permission to remove him from the kidney dialysis treatments that were sustaining his life. The court granted the petition, but several nurses and aides from the center, with the approval of the center's administrator, wrote a letter to a local newspaper protesting the decision. The letter appeared on the front page of the paper. A jury awarded the plaintiff's widow and estate $1 million for violation of a statute that prohibits release of personal information. The case clearly shows the danger of disclosing confidential patient information without proper authority, and it was decided in 1985—11 years before HIPAA brought further attention to the subject of privacy and stricter enforcement activity.

In many situations, state or federal law requires disclosure of confidential information. For example, confidential information from a patient's medical record may be disclosed for purposes of quality assurance and peer review activities and to state authorities in cases of suspected child abuse. Other reporting requirements include those relating to communicable disease, abortion, birth defect, injury or death resulting from use of a medical device, environmental illness and injury, injuries (such as knife or gunshot wounds) resulting from suspected criminal activities, and conditions (such as epilepsy) affecting one's ability to drive safely or operate heavy machinery.

Disclosures made in conformity with the law are not wrongful, and no liability will attach. Similarly, there is no liability for disclosing patient information when the patient (or the patient's guardian) has given permission or when a search warrant or other legal procedure requires it. Healthcare facilities must be aware of the federal and state requirements regarding confidentiality of medical records and must have policies and procedures in place to protect the information contained in them. (All of these requirements are discussed in more detail in chapter 9.)

Misrepresentation

Misrepresentation is another intentional tort for which physicians can be held liable. Misrepresentation is either intentional (fraudulent or deceitful) or negligent. Either way, the person claiming injury must show that a fact was falsely represented and that he based decisions on the misrepresentation. Misrepresentation cases involving physicians are of two types: (1) misrepresentation to persuade a patient to submit to treatment and (2) misrepresentation of a prior treatment or its results.

Physicians who misrepresent the nature or results of treatment they have given are liable for fraud even if the treatment was done carefully. In *Johnson v. McMurray*,[50] Dr. McMurray had performed surgery on Lavoid Johnson and had left a surgical sponge in his body. Johnson specifically asked that Dr. McMurray not participate in the follow-up surgery needed to remove the sponge, and he sought out Dr. Griffith to operate. Unknown to Johnson, Dr. Griffith intended to have Dr. McMurray assist in the surgery anyway, which he did. More complications arose, and the patient eventually lost his leg. The court decided that the two doctors had fraudulently concealed a significant fact and a jury could award damages.

Misrepresentation sometimes allows a patient to bring suit after the **statute of limitation** expires. In *Hundley v. Martinez*, the patient suffered vision problems for a number of months after cataract surgery. On numerous occasions he returned to his ophthalmologist for follow-up and was repeatedly assured that his "eye was all right, getting along fine."[51] Eventually, the patient (an attorney) became virtually blind in the affected eye. More than two years later, he consulted another ophthalmologist about cataract formation in the other eye. Only then did he learn that the first eye had been permanently damaged by the earlier surgery. The court held that the two-year limitation period should be disregarded if the jury found that the physician had obstructed the plaintiff's case by fraud or in other ways. Accordingly, a new trial was ordered.

statute of limitation
a law setting the maximum period one can wait before filing a lawsuit, depending on the type of case or claim

Outrage

The tort of outrage—sometimes called "intentional infliction of emotional distress"—arises from extreme and offensive conduct by the defendant. *Rockhill v. Pollard* is a graphic example of a case involving outrage.[52] The plaintiff, her mother-in-law, and her ten-month-old daughter were injured in an automobile accident on a wintry evening in Oregon shortly before Christmas; the accident knocked the baby unconscious. A passing motorist picked them up and arranged for a physician to meet them at the doctor's office. Here is a portion of the court's opinion describing the encounter with the defendant, Dr. Pollard:

> Both plaintiff and [her mother-in-law] Christine Rockhill testified that defendant was rude to them from the moment they met him. Plaintiff testified:
>
> "And the first thing, he looked at us, and he had a real mean look on his face, and this is what he said. He said, 'My God, women, what are you doing out on a night like this?' . . . and my mother-in-law tried to explain to him why we were on the road, and her and I both pleaded to him."
>
> Without making any examination, defendant told them there was nothing wrong with any of them. [The baby] was still unconscious at this time. According to plaintiff:
>
> "She was very lifeless. I was saying her name, and she wouldn't respond at all. Her eyelids were a light blue. She was clammy, very cold.
>
> "In fact, I thought she was dead at the time."[53]

After repeated requests to do so, the doctor finally gave the child a cursory examination and said there was nothing wrong with her. The baby had vomited, and both the adults had blood and vomit on them. The opinion states that the doctor told the mother-in-law, "Get in there and clean yourself up. You are a mess." The opinion continues, quoting from the transcript:

> "The doctor was out of the room, and I told her [Christine Rockhill, the mother-in-law], I says, 'We have got to get help for this baby,' and she said, 'Well, what are we going to do?'
>
> "And the doctor came back in the room, and she asked the doctor, she says, 'What are we going to do?' And he just shrugged his shoulders and said he didn't know."
>
> When Christine Rockhill suggested that her brother would pick them up at defendant's office, defendant said, "My God, woman, I can't stay here until somebody comes and gets you." Although the temperature was below freezing and [the baby's] clothing and blanket were wet with vomit, he told them to wait outside by a nearby street light while someone came . . . to get them.

After a 20-minute wait in the cold, the group was taken to a hospital. By the time they arrived, the baby was apparently semiconscious and suffering from shock. The women were given emergency treatment and released. The child had surgery to repair a depressed skull fracture and was released after a week in the hospital.

The trial court had dismissed the lawsuit, thinking that the plaintiff had not presented a **prima facie** case (enough evidence to win unless the defendant presents contradictory evidence). The Supreme Court of Oregon disagreed, stating, "We think the issue should have been submitted to the jury."[54]

It is not hard to see why a jury could find that the defendant's conduct was "outrageous" and thus an intentional tort.

prima facie
containing enough evidence to win unless the defendant presents contradictory evidence

Violation of Civil Rights

For 50 years now, courts have recognized causes of action for violations of patients' civil rights. Violation of federal civil rights statutes—such as committing discrimination on the basis of race, religion, ethnicity, and other protected categories—is an obvious example.[55] Less apparent discrimination is shown in *Widgeon v. Eastern Shore Hospital Center*.[56] In this unusual case, the plaintiff was involuntarily committed to a Maryland hospital after an **ex parte hearing** (one in which only one party is present), in which the plaintiff's wife testified that he had exhibited abnormal and violent behavior.

ex parte hearing
a hearing in which only one party is present

Two physicians examined the plaintiff on his arrival at the hospital, and although he showed no outward signs of mental illness, the doctors ordered that he be held at the hospital. The plaintiff maintained that his wife lied about his behavior because she wanted to be free to join her male friend in Florida. As soon as she met up with her "friend," the hospital released the plaintiff. He promptly sued his wife, the physicians, and the hospital for violation of federal and state civil rights statutes, negligence, false imprisonment, false arrest, defamation, intentional infliction of emotional distress, and conspiracy to commit these wrongs. The court held that the complaint stated a valid cause of action under federal law and the Maryland Declaration of Rights: "That no man ought to be taken or imprisoned or disseized of his freehold, liberties or privileges, or outlawed, or exiled, or, in any manner, destroyed, or deprived of his life, liberty or property, but by the judgment of his peers, or by the Law of the land."[57]

Summary

This chapter addresses the essential elements of a valid contract (competent parties, a "meeting of the minds," consideration, legality of purpose) and the importance of contracts law in the relationships between patients and their physicians and between patients and hospitals. The chapter also briefly discusses issues relating to workers' compensation and intentional tort, pointing out that both can affect doctor–patient and hospital–patient relationships.

Discussion Questions

1. In *Oliver v. Brock*, what factors did the court consider most significant in determining whether Dr. Brock had a contractual relationship with Oliver?

2. Why are workers' compensation benefits the sole remedies for workplace injuries of employees, as discussed in *Guy v. Arthur H. Thomas Co.* and *Suburban Hospital v. Kirson*? What is the "social contract" referred to in the latter opinion?

3. Explain why a case alleging a breach of contract, such as *Guilmet v. Campbell*, might be easier to prove than a standard case alleging negligence.

4. In what ways can intentional torts occur in the healthcare field?

The Court Decides

Stowers v. Wolodzko
386 Mich. 119, 191 N.W.2d 355 (1971)

Swainson, J.

[In court opinions a jurist's position is often given by the addition of "J" or "CJ" behind the name. The initials stand for Judge *or* Justice, *or* Chief Judge *or* Chief Justice, *depending on the title of the position in the particular jurisdiction. Members of the Michigan Supreme Court are known as* justices, *thus the* Stowers *decision was written by Justice Swainson.]*

This case presents complicated issues concerning the liability of a doctor for actions taken subsequent to a person's confinement in a private mental hospital pursuant to a valid court order. . . .

Plaintiff, a housewife, resided in Livonia, Michigan, with her husband and children. She and her husband had been experiencing a great deal of marital difficulties and she testified that she had informed her husband . . . that she intended to file for a divorce.

On December 6, 1963, defendant appeared at plaintiff's home and introduced himself as "Dr. Wolodzko." Dr. Wolodzko had never met either plaintiff or her husband before he came to the house. He stated that he had been called by the husband, who had asked him to examine plaintiff. Plaintiff testified that defendant told her that he was there to ask about her husband's back. She testified that she told him to ask her husband, and that she had no further conversation with him or her husband. She testified that he never told her that he was a psychiatrist.

Dr. Wolodzko stated in his deposition . . . that he told plaintiff he was there to examine her. However, upon being questioned upon this point, he stated that he

could "not specifically" recollect having told plaintiff that he was there to examine her. He stated in his deposition that he was sure that the fact he was a psychiatrist would have come out, but that he couldn't remember if he had told plaintiff that he was a psychiatrist.

Plaintiff subsequently spoke to Dr. Wolodzko at the suggestion of a Livonia policewoman, following a domestic quarrel with her husband. He did inform her at that time that he was a psychiatrist.

On December 30, 1963, defendant Wolodzko and Dr. Anthony Smyk, apparently at the request of plaintiff's husband and without the authorization, knowledge, or consent of plaintiff, signed a sworn statement certifying that they had examined plaintiff and found her to be mentally ill. Such certificate was filed with the Wayne County Probate Court on January 3, 1964, and on the same date an order was entered by the probate court for the temporary hospitalization of plaintiff until a sanity hearing could be held. The Judge ordered plaintiff committed to Ardmore Acres, a privately operated institution, pursuant to the provisions of [Michigan law].

Plaintiff was transported to Ardmore Acres on January 4, 1964. . . .

. . .

The parties are in substantial agreement as to what occurred at Ardmore Acres. Defendant requested permission to treat the plaintiff on several different occasions, and she refused. For six days, she was placed in the "security room," which was a bare room except for the bed. The windows of the room were covered with wire mesh. During five of

(continued)

(continued from previous page)

the six days, plaintiff refused to eat, and at all times refused medication. Defendant telephoned orders to the hospital and prescribed certain medication. He visited her often during her stay.

When plaintiff arrived at the hospital she was refused permission to receive or place telephone calls, or to receive or write letters. Dr. Wolodzko conceded at the trial that plaintiff wished to contact her brother in Texas by telephone and that he forbade her to do so. After nine days, she was allowed to call her family, but no one else. Plaintiff testified on direct examination that once during her hospitalization she asked one of her children to call her relatives in Texas and that defendant took her to her room and told her, "Mrs. Stowers, don't try that again. If you do, you will never see your children again." It is undisputed that plaintiff repeatedly requested permission to call an attorney and that Dr. Wolodzko refused such permission.

At one point when plaintiff refused medication, on the written orders of defendant, she was held by three nurses and an attendant and was forcibly injected with the medication. Hospital personnel testified at the trial that the orders concerning medication and deprivation of communication were pursuant to defendant's instructions.

Plaintiff, by chance, found an unlocked telephone near the end of her hospitalization and made a call to her relatives in Texas. She was released by court order on January 27, 1964.

Plaintiff filed suit alleging false imprisonment, assault and battery, and malpractice, against defendant Wolodzko, Anthony Smyk and Ardmore Acres. Defendants Ardmore Acres and Smyk were dismissed prior to trial. At the close of plaintiff s proofs, defendant moved for a directed verdict. The court granted the motion as to the count of malpractice only, but allowed the counts of assault and battery and false imprisonment to go to the jury. At the Conclusion of the trial, the jury returned a verdict for plaintiff in the sum of $40,000. . . .

Defendant has raised five issues on appeal. . . .

. . .

The second issue involves whether or not there was evidence from which a jury could find false imprisonment.

"False imprisonment is the unlawful restraint of an individual's personal liberty or freedom of locomotion." [Citation omitted.] It is clear that plaintiff was restrained against her will. Defendant, however, contends that because the detention was pursuant to court order (and hence not unlawful), there can be no liability for false imprisonment. However, defendant was not found liable for admitting or keeping plaintiff in Ardmore Acres. His liability stems from the fact that after plaintiff was taken to Ardmore Acres, defendant held her incommunicado and prevented her from attempting to obtain her release, pursuant to law. Holding a person incommunicado is clearly a restraint of one's freedom, sufficient to allow a jury to find false imprisonment.

Defendant contends that it was proper for him to restrict plaintiff's communication with the outside world. Defendant's witness, Dr. Sidney Bolter, testified that orders restricting communications and visitors are customary in cases of this type. Hence, defendant contends these orders were lawful and could not constitute the basis for an action of false imprisonment. However, the testimony of Dr. Bolter is not conclusive on this point.

. . . Psychiatrists have a great deal of power over their patients. In the case of a person confined to an institution, this power is virtually unlimited. All professions (including the legal profession) contain unscrupulous individuals who use their position to injure others. The law must provide protection against the torts committed by these individuals. In the case of mental patients, in order to have this protection, they must be able to communicate with the outside world.

In our country, even a person who has committed the most abominable crime has the right to consult with an attorney.

Our Court and the courts of our sister States have recognized that interference with attempts of persons incarcerated to obtain their freedom may constitute false imprisonment. Further, we have jealously protected the individual's rights by providing that a circuit Judge "who willfully or corruptly refuses or neglects to consider an application, action, or motion for, habeas corpus is guilty of malfeasance in office." [Citation omitted.]

... [P]laintiff was ... attempting to communicate with a lawyer or relative in order to obtain her release. Defendant prevented her from doing so. We ... hold that the actions on the part of defendant constitute false imprisonment. . . .

A person temporarily committed to an institution pursuant to statute certainly must have the right to make telephone calls to an attorney or relatives. We realize that it may be necessary to restrict visits to a patient confined to a mental institution. However, the same does not apply to the right of a patient to call an attorney or relative for aid in obtaining his release. This does not mean that an individual has an unlimited right to make numerous telephone calls, once he is confined pursuant to statute. Rather, it does mean that such an individual does have a right to communicate with an attorney and/or a relative in attempt to obtain his release.

Dr. Bolter was unable to give any valid reason why a person should not be allowed to consult with an attorney. We do not believe there is such a reason. While problems may be caused in a few cases because of this requirement, the facts in the instant case provide cogent reasons as to why such a rule is necessary. Mrs. Stowers was able to obtain her release after she made the telephone call to her relatives and they, in turn, obtained an attorney for her. Prior to this, because of the order of no communications, she was virtually held a prisoner with no chance of redress. We, therefore, agree with the Court of Appeals that there was sufficient evidence from which a jury could find that Dr. Wolodzko had committed false imprisonment. The Court of Appeals is affirmed. ■

Discussion Questions

1. Note that this case was decided in 1971 on facts that occurred in the early 1960s. The case may remind readers of the classic movie *One Flew Over the Cuckoo's Nest*. At the time, laws addressing involuntary psychiatric commitment were not common or were nonexistent in some jurisdictions. Research your state's standards for involuntary commitment and determine how these cases would be handled today.
2. What other information would you like to have to fully consider this case?
3. According to the opinion, Stowers was committed on the strength of the statement of two physicians that she was "mentally ill." What additional evidence would be sufficient today to have someone committed involuntarily? What would the evidence have to prove? Why?
4. What are the procedural steps to follow under the commitment laws of your state?

Notes

1. Some physicians and hospitals believe they have full professional liability coverage under their malpractice insurance policies, but in fact they are covered only for negligent acts. For example, in *Security Ins. Group v. Wilkinson*, 297 So. 2d 113 (Fla. App. 1974), the court held that a hospital's professional liability policy did not cover a breach of contract to treat the plaintiff's wife.

2. Courts can and often do find legal duties where none existed previously. In *Tarasoff v. Regents of the Univ. of Cal.*, 17 Cal. 3d 425, 131 Cal. Rptr. 14, 551 P.2d 334 (1976), the court found that a psychiatrist had a duty to warn the person whom the patient had threatened to kill, even though there was no relationship between the doctor and the threatened person and in spite of the fact that doctor–patient communications are normally confidential. This case is discussed further in chapter 9.

3. For example, in *Hurley v. Eddingfield*, 156 Ind. 416, 59 N.E. 1058 (1901), the only physician available to aid a critically ill person refused to assist, for no apparent reason. The court stated that, unless some special contract or other commitment exists, physicians have no legal duty to treat people. Vermont and Minnesota have statutes that require a bystander to render aid in an emergency and provide a measure of immunity for doing so. *See* Vt. Stat. Ann. Tit. 12, § 519 (1968) *and* Minn. Stat. Ann. § 604A.01 (2010).

4. 440 S.W.2d 104 (Tex. Civ. App. 1969). This case is discussed in greater detail in chapter 10.

5. 342 So. 2d 1 (Ala. 1976).

6. *Id.* at 5.

7. Am. Jur. 2d, *Physicians, Surgeons, and Other Healers*, § 96 (2012).

8. Angela R. Holder, Medical Malpractice Law at 6 (2nd ed. 1978).

9. 483 F. Supp. 581 (1980).

10. *See, e.g.*, Young v. St. Elizabeth Hosp., 131 Ill. App. 3d 193, 475 N.E.2d 603 (1985) (the plaintiff alleged negligent treatment of injuries sustained on the job; suit dismissed); McAlister v. Methodist Hosp. of Memphis, 550 S.W.2d 240 (Tenn. Sup. Ct. 1977) (a hospital employee alleged negligent treatment of work-related back injury).

11. Guy v. Arthur H. Thomas Co., 55 Ohio St. 2d 183 at 190, 378 N.E.2d 488 at __ (1978).

12. 362 Md. 140, 763 A.2d 185 (2000).

13. 763 A.2d at 202.

14. *Id.* at 195–96.

15. *Id.* at 198.

16. 36 Cal. App. 2d 199, 97 P.2d 503 (1939).

17. 210 N.W.2d 576 (Iowa 1973). *See also* Kaiser v. Suburban Transp. Sys., 65 Wash. 2d 461, 398 P.2d 14 (1965), *amended by* 65 Wash. 2d 461, 401 P.2d 350 (1965) (passengers on a patient bus were allowed to recover damages from the defendant physician); Duvall v. Goldin, 139 Mich. App. 342, 362 N.W.2d 275 (1984) (physician owed a duty to third persons injured in an auto accident after the physician failed to warn his patient not to operate a motor vehicle).

18. *Supra* note 2. *See also* Davis v. Lhim, 124 Mich. App. 291, 335 N.W.2d 481 (1983) (a psychiatrist was held liable for discharging a patient who subsequently killed his mother and for failing to warn the patient's mother). *But see* Soto v. Frankford Hosp., 478 F. Supp. 1134 (E.D. Pa. 1979).

19. 751 F.2d 329 (10th Cir. 1984).

20. David W. Louisell & Harold Williams, Medical Malpractice § 8.08 at 219 (1973).

21. 92 Ga. App. 727, 89 S.E.2d 809 (1955).

22. 370 S.W.2d 591 (Ky. 1963).

23. *Id.* at 596.

24. 131 Cal. App. 3d 38, 182 Cal Rptr. 225 (1982).

25. Cal. Health & Safety Code § 1317 (West 1979).

26. *See* Sallie T. Sanford, *What Scribner Wrought: How the Invention of Modern Dialysis Shaped Health Law and Policy*, 13 Rich. J. L. & Pub. Int. 337 (2010). A 2009 case involving Grady Memorial Hospital in Atlanta raises a larger issue in the context of undocumented immigrants with ESRD who are not eligible for Medicare or Medicaid and whose clinic at Grady had closed. *See* Kevin Sack, *Hospital Falters as Refuge for Illegal Immigrants* (published November 21, 2009), at http://www.nytimes.com/2009/11/21/health/policy/21grady.html.

27. 144 Cal. App. 3d 362, 192 Cal. Rptr. 650 (1983).

28. Cal. Civ. Code § 51.

29. 86 Cal. App. 3d 656, 150 Cal. Rptr. 384 (1978).

30. *Id.* at 672, 150 Cal. Rptr. at 394.

31. 388 F.2d 829 (1st Cir. 1968).

32. 349 Mich. 459, 84 N.W.2d 816 (1957).

33. 363 Mass. 579, 296 N.E.2d 183 (1973).

34. 385 Mich. 57, 68, 188 N.W.2d 601, 606 (1971).

35. Mich. Comp. Laws Ann. § 566.132(1)(g) (2009).

36. For the subject of torts generally, *see* Restatement (Second) Of Torts. For intentional torts specifically, *see* Restatement §§ 13–62.

37. 123 So. 2d 766 (La. Ct. App. 1960).

38. 194 A.2d 307 (D.C. Ct. App. 1963).

39. 211 N.Y. 125, 105 N.E. 92 (1914).

40. Perna v. Pirozzi, 92 N.J. 446, 438, 457, A.2d 431, 461 (1983). Against the urologist, the plaintiff had a cause of action for breach of contract, breach of fiduciary duty, and malpractice.

41. *Id.* at 461, 457 A.2d at 439.

42. 95 Minn. 261, 104 N.W. 12 (1905).

43. 34 A.2d 626 (D.C. Mun. Ct. App. 1943).

44. *See generally* 53 C.J.S., Libel & Slander §§ 1–9.

45. 80 Cal. App. 2d 911, 916, 183 P.2d 318, 322 (1947).

46. 178 N.C. 589, 101 S.E. 99 (1919).

47. 386 Mich. 119, 191 N.W.2d 355 (1971). The court also held the psychiatrist liable for assault and battery for giving the patient involuntary medication beyond what was permitted by the statute.

48. 492 A.2d 580 (D.C. App. 1985). The department store was not liable because it had obtained assurances from the physician that the plaintiff had given her consent.

49. Spring v. Geriatric Authority of Holyoke, 394 Mass. 274, 475 N.E.2d 727 (1985).

50. 461 So. 2d 775 (Ala. 1984).

51. 151 W. Va. 977, 158 S.E.2d 159 (1967).

52. 259 Or. 54, 485 P.2d 28 (1971).

53. 259 Or. at 55, 485 P.2d at 29.

54. *Id.*

55. *See, e.g.*, Washington v. Blampin, 226 Cal. App. 2d 604, 38 Cal. Rptr. 235 (1964).

56. 479 A.2d 921 (Md. 1984).

57. Md. Declaration Of Rights, Art. 24.

NEGLIGENCE

After reading this chapter, you will

- understand that four essential elements must be proven for a plaintiff to prevail in a negligence case;
- know that the standard of care (the duty) can be proven by expert testimony, published principles, or the jury's common experience of what is reasonable;
- grasp that the plaintiff's injuries must be caused by the defendant's breach of the duty; and
- see why, under the concept of vicarious liability, one can be liable for the actions of someone else.

As mentioned in chapter 4, a *tort* is a civil wrong not based on contract. The most common type of tort case involves *negligence*, the unintentional failure to live up to accepted standards of behavior. Four elements are essential to a case alleging a negligent tort: (1) the duty of care, (2) breach of that duty, (3) injury, and (4) causation.

> *Even a dog distinguishes between being stumbled over and being kicked.*
>
> —Oliver Wendell Holmes Jr.[87]

Duty

Duty refers to a legal obligation the defendant (the alleged tortfeasor) owes to the plaintiff. Although in some cases there are very precise standards by which to determine duty, most commonly it is expressed as a general obligation to act with *due care*—in other words, to conduct oneself as a reasonably prudent person would in similar circumstances. A breach of duty imposes liability if it results in injury to property or another person.

standard of care the caution and prudence that a reasonable person would exercise under the circumstances or that are required by appropriate authority for such situations

The most common negligent tort is a motor vehicle accident. The duty—the **standard of care**—in such cases may be relatively easy to prove by relying on such measures as

- traffic laws (e.g., speed limits, traffic lights);
- the driver's physical or mental condition (e.g., intoxication, physical impairment); and
- common sense about what an average, reasonable driver would have done.

Common sense or due care is often called the *reasonable man* or *reasonably prudent person* standard, and it suffices in many tort cases. But the most common negligent tort in healthcare—medical malpractice—usually cannot be judged on the basis of such simple criteria. Because most jurors are not competent to judge whether a healthcare provider has acted reasonably, the courts have adapted the reasonably prudent person standard for medical malpractice cases so that a **physician** is measured against other physicians, not against the average person.

One case stated the rule as follows: "A physician is bound to bestow such reasonable and ordinary care, skill and diligence as physicians and surgeons in good standing in the same neighborhood, in the same general line of practice, ordinarily have and exercise in like cases."[1] Courts generally agree with this concept, but like all legal standards, it is subject to interpretation when applied to specific facts. Interpretation is usually required when determining four aspects of duty in malpractice cases:

1. Who is a "reasonable" physician?
2. What "neighborhood" should be considered?
3. What school of medicine ("school rule") do other physicians follow?
4. Are the profession's standards adequate?

These questions are considered in the following paragraphs. Expert witnesses, whose role will be discussed in more detail later in the chapter, are used to help the jury answer these questions and to opine about whether the defendant has met the duty that has thus been established—that is, whether the physician has met the standard of care.

physician
for purposes of federal healthcare programs (42 U.S.C. § 1395x(r)), doctors of medicine (MD), doctors of osteopathy (DO), doctors of dental surgery or dental medicine (DDS or DMD), doctors of podiatric medicine (DPM), doctors of optometry (OD), and chiropractors (DC)

The Reasonable Physician

In general terms, physicians are required to provide only "reasonable and ordinary" treatment. Their actions are not typically judged against those of their most knowledgeable and highly skilled colleagues but against the knowledge and skill of average physicians in the same line of practice.

For example, if various methods of treatment for a patient's condition are available, a physician's treatment would not be considered malpractice if he chose an option that seemed to best meet the patient's needs, even though other physicians might have opted for a different course of treatment. Thus, the courts usually hold that the physician is not liable if the chosen treatment would be recognized by a "respectable minority" of the medical profession, even if most physicians would have adopted another treatment plan.[2]

In one case, a surgeon damaged the patient's laryngeal nerves while performing a thyroidectomy.[3] In her subsequent lawsuit the patient did not claim that the physician was reckless; rather, she claimed that the medical community recognized two possible surgical procedures for her condition and that the defendant should have chosen the other one. The court rejected this argument because the evidence showed that the two methods were equally acceptable, the risk of nerve damage was roughly the same with each procedure, and the choice of method was a matter of the physician's professional judgment.

A more difficult problem arises when the physician treats the patient by a method that even a respectable minority would deem unacceptable because it verges on experimentation. However, physicians are clearly right to use innovative techniques when standard methods have failed and the condition is serious. In one case, a surgeon performed an unorthodox operation on an ankle after trying standard techniques and when other physicians had advised amputation.[4] The court held that the operation was justified as a last resort. But a doctor who follows an experimental procedure before attempting standard methods is likely to be considered negligent. In one instance, a physician treating an infant for a curvature of the spine used a surgical procedure he had developed but no one else had used. The child died after suffering a severe hemorrhage. In the lawsuit that followed, the court found both the doctor and the hospital liable for not disclosing to the child's parents that the procedure was unorthodox.[5]

The Neighborhood: Local, State, or National

The second aspect of duty compares the treatment in question with that used by physicians and surgeons "in the same neighborhood." Originally, the *neighborhood* was considered to be the town or small region in which the physician practiced and similar areas elsewhere in the state or the nation. This principle is called the *locality rule* because it measures the standard of care in a given instance solely by the practices of other physicians in the same or a similar locality.

The traditional locality rule was based on the theory that doctors in remote areas should not be held to the same standards of medical expertise as doctors in urban areas because of difficulties of communication and travel and because they had limited opportunities to keep abreast of medical advances. It also relied on the fact that in such areas, physicians were often forced to practice in inadequate hospital facilities.[6] In most states, the traditional locality rule has given way to a broader standard because the original reasons for the rule have all but disappeared.[7] As one court stated:

> Locality rules have always had the practical difficulties of: (1) a scarcity of profes-
> sional people . . . qualified [or willing] to testify; and (2) treating as acceptable a
> negligent standard of care created by a small and closed community of physicians
> in a narrow geographical region. Distinctions in the degree of care and skill to be
> exercised by physicians in the treatment of patients based upon geography can no
> longer be justified in light of the presently existing state of transportation, com-
> munications, and medical education and training which results in a standardiza-
> tion of care within the medical profession. There is no tenable policy reason why
> a physician should not be required to keep abreast of the advancements in his
> profession.[8]

For these reasons, the court in that case held that "the language 'same
neighborhood' . . . refer[s] to the national medical neighborhood or national
medical community, of reasonably competent physicians acting in the same
or similar circumstances."[9]

This newer, broader standard is all the more reasonable given national
accreditation standards for medical education, national certification for medical board specialties, and advances in communications technology, including
the Internet. Today, a majority of jurisdictions employ the "national standard" in malpractice cases.[10]

For physicians who practice under conditions that are less than ideal,
the burden of meeting a national standard is alleviated somewhat by permitting "justifiable circumstances" as a defense.[11] For example, a physician
would not be responsible for providing a higher level of care if the necessary
facilities or resources for that care are not available. The test is what is reasonable under the circumstances. All surrounding circumstances are to be considered in determining whether there was a breach of the standard of care.

The School Rule

The third consideration is whether the care is comparable to that of physicians
and surgeons "in the same general line of practice." This principle, sometimes
called the **school rule**, is a throwback to the days when the schools of treatment were strictly divided. For example, traditional Western medicine as
practiced by MDs—the *allopathic school*—treats disease by using agents, such
as antibiotics, that oppose the patient's symptoms. The *homeopathic school*
posits that to cure a patient's symptoms, the doctor should give medicine that
would cause in healthy people the same set of symptoms the patient exhibits.
Practitioners of *osteopathic* medicine and *chiropractic* medicine, at least in
the "pure" form of their art, emphasize manipulative techniques to correct
bodily anomalies thought to cause disease and inhibit recovery.

Although still recognized, the distinctions among these schools have
blurred, leaving what is sometimes called the "regular practice of medicine."

school rule
the principle
that healthcare
practitioners are
judged by the
standards of their
own branch of
medicine

For example, for many years osteopathy was not considered regular medicine in some states, and osteopaths were not allowed to prescribe drugs or perform surgery; they were judged only by the standards prevailing in their own discipline.[12] Today, however, all states allow osteopaths to perform surgery and prescribe drugs,

> **Legal Brief**
>
> The school rule becomes significant in cases involving complementary and alternative medicine. See further discussion on this topic in chapter 8.

and they are regarded as part of the regular practice of medicine. The school rule remains important, however, because a few branches of medicine remain and the trend is toward specialization.

Alternative remedies (see Legal Brief), such as acupuncture, herbal medicine, faith healing, naturopathy, massage, and music and aroma therapies, claim numerous adherents. These techniques are known to improve psychological and physical well-being, and their practitioners, who usually do not have medical degrees, generally apply them without promising or implying that they are practicing medicine. Therefore, they are not judged by the standards of medical practice. However, if they stray from their area of expertise, they may be judged against the standards taught in traditional medical schools and may be accused of practicing medicine without a license.

Similarly, practitioners may be considered proficient only in their discipline. For example, in a case in Hawaii, a physician who often employed alternative medicine in his general practice was deemed unqualified to testify as an expert witness on the cause of his patient's symptoms following breast implantation by a general surgeon. The court noted:

> Dr. Arrington does not possess any education, training, or experience with silicone. He is a general practitioner with an orientation toward holistic medicine and alternative therapies, such as nutritional, vitamin, and herbal remedies. He is not a pathologist, general surgeon, plastic surgeon, or an immunologist. Prior to moving to Hawaii, Dr. Arrington practiced with chiropractic, naturopathic, and holistic medicine specialists. Nothing in Dr. Arrington's background or experience suggested that he would be competent to testify regarding the effects of silicone on the human body.[13]

In applying the school rule, courts must decide whether the school is legitimate. Legitimacy generally depends on whether rules and principles of practice have been set up to guide the school's members in treating patients. When standard of care is in question, the existence of licensing requirements will usually suffice as recognition of a separate school.[14] In one early case, the court did not recognize a spiritualist's practice as following a school of treatment because the practitioner's only principle was to diagnose and treat the disease by means of a trance. Because there was no legitimate school, the practitioner was held to the standards of mainstream medical practice.[15] In the case of a Christian Science practitioner, however, the court held the defendant to the standard of care, skill, and knowledge of ordinary Christian Science healers because he belonged to a recognized school.[16]

The school rule standards also hold nonphysician practitioners responsible for knowing which diagnoses are in their area of practice and which cases should be referred to a licensed physician for standard treatment. For example, in *Mostrom v. Pettibon*, a chiropractor was held liable for not identifying medical problems for which chiropractic treatment was not appropriate.[17]

Even allopathic physicians can be held responsible for failing to refer a case to a specialist if the problem is beyond their training and experience. For example, a general practitioner was held liable for negligence when a patient died of a hemorrhage after coughing up blood for two days. The court found that the physician should have grasped the seriousness of the patient's condition and called in a thoracic surgeon, who might have saved the patient's life.[18]

Assuming that a general practitioner remains in her area of expertise and does not fail to refer a patient to a specialist when required, most courts hold the physician to the standards of other general practitioners and not to the standards of specialists.[19] Physicians who present themselves as specialists, however, are held to a higher standard of care than that to which general practitioners are held.[20]

Practitioners who are licensed, trained, or credentialed only in certain fields of medicine are held to higher standards of care if they go beyond their ken. This situation has arisen not only with licensed practitioners such as chiropractors and podiatrists but also with nurses, medical students, and other clinical personnel. In *Thompson v. Brent*, a medical assistant working in an orthopedist's office was held to the standard of care required of physicians when using a Stryker saw to remove a cast.[21]

The Substandard Profession: Helling and Mammograms

A final aspect of duty concerns the profession itself. Physicians are usually judged by what other physicians would do under the circumstances; however, courts sometimes find the profession's own standard inadequate. In so doing, they have found negligence "as a matter of law" from the facts of the case.

In *Favalora v. Aetna Casualty & Surety Co.*, a 71-year-old patient fell while being x-rayed. She suffered numerous injuries, including a fractured femur.[22] The patient's subsequent prolonged hospitalization brought on a pulmonary embolism and a kidney infection. In bringing suit, the patient claimed that the fall would not have occurred if her radiologist had examined her medical records, which documented her history of sudden fainting spells. It was not the practice of radiologists to review a patient's medical history; their role was merely to take and interpret "pictures." When the judge explained the legal standard to the jury in this way, they returned a verdict for the defendant. The appellate court reversed the decision, however, believing that the accepted practices of the radiology profession were inadequate. In reaching this decision, the court looked to the custom of teaching hospitals, which did require radiologists to examine patients' histories.

Favalora received little attention, perhaps because the case was decided in Louisiana, a state not often considered a legal bellwether. But 12 years later, in 1974, a landmark case from the state of Washington caused a furor in medicolegal circles.

Barbara Helling, the plaintiff, had been treated by two ophthalmologists from 1959 until 1968 for difficulties with her contact lenses. After Helling was diagnosed with glaucoma in 1968, she sued her erstwhile ophthalmologists and alleged that her vision was permanently damaged because they did not conduct some simple tests nine years earlier.

According to expert witnesses for the defense, the standard of practice at the time did not require routine testing for glaucoma in patients younger than age 40, and thus both the trial and appellate courts found for the ophthalmologists. The Supreme Court of Washington disagreed, however; it held that reasonable prudence may require a standard of care higher than that actually practiced by the profession, and it reversed the trial court's decision and remanded the case for a new trial on the issue of damages. (See The Court Decides: *Helling v. Carey* at the end of this chapter).

Reaction to *Helling*

This decision sent shock waves through the physician community, and many assailed *Helling* as judicial impertinence toward the medical profession. In response, the Washington legislature passed a statute that purported to overturn the *Helling* rule:

> In any civil action for damages based on professional negligence against a hospital . . . or against a member of the healing arts . . . the plaintiff in order to prevail shall be required to prove by a preponderance of the evidence that the defendant or defendants failed to exercise that degree of skill, care, and learning possessed at that time by other persons in the same profession, and that as a proximate result of such failure the plaintiff suffered damages.[23]

Despite the statute, a later case, *Gates v. Jensen*, held that *Helling*'s rule was still in effect.[24] The *Gates* court noted that the original bill had used the word "practiced" rather than "possessed," as in the version that passed

Legal Brief

As an example of positive predictive value at work, suppose epidemiology predicts the prevalence of a hypothetical disease to be 1 percent. In a population of 25,000, there should be 250 actual cases. If the diagnostic test is 95 percent accurate, it will accurately diagnose about 237 of those cases (95 percent × 250), but it will falsely diagnose as positive 1,238 others (5 percent × the remaining 24,750), whom we postulate do not have the disease. Thus, there will be a total of 1,475 positive test results, but only about 16 percent of them will be true positives (237 ffi 1,475). Each positive test result will require further diagnostic procedures, which undoubtedly contribute to a higher cost and a heightened level of patient anxiety. Negative test results are similarly unrealistic and may lead to a false sense of security in the 13 persons who have the disease but tested negative.

positive predictive value
the probability that subjects with a positive screening test truly have the disease

the legislature (quoted earlier). According to the court, the change in the bill prior to enactment showed that the standard was not limited to what members of the profession actually did but could be extended to what they *ought to have done*.

The reaction to the *Helling* decision might have been different—and the case itself might have been decided differently—had more critical analysis been undertaken at trial. Tonometry, the test Mrs. Helling argued should have been used, measures intraocular pressure and produces a relatively high number of false positives. In other words, its **positive predictive value** is low, perhaps as low as 5 percent according to a 1989 report by the US Preventive Services Task Force (PSTF), an independent advisory panel charged with conducting impartial assessments of scientific evidence (see Legal Brief).[25]

Given the inaccuracy of tonometry tests, the relatively low incidence of the disease in younger persons, and some disagreement about the effectiveness of existing treatment options, there is an issue as to whether universal glaucoma screening makes good sense as public policy—irrespective of *Helling*'s outcome. Similar issues of false-positive and false-negative results attend other diagnostic tests, such as prostate-specific antigen (PSA) screening for prostate cancer.

Science Versus Politics

The Washington legislature's involvement in the issue is an example of political interference in what should be a scientific issue. Another example occurred in late 2009 when the PSTF recommended changes to the standards for mammography screening. After reviewing the efficacy of five types of breast cancer screening, the group recommended against routine screening mammography for women younger than age 50. Rather, the PSTF stated, "The decision to start regular, biennial screening mammography before the age of 50 years should be an individual one and [should] take into account patient context, including the patient's values regarding specific benefits and harms."[26]

The mammogram issue was virtually the opposite of the question about glaucoma testing in the *Helling* case 25 years earlier. In *Helling*, the professional practice was *not* to screen routinely, and the court thought it too loose a standard. However, in regard to mammography, the regular practice to require screening was considered too strict a rule. Whereas ocular tonometry is a relatively risk-free procedure, certain harms can attend frequent mammograms. According to the US Preventive Services Task Force, these harms include

> psychological harms, unnecessary imaging tests and biopsies in women without cancer, and inconvenience due to false-positive screening results. Furthermore, one must also consider the harms associated with treatment of cancer that would not become clinically apparent during a woman's lifetime (overdiagnosis), as well as the harms of unnecessary earlier treatment of breast cancer that would have become clinically apparent but would not have shortened a woman's life. Radiation exposure (from radiologic tests), although a minor concern, is also a consideration.[27]

The timing of the mammogram recommendations was unfortunate; they were issued during the debate over President Barack Obama's health reform initiative, the Affordable Care Act of 2010 (ACA). The thoughtful and nuanced approach taken by the group of scientists was lost on politicians, much of the media, and virtually all of the public. The report thus became a political football and an occasion for demagoguery, partisan posturing, and political interference in medical practice. Nevertheless, opinions such as that of the PSTF provide evidence to consider when determining the standard of care in malpractice cases.

Breach of Duty

Once the duty (the standard of care) has been established, the plaintiff must show that it was breached by presenting evidence of the facts of the case *and* testimony from expert witnesses regarding whether the standard was met. Typically, these are the same witnesses who helped establish the duty in the first place.

Expert Witnesses

Unlike lay witnesses, experts are not limited to testifying about facts; they may express opinions about the nature and cause of a patient's illness or injury and whether the defendant treated it properly. An expert witness must have two qualifications. First, he must be familiar with the practice of medicine in the area in question. If the court follows the locality rule, the witness must practice in or be knowledgeable about local practices.[28] Finding

Legal Brief

In an Ohio case, the court noted that "locating an expert to testify for the plaintiff in a malpractice action is known to be a very difficult task, mainly because in most cases one doctor is reluctant and unwilling to testify against another doctor. Although doctors may complain privately to each other about the incompetence of other doctors, they are extremely reluctant to air the matter publicly."[88]

physicians in a particular town to testify against their colleagues and friends can be a daunting task; among trial lawyers, this situation is sometimes referred to as the "conspiracy of silence" (see Legal Brief). If a national standard applies, any otherwise qualified expert in the country is acceptable. A national standard of care therefore eases the plaintiff's burden of finding a willing expert and is another reason the "locality rule" was relaxed.

Second, the expert witness must be professionally qualified. The basic requirement is knowledge of the standard practice involved in treating the patient's condition. The witness need not practice the same specialty or even follow the same school of medicine, but she must be familiar with the type of treatment involved in the patient's case. For example, specialists may testify about the standards for general practitioners if they are knowledgeable about them even though they themselves do not practice as general practitioners.[29] The plaintiff must lay a foundation for expert testimony by persuading the judge that the witness has the appropriate training and experience to qualify as an expert. If the judge decides that the witness meets the qualifications, the testimony is allowed and the jury decides what weight to give it.

For example, in *Gilmore v. O'Sullivan*, an obstetrician/gynecologist's negligence was alleged in the prenatal care and delivery of the plaintiffs' son. The court refused to permit the plaintiffs' expert to testify because he was not board certified in obstetrics and gynecology, there was no evidence of the number or types of maternity cases he had handled, he had not delivered a baby in more than 20 years and had not performed surgery in 14 years, and he had pursued no research in or study of obstetrics and gynecology in recent years.[30]

Sometimes even the defendant will be called as an expert witness. Unlike criminal defendants, who can invoke the constitutional privilege against self-incrimination, defendants in a civil case must testify to facts within their knowledge if called on to do so. Most courts have thought it unfair to require the physician not only to testify regarding such facts but also to provide the expert testimony needed to establish the standard of care, but the New York decision in *McDermott v. Manhattan Eye, Ear and Throat Hospital* illustrates a contrary view.[31] The defendants, one of whom was one of the world's leading ophthalmologists, advised the plaintiff to undergo a series of operations to correct a condition of the cornea in her left eye. The operations resulted in blindness, and the plaintiff claimed that the surgery was not approved by accepted medical practice for the original diagnosis. At the trial, the plaintiff presented no expert witness of her own but called on the defendant to testify to the standard of care required and the deviation from that standard. The appellate court stated that the plaintiff had the right to require the defendant to testify both to his actual knowledge of the case and as an expert to establish the generally accepted medical practice.

Even though statements made out of court are **hearsay** and normally excluded from evidence, in some circumstances a physician's out-of-court statements may be used as evidence of breach of the standard of care. Courts face a difficult task in determining whether a given statement was an admission of negligence or merely an expression of sympathy. After the death of one patient, for instance, the physician said, "I don't know; it never happened to me before. I must have gone too deep or severed a vein." The court said this statement was too vague to be an admission of negligence.[32]

hearsay
an out-of-court statement offered into evidence to prove the truth of the matter asserted in the statement

On the other hand, in a case involving a sigmoidoscopy—a visual examination of the colon in search of polyps—a physician tore the patient's large intestine.[33] On the way out of the operating room, the physician said to another physician, "Boy, I sure made a mess of things," and the patient's husband overheard him. To the husband he said, "In inserting the sigmoidoscope into the rectum, I busted the intestine."[34] The court held that this admission could take the place of expert testimony because a jury could infer that the physician had not exercised the requisite degree of care.

For these reasons, when adverse results occur, health lawyers often advise clients to comment only—if at all—on the facts of what happened without making value judgments as to their own or others' actions. Each case is different and must be judged on its own merits.

Other Evidence of the Standard

In some instances, a plaintiff is permitted to introduce medical treatises as evidence to prove the standard of care. Because medical publications are hearsay—out-of-court statements offered to prove the truth of the matter asserted—most states limit their use to impeaching (i.e., challenging) the credibility of an expert witness or reinforcing the opinion given in an expert's testimony.[35] A few states, however, permit medical treatises to be used as direct evidence to prove the standard of care. In a Wisconsin case, the court took "judicial notice" of the standard of care set forth in a loose-leaf reference service, *Lewis' Practice of Surgery*, to determine whether an orthopedic surgeon was negligent in performing surgery for a ruptured disk.[36] In states that use the Wisconsin approach, the author must be proved to be a recognized expert or the publication to be a reliable authority.

Written rules or procedures of the hospital, regulations of governmental agencies, standards of private accrediting agencies, and similar published material may be admissible to show the requisite standard of care. The landmark decision of *Darling v. Charleston Community Memorial Hospital* held, among other things, that the standards of The Joint Commission on Accreditation of Hospitals (now The Joint Commission) and provisions of the hospital's medical staff bylaws were admissible as evidence of negligence.[37]

Similarly, a statute or other law may be used to establish the standard of care.[38] Negligence that is established by showing a violation of law is *negligence per se*. This doctrine requires that several elements be proven, including that

1. violation of the statute occurred and an injury resulted,
2. the injured person was one whom the statute was meant to protect, and
3. the harm was the type that the statute was enacted to prevent.[39]

In *Landeros v. Flood*, the defendant physician examined an 11-month-old child. She was suffering from a fracture of the right tibia and fibula, an injury that appeared to have been caused by a twisting force. Her mother gave no explanation for the injury, but in fact she and her common-law husband had abused the child repeatedly. The physician failed to diagnose battered child syndrome, and he did not take X-rays that would have revealed a skull fracture and other injuries. The child returned home where she was again severely injured.

guardian ad litem
a guardian appointed by a court to represent the interests of a minor or an incompetent person

Because the matter was not reported to the authorities as required by law, the court allowed the child's **guardian ad litem** (from Latin *litem*, meaning "lawsuit") to bring suit on her behalf against the doctor and the hospital. "Plaintiff is entitled to prove by expert testimony that defendants should reasonably have foreseen that her caretakers were likely to resume their physical abuse and inflict further injuries on her if she were returned directly to their custody."[40] Similar laws require that abuse of other vulnerable persons also be reported.

Inexcusable Outcomes ("Adverse" or "Never" Events)

In some cases, such as when the outcome is so egregious that it is indefensible, no expert testimony is required to establish professional negligence.[41] One example is amputation of the wrong limb. Another is shown by *Hammer v. Rosen*, in which three lay witnesses testified that the defendant had beaten an incompetent psychiatric patient. The defendant physician claimed that without expert testimony, the plaintiff could not prove that the beatings deviated from standard treatments, but the court held otherwise because "the very nature of the acts complained of bespeaks improper treatment and malpractice."[42] (Why experts were not asked to testify is not clear from the opinion, but the plaintiff's attorneys may have thought it unnecessary. As things turned out, they were right.)

In 1999, the Institute of Medicine issued *To Err Is Human*, which estimated that as many as 98,000 people die in US hospitals each year as a result of serious medical errors. This number may seriously underestimate the problem, however; the latest estimate is that more than four times that many persons may die each year from hospital errors.[43] At least two dozen serious events—*adverse events* or *never events*—result from failure to follow standard medical practices and policies. The *Adverse Events in Hospitals: National Incidence Among Medicare Beneficiaries* report lists 29 such occurrences and groups them as follows:

1. **Surgical or Invasive Procedure Events**
   A. Surgery or other invasive procedure performed on the wrong site
   B. Surgery or other invasive procedure performed on the wrong patient
   C. Wrong surgical or other invasive procedure performed on a patient
   D. Unintended retention of a foreign object in a patient after surgery or other invasive procedure
   E. Intraoperative or immediately postoperative/postprocedure death in an ASA Class 1 patient

2. **Product or Device Events**
   A. Patient death or serious injury associated with the use of contaminated drugs, devices, or biologics provided by the healthcare setting
   B. Patient death or serious injury associated with the use or function of a device in patient care, in which the device is used or functions other than as intended
   C. Patient death or serious injury associated with intravascular air embolism that occurs while being cared for in a healthcare setting

3. **Patient Protection Events**
   A. Discharge or release of a patient/resident of any age, who is unable to make decisions, to other than an authorized person
   B. Patient death or serious injury associated with patient elopement (disappearance)
   C. Patient suicide, attempted suicide, or self-harm that results in serious injury, while being cared for in a healthcare setting

4. **Care Management Events**
   A. Patient death or serious injury associated with a medication error (e.g., errors involving the wrong drug, wrong dose, wrong patient, wrong time, wrong rate, wrong preparation, wrong route of administration)
   B. Patient death or serious injury associated with unsafe administration of blood products
   C. Maternal death or serious injury associated with labor or delivery in a low-risk pregnancy while being cared for in a healthcare setting
   D. Death or serious injury of a neonate associated with labor or delivery in a low-risk pregnancy

E. Patient death or serious injury associated with a fall while being cared for in a healthcare setting

F. Any Stage 3, Stage 4, and unstageable pressure ulcers acquired after admission/presentation to a healthcare setting

G. Artificial insemination with the wrong donor sperm or wrong egg

H. Patient death or serious injury resulting from the irretrievable loss of an irreplaceable biological specimen

I. Patient death or serious injury resulting from failure to follow up or communicate laboratory, pathology, or radiology test results

5. **Environmental Events**

A. Patient or staff death or serious injury associated with an electric shock in the course of a patient care process in a healthcare setting

B. Any incident in which systems designated for oxygen or other gas to be delivered to a patient contain no gas, contain the wrong gas, or are contaminated by toxic substances

C. Patient or staff death or serious injury associated with a burn incurred from any source in the course of a patient care process in a healthcare setting

D. Patient death or serious injury associated with the use of physical restraints or bedrails while being cared for in a healthcare setting

6. **Radiologic Events:** Death or serious injury of a patient or staff associated with the introduction of a metallic object into the MRI area

7. **Potential Criminal Events**

A. Any instance of care ordered by or provided by someone impersonating a physician, nurse, pharmacist, or other licensed healthcare provider

B. Abduction of a patient/resident of any age

C. Sexual abuse/assault on a patient or staff member within or on the grounds of a healthcare setting

D. Death or serious injury of a patient or staff member resulting from a physical assault (i.e., battery) that occurs within or on the grounds of a healthcare setting[44]

These types of incidents are generally considered negligence per se and do not require expert testimony to establish the standard of care.

Res Ipsa Loquitur

res ipsa loquitur
a rule of law that one is presumed to be negligent if one had exclusive control of the cause of the accident or injury, even though there is no specific evidence of negligence

Perhaps the most complex exception to the need for expert testimony is the doctrine of **res ipsa loquitur** (Latin for "the thing speaks for itself"). Res ipsa, as it is commonly known, dates back to *Byrne v. Boadle*, an English case decided more than a century and a half ago.[45] Plaintiff Byrne was walking down the street when he was hit by a barrel of flour that had rolled out of the upper level of a warehouse owned by defendant Boadle. The precise negligent act or omission was never determined, but the court found Boadle responsible because barrels of flour do not fall out of buildings unless some-one has been negligent. The fact that this one did so "spoke for itself."

Three conditions must be present for res ipsa to apply:

1. The accident or injury must be of a type that normally would not occur without someone's negligence.
2. The defendant must have had sole control of the apparent cause of the accident or injury.
3. The plaintiff could not have contributed to the accident or injury.

The judge determines whether the doctrine applies in a particular case. Once a judge decides that res ipsa applies, an *inference* of negligence has been created, meaning the case must go to the jury, who can then decide for the plaintiff or the defendant.

Res ipsa can be helpful in medical malpractice cases because it is sometimes impossible for patients to know the precise cause of their adverse outcome, particularly if they were anesthetized during the treatment. If a plaintiff is permitted to invoke res ipsa, she can prevail even without proving that the defendant committed specific negligent acts. (Plaintiffs' attorneys would prefer, however, to point to specific negligent acts in making their case rather than to rely on res ipsa, because proving specific negligence has a more dramatic effect on the jury.)

Requirement 1

The primary difficulty for malpractice plaintiffs in res ipsa cases has been the first requirement: The accident or injury must be of a type that normally would not occur without someone's negligence. The general test is whether on the basis of common knowledge and ordinary experience someone could infer that the defendant was negligent. In one example, a patient underwent surgery for removal of part of his colon.[46] The incision was closed with sutures, but eight days later it opened and a second operation was required to close it. The court held that res ipsa did not apply because a layperson would not know whether the incision failed to close because of the physician's negligence or for some other reason. Thus, the doctrine cannot be based simply on bad treatment outcomes.

In contrast, laypersons clearly understand that leaving foreign objects in a patient after surgery is negligence, and res ipsa is frequently used in such cases. In *Jefferson v. United States*, the plaintiff was a soldier who had under-gone a gallbladder operation.[47] Eight months later, after he had been suffer-ing spells of nausea and vomiting, another operation disclosed that a towel had eroded his small intestine. It was 30 inches long and 18 inches wide and was marked "Medical Department US Army." In this case, the thing almost literally "spoke" for itself!

Requirement 2

In addition to showing that the accident or injury would not normally occur without someone's negligence, the plaintiff must show that the defendant must have had sole control of the apparent cause of the accident or injury. This requirement can be a problem for malpractice plaintiffs. In cases involving surgery, there is often more than one defendant, and traditionally res ipsa cannot be applied in an action against several defendants because any one of them could have caused the plaintiff's injury.[48]

A major departure from the rule, however, was the California case of *Ybarra v. Spangard*.[49] After an appendectomy, the plaintiff felt sharp pains in his right shoulder and later suffered paralysis and atrophy of the shoulder muscles. The subsequent suit went to a California appellate court, which allowed the use of res ipsa against all of the defendants who had any control over the patient while he was anesthetized. They included the surgeon, the consulting physician, the anesthesiologist, the owner of the hospital, and several hospital employees. The court held that

> where a plaintiff receives unusual injuries while unconscious and in the course of medical treatment, all those defendants who had any control over his body or the instrumentalities which might have caused the injuries may properly be called upon to meet the inference of negligence by giving an explanation of their conduct.[50]

Requirement 3

The third requirement for use of res ipsa is showing that the plaintiff could not have contributed to the accident or injury. In many cases, this requirement is not difficult; if the plaintiff was under anesthesia, for example, he clearly had no responsibility. However, if the misadventure could have been caused by the plaintiff's negligence, res ipsa loquitur will not apply. In *Rice v. California Lutheran Hospital*, a hospital employee left a cup, saucer, tea bag, and hot water on a table beside a patient who was recovering from surgery and was under the influence of painkilling drugs.[51] Scalding water spilled on the patient, who claimed that res ipsa should apply because the injury occurred while she was under sedation and did not understand what was going on. The court held that the doctrine did not fit this case because witnesses testified that the plaintiff confessed to spilling the water on herself and that she was awake and alert at the time. As this case shows, the third requirement for res ipsa is based on the facts of a particular case.

Strict Liability

By definition, strict liability does not fit into a discussion of negligence; rather, strict liability imposes liability *without* any showing of negligence. A brief discussion is nevertheless relevant here because the concept is closely tied to the doctrine of res ipsa loquitur and the standard of reasonable prudence discussed earlier.

A showing of fault was not required to impose liability until the mid-nineteenth century, when society decided that some wrongdoing must be shown before persons could be held responsible for injuries caused by their actions. Thus, negligence must be proven in most tort cases. Strict liability is imposed, however, on those whose activities—such as using dynamite or keeping dangerous animals—entail a high degree of risk to others. The rationale behind strict liability is to place the burden of inevitable losses on those best able to bear them, even if they dealt with the danger as carefully as possible.

Developments in product liability law have imposed strict liability on the manufacturers and vendors of various dangerous products. The doctrine imposes liability on those responsible for defective goods that pose an unreasonable risk of injury and do in fact result in injury, regardless of how much care was taken to prevent the dangerous defect.[52] Accidents caused by defective automobile parts are good examples, and product recalls are a direct result of developments in the law of product liability.

The doctrine does not apply to services, only to products. For example, courts have generally held that when giving blood, hospitals are providing a service—not a product—and therefore strict liability does not apply.[53]

Injury and Causation

For a plaintiff to prevail, proving that a physician failed to meet the standard of care and that the patient was injured is not enough. The plaintiff must show that the injury was the **proximate cause** of the negligence. The law considers an injury to be the proximate result of a negligent act if

- the injury would not have occurred but for the defendant's act, or
- it was a foreseeable result of the negligent conduct.

The purpose of a malpractice trial is not to "convict" the defendant but to decide whether the plaintiff's loss is more likely than not the result of substandard conduct on the part of the defendant. Therefore, the plaintiff's burden of proof is lower than that of the government in a criminal prosecution, where proof beyond a reasonable doubt is required. The plaintiff in a civil trial needs only to prove that there is a strong likelihood (a "preponderance of the evidence") that negligence caused the result, and the negligence need not be the sole cause of, but only a significant factor in, the injury.

proximate cause the act or omission from which an injury results as a natural, direct, uninterrupted consequence and without which the injury would not have occurred; the legal cause of the damages to the plaintiff; the cause that immediately precedes and produces the effect (as contrasted with a remote or an intermediate cause)

If a physician has failed to meet the standard of care, the injuries that result from that lapse (if any) may be difficult to determine. This element is especially difficult to determine in healthcare cases because the patient presumably already had some illness or impairment. Physicians can be absolved from liability, despite their negligence, if there is inadequate proof of causation. For example, in *Henderson v. Mason*, the defendant physician negligently failed to discover a small piece of steel embedded in the patient's eye. The steel was eventually discovered and removed by another physician.[54] The court denied recovery because testimony showed that the patient would have suffered infection and loss of vision even if the defendant's diagnosis had been correct.

A court may determine that only some of a patient's injuries resulted from negligence. In one case, a woman and her obstetrician lived near each other. In the sixth month of pregnancy, she experienced labor pains, and her husband summoned the doctor. The doctor did not arrive for several hours, however, and the patient miscarried. In the suit charging him with negligence, the court decided that the obstetrician's failure to treat the patient did not cause the miscarriage because his presence in the house would not have prevented it. He was nevertheless held liable for the patient's pain and suffering, which he might have eased or prevented had he arrived sooner.[55]

Loss of a Chance

Sometimes the nature of a disease means that a patient has virtually no chance of long-term survival, but an early diagnosis may prolong the patient's life or permit a slim chance of survival. Should a practitioner who fails to make that early diagnosis be liable for negligence even though the chances are great that she could not have prevented the patient's death? The courts have been divided on this question. Some jurisdictions have held that the defendant should not be liable if the patient more likely than not would have died anyway.[56] Other courts have concluded that if the defendant increased the risk of death by lessening the chance of survival, such conduct was enough to permit the jury to decide the proximate-cause issue, at least when the chance of survival was significant.[57] In one case, the Supreme Court of Washington summarized this point as follows: "It is not for the wrongdoer, who put the possibility of recovery beyond realization, to say afterward that the result was inevitable."[58]

In another Washington case, the defendants allegedly failed to diagnose the patient's lung cancer in its early stage, and the patient eventually died.[59] The defendants offered evidence that, given that type of lung cancer, death within several years was virtually certain regardless of how early the cancer was diagnosed. The defendants moved for summary judgment. Because the plaintiff could not produce expert testimony that the delayed diagnosis more likely than not caused her husband's death, the trial court dismissed the suit. For purposes of appeal, both parties stipulated that if the cancer had been diagnosed when the defendants first examined the patient, his chances of surviving five years would have been 39 percent, but at the time the cancer was actually diagnosed, his chances were 25 percent. Thus, the delayed diagnosis may have reduced the chance of a five-year survival by 14 percent. The appellate court held that the reduction was sufficient evidence of causation to allow the issue to go to the jury, who would then decide whether the negligence was a substantial factor in producing the injury. "To decide otherwise would be a blanket release from liability for doctors and hospitals any time there was less than a 50 percent chance of survival, regardless of how flagrant the negligence."[60] The court also noted, however, that if the jury found the defendants liable, they would not necessarily be liable for all damages caused by the patient's death but only for those resulting from the early death.

Damages

The question of damages is closely related to the element of causation. In addition to proving that the injury was caused by negligence, the plaintiff must prove which injuries resulted from the negligent conduct and what those injuries are worth. Punitive damages are seldom awarded in negligence cases; the most common damages are called *actual* or *compensatory damages*. They compensate the plaintiff for out-of-pocket loss (such as the cost of medical and rehabilitation treatments and lost earnings) and for noneconomic loss (such as pain and suffering). While economic losses can be fairly accurately demonstrated, it can be difficult to attach dollar values to pain and suffering. Nevertheless, juries do assign dollar values to noneconomic injuries, sometimes in large amounts. For this reason, people who argue for reform in the tort system often suggest limitations on recovery for pain and suffering; several states have statutes that limit noneconomic damages, and these statutes have often been upheld as constitutional.[61] (Reform of the tort system is discussed at the end of this chapter.)

Defenses

Malpractice defendants may have legal defenses that can clear or reduce their liability even if a plaintiff can prove all the elements of the case. For example, a statute of limitations can prevent a case from going to trial. Other defenses, such as comparative negligence, require a decision by the trier of fact (the jury or the judge in nonjury trials). Defenses especially relevant in malpractice actions are discussed in the following sections. Other legal defenses, such as res judicata (discussed in chapter 1), can also be used but have no greater significance in malpractice cases than in any other civil litigation.

Assumption of Risk

In many jurisdictions, people who perceive a risk and still voluntarily expose themselves to that risk are precluded from recovering damages if injury results. In medical malpractice cases, the risk often involves a new method of treatment, and an important issue is whether the possible effects of such treatment were made known to the patient. (This issue is closely related to informed consent, discussed in chapter 11.) In *Karp v. Cooley*, for example, the surgeon was not held liable for the patient's death after a heart transplant because he had fully informed the patient of the risks and had obtained consent to perform the operation.[62]

assumption of risk
a situation that is so obviously dangerous that the individual knows he could be injured but might (or did) take the chance anyway

Assumption of risk does not usually include the risk of a physician's negligence. In the *Karp* case, if death had been caused by an error unrelated to the novelty of the surgery (e.g., a mishap in administering anesthesia), the defendants could have been held liable.

Contributory and Comparative Negligence

Even if a physician has been negligent, **contributory negligence** is a complete defense in many states. Under this theory, if the patient failed to act as a reasonably prudent person would have done, and if the patient's negligence contributed in any way to the injury, she cannot recover damages for the physician's negligence. In one case, a physician who was grossly intoxicated treated a patient negligently.[63] The court refused to hold the doctor liable on the ground that the patient was negligent in accepting treatment from a physician who was obviously drunk.

There are cases, however, in which the patient's contributory negligence merely aggravated an injury caused by the physician's negligence. If the injury would have occurred despite due care by the patient, the patient will be allowed at least a partial recovery. In *Schultz v. Tasche*, an 18-year-old Wisconsin woman was treated negligently for a fracture of the femur. As a result, the ends of the broken bone were not put in apposition, but were negligently allowed to override and unite, thus causing a shortening, lameness, weakness, and pain in the leg.[64] The appellate court decided that the patient could recover for the doctor's negligence despite her own negligence in leaving the hospital early, driving 15 miles to her home, and failing to return for additional treatment. The plaintiff's negligence, the court decided, merely aggravated the existing injury, and its only relevance was to reduce the damages awarded.

contributory negligence and **comparative negligence**
common-law doctrines relating to allocation of responsibility when the plaintiff was partially at fault

Although nominally a contributory negligence case, *Schultz* — decided a century ago — illustrates the **comparative negligence** approach adopted by many states because of the harsh "all or nothing" requirement of traditional contributory negligence. Several theories of comparative negligence exist, but all attempt to compensate the injured party in some way despite the injured party's own negligence. A later Wisconsin case illustrates one variation.[65] A hospital patient slipped while taking a shower and was injured. The jury decided that the hospital was 20 percent negligent—possibly for failing to install safety devices in the shower—but the patient was found 80 percent negligent and was awarded only $4,500.

Exculpatory Contracts

Historically, defendant physicians could raise exculpatory contracts as a defense. An *exculpatory contract* is one in which a party forfeits in advance the right to sue; in other words, it is a release from liability for the other party's future negligence. Absent separate consideration and the releasor's clear understanding of the effect of the agreement, exculpatory contracts are invalid in most contexts, including in healthcare. The landmark case is *Tunkle v. Regents of the University of California*, in which more than 50 years ago the Supreme Court of California held that a contract between a hospital and a patient that attempted in advance to release the hospital from malpractice liability was contrary to **public policy**.[66] The key provision of the contract read:

> RELEASE: The hospital is a nonprofit, charitable institution. In consideration of the hospital and allied services to be rendered and the rates charged therefor, the patient or his legal representative agrees to and hereby releases The Regents of the University of California, and the hospital from any and all liability for the negligent or wrongful acts or omissions of its employees, if the hospital has used due care in selecting its employees.[67]

public policy
the common sense and common conscience of the citizenry as a whole that is applied to matters of public health, safety, and welfare; the general, well-settled (and usually unwritten) sense of public opinion relating to the duties of citizens to one another

The court held that this provision was not part of a fair bargain. It essentially says, "If you want to get treated, you must sign on the dotted line." In a footnote, the opinion points out that when the plaintiff signed the release, he "was in great pain, under sedation, and probably unable to read."[68] This fact was not the underlying rationale for the decision, however.

Release

In contrast to an exculpatory contract, a release executed by a patient *following* treatment may operate as a defense. If a physician and his patient reach a settlement on a malpractice claim, for example, a release signed by the patient will bar a later suit for injuries arising from the same negligent act. The situation is more complicated when a person wrongfully injures a patient and a physician's treatment aggravates the injury later. If the patient settles with the original tortfeasor and releases that person, does the release also cover the physician? It depends.

In *Whitt v. Hutchison*, the plaintiff—who was injured at a ski resort—claimed that his injuries were aggravated by the negligence of the physicians who treated him. Three and a half years after the original injury, the plaintiff had settled with the ski resort and signed a form releasing

> the resort from any and all liability . . . and any and all other loss and damages of every kind and nature sustained by or hereafter resulting to the undersigned . . . from an accident which occurred on or about the first day of March, 1969, at Clear Fork Ski Resort . . . and from all liability, claims, demands, controversies, damages, actions, and causes of action whatsoever, either in law or equity, which the undersigned, individually or in any other capacity . . . may have by reason of or in any wise incident [to] or resulting from the accident hereinbefore mentioned.[69]

The court held that this release was broad enough to include the subsequent malpractice claims and dismissed the suit against the physicians and the hospital. The reasoning was that the injury created the need for the medical treatment and therefore the malpractice was a proximate result of the ski resort's negligence. The physicians and the hospital were not excluded from the terms of the release, so the release was considered to extinguish all claims for all parties jointly liable for the injury. The court stated, "Such a release is presumed in law to be a release for the benefit of all the wrongdoers who might also be liable."[70]

The outcome in other states may vary, and even in this case the harsh result might have been avoided by more precise crafting of the release document to clarify the parties' intentions. Nevertheless, the case is an example of a release being used successfully as a defense to a negligence claim.

Good Samaritan Statutes

Good Samaritan statutes, discussed more completely in chapter 10, provide a defense if the physician has rendered aid at the scene of an accident (see Legal Brief). These statutes, which most states have in some form, commonly provide that a physician rendering emergency care will not be held liable for negligence unless she is grossly negligent or acts in a reckless manner.[71] Most of these statutes do not require doctors to assist in emergencies but protect those who volunteer their aid. Some states, however, have created a duty to assist with immunity from civil suit for persons who comply with the law.[72] References to a Good Samaritan statute may thus indicate either immunity or a duty to assist or both.

Legal Brief

One might question the need for Good Samaritan statutes. Given that negligence is judged according to the standard of "due care under the circumstances," it can be argued that nothing short of gross negligence could lead to liability for rendering care in a true emergency.

In fact, research fails to reveal any cases in which Good Samaritan statutes have been applied to traditional emergency situations, such as when a physician happens on the scene of an automobile accident and renders first aid.

Workers' Compensation Laws

Workers' compensation statutes may provide a defense to an employed physician who is sued by fellow employees he treats in the course of their employment. In many states, workers' compensation laws are the exclusive remedy for employees, and a malpractice suit against the physician will not be permitted. Some courts, however, have allowed such suits.

Governmental Immunity

Statutes grant immunity to many individuals, including physicians, who are employed by government agencies. This immunity is based on the historical concept of **sovereign immunity**, a principle derived from early English law that holds that the sovereign—in the United States, a state or the federal government—cannot commit a legal wrong and is immune from suit or prosecution. This immunity has been waived in most jurisdictions today to allow suits for discretionary acts of government agents.

sovereign immunity
an ancient legal doctrine exempting the sovereign (monarch or state) from liability for wrongs

Statutes of Limitation

Statutes of limitation specify a period during which lawsuits must be filed. The time allowed for malpractice actions—often, two years—is generally shorter than for other actions, although the statutory provisions vary greatly from state to state.

Statutes of limitation generally specify that the period begins when the cause of action "accrues." A cause of action in an assault and battery case, for example, accrues the moment the defendant threatens or touches the plaintiff. In many malpractice cases, however, the beginning of the statutory period is difficult to determine, particularly if the adverse result appears much later. There are three specific times at which the statute might begin, depending on the state's law and the particular circumstances:

1. When the alleged negligent treatment is rendered[73]
2. When the patient discovers or should have discovered the alleged malpractice (the "discovery rule")[74]
3. When the treatment ends or, in a few states, when the physician–patient relationship ends[75]

Particular circumstances create other possibilities. For example, if a physician fraudulently conceals malpractice, the limitation period begins only at discovery of the negligence.[76] Likewise, the period is often delayed in the case of patients who are minors. In one old case, for example, a physician's negligent use of forceps during a birth caused an almost complete loss of sight in the child's right eye.[77] Suit was allowed 22 years later because it was brought after the injured person reached the age of majority, which was then

21. Moreover, some courts have decided, despite the discovery rule, that an action for wrongful death accrues at the date of the death.[78] The limitation periods vary by state, especially with regard to age-related legal disability and medical malpractice cases, and they are never as long today as in the old case mentioned earlier.

Liability for Acts of Others: Vicarious Liability

vicarious liability
attachment of responsibility to a person whose agent caused the plaintiff's injuries

A healthcare provider can be held liable for the negligence of others, even though he has not been personally negligent. **Vicarious liability** is based on the principle of **respondeat superior**—"let the superior respond"— for the negligence of agents or employees. Thus, hospitals, physicians, and other providers are responsible for the negligent acts of their nurses, paramedics, X-ray technicians, and other persons in their employ.[79]

respondeat superior
a doctrine in the law of agency that provides that a principal—the employer (superior)—is responsible for the actions of her agent done in the course of employment

Liability under the theory of respondeat superior does not depend on whether the negligent person was an employee of the superior (although employment is a consideration) but on whether the person was under the *direction and control* of the superior. In *Baird v. Sickler*, a surgeon was held liable for the acts of a nurse anesthetist employed by the hospital.[80] The court judged that the close relationship between the surgeon and the anesthetist resembled that of an employer and employee in that the former had the right of control over the latter. A significant factor in this case was that the surgeon had instructed the anesthetist in some of the procedures and participated in positioning the patient and administering the anesthetic. This cooperation created the appearance of a "master–servant" (employer–employee) relationship; thus, the physician had to answer for the servant's failures. In contrast, in *Honeywell v. Rogers*, a nurse had negligently administered an injection ordered by a physician, but the physician was found not vicariously liable for the negligent act because he did not control the administration of the medicine.[81] (The liability of hospital employees is discussed in chapter 7.)

In addition to being liable for the acts of employees, physicians who refer cases to physicians not in their employ may be held liable in limited circumstances. In general, physicians are not liable when a substitute physician or a specialist takes over a case, but if they are careless in selecting that substitute or specialist, they will be liable for their own negligence. Of course, physicians who are in a legal partnership with other physicians are liable for the torts of the partners (as long as they acted in the scope of the partnership) because every partner is legally an agent of the other partners.

In some situations, an individual can be found to be the employee of two employers at once. This "dual" or "joint" employer concept was at play in a 2015 labor relations case involving a recycling company that contracted with an outside firm to augment its work-force. The contract agency chose and supplied manual laborers who sorted recyclable materials from regular trash; the recycling company set shift times, performance standards, and maximum wages. The labor relations board held that the companies are joint employers, that each is liable for the other's unfair labor practices, and that they must bargain jointly with the employees' unions. Although the immediate effect of the case is limited to the two named companies, the concept, if expanded, could have implications for hospitals and other healthcare providers who use staffing agencies.[82]

Legal Decision Point

Suppose that your hospital has a laboratory that provides services to physician practices. You have drivers who travel a route to pick up specimens for lab work. One day, a courier deviates from his assigned route for a two-hour lunch with his girlfriend. Afterward, he is involved in an accident on his way to the next assigned pickup point. Is the hospital liable to the other driver? What additional facts, if any, do you need to know to answer this question? What, if anything, should be done about the courier?

Determining whether an individual was acting in the scope of the employer's business can be tricky. Suppose a sailor receives orders to report to a new duty station across the country by a date 30 days in the future. The sailor takes leave in the interim. He is not told by what means to travel or what route to take, just to be at the Navy base by a certain time. He drives his own car and detours to visit friends and family for a few days. While in his hometown, he is involved in a motor vehicle accident. The occupants of the other car sue the US government, claiming that the sailor is the government's agent carrying out its orders and therefore the government should be liable on the basis of respondeat superior. How do you think this case should be decided? Develop the arguments for each side of the case. (For a similar situation in healthcare, see Legal Decision Point.)

Countersuits by Physicians

For physicians, being the defendant in a lawsuit is usually an expensive proposition. Even if insurance covers attorneys' fees and other expenses, patients and work time are lost, anxiety increases, reputation suffers, and malpractice insurance premiums may rise. When a defendant who prevailed in a lawsuit asks years later, "Can I now sue the plaintiff or the plaintiff's lawyer to get back at them for this outrage?" in most cases the answer is, "Yes, you can, but you will lose." Even if the original suit was frivolous, a physician will have difficulty recovering damages in most states. Besides, the expense in time, money, and angst hardly seem worth the possibility of revenge (see Legal Brief on p. 166).

Legal Brief

The revenge-seeking defendant would be well advised to heed Justice Learned Hand's remark: "After some dozen years of experience I must say that as a litigant I should dread a lawsuit beyond almost anything else short of sickness and death."[89]

The legal theories on which physicians have based countersuits in malpractice cases include defamation, negligence, abuse of process, and malicious prosecution. Claims of defamation are rarely successful because statements made in the course of legal proceedings are privileged.[83] Furthermore, courts have held that an attorney owes no duty to an adverse party in litigation, so a negligence theory will not help a physician's countersuit.[84] Abuse of process is difficult to prove because, in itself, filing suit is not sufficient to sustain the cause of action.

Physicians have, however, sometimes successfully sued for *malicious prosecution*, an intentional tort. In such cases, they generally must show that

- the malpractice suit was decided in the physician's favor,
- there was no probable cause to believe that the physician was liable, and
- the plaintiff or her attorney acted with malice in bringing the suit.

Although these cases are difficult for a physician to win, ill will or the lack of any reasonable possibility of success may support an allegation of malice. Most states require that actual damages be shown, and in some states, special damages must be proved—for example, damages that arise from an arrest of the person or seizure of property.[85] Damages common to anyone involved in litigation—such as attorneys' fees, injury to reputation, and mental distress— are not sufficient to uphold such an allegation.

Reforming the Tort System

Periodically, the healthcare system encounters a "malpractice crisis," during which the cost of professional liability insurance rises steeply. These crises have multiple causes, but they are usually triggered by economic factors. Drops in the stock market cause insurance companies to lose investment income, which prompts them to raise their premiums, which causes physicians to call for reform of the medical liability system. State legislatures have responded by taking such reform measures as the following:

- Limiting awards for "pain and suffering"
- Shortening the statute of limitations

- Eliminating "joint and several" liability so that any one of multiple defendants is liable only for his percentage fault
- Requiring pretrial screening of claims
- Requiring arbitration or mediation in lieu of civil litigation
- Limiting attorneys' contingency fees
- Allowing the defendant to deduct from the jury's award any payments made to the plaintiff by other sources (such as health insurance)
- Creating joint underwriting associations to spread malpractice risks among various insurance carriers
- Establishing "secondary" insurance plans to cover judgments beyond the limit of the primary insurance
- Improving peer review measures to identify incompetent physicians
- Allowing insurers to pay out the award over time rather than in a lump sum (i.e., structured settlements, which are discussed later in this chapter).

These attempts at tort reform have been only moderately successful. Physicians and others continue to blame malpractice suits for rising healthcare costs, doctors continue to practice defensive medicine, and the courts have struck down some of the reforms. For example, in 2010 the Supreme Court of Georgia ruled that the legislature had no constitutional authority to limit pain and suffering awards.[86] The ACA includes no real tort reforms, but it does include $25 million in grants for states to test new alternatives. It remains to be seen whether these studies will uncover effective means of reducing the consequences of defensive medicine and holding down the cost of healthcare.

If a defendant (or insurance company) wants to resolve a case without trial, there are numerous ways to design a settlement agreement. *Structured settlements* are financial arrangements that compensate the plaintiff through periodic payments rather than in the traditional form of a lump sum. A structured settlement incorporated into a trial judgment by agreement of the parties and with the approval of the court is a *periodic payment judgment*. Structured settlements are advantageous for the defendant in that they compensate the plaintiff for her damages without creating the possibility of a windfall. One kind of structured settlement is illustrated in *Perin v. Hayne* (see The Court Decides at the end of this chapter).

My personal experience with a structured settlement stems from a negligence case at a US Navy hospital in the 1970s. A baby suffered severe brain damage because of lack of oxygen during delivery, but with proper care she was expected to have a normal life expectancy. The parents and the government settled the case by creating a "reversionary trust" to care for the

EXHIBIT 5.1
Example of
a Structured
Settlement

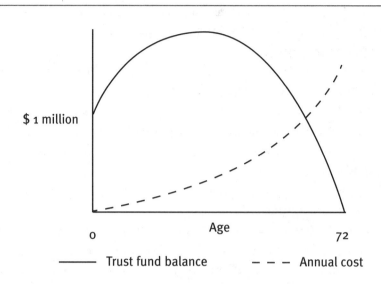

$ 1 million

Age

0   72

———— Trust fund balance   – – – Annual cost

child as long as she lived. Calculations showed that a principal amount of $1 million, plus reinvested earnings, would cover the expected cost of custodial care for 72 years, the life expectancy of a newborn at the time. To prevent the parents from receiving a windfall, the government provided in the language of the trust document that the funds would revert to the government if the child died before age 72. (See exhibit 5.1 for a graph depicting this type of structured settlement.)

Forty years after the settlement was approved, I spoke with the father of the child and learned that she was still living and was in a facility that provides round-the-clock care. He reported that the trust was functioning as planned and that its principal and accumulated interest seem to be sufficient.

Summary

This chapter outlines the four basic elements of proof in a tort case—duty, breach, injury, and causation. The duty (standard of care) can be proven in various ways, and the plaintiff's injuries must have been caused by the defendant's (or defendant's agent's) breach of that duty. In the case of an agency relationship, the concept of respondeat superior (vicarious liability) applies. In the case of a physician's negligence (medical malpractice), the standards of different schools of practice (traditional medicine vs. osteopathy, for example) might determine the standard of care. When proof of specific negligence is difficult to demonstrate, res ipsa loquitur might be applied. Also explored in this chapter are a number of defenses to malpractice suits as well as reform of and alternatives to the tort system.

Discussion Questions

1. What are the four elements of proof necessary for a plaintiff to succeed in a negligence case?
2. Explain the significance of *Helling v. Carey* in relation to the standard of care in medical malpractice cases.
3. How can the standard of care be proven?
4. What is an exculpatory contract, and when is one held to be enforceable?
5. What is the principle of vicarious liability (respondeat superior)?
6. What are some examples of tort reform, and how successful have they been?
7. How might the ACA affect the field of medical malpractice?

The Court Decides

Helling v. Carey
83 Wash. 2d 514, 519 P.2d 981 (1974)

Hunter, J.

We find this to be a unique case. The testimony of the medical experts is undisputed concerning the standards of the profession for the specialty of ophthalmology. . . . The issue is whether the defendants' compliance with the standard of the profession of ophthalmology, which does not require the giving of a routine pressure test to persons under 40 years of age, should insulate them from liability under the facts of this case. . . .

[The court points to evidence that the incidence of glaucoma in persons under the age of 40 was about 1 in 25,000.] However, that one person, the plaintiff in this instance, is entitled to the same protection, as afforded persons over 40, essential for timely detection of the evidence of glaucoma where it can be arrested to avoid the grave and devastating result of this disease. The test is a simple pressure test, relatively inexpensive. There is no judgment factor involved, and there is no doubt that by giving the test the evidence of glaucoma can be detected. . . .

Justice Holmes stated in *Texas & Pac. Ry. v. Behymer*:

What usually is done may be evidence of what ought to be done, but what ought to be done is fixed by a standard of reasonable prudence, whether it usually is complied with or not.

In [another case,] Justice [Learned] Hand stated:

[I]n most cases reasonable prudence is in fact common prudence; but strictly it is never its measure; a whole calling may have unduly lagged in the adoption of new and available devices. It never may set its own tests, however persuasive be its usages. Courts must in the end say which is required; there are precautions so imperative that even their universal disregard will not excuse their omission.

Under the facts of this case reasonable prudence required the timely giving of the pressure test to this plaintiff. The precaution of giving this test to detect the incidence of glaucoma to patients under 40 years of age is so imperative that irrespective of its disregard by the standards of the ophthalmology profession, it is the duty of the courts to say what is required to protect patients under 40 from the damaging results of glaucoma.

We therefore hold, as a matter of law, that the reasonable standard that should have been followed under the undisputed facts of this case was the timely giving of this simple, harmless pressure test to this plaintiff and that, in failing to do so, the defendants were negligent, which proximately resulted in the blindness sustained by the plaintiff for which the defendants are liable.

. . .

The judgment of the trial court and the decision of the Court of Appeals [are] reversed. . . . ■

Discussion Questions

1. The Supreme Court of Washington is often viewed as nontraditional—liberal, activist, or bellwether, depending on one's point of view. Do you agree with the court's decision in this case to abandon a traditional, physician-determined standard of care? Why or why not?

2. Is this decision an example of "judge-made law"? Is it "judicial activism"? Is it to be admired or disdained? Fashion an argument supporting each point of view.

3. The legislation that attempted to overturn the *Helling* precedent has been on the books since 1974 but has had little effect. Why do you suppose this is so, and why has the legislature not seen fit to reinforce it?

4. Consider the discussion in the text concerning whether *Helling* is good public policy. Explain how a test that is 95 percent accurate can result in positive test results that are truly positive only 16 percent of the time.

The Court Decides

Perin v. Hayne
210 n.W.2d 609 (Iowa 1973)

McCormick, J.

This is an appeal from a directed verdict for a doctor in a malpractice action. We affirm.

The claim arose from an anterior approach cervical fusion performed on plaintiff Ilene Perin by defendant Robert A. Hayne. . . . The fusion was successful in eliminating pain, weakness and numbness in plaintiff's back, neck, right arm and hand caused by two protruded cervical discs, but plaintiff alleged she suffered paralysis of a vocal chord [*sic*] because of injury to the right recurrent laryngeal nerve during surgery. . . . The injury reduced her voice to a hoarse whisper.

She sought damages on four theories: specific negligence, res ipsa loquitur, breach of express warranty and battery or trespass. After both parties had rested, the trial court sustained defendant's motion for directed verdict, holding the evidence insufficient to support jury consideration of the case on any of the pleaded theories. Plaintiff assigns this ruling as error. We must review each of the pleaded bases for recovery in the light of applicable law and the evidence.

I. Specific negligence. Plaintiff alleges there was sufficient evidence to support jury submission of her charge [that] defendant negligently cut or injured the recurrent laryngeal nerve. Plaintiff had protruded discs at the level of the fifth and sixth cervical interspaces. The purpose of surgery was to remove the protruded discs and fuse the vertebrae with bone dowels from her hip. Removal of a disc ends the pinching of the nerve in the spinal column which causes the patient's pain. The bone supplants the disc.

The procedure involves an incision in the front of the neck at one side of the midline at a level slightly below the "Adam's apple." Four columns run through the neck. The vertebrae and spinal cord are in the axial or bone column at the rear. In order to get to the axial column the surgeon must retract the visceral column which lies in front of it. The visceral column, like the vascular columns on each side of it, is covered with a protective fibrous sheath, called fascia. It contains the esophagus and trachea. The recurrent laryngeal

(continued)

(continued from previous page)

nerve, which supplies sensitivity to the muscles that move the vocal chord [*sic*], is located between the esophagus and trachea.

The surgeon does not enter the visceral column during the cervical fusion procedure. The same pliancy which enables the neck to be turned enables the visceral column to be retracted to one side to permit access to the axial column. The retraction is accomplished by using a gauze-padded retractor specifically designed for retraction of the visceral column during this surgery.

The record shows the defendant used this procedure in the present case. Plaintiff was under general anesthetic. The anesthesia record is normal, and there is no evidence of any unusual occurrence during surgery. Defendant denied any possibility the laryngeal nerve was severed. He said it could not be severed unless the visceral fascia was entered, and it was not. He also believed it would be impossible to sever the nerve during such surgery without also severing the esophagus or trachea or both.

[An expert witness for the plaintiff testified that it would be unusual to specifically encounter the laryngeal nerve during this surgery but that "the injury could occur despite the exercise of all proper skill and care."]

Defendant testified he did not know the cause of the injury but presumed it resulted from contusion of the nerve incident to retraction of the visceral column. He thought plaintiff's laryngeal nerve may have been peculiarly susceptible to such injury. He insisted the surgery was done just as it always was and if he were doing it again he would do it the same way. He said one study has shown the surgery will result in paralysis of a vocal chord [*sic*] in two or three-tenths of one percent of cases in which it is used. He also said there is no way to predict or prevent such instances.

. . .

In considering the propriety of the verdict directed for defendant we give the evidence supporting plaintiff's claim the most favorable construction it will reasonably bear.

We recognize three possible means to establish specific negligence of a physician. One is through expert testimony, the second through evidence showing [that] the physician's lack of care is so obvious as to be within comprehension of the layman, and the third (actually an extension of the second) evidence that the physician injured a part of the body not involved in the treatment. The first means is the rule and the others are exceptions to it.

In this case plaintiff asserts [that] a jury question was generated by the first and third means. We do not agree.

Plaintiff alleges the laryngeal nerve was negligently cut or injured. The record is devoid of any evidence the nerve was severed during surgery. . . .

The doctors agree the technique employed by defendant was proper. The sole basis for suggesting the expert testimony would support a finding of specific negligence is that the nerve was injured during retraction. Where an injury may occur despite due care, a finding of negligence cannot be predicated solely on the fact it did occur. . . .

Plaintiff also maintains there is evidence of negligence from the fact this is a case of injury to a part of the body not involved in the treatment. However, that is not so. The surgical procedure did include retraction of the visceral column. It was very much in the surgical field. . . .

Trial court did not err in directing a verdict for defendant on the issue of specific negligence.

II. Res ipsa loquitur. Plaintiff also alleges the applicability of the doctrine of res ipsa loquitur. Our most recent statement of the doctrine appears in [a 1973 case]:

Under the doctrine of res ipsa loquitur, where (1) injury or damage is caused by an instrumentality under the exclusive control of defendant and (2) the occurrence is such as in the ordinary course of things would not happen if reasonable care had been used, the happening of the injury permits, but does not compel, an inference defendant was negligent.

The contest in this case concerns presence of the second foundation fact [from the quoted paragraph].

. . .

Defendant argues the second foundation fact for res ipsa loquitur is absent because it does not lie in the common knowledge of laymen to say injury to the laryngeal nerve does not occur if due care is exercised in anterior approach cervical fusion surgery.

We must initially decide what has previously been an open question in this jurisdiction: may the common experience to establish the second foundation fact for res ipsa loquitur be shown by expert testimony?

[The court proceeds to review cases from Wisconsin, California, Oregon, and Washington, plus three legal treatises on the subject. It quotes with favor the following:]

In the usual case the basis of past experience from which this conclusion may be drawn is common to the community, and is a matter of general knowledge, which the court recognizes on much the same basis as when it takes judicial notice of facts which everyone knows. It may, however, be supplied by the evidence of the parties; and expert testimony that such an event usually does not occur without negligence may afford a sufficient basis for the inference.

Thus we disagree with defendant's contention [that] the second foundation fact must be based exclusively on the common knowledge of laymen.

In this case, however, even considering the expert testimony, the record at best only supports an inference [that] plaintiff suffered an extremely rare injury in anterior approach cervical fusion surgery which may occur even when due care is exercised. Rarity of the occurrence is not a sufficient predicate for application of res ipsa loquitur. . . . There is no basis in the present case, in expert testimony or otherwise, for saying plaintiff's injury is more likely the result of negligence than some cause for which the defendant is not responsible.

. . .

We do not believe there was any basis in this case for submission of res ipsa loquitur. Trial court did not err in refusing to submit it.

III. Express warranty. *[The court dismisses this count, saying that the evidence supporting her argument that the physician guaranteed a good result was equivocal in nature: "There comes a point when a question of fact may be generated as to whether the doctor has warranted a cure or a specific result. However, in the present case the evidence does not rise to that level."]*

IV. Battery or trespass. Plaintiff contends there was also sufficient evidence to submit the case to the jury on the theory of battery or trespass. In effect, she alleges she consented to fusion of two vertebrae (removal of only one protruded disc) thinking there would be a separate operation if additional vertebrae had to be fused. She asserts the fact four vertebrae were fused combined with defendant's assurances and failure to warn her of specific hazards vitiated her consent and makes the paralyzed vocal chord [sic] the result of battery or trespass for which defendant is liable even without negligence. There was no evidence or contention by her in the trial court nor is there any assertion here that she would not have consented to the surgery had she known those things she says were withheld from her prior to surgery.

(continued)

(continued from previous page)

Defendant testified plaintiff was fully advised as to the nature of her problem and the scope of corrective surgery. He acknowledges he did not advise her of the hazard of vocal chord [*sic*] paralysis. He believed the possibility of such occurrence was negligible and outweighed by the danger of undue apprehension if warning of the risk was given.

[The court next begins a discussion of the distinction between consent and informed consent, quoting with approval from its own landmark case Cobbs v. Grant:*]* Where a doctor obtains consent of the patient to perform one type of treatment and subsequently performs a substantially different treatment for which consent was not obtained, there is a clear case of battery. However, when an undisclosed potential complication results, the occurrence of which was not an integral part of the treatment procedure but merely a known risk, the courts are divided on the issue of whether this should be deemed to be a battery or negligence.

. . .

We agree with the majority trend. The battery theory should be reserved for those circumstances when a doctor performs an operation to which the patient has not consented. When the patient gives permission to perform one type of treatment and the doctor performs another, the requisite element of deliberate intent to deviate from the consent given is present. However, when the patient consents to certain treatment and the doctor performs that treatment but an undisclosed inherent complication with a low probability occurs, no intentional deviation from the consent given appears; rather, the doctor in obtaining consent may have failed to meet his due care duty to disclose pertinent information. In that situation the action should be pleaded in negligence.

From our approval of this analysis it should be clear we believe the battery or trespass theory pleaded by plaintiff in this case is limited in its applicability to surgery to which the patient has not consented. There must be a substantial difference between the surgery consented to and the surgery which is done. Plaintiff asserts she consented to only one fusion rather than two. Assuming this is true, the most that could be argued is [that] the second fusion was a battery or trespass. But she does not claim damages for a second fusion. She asks damages because of injury to the laryngeal nerve during surgery. The evidence is undisputed that whether one or two fusions were to be done the path to the axial column had to be cleared by retraction of the visceral column. Hence, any injury caused by such retraction occurred during a procedure to which consent had been given. Retraction of the visceral column during the surgery was not a battery or trespass.

We have no occasion to reach the question whether failure to advise plaintiff of the risk of laryngeal nerve injury would in the circumstances of this case have generated a jury issue on negligence, but we do point out that recovery on such basis is precluded unless a plaintiff also establishes he would not have submitted to the procedure if he had been advised of the risk. . . . There is no evidence plaintiff would have withheld her consent in this case.

. . .

Affirmed. ■

Discussion Questions

1. Has due care been shown? Does it need to be?
2. What is the "second foundation fact," and how does "common experience" matter in relation to it?

3. The opinion states, "There must be a substantial difference between the surgery consented to and the surgery which is done [for a battery case to be made]." What would amount to a "substantial difference" in your mind? What if throat cancer had been discovered and cleanly removed with no aftereffects? Would that procedure be a substantial difference justifying damages for battery even though no other injury (and, in fact, a benefit) had resulted?

4. Why did the court "have no occasion" to decide whether failure to advise the plaintiff of the risk of nerve injury raised a negligence issue?

Notes

1. 61 Am. Jur. 2d, *Physicians and Surgeons* § 205 (1981).
2. Baldor v. Rogers, 81 So. 2d 658 (Fla. 1954), *reh'g denied*, 81 So. 2d 661 (Fla. 1955); Angela R. Holder, Medical Malpractice Law 47 (2d ed. 1978).
3. DeFilippo v. Preston, 53 Del. 539, 173 A.2d 333 (1961).
4. Miller v. Toles, 183 Mich. 252, 150 N.W. 118 (1914).
5. Fiorentino v. Wenger, 272 N.Y.S.2d 557, 26 A.D.2d 693 (1966), *rev'd on other grounds*, 19 N.Y.2d 407, 227 N.E.2d 296 (1967).
6. Faulkner v. Pezeshki, 44 Ohio App. 2d 186, 337 N.E.2d 158 (1975).
7. Small v. Howard, 128 Mass. 131, 35 Am. R. 363 (1880) was overruled by Brune v. Belinkoff, 235 N.E.2d 793 (Mass. 1968).
8. Zills v. Brown, 382 So. 2d 528, 532 (Ala. 1980).
9. *Id*. at 532. *See also* Morrison v. MacNamara, 407 A.2d 555 (D.C. 1979).
10. C. J. Willis, *Establishing Standards of Care: Locality Rules or National Standards*, AAOS Now (published February 2009), at http://www.aaos.org/news/aaosnow/feb09/managing9.asp.
11. Drs. Lane, Bryant, Eubanks & Dulaney v. Otts, 412 So. 2d 254 (Ala. 1982).
12. Jon R. Waltz & Fred E. Inbau, Medical Jurisprudence 54 (MacMillan 1971).
13. Craft v. Peebles, 893 P.2d 138 (Haw. 1995).
14. *See, e.g.*, Dolan v. Galluzzo, 77 Ill. 2d 279, 396 N.E.2d 13 (1979) (a podiatrist was held to standards of podiatrists; physician testimony excluded).
15. Nelson v. Harrington, 72 Wis. 591, 40 N.W. 228 (1888). *See also* Hansen v. Pock, 57 Mont. 51, 187 P. 282 (1920) (an herbologist was

held to standards of surgical and medical practice in the absence of a school of practice).

16. Spead v. Tomlinson, 73 N.H. 46, 59 A. 376 (1904).

17. 25 Wash. App. 158, 607 P.2d 864 (1980). *See also* Kelly v. Carroll, 36 Wash. 2d 482, 219 P.2d 79 (1950), *cert. denied*, 340 U.S. 892 (1950) (a naturopath was liable for a patient's death from appendicitis; the naturopath must know when treatment is ineffective and when standard medical care is needed).

18. Pittman v. Gilmore, 556 F.2d 1259 (5th Cir. 1977). *See also* Lewis v. Soriano, 374 So. 2d 829 (Miss. 1979) (a general practitioner had a duty to refer a complicated fracture to an orthopedic specialist).

19. *See, e.g.*, Sinz v. Owens, 33 Cal. 2d 749, 205 P.2d 3 (1949) (a physician who did not use skeletal traction in treating a double comminuted fracture of a patient's leg would be held to the skill of a specialist only if he should have known that greater skill than a general practitioner's was necessary); Reeg v. Shaughnessy, 570 F.2d 309 (10th Cir. 1978) (physicians are held to the degree of care commensurate with their training and experience).

20. *See, e.g.*, Lewis v. Soriano, 374 So. 2d 829 (Miss. 1979).

21. 245 So. 2d 751 (La. App. 1971).

22. 144 So. 2d 544 (La. App. 1962).

23. Wash. Rev. Code § 4.24.290 (1975, as amended).

24. 92 Wash. 2d 246, 595 P.2d 919 (1979).

25. US Preventive Services Task Force, Guide to Clinical Preventive Services (1989) at 124. The report states, "There is insufficient evidence to recommend routine performance of tonometry by primary care physicians as an effective screening test for glaucoma. . . . The limited specificity of tonometry combined with the low prevalence of [glaucoma] results in a positive predictive value of only 5% in asymptomatic populations."

26. US Preventive Services Task Force, *Screening for Breast Cancer*, 151 Ann. Int. Med. 716–26 (November 2009), at http://www.annals.org/content/151/10/716.full.

27. *Id.*

28. *See, e.g.*, Johnson v. Richardson, No. W2009-02626-COA-R3-CV (Tenn. Ct. App., Aug. 12, 2010); Callahan v. William Beaumont Hosp., 400 Mich. 177, 254 N.W.2d 31 (1977).

29. *See, e.g.*, Siirila v. Barrios, 398 Mich. 576, 248 N.W.2d 171 (1976).

30. 106 Mich. App. 35, 307 N.W.2d 695 (1981).

31. 15 N.Y.2d 20, 255 N.Y.S.2d 65, 203 N.E.2d 469 (1964), *aff'd*, 18 N.Y.2d 970, 278 N.Y.S.2d 209, 224 N.E.2d 717 (1966). *See* Waltz & Inbau, *supra* note 12 at 82.

32. Scacchi v. Montgomery, 365 Pa. 377 at 380, 75 A.2d 535 at 537 (1950).

33. Wickoff v. James, 159 Cal. App. 2d 664, 324 P.2d 661 (1958).

34. Both quotes found at 159 Cal. App. 2d at 667, 324 P.2d at 663.

35. R. P. Bergen, *Law & Medicine: Medical Books as Evidence*, 217 J. AM. MED. ASS'N 527 (1971), at http://jama.ama-assn.org/content/217/4/527.full.pdf+html?sid=44bd6566-35de-445e-be4c-5057e577a050.

36. Burnside v. Evangelical Deaconess Hosp., 46 Wis. 2d 519, 175 N.W. 2d 230 (1970).

37. 33 Ill. 2d 326, 211 N.E.2d 253, 14 A.L.R.3d 860 (1965), *cert. denied*, 383 U.S. 946 (1966).

38. Darling v. Charleston Community Memorial Hosp., 33 Ill. 2d 326, 211 N.E.2d 253 (1965).

39. *See, e.g.*, Cal. Evid. Code § 669 (Supp. 1985).

40. 17 Cal. 3d 399, 131 Cal. Rptr. 69, 551 P.2d 389, 97 A.L.R. 3rd 324 (1976).

41. 43. *See, e.g.*, Sinz v. Owens, 33 Cal. 2d 749, 205 P.2d 3, 8 A.L.R.2d 757 (1949).

42. 7 N.Y.2d 376, 380, 165 N.E.2d 756, 757 (1960).

43. INSTITUTE OF MEDICINE, TO ERR IS HUMAN: BUILDING A SAFER HEALTH SYSTEM (National Academies Press 1999). For a 2013 report estimating the number to be upward of 440,000 deaths annually, *see* Sally Robertson, *Medical Error Is the Third Biggest Cause of Death in the United States, According to Experts* (published May 5, 2016), at http://www.news-medical.net/news/20160505/Medical-error-is-the-third-biggest-cause-of-death-in-the-US-according-to-experts.aspx.

44. These never events were the subject of a US Department of Health and Human Services report, *Adverse Events in Hospitals: National Incidence Among Medicare Beneficiaries* (published November 2010), at http://oig.hhs.gov/oei/reports/oei-06-09-00090.pdf, which provides updated statistics on their incidence. Medicare denies hospitals higher payments for complications caused by these events. *See, e.g.*, FY 2009 Inpatient PPS Final Rule, 73 Fed. Reg. 48434, 48471–4891 (August 19, 2008).

45. 2 H. & C. 722, 159 Eng. Rep. 299 (1863).

46. Jamison v. Debenham, 203 Cal. App. 2d 744, 21 Cal. Rptr. 848 (1962).

47. 77 F. Supp. 706 (Md. 1948), *aff'd*, 178 F.2d 518 (4th Cir. 1949), *aff'd*, 340 U.S. 135 (1950).

48. WALTZ & INBAU, *supra* note 12 at 100.

49. 25 Cal. 2d 486, 154 P.2d 687 (1944), 162 A.L.R. 1258.

50. *Id.* at 493, 154 P.2d at 691. *Ybarra v. Spangard* has been followed in California; *see, e.g.*, Hale v. Venuto, 137 Cal. App. 3d 910, 187

Cal. Rptr. 357 (1982)—it has also been cited with approval in various jurisdictions; *see* DAVID W. LOUISELL & HAROLD WILLIAMS, MEDICAL MALPRACTICE § 14.02, at 14–18 (Matthew Bender 1984).

51. 158 P.2d 579 (Cal. App. 1945), *rev'd on other grounds*, 27 Cal. 296, 163 P.2d 860 (1945).

52. *See* RESTATEMENT (SECOND) OF TORTS § 402A.

53. *See, e.g.*, Perlmutter v. Beth David Hosp., 308 N.Y. 100, 123 N.E.2d 792 (1954). Many states have dealt with this issue by legislation; *see, e.g.*, Wis. Stat. § 146.31(2) (West Supp. 1986).

54. 386 S.W.2d 879 (Tex. Civ. App. 1964).

55. Mehigan v. Sheehan, 94 N.H. 274, 51 A.2d 632 (1947).

56. *See, e.g.*, Cornfeldt v. Tongen, 295 N.W.2d 638 (Minn. 1980); Hanselmann v. McCardle, 275 S.C. 46, 267 S.E.2d 531 (1980); Hiser v. Randolph, 126 Ariz. 608, 617 P.2d 774 (Ct. App. 1980); Cooper v. Sisters of Charity of Cincinnati, Inc., 272 N.E.2d 97 (1971).

57. *See, e.g.*, Hamil v. Bashline, 481 Pa. 256, 392 A.2d 1280 (1978); McBride v. United States, 462 F.2d 72 (9th Cir. 1972).

58. Herskovits v. Group Health Cooperative of Puget Sound, 99 Wash. 2d 609, 614, 664 P.2d 474, 476 (1983).

59. *Id. See also* Glicklich v. Spievack, 16 Mass. App. 488, 452 N.E.2d 287 (1983), *appeal denied*, 454 N.E.2d 1276 (1983) (diagnosis of breast cancer delayed for nine months; jury verdict for plaintiff upheld).

60. Herskovits, *supra* note 58, 99 Wash. 2d at 614, 664 P.2d at 477.

61. *See, e.g.*, Johnson v. St. Vincent Hospital, Inc., 273 Ind. 374, 404 N.E.2d 585 (1980).

62. 349 F. Supp. 827 (S.D. Tex. 1972), *aff'd*, 493 F.2d 408, *cert. denied*, 419 U.S. 845. This case is discussed in greater detail in chapter 11. *See also* HOLDER, *supra* note 2 at 306–9.

63. Champs v. Stone, 74 Ohio App. 344, 58 N.E.2d 803 (1944).

64. 166 Wis. 561, 165 N.W. 292 (1917).

65. Schuster v. St. Vincent Hosp., 45 Wis. 2d 135, 172 N.W.2d 421 (1969).

66. 60 Cal. 2d 92, 32 Cal. Rptr. 33, 383 P.2d 441 (1963).

67. *Id.*

68. 383 P.2d at 449.

69. 43 Ohio St. 2d 53, 330 N.E.2d 678 (Ohio 1975).

70. 43 Ohio St. at 61.

71. *See, e.g.*, Vt. Stat. Ann. tit. 12, § 519(b) (1973).

72. Vt. Stat. Ann. tit. 12, § 519 (1973); Minn. Stat. Ann. § 604.05 (as amended 1984) (West Supp. 1985).

73. ALAN RICHARDS MORITZ & R. CRAWFORD MORRIS, HANDBOOK OF LEGAL MEDICINE 211 (Mosby 1970); Hill v. Hays, 193 Kan. 453, 395 P.2d 298 (1964).

74. *See, e.g.*, Cates v. Bald Estate, 54 Mich. App 717, 221 N.W.2d 474 (1974).

75. *The Statute of Limitations in Medical Malpractice Actions*, WIS. L. REV. (1970) 915, 918; 6 AKRON L. REV. 265, 267–68 (1973).

76. Bauer v. Bowen, 63 N.J. Super. 225, 164 A.2d 357 (1960).

77. Chaffin v. Nicosia, 261 Ind. 698, 310 N.E.2d 867 (1974).

78. Hubbard v. Libi, 229 N.W.2d 82 (N.D. 1975).

79. *See, e.g.*, Thompson v. Brent, 245 So. 2d 751 (La. App. 1971) (the physician was liable because a medical assistant in his employ was negligent in removing a cast with a Stryker saw).

80. 69 Ohio St. 2d 652, 433 N.E.2d 593 (Ohio 1982).

81. Honeywell v. Rogers, 251 F. Supp. 841 (W.D. Pa. 1966). Vicarious liability is discussed in greater detail under the captain-of-the-ship and borrowed-servant doctrines in chapter 7.

82. Browning-Ferris Industries of California, Case. No. 32-RC-109684, 362 NLRB No. 186 (August 27, 2015).

83. Huene v. Carnes, 121 Cal. App. 3d 432, 175 Cal. Rptr. 374 (1981).

84. *See, e.g.*, Friedman v. Dozorc, 412 Mich. 1, 312 N.W.2d 585 (1981), *and* Hill v. Willmott, 561 S.W.2d 331 (Ky. App. 1978).

85. *See, e.g.,* Dakters v. Shane, 64 Ohio App. 2d 196, 412 N.E.2d 399 (1978); Berlin v. Nathan, 64 Ill. App. 3d 940, 381 N.E.2d 1367 (1978), *cert. denied*, 444 U.S. 828, *reh'g denied*, 444 U.S. 974 (1979).

86. Atlanta Oculopic Surgery, P.C. v. Nestlehutt, 691 S.E.2d 218 (Ga. 2010).

87. OLIVER WENDELL HOLMES JR., THE COMMON LAW at 7 (1881).

88. Faulkner v. Pezeshki, 44 Ohio App. 2d 186 at 193, 337 N.E.2d 158 at 164 (1975).

89. Quoted in RICHARD A. POSNER, LAW AND LITERATURE at 135 (Harvard University Press 1998).

THE ORGANIZATION AND MANAGEMENT OF A CORPORATE HEALTHCARE INSTITUTION

6

After reading this chapter, you will

- understand that a corporation is a "person" for many legal purposes, but not an "individual" or a "citizen"; therefore, laws that apply to persons also apply to corporations, but laws that specify individuals or citizens do not;
- appreciate that incorporation has many advantages, the most significant of which is limiting the liability of the individuals who own it;
- know that the powers of a corporation are limited to those specified in state law and the corporate charter;
- be able to explain why the governing board must be actively involved in overseeing the affairs of the company without meddling in management's control of day-to-day operations;
- realize that various factors have led to the development of multi-institutional healthcare systems rather than stand-alone hospital corporations; and
- see that health reform legislation has provided an impetus for another round of corporate reorganization, especially in the area of hospital–physician relations.

Most institutional healthcare providers are corporations, thus this chapter focuses primarily on the fundamental nature of the corporate form of organization. However, healthcare is also provided by sole proprietorships, partnerships, and other types of business entities.

In a *sole proprietorship*, an individual (e.g., a family physician in solo practice) assumes all organizational roles: employer, employee, and owner. The proprietor usually retains any profits or suffers any losses and bears the full risks of the enterprise.

A *partnership* exists if someone joins the proprietor and shares in the rewards and risks. Partnerships are governed by state law and by an agreement between the parties.[1] The parties have great latitude to develop an agreement that suits their needs.

The simplest kind of partnership is a *general partnership*. In this arrangement, the partners usually receive equal shares of profits or losses, are entitled to equal voting rights, and are personally liable for the debts of the venture. On the death or departure of a partner, the partnership is automatically dissolved, but the business operation does not necessarily end. General partners ordinarily control the business by consensus; however, as the volume of business and number of partners increase, this arrangement may become cumbersome. As a result, the owners often change the business to a limited partnership or a corporate structure.

A *joint venture* is a special form of partnership created by contract for a specific purpose and for a limited duration. A joint venture is thus one way of integrating two or more business organizations. In joint ventures, the parties have fiduciary responsibilities to each other, and depending on the contractual terms, each usually has a right to participate in management. Profits and losses are shared according to the agreement, and each participant may be liable to third parties. Although somewhat similar, a joint venture differs from a general partnership in that its participants are not agents of each other.

Because of their flexibility, joint ventures have become popular in the healthcare sector and have been used, for example, to effect hospital–physician integration (discussed later). The rest of this chapter focuses primarily on corporations, the predominant form of healthcare organization.

Other organizational forms such as *limited partnership*, *limited liability company*, *professional limited liability company*, and *professional corporation* may also be used by licensed individuals such as physicians, psychologists, midwives, and others to protect their personal assets from lawsuits brought against their practices. The requirements for creating these entities vary from state to state, and the implications for taxation and tort liability may differ from one type to another. The details are too many to describe here, and it is sufficient to say that competent legal and accounting advice should be sought before creating any business entity.

corporation
an organization formed with governmental approval to act as an artificial person to carry on business (or other activities), which can sue or be sued and (unless not-for-profit) can issue shares of stock to raise capital

Formation and Nature of a Corporation

A **corporation** is "an artificial being, invisible, intangible, and existing only in contemplation of law. Being the mere creature of the law, it possesses only those properties which the charter confers on it, either expressly or as incidental to its very existence."[2] In England and the United States, early corporations were ecclesiastical, educational, charitable, or even governmental in purpose and were usually created by special act of the legislature.

The American Red Cross, for example, is a corporation chartered by the US Congress.

The modern corporation came into prominence in the late nineteenth century with the passage of state statutes regarding business incorporation. These laws allow any group of persons (or in some states, a single individual) to incorporate an enterprise for any lawful purpose, as long as it meets statutory requirements. These corporation laws eliminate the need for special legislative action each time a corporation is created.

General business corporation acts provide for the formation and operation of a wide range of commercial activities, such as manufacturing, wholesaling, and retailing. Most states have a separate corporate statute for not-for-profit organizations and separate laws governing particular types of business, such as banking; public utilities; and the practice of law, medicine, dentistry, accountancy, and similar professions.

Corporate executives need to know the relevant statute under which they operate because it will limit the conduct of the corporation's affairs. The organization has only the powers granted to it by its charter and as specified or implied in the relevant statute.

The Corporation Is a "Person"

Because corporations are legal entities distinct from the individuals who created or manage them, they fall within the definition of "person" for most constitutional and statutory purposes. For example, the Fifth and Fourteenth Amendments to the US Constitution provide that no person shall be deprived of "life, liberty, or property without the due process of law." Similarly, the Fourteenth Amendment provides that no state "shall deny to any person . . . the equal protection of the laws." Corporations are protected by these fundamental doctrines (see Legal Brief). Personhood also enables a corporation to acquire, own, and dispose of property (including stock in other corporations) and to sue and be sued. In short, a corporation is an independent entity with rights and responsibilities of its own.

On the other hand, a corporation is not a "citizen." It cannot vote in an election and is not protected by the Fourteenth Amendment's provision that "no state shall make or enforce any law which shall abridge the privileges or immunities of citizens of the United States." Neither is a corporation protected by the Fifth Amendment's prohibition against self-incrimination because that right applies only to real people (individuals). Similarly, a corporation is not a person for

Legal Brief

Corporations' constitutional rights were confirmed again in the 2010 *Citizens United* case when the US Supreme Court held that corporate funding of political broadcasts during election campaigns is a form of free speech protected by the First Amendment. "Political speech does not lose First Amendment protection 'simply because its source is a corporation.'"[36]

the purpose of licensure statutes because it cannot meet the educational requirements or standards of personal character required for professional licensure.

Forming a Corporation

A corporation is formed by filing *articles of incorporation* with the secretary of
state or other designated official of the state in which incorporation is sought.
On approval, a **corporate charter** is issued. Although requirements regarding the specific content of the articles differ from state to state, the articles
must typically include the following:

corporate charter
the fundamental
document
(usually articles of
incorporation) of a
corporation's legal
authority

- Name of the corporation
- Address of the corporation's office
- Name of the registered agent authorized to receive service of process
- Names and addresses of the incorporators
- Duration of corporate existence (which is usually unlimited)
- Purpose of the corporation
- Names of the initial members of the governing board (also known as
  board of directors and board of trustees)
- Number and classification of shares of stock (in a for-profit
  corporation) or the designation of members, if any (in a not-for-profit
  organization)

The incorporators are those who prepare, sign, and file the articles
of incorporation. Some states require a minimum number of incorporators,
while others permit an individual to act as the incorporator.

Advantages of the Corporate Form of Organization

There are five principal advantages to incorporation:

1. *Limited liability.* Normally, the owners of a corporation are not
   personally liable for the corporation's contracts or torts. A shareholder
   of a for-profit corporation is not personally liable, with a few
   exceptions, for corporate debts beyond the extent of the shareholder's
   investment in the corporation's stock. Similarly, employees generally
   are not personally liable for corporate obligations as long as they act in
   the scope of delegated authority.
2. *Perpetual existence.* Unlike a sole proprietorship or partnership, a
   corporation's continued legal existence and operational capabilities in
   most instances are not affected by the death or disability of an owner.
3. *Free transfer of ownership interests* (at least if the corporation is for-
   profit). Shareholders in the organization can sell their interests to

fellow shareholders or the general public (unless special provisions are made and noted on the stock certificates). Free transferability increases the liquidity and value of corporate investments. State statutes usually provide that membership interests in not-for-profit corporations may not be transferred.

4. *Taxation separate from individual income taxes.* The corporate tax rate is generally lower than the personal income tax rate, and the persons who own the corporation are taxed only on the distributions of income (dividends) they receive, not on their proportionate shares of the entire corporate profit.

5. *Ability to raise capital.* Access to equity capital, as distinct from borrowing and creating debt, is a major consideration when undertaking new or expanded ventures.

Powers of a Corporation

A corporation may act only within its corporate authority, and its powers are limited to those consistent with its charter (articles of incorporation) and the statute under which it was formed.

There are two kinds of powers: express and implied. *Express powers* are those specifically designated by charter or statute. The relevant statute under which the corporation is formed enumerates express powers, such as the power to buy, lease, or otherwise acquire and hold property and the power to make contracts to effectuate corporate purposes. *Implied powers* are those reasonably necessary to carry out the express powers and achieve the corporation's purposes and objectives.

Any departure from express or implied corporate power is said to be *ultra vires* (Latin for "beyond the power" of the corporation). For example, *Charlotte Hungerford Hospital v. Mulvey*, although not involving a typical corporate charter, illustrates the importance of knowing the limits of corporate power. (To read this case, see The Court Decides at the end of this chapter.) Therefore, in planning for the future and in making commitments, the governing body of the corporation must keep a close eye on the corporation's legal authority, and legal advice regarding this issue is of utmost importance. For example, if a not-for-profit corporation makes a donation or transfers assets to another institution for a purpose not included in its own charter, the donation or transfer is ultra vires. As such, it could be challenged in a suit for an injunction and would likely be held void.

An ultra vires transaction is distinguished from an illegal act. The latter is an absolutely void transaction; an example is employment by the hospital of an unlicensed professional person to act in that professional capacity.[3]

Some hospital transactions that may raise questions about corporate power include the following:

- Lending credit or guaranteeing the debts of another corporation
- Issuing loans to its corporate trustees, officers, or members
- Forming a partnership with another corporation or an individual
- Consolidating or merging with another corporation[4]
- A public hospital leasing facilities to a private corporation[5]
- A public hospital engaging in independent private business enterprises without statutory authority to do so[6]

These transactions are not necessarily ultra vires, but the authority to engage in them must be verified with legal counsel. (Corporate consolidations and mergers are discussed later in this chapter.)

Not-for-Profit Corporation

not-for-profit (or nonprofit)
a type of organization in which legal and ethical restrictions prohibit distribution of profits to owners or shareholders

A general business corporation is owned by shareholders, who are entitled and expect to receive dividends from the earnings of the corporation and to share in assets should the corporation be dissolved. But no part of the net earnings of a **not-for-profit** corporation may be distributed for the private gain of its members, directors or trustees, officers, or other private individuals. However, a not-for-profit corporation can earn income and make a profit (see Legal Brief) without sacrificing its not-for-profit status, as long as it uses that profit for institutional purposes. Moreover, it can, without question, pay its employees; as long as the compensation paid is reasonable, it is not "private gain" that would jeopardize the corporation's not-for-profit status.[7]

Motive is important in determining not-for-profit status. In a not-for-profit institution, motives of ethical, moral, or social purposes predominate and profit is secondary to the overall purpose. But a mere declaration of not-for-profit purpose in a corporate charter is never conclusive if the entity is being used as an alter ego for private gain.[8] For this reason, the purpose clause in the articles of incorporation of a not-for-profit corporation is usually restrictive. Although a not-for-profit corporation can be organized for many lawful aims, the incorporators normally state a specific purpose, such as establishing a hospital, a symphony orchestra, or a museum of fine arts.

Although charitable status is contingent on not-for-profit status, a not-for-profit corporation need not have a charitable purpose. Many social clubs and similar organizations that provide services exclusively to members are organized and operated as legitimate not-for-profit

Legal Brief

The terms *not-for-profit* and *nonprofit* are synonymous. The former expression is preferred, however, because it emphasizes that the purpose of the corporation is not to make a profit even though it may (and usually does) do so. Clearly, no corporation can long survive with a negative bottom line.

corporations without charitable or benevolent purposes. Such corporations do not qualify for the tax-exempt status that charitable corporations enjoy (see chapter 12).

Not-for-profit status is a prerequisite to tax exemption not only under federal law but also under the various state statutes providing for taxes on sales, income, and real or personal property.[9]

Not-for-profit corporations do not have shareholders, but they may or may not have "corporate members" (depending on the provisions of the law under which they are incorporated). These members are roughly equivalent to a business corporation's shareholders, but they are not entitled to receive dividends. Like shareholders, however, they hold certain *reserved powers*, such as the authority to

- elect directors to the governing body;
- approve merger or dissolution of the corporation;
- amend the articles of incorporation and bylaws, including the corporate purpose;
- set the corporate philosophy and mission; and
- adopt annual budgets, unless the board of directors is given this power.

In most states, members must meet at least annually to conduct business. In a corporation without members, the board of directors is the sole governing authority, and it has the statutory power to exercise the reserved powers. In any event, the reserved powers are set forth in the not-for-profit corporation law and the articles of incorporation.

Upon the dissolution or merger of a not-for-profit corporation, the assets of the corporation must be distributed in accordance with state law and the provisions of the articles of incorporation.

Internal Management of a Corporation

Corporate bylaws contain rules for the internal management and governance of corporations. Unless state statutes or a corporation's articles of incorporation provide otherwise, the power to adopt and amend a corporation's bylaws lies with its members or shareholders. In short, the governing body of a corporation cannot adopt or amend corporate bylaws unless state statutes or the corporation's charter has specifically granted it this power. The bylaws define the rights and duties of the corporate members or shareholders, the powers and responsibilities of the governing body, and the rights and duties of the major corporate officers. Corporate bylaws are an internal document; hence, they need not be filed in any public office or otherwise made available for public inspection (unless state law so requires).

As noted earlier, certain extraordinary matters normally require the vote of members or shareholders. As discussed in the following section, other major powers reside with the governing board. Otherwise, the day-to-day management of the corporation is the responsibility of its CEO and other management staff.

Responsibilities of the Governing Board

The governing body of a healthcare institution has four major functions:

1. Develop policy and strategic plans
2. Appoint senior administration and medical staff members
3. Delineate clinical privileges
4. Oversee the professional performance of lay administrators and the medical staff

To fulfill these functions properly, the board must ensure the proper organization of its own committee structure. For example, the board must ensure that the executive committee is properly executing corporate policy in the interval between board meetings, and this committee must not assume the decision-making power legally reserved for the whole board or for corporate members or shareholders. Moreover, the executive committee is usually not permitted to delegate its responsibilities to any single member of the committee.

In addition to the executive committee, other standing committees often include committees on finance, medical staff relations, corporate compliance, buildings and grounds, personnel, public relations, and education.

Having set policy for the institution, the board must ensure that the medical staff and management execute it effectively. The board should not become involved in the details of day-to-day operations—these responsibilities should be delegated to hospital administration and the medical staff—but it must have mechanisms in place to review performance and hold accountable the corporation's agents (employees or others authorized to act on the organization's behalf). When authority for implementing policy is delegated, it can be revoked if performance is unsatisfactory. The board must monitor delegated powers; it cannot abdicate its oversight responsibilities.

Board Composition and Meetings

The board's size is determined by the articles of incorporation or bylaws. Some states require a minimum number of directors—usually three—while others allow as few as one board director.[10] In a not-for-profit corporation of the membership type, the corporate members elect the governing board. In a not-for-profit corporation without corporate members, the board may select new directors; boards that do so are referred to as "self-perpetuating." In some situations, such as in a state or county hospital, a public official or body may appoint the directors. Terms of office and qualifications of these directors are determined by charter or bylaw provisions drafted in accordance with statutory requirements. For example, local statutes may require that directors be of majority age and that a certain number be residents of the state of incorporation.[11]

Removal of directors for cause and special elections to fill vacancies on the board are governed by provisions of state law and the corporate charter. Legal counsel should be sought in such situations.

Directors usually cannot be paid or compensated for their services unless local law and the corporate charter permit it. This rule is particularly relevant to not-for-profit corporations because of the fundamental doctrine that members and directors of not-for-profits must not derive personal financial gain from the corporation. (This prohibition does not exclude the salary paid to a director who is also a corporate employee.)

A unique provision exists in West Virginia. A licensing statute enacted in 1983 requires that at least 40 percent of the governing boards of local government and not-for-profit hospitals be equal numbers of individuals who operate small businesses, belong to labor organizations, are elderly, and are low income. The statute was meant to control healthcare costs, but there is no evidence that the presence of consumer representatives on healthcare organizations' boards helps reduce healthcare expenditures. Only one reported case exists in which the law was much of an issue, and even then it was not especially significant.[12]

In managing the affairs of the corporation, the board must act in properly constituted, formal meetings. Independent action by one or even by a majority of directors does not bind the corporation. Except for regular meetings provided for in the articles of incorporation or corporate bylaws, proper notice (usually in writing) of a meeting must be given to each director. Unless such notice is given, the meeting is invalid. There is one exception: If all directors attend a meeting that was called without proper notice, they have, in effect, waived the notice requirement. Even so, decisions made at a casual, unannounced gathering of the board may lack legal effect. If the statutes permit, meetings can be held by teleconference; otherwise, directors must attend in person.[13]

A written record (minutes) should be made of the actions taken at each board meeting. Directors who object to a proposed action should make certain that their dissents are noted in the record. The frequency of meetings depends on provisions in the charter or bylaws and on particular circumstances. Unless the local statutes, charter, or bylaws provide otherwise, the location of the board meeting may be at the discretion of the board.

Meetings may even occur outside the state of incorporation, as long as the place is a reasonably convenient destination.

The charter or bylaws fix the number of directors necessary for a quorum. In the absence of a provision, the rule is that a quorum is a simple majority of the board and that a majority vote is sufficient to bind the corporation. Directors may not vote by proxy in the absence of a specific statutory or bylaw provision because each director has a fiduciary duty to attend meetings personally and exercise independent judgment.

The foregoing general principles of corporate law are reflected in the hospital accreditation standards published by The Joint Commission. Note also that many public hospitals (e.g., those owned by counties, cities, tax districts) are governed by the provisions of open-meetings legislation ("*sunshine laws*") as to the frequency, location, and public notice of meetings and the public's right to attend.

The Governing Board's Duties

Directors have *fiduciary* duties—special responsibilities owed to the corporation, its members (if any), and its intended beneficiaries. For the governing board of a hospital corporation, these duties include the following:

- Acting with loyalty and due care
- Protecting hospital property
- Not engaging in self-dealing and conflicts of interest
- Establishing and overseeing the hospital's strategic goals
- Selecting the CEO
- Selecting a qualified medical staff
- Monitoring the quality of medical care
- Establishing operating budgets

Fiduciary duties can be summarized in two words: loyalty and responsibility.

Members of the governing board of charitable corporations are frequently called *trustees*. They are not trustees in the formal sense, however, because a traditional trustee holds legal title to property and manages that property for the benefit of others. In a corporation, however, the title to property is vested in the corporation itself. Furthermore, under trust law, the duty of a trustee is generally higher than the duty of a corporate director. For example, the trustee of a trust may be liable for poor business judgments in the management of the property held for the beneficiaries' benefit. A corporate director would generally be held liable only for actual negligence, willful disregard of duty, or wrongful acts.

Throughout the following discussion we use the term *director* to encompass board members of charitable corporations generally.

Duty of Loyalty

Loyalty to the organization is the paramount duty. It requires the individual to put the interests of the corporation before self-interest. Specifically, no director is permitted to gain personally, accept bribes, or compete with the corporation.[14]

The duty of loyalty also raises the question of whether a director can personally contract with the corporation. Can directors, for instance, sell supplies or services to the hospital? The answer is yes if certain high standards are met. A director may usually contract with the corporation if the contract is fair, if full disclosure of all personal interest is made, and if utmost good faith is exercised. A director should never vote on or participate in the board's decision to approve or veto the transaction, either directly or through an agent. Competitive bids should be solicited to establish the fairness of the contract. The burden of proving the fairness of a contract and disclosing self-interest is always on the individual director, and the court will closely scrutinize the transaction if the matter is challenged. For a director, buying from a hospital and then reselling at a personal profit is riskier than selling personal property or services to the institution at fair market value. A contract with a director that does not meet the aforementioned standards is not void, but it is voidable.[15]

There may be specific state statutes pertaining to directors' contracts with the corporation they serve.[16] In a government hospital, state law may prohibit all transactions between a director and the corporation, even if full disclosure is made and the contract is fair. Whenever directors wish to contract with the corporation they serve, they and the board should seek careful legal advice based on local law.

Every hospital should have and follow conflict-of-interest policies. Each director must be required to file a written declaration of possible conflicts of interest and disclose gifts, gratuities, and lavish entertainment offered by companies that do business with the hospital.

Duty of Responsibility

The duty of responsibility is to act with due care in every activity of the board. Good faith and honesty are the major tests in determining whether due care has been exercised. This same standard of care is imposed on the director of a business corporation.[17]

Directors of a hospital corporation must take an active role in directing the company. Merely preserving corporate property as caretakers is not enough; they must use corporate property to achieve corporate objectives. Directors must attend meetings of the board and actively participate in decision making by learning about the issues, asking appropriate questions, and demonstrating complete rectitude in their decisions.

The duty of responsibility also includes exercising reasonable care in selecting and appointing the CEO and other corporate agents, such as outside legal counsel.[18] Directors must use reasonable care in supervising the agents they appoint and in holding them accountable, and they have a duty to remove an incompetent CEO or other agent.

Directors also have a duty to use reasonable care in appointing individuals to the medical staff. Per case law, a corporate duty exists to restrict clinical privileges or to terminate an appointment when the board knows, or should have known, of incompetence on the part of a medical staff member (see chapters 7 and 8). A corporation may be held liable if the board knew of professional malpractice—or should have known about it from the managers and medical staff departments charged with reviewing each staff physician's clinical performance—but did not take action.

In reaching their decisions, directors may rely on written, documented reports and recommendations from responsible professional sources such as medical staff committees, accountants, and legal counsel. They need not personally verify all items in these reports if no activity arouses suspicion or question,[19] but they face potential liability if they fail to obtain professional advice when a problem becomes apparent—for example, if they fail to obtain competent legal counsel when the hospital has a recognizable legal issue.

In general, directors are not personally liable for honest errors in business judgment. This standard is consistent with that applicable to the directors of for-profit corporations and means that board members must exercise the judgment that reasonably prudent directors or trustees would be expected to exercise under similar circumstances. An example of dishonest business judgment that could render a director personally liable is permitting institutional funds to remain in a bank that she knew or ought to have known was in financial straits.[20]

A famous case involving Sibley Memorial Hospital in Washington, DC, illustrates the kinds of responsibilities board directors carry and the difficulties that can arise when directors do not adhere to them (see The Court Decides: *Stern v. Lucy Webb Hayes National Training School for Deaconesses and Missionaries* at the end of this chapter). As you read this case, remember that its facts occurred more than 50 years ago. For this reason, the sanctions the court meted out are mild compared with what would be ordered if a board today abdicated its responsibilities in the way Sibley Memorial's board did.

Protection Against Liability

In general, hospital directors' personal liability is not a serious financial risk as long as they regularly attend board meetings, vote personally, avoid conflicts of interest, and exercise utmost good faith and honesty in overseeing the corporation's affairs. The best means of establishing good faith and honesty is a written record of all the board's deliberations, including the votes of individual directors on transactions that involve personal interests. Any director who dissents from majority action of the board should make sure that his dissent is part of the written record.

Individual directors and corporate officers have two means of protecting themselves: (1) purchasing liability insurance and (2) making sure that the corporation has appropriate indemnification provisions to protect them in the event they suffer personal loss as a result of exercising their (good faith) board responsibilities.

Many not-for-profit corporations favor indemnification plans or a combination of insurance and indemnity. Insurance for directors and officers (D&O coverage) may exclude coverage for gross negligence, intentional acts, and criminal activity. *Indemnification* is corporate reimbursement of a trustee's personal expenses in the event the trustee faces a civil suit or criminal prosecution for alleged violation of fiduciary responsibilities. The trustee may be reimbursed for attorneys' fees and possibly for amounts paid as a result of a judgment against the individual. The hospital may, in turn, purchase insurance covering the costs of indemnification. Careful legal advice is necessary to ensure that directors understand the circumstances under which insurance and indemnification can and cannot be provided. Drafting the corporate charter or bylaw provisions covering these issues with utmost care is imperative.

Responsibilities of Management

Under the overall guidance of the governing board, a group of people known as "management" (see Legal Brief) run the day-to-day operations of the corporation. Management is an art, and like art, it is hard to define. From Adam Smith and John Stuart Mill in the eighteenth and nineteenth centuries, to Frederick Winslow Taylor and Henri Fayol around the turn of the twentieth century, and through Peter Drucker more recently, many have tried to define management in scientific terms. All have failed to some degree. But no matter how one describes management, it is the function of an organization that is

Legal Brief

The word *management* comes from the Latin *manu agere*, meaning "to lead by the hand"—as in training horses, for example. We prefer to think of enlightened managers as people who set goals and empower others to reach those goals, not as taskmasters who pull employees along by the bridle. Regardless of the metaphor, the fact remains that the job of management (or leadership, if you prefer) is to enable people to get things done. *Administration* is derived from the Latin *administratio*, a compound of *ad* ("to") and *ministratio* ("serve"). The term is also the source of the verb *to minister*.

concerned with setting goals (strategy), creating an action plan to achieve those goals (tactics), measuring outcomes, and reassessing the strategy and tactics on the basis of those outcomes.

In a healthcare organization, management functions begin with senior administrative positions, including those of CEO, vice president, and department director (or similar titles). Their responsibilities include the following:

- Supporting the governing board in its strategic planning and policymaking activities
- Carrying out (implementing, administering, executing) the board's policies and strategic goals
- Communicating board policies and the strategic plan to employees and the medical staff
- Overseeing day-to-day operations, including personnel functions and personnel records
- Measuring the quality of patient care
- Managing operating funds
- Selecting qualified junior executives
- Conducting necessary business transactions

Management must report regularly to the governing board on the general status of these activities while maintaining a distinction between the board's governance role and management's day-to-day operations.

Because corporations can act only through people, most members of management find they spend large portions of their time dealing with personnel issues, such as recruitment, performance reviews, discipline, dispute resolution, terminations, and myriad related subjects. Employment law comes in the form of statutes, regulations, and a large body of common law addressing such topics as the following:

- Nondiscrimination
- Sexual harassment
- Minimum wage and maximum hours standards (Fair Labor Standards Act)
- Collective bargaining
- Unemployment compensation
- Employment at will
- Union activities
- Retaliatory discharge
- Pension plans (Employee Retirement Income Security Act)
- Equal employment opportunity laws

- Occupational safety (Occupational Safety and Health Administration)
- Privacy and confidentiality
- Immigration standards
- Disabilities laws (Americans with Disabilities Act)
- Whistle-blower protections

Education in human resource (HR) management is a full graduate program, and employment law is a full course of its own in many graduate programs. For these reasons, this text cannot do justice to the subject in a few pages. Nevertheless, students must be aware that healthcare executives encounter many situations that implicate labor and employment laws, and dealing with these situations will take up much of their time. The legal principles are complex, and management personnel are advised to rely on their HR professionals and on attorneys who specialize in the type of law involved in the individual situation.[21]

Piercing the Corporate Veil

A corporation is a legal entity that has rights and responsibilities separate from those of its owners. It is a convenient legal fiction, and because it can limit legal and financial liability, it has been an invaluable vehicle for encouraging investment in for-profit and not-for-profit activities. On the other hand, if a corporation is used to "defeat public convenience, justify wrong, protect fraud, or defend crime," the law will disregard the corporate fiction and place liability on the owners of the corporation.[22] This action is known as *piercing the corporate veil*. Most litigated cases in which the corporate veil has been pierced have involved closely held corporations or parent–subsidiary relationships.

For a court to pierce the corporate veil, the party challenging the corporation normally must prove three elements:

1. The corporation's owners dominated it completely.
2. The owners used their control of the corporation to commit fraud or perpetrate a wrong, violate a statutory or other duty, or commit a dishonest or unjust act.
3. Corporate control was the proximate cause of the injury that is the subject of the suit.[23]

Although precedent for piercing the corporate veil is more than a century old, courts are reluctant to look beyond the corporate form.[24] Accordingly, as a general rule, all three elements must be proved to the satisfaction of the "trier of fact" (the judge or the jury, as appropriate).

Complete domination of the corporation means domination of finances, business practices, and corporate policies to such an extent that the entity has no mind or will of its own. Mere directorship of the corporation by a sole shareholder entitled to corporate profits is not enough to justify piercing the veil. Courts look, on a case-by-case basis, for unity of interest and ownership sufficient to destroy the separate identities of the owner or owners and the corporation. Evidence of this unity is found in such factors as the following:

- Mingling of corporate assets with the owner's personal funds
- Neglect of business formalities, such as failure to file separate tax returns, hold regular board meetings, and keep adequate corporate minutes
- Having a mere "paper corporation" with nonfunctioning officers and directors listed in the articles of incorporation
- Insufficient investment of capital in the corporation[25]

The decision whether to disregard the corporate fiction, however, does not rest on a single factor. Courts most often look for several factors suggesting that the corporation and owner should be treated as one and the same.[26] *United States v. Healthwin-Midtown Convalescent Hospital* is a good example.[27] Defendant Israel Zide owned half of the stock of Healthwin, a convalescent center that provided skilled nursing care in return for payments from Medicare. Zide also had a 50 percent interest in a partnership that held title to the real estate occupied by Healthwin and the furnishings of the nursing home. Concluding that the nursing home had been overpaid, the government brought suit against Healthwin and against Zide for the amount of the alleged overpayment. Zide defended the claim against him on the basis that the debt was solely the corporation's and that he was entitled to limited liability.

In rejecting Zide's defense, the court noted these factors:

- He alone controlled the corporation's affairs.
- He was a member of the board, the president of the corporation, and the administrator of the nursing facility.
- He alone signed corporate checks without concurrence of another corporate officer.
- The governing board did not meet regularly.
- He failed to maintain an arm's-length relationship with the corporation by permitting Healthwin's funds to be "inextricably intertwined" with his personal accounts and other business transactions.
- The corporation was seriously undercapitalized, having liabilities consistently in excess of $150,000 and an initial capitalization of only $10,000.
- He diverted corporate funds to the detriment of creditors.

In the court's opinion, these facts demonstrated that Zide used the corporation to accommodate his personal business dealings. The court held that to allow him to escape liability in these circumstances would be unfair to his creditors (including Medicare). Accordingly, Zide was found personally liable for the amount due the federal government because the corporation was a mere alter ego of its principal shareholder.

In addition to the various factors showing a unity of interest and ownership strong enough to outweigh the separate identity of the corporation, for the corporate veil to be pierced, limited liability must result in an inequity. An inequitable result is often found when a statutory duty has been violated or fraud or other wrongful action has been perpetrated (see The Court Decides: *Woodyard, Insurance Commissioner v. Arkansas Diversified Insurance Co.* at the end of this chapter for another case that illustrates judicial application of the doctrine of piercing the corporate veil).

Multi-institutional Systems and Corporate Reorganization: The Independent Hospital as Anachronism

For many years the hospital was a single legal entity, and its purpose was merely to provide doctors with a building, equipment, and supplies so they could treat medical and surgical patients. Today, however, these former "doctors' workshops" operate as multifaceted organizations with teams of people who work together to improve the health and quality of life of the individuals and communities they serve.

This new organizational vision—a focus on promoting health rather than merely treating illness—involves activities that are unfamiliar to a traditional hospital corporation (see Legal Brief). It requires not only different leadership skills but a different corporate structure as well. Therefore, the independent hospital entity is becoming less and less common, and the landscape is now populated with multi-institutional systems that are better suited to the vision of healthcare today. As noted in the next section, corporate reorganization (restructuring) takes several forms; the particular form is determined by the needs of each situation.

Healthcare is now a giant sector (see chapter 2). Beginning in the 1980s, a huge number of corporate reorganizations (and re-reorganizations) enabled hospitals to

- add new service lines,
- maximize revenues,
- reduce costs,

Legal Brief

The vision statement of the American Hospital Association (AHA) is typical of healthcare organizations' modern focus: Our "vision is of a society of healthy communities, where all individuals reach their highest potential for health."[37]

- increase market share,
- partner with physicians or other organizations, and
- obtain freedom from governmental regulation (to the extent possible).

A multiorganizational system can diversify operations and engage in a wide range of activities that a single institution cannot undertake. Subsidiary entities can provide special services or perform functions not related to healthcare without being hampered by certificate-of-need regulations, restrictive corporation laws, and third-party reimbursement regulations.

Multi-institutional system and *corporate reorganization* are generic terms, and no single definition, model, or form exists that describes either concept. The AHA defines *multihospital systems* as "two or more acute care hospitals that are owned, leased, sponsored, or contract-managed by a central organization," and it distinguishes them from *networks*, which are "group[s] of hospitals, physicians, other providers, insurers and/or community agencies that work together to coordinate and deliver a broad spectrum of services to their community."[28] This distinction reminds us that healthcare systems now include skilled nursing facilities, extended care facilities, ambulatory care centers, outpatient surgical centers, hospital-owned physician practices, home health agencies, managed care plans, and various other health-related organizations (see exhibit 6.1 for an example of a multi-institutional healthcare system).

Systems may comprise not-for-profit, proprietary (for-profit), or both types of organizations. For example, a not-for-profit system corporation may own not-for-profit and for-profit subsidiaries. A system may also be owned and managed by state or local government. Whether consisting of multiple corporate entities or a single corporation with multiple divisions, all multi-institutional systems have a corporate office responsible for activities that are best performed centrally, thus providing efficiency and economies of scale. Some functions commonly managed at the corporate level include the following:

- Finance and billing
- Legal and risk management
- Quality assurance
- Compliance
- Legislative advocacy
- Human resources
- Health information management
- Strategic planning
- Education
- Health plan administration

EXHIBIT 6.1
XYZ Regional Health System Organization Chart

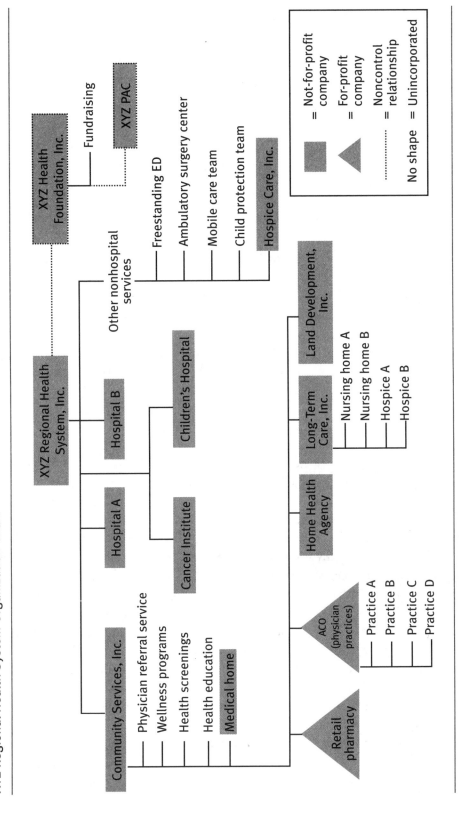

Note: ACO = accountable care organization; PAC = political action committee.

Alternative Corporate Strategies
Sale of Assets

For various reasons, corporations sometimes sell all or a substantial portion of their assets to another corporation. This transaction is relatively straight-forward except that local law must be followed carefully when the seller is a charitable corporation. Normally, the stockholders or members and the governing boards of both the buyer and the seller must approve the terms of the sale. If the seller is a charitable corporation, state laws may require that a designated state officer approve the final arrangement because the state has the ultimate responsibility to enforce the terms of charitable trusts. After the sale is completed, the selling corporation may dissolve or may continue to operate on a restricted scale.

merger or **acquisition** the joining of two or more corporations, whereby one or more of the organizations transfers assets to another (the survivor) and then is dissolved

Merger and Consolidation

Corporations also sometimes wish to join forces with others. They can do so in various ways, including merger, consolidation, and joint venture.

In a **merger** or **acquisition**, two or more corporations are joined, whereby one or more of the organizations transfers assets to another (the survivor) and then is dissolved. A **consolidation**, in contrast, is a transaction in which two or more organizations combine to form a new corporation, thereby dissolving the predecessor companies. The terms are often used interchangeably in casual conversation, but keeping this distinction in mind is advisable: In a merger or acquisition, one company survives after taking over one or more other corporations; in a consolidation, two companies blend into a completely new entity.

consolidation a transaction in which two or more organizations combine to form a new corporation, thereby dissolving the predecessor companies; sometimes used as a general term inclusive of *merger* and *acquisition*

Before completing any type of corporate integration, each party must carefully scrutinize state corporation law; certificate-of-need legislation; the state and federal statutes relevant to charitable organizations, if applicable; and other regulatory requirements. Normally, the governing boards of the corporations involved and the shareholders or members must approve the plan. The terms of any bond documents may require approval of the bond-holders. When the interested parties approve the plan, articles of merger or consolidation are prepared and filed with the appropriate state officer responsible for enforcing the relevant corporate law, who then issues a cer-tificate authorizing the transaction. Once the certificate is issued, the new corporation owns all the property of the former entities, has all their rights and privileges, and is liable for all their debts.[29]

If the merger or consolidation significantly affects competition in the relevant market, it may invite charges of antitrust law violation. (The antitrust aspects of asset acquisitions, consolidations, and mergers are thoroughly dis-cussed in chapter 13.) Most consolidations and mergers, however, benefit the community at large and the institutions involved. Such arrangements not only enhance competition but also enable the surviving corporation(s) to provide a wider range of services, improve quality assurance and risk management, and have greater economies of scale. These arrangements are especially beneficial when one or more of the corporations would have failed had they not combined.

Joint Venture

In contrast to a merger or consolidation, a **joint venture** is a mutual endeavor by two or more organizations for a specific purpose or for a limited duration. This term is loosely applied to a variety of relationships (e.g., between a hospital and a physician practice) for purposes such as

joint venture
a mutual endeavor by two or more organizations for a specific purpose or for a limited duration

- diversifying their activities,
- providing new or additional services to the community,
- seeking capital from interested investors,
- maximizing their reimbursement from Medicare and other governmental healthcare programs, and
- gaining tax benefits.

Although the participants are not agents of each other, other rules of a general partnership normally apply:

- The parties owe fiduciary duties to each other.
- Each has a right to participate in management.
- Property is owned jointly.
- Profits and losses are shared according to an agreement.
- Each participant has unlimited liability to third parties.

As discussed in the following sections, outright employment of physicians is on the rise, but historically joint ventures have been the most common form of hospital–physician collaboration.

Collaborative Strategies with Physicians
Medicare as a Driver

At its inception, Medicare basically paid hospitals and physicians their usual rates for the services they provided. Obviously, under such a system, the more services you provide, the more you get paid. This arrangement was an advantage for both hospital and physician providers, and Medicare spending rose at an annual rate more than twice that of inflation during the 1970s and early 1980s.[30]

Concerned about these sharply rising costs, Congress in 1983 replaced Medicare Part A's cost-based reimbursement system with a *prospective*

Legal Brief

Medicare Part A pays for medically necessary hospitalization, hospice care, skilled nursing, and home health care. It is premium-free to individuals aged 65 or older.

Medicare Part B functions as a health insurance plan, paying for physician visits, outpatient care, medical supplies, and other necessary services. Part B is funded by contributions from the federal government and by monthly enrollee premiums.

Medicare Part C (also known as *Medicare Advantage*) is an alternative to the parts A and B combination.

Medicare Part D covers prescription drugs.

payment system (PPS). (See Legal Brief for a summary of the various "parts" of Medicare.) Under PPS, hospitals were paid a fixed amount per diagnosis as assigned to a diagnosis-related group (DRG), regardless of the length of the patient's stay or the complexity of the treatment rendered. In theory this change would give hospitals reasons to provide services more efficiently and shorten inpatient stays, but it actually created an incentive to increase the number of hospital admissions and diagnoses.

Furthermore, the theory of PPS overlooked certain basic principles. First, physicians—not hospitals—determine most Medicare spending; only physicians can decide when a patient will be admitted or discharged, and only they can order the services the hospital will provide. Second, physicians have traditionally been independent members of hospital medical staffs; they have admitting privileges and may order services, but they are not under the hospital's direct control (see chapter 8).

When Congress imposed PPS on hospitals, it made no fundamental changes to Medicare Part B (the physician payment system). It placed some minor limitations on the physician fee schedule, but the net result of the Medicare amendments of the early 1980s was a set of perverse incentives (see Legal Decision Point): Hospitals were encouraged to be more efficient, but physicians had few reasons to limit—and many reasons to increase—the number of services provided. As the Congressional Budget Office noted in 1986:

> Although part of the increased volume of services provided per enrollee that has occurred since Medicare's inception has been a desirable response to the greater needs of an aging population, aided by remarkable improvements in medical technology, some increases may have been motivated more by physicians' attempts to maintain revenues in the face of fee constraints or insufficient patient-initiated demand for services than by expected benefits for patients.[31]

Congress attempted to address these problems when, in the Balanced Budget Act of 1997, it mandated the *sustainable growth rate* (SGR) method to control the cost of physician services. Under SGR, the physician fee schedule was to be adjusted each year on the basis of the previous year's gross domestic product. If Medicare's expenditures exceeded the target amount,

SGR mandated a corresponding decrease in payments for the following year. Reductions in physician payments were predicted to occur every year as a result.

Implementation of the SGR formula could be suspended by Congress, and in fact, physician groups, including the American Medical Association, successfully lobbied for its suspension and even a modest pay *increase* each year from 1997 onward. This annual "doc fix," as it was called, ultimately led to the SGR being permanently repealed in 2015. In return, policymakers hope that under the Affordable Care Act (ACA), accountable care organizations (more about this later in the chapter) will help reduce Medicare costs by promoting prevention and primary care.

Legal Decision Point

Consider the unfairness (from a hospital's perspective, at least) of the perverse incentives that resulted from the Medicare Part A reforms of the early 1980s. What might have caused this outcome? What political factors do you suppose were involved?

The First Wave of Hospital–Physician Integration

Recognizing the difficult situation they faced, and considering the increasingly competitive and cost-conscious environment of the late 1980s, many healthcare institutions attempted to develop business arrangements with groups of physicians to share risk and reap economic rewards. Most common, hospitals integrated with members of their own medical staffs, but sometimes hospitals acquired the practices of previously unrelated physicians—either by contracted services or through direct employment. Typically, the goals of these collaborative efforts were as follows:

- Reduce costs
- Provide a full range of services along the continuum of care
- Provide practice management and administrative support
- Negotiate contracts with payer organizations
- Generate economies of scale
- Provide access to capital
- Improve quality
- Conduct utilization reviews
- Provide staffing for particular hospital departments (e.g., radiology, anesthesiology, emergency)

The arrangements took different names, such as *management services organization, physician–hospital organization, integrated delivery system,* and *health maintenance organization.* They were often organized as joint ventures but were sometimes corporations, partnerships, or simple contractual arrangements.

Regardless of their organizational form, many well-intentioned hospital–physician collaborations met with limited success, if not outright failure. Hospital executives discovered that managing a physician practice is different from running a hospital and that salaried physicians sometimes do not work as many hours as their contracts require. Physicians, on the other hand, discovered that hospitals are large bureaucracies that can stifle their independence and limit their autonomy. For various reasons, each side was often skeptical of the other; thus, many of the arrangements fell apart.

To be successful, collaboration between physicians and hospitals requires more than a written contract or a lofty mission statement. It requires true congruence of interests. Both groups must have common values, shared governance and management, and common data systems. Full openness and complete trust must exist. Physicians and hospitals learned this lesson the hard way in the 1990s, and interest in hospital–physician collaboration waned.

The Second Wave of Hospital–Physician Integration: Integration Under the ACA

concierge medicine
a relationship between a patient and a primary care physician in which the patient pays an annual fee in return for direct, personalized care; also known as *boutique medicine*

accountable care organizations (ACOs)
organizations of hospitals, physicians, and other providers who—under a shared governance structure—coordinate patient care, are accountable for the quality and cost of that care, and receive bonuses when they deliver care more efficiently

The healthcare environment changed as the twenty-first century arrived, and for various reasons there was a second wave of interest in hospital–physician cooperation. First, declining incomes and the increased administrative stress of private practice prompted many older physicians to retire or switch to **concierge medicine**. Second, during the Great Recession of 2008–2010, younger physicians became more open to hospital employment than had been their counterparts of a few years earlier.[32] Third, in anticipation of medical staff shortages, hospitals made physician recruitment and retention a top priority. Fourth, and perhaps most significant, health reform legislation provided a strong incentive.

The ACA created a new incentive for physicians and hospitals to work together and thus to invent new organizational arrangements by which to do so. The ACA's shared Savings Program encourages creation of provider networks that manage the full continuum of care for their Medicare patients in return for bonuses based on cost savings.[33] These networks—called **accountable care organizations (ACOs)**—come in three forms. The first and largest group consists of organizations that participate in the basic Medicare Shared Savings Program. They are not at risk for failure to meet program goals but are eligible only for lower bonuses. The second group, the Advance Payment Model ACO, is designed for select physician-based and rural providers; they receive up-front and monthly payments that they use to invest in their care coordination efforts. The third and smallest group, the Pioneer Model ACOs, consists of high-performing health systems that are already experienced in coordinating care for patients across care settings. They assume greater risk but also are eligible for higher levels of bonuses. As of early 2016 there were only nine Pioneer Model ACOs.[34]

All ACOs are accountable for the quality and cost of the care they provide to Medicare beneficiaries. They must agree to participate for at least three years, and by statute they must have a "formal legal structure that would allow the organization to receive and distribute payments for shared savings."[35]

From a public policy standpoint, the goal of the ACO program is to "bend the cost curve"—that is, to slow the growth of Medicare expenditures. As this text was being prepared, however, the jury is still out whether ACOs are achieving their intended purpose.

Legal Decision Point

Because some provisions of the ACA are not scheduled to take effect until 2019 at the earliest, the ultimate outcome of its reforms is impossible to predict. Furthermore, the law and the regulations likely will be amended from time to time to correct for unintended consequences or because of changes in the political climate.

Students should be alert for these changes and should monitor developments in all areas of the US healthcare delivery system, particularly how those changes may affect the organization and management of the corporate healthcare institution.

Nevertheless, as ACOs take hold and the ACA becomes fully operative (if it survives various political challenges), the organization and management of corporate healthcare institutions will undoubtedly be greatly affected (see Legal Decision Point). Healthcare executives will need to work closely with their attorneys and other consultants to analyze carefully both the business arguments and the legal reasons for undertaking a particular venture before embarking on it.

Summary

This chapter reviews some basic concepts of corporation law, including a corporation's status as a legal "person," its ability to shield owners from personal liability, the foundation of corporate power, and the duties of a corporation's governing board. The concept of piercing the corporate veil and the various reasons for and methods of restructuring a healthcare corporation are also explored.

The powers of a corporation are limited by state corporation law and the company's organizing documents (the corporate charter). Healthcare executives must be aware of those powers and help—within their limits—the governing board accomplish corporate objectives.

Particular attention is given to the phenomenon of hospital–physician joint ventures, the wax and wane of the trend in the 1990s, and its potential for renewal in the coming years because of the effects of the Affordable Care Act.

Discussion Questions

1. Why is a corporation considered an "artificial person" under the law? What are the consequences of this concept?
2. Describe the advantages of incorporation as opposed to organization as a partnership.
3. Where does one look to find the powers of a corporation?
4. What are the functions and responsibilities of the governing board of a healthcare corporation?
5. Why is the concept of piercing the corporate veil important to any corporation and its subsidiaries?
6. What are the pros and cons of hospital–physician joint ventures?
7. How has health reform legislation affected the organization and management of corporate health institutions?

The Court Decides

Charlotte Hungerford Hospital v. Mulvey
26 Conn. Supp. 394, 225 A.2d 495 (1966)

MacDonald, J.

The plaintiff in this action for a declaratory judgment is a nonstock corporation which for many years has owned and operated a voluntary general hospital in a complex of buildings located on a 120-acre tract of wooded land about one mile from the center of the city of Torrington. The land was acquired under a deed of trust providing that the premises thus conveyed "are to be held and used by said grantee for the purpose of maintaining and carrying on a general hospital and, if a majority of corporators so elect, a training school for nurses in connection therewith may be established, and for no other purpose whatsoever." The deed of trust in question, executed in 1917, specifically provided that "if the land herein granted shall cease to be used for the [stated] purposes, title . . . shall thereupon pass to and vest in said town of Torrington . . . to be used forever as a public park." *[A state statute later chartered the hospital subject to the "terms, conditions, restrictions and provisions" of the deed of trust.]*

Plaintiff [now wants to erect] a medical office building on the hospital grounds [because it] would be of great convenience and advantage both to the individual doctors and to the hospital. . . .

. . . [However,] various questions have arisen with respect to the right, power and authority of plaintiff, under the terms of said deed of trust and special act, to proceed with such a project. . . . The specific questions which the court is requested to answer . . . are (a) whether plaintiff is authorized . . . to construct and operate, as an integral part of its general hospital complex, a medical office

building for members of its medical staff; (b) whether such a medical office building may, under the terms of the aforesaid deed of trust, be located on a portion of the land held by plaintiff thereunder; (c) whether . . . the plaintiff is authorized and empowered to lease . . . a portion of the land included in the aforesaid deed of trust [to a subsidiary corporation that will operate the medical office building]; [and] (d) whether, in addition to offices and office suites for members of plaintiff's medical staff, said building may contain facilities related to or supporting such offices and suites, such as medical laboratories, pharmacies and dispensaries.

The court, after hearing the evidence and the arguments of counsel with full participation by counsel representing the only interested parties, namely, the attorney general of the state of Connecticut, as representative of the public interest in the protection of trusts for charitable uses and purposes . . . and the city of Torrington, contingent beneficiary, has no hesitation in answering all four of the questions posed in the affirmative. It is clear . . . that the proposed project would materially aid the plaintiff in more efficiently carrying out the stated purposes of the trust deed under which it was founded. . . . It is equally clear from the extremely impressive testimony of [the president of the AHA and another witness] that the modern trend is almost universally toward the practice of having nonprofit hospitals provide physicians' private offices for rental to staff members, either in the hospital buildings themselves or on the hospital grounds. . . .

(continued)

(continued from previous page)

The language of the deed of trust is to be construed in light of the settlor's purpose. And reasonable deviations and expanded interpretations must be made from time to time in order to keep pace with changes in recognized concepts of the proper sphere of general hospital operations. . . . Such

deviations are recognized by our Connecticut courts even though the elements for applying cy pres principles are not present.

A decree may enter advising plaintiff of its rights, powers and authority herein by answering the four questions propounded in the affirmative. ■

Discussion Questions

1. Why is the state attorney general an "interested party" to these proceedings?
2. What is a *settlor*?
3. What are *cy pres* principles?
4. How does this case enhance your understanding of the limits of corporate power?

The Court Decides

Stern v. Lucy Webb Hayes National Training School for Deaconesses and Missionaries
381 F. Supp. 1003 (D. D.C. 1974)

Gesell, J.

[This case is a class action suit in which patients of Sibley Memorial Hospital, known officially by the name shown, challenged various aspects of the hospital's management and governance. The defendants were certain members of the hospital's board of trustees and the hospital itself. For a summary of the differences between trustees of a trust and directors of a corporation, see the discussion in this chapter.]

The two principal contentions in the complaint are that the defendant trustees conspired to enrich themselves and certain financial institutions with which they were affiliated by favoring those institutions in financial dealings with the Hospital, and that they breached their fiduciary duties of care

and loyalty in the management of Sibley's funds. . . .

[The court explains that the hospital was begun by the Methodist Church–affiliated Lucy Webb Hayes School in 1895 and eventually became the school's main activity.]

In 1960 . . . the Sibley Board of Trustees revised the corporate by-laws. . . . Under the new by-laws, the Board was to consist of from 25 to 35 trustees, who were to meet at least twice each year. Between such meetings, an Executive Committee was to represent the Board [and in effect had full power to run the hospital]. . . .

In fact, management of the Hospital from the early 1950s until 1968 was handled almost exclusively by two trustee officers: Dr. Orem, the Hospital Administrator, and Mr. Ernst, the Treasurer. Unlike most of their fellow trustees, to whom membership on the Sibley Board was a charitable service incidental to their principal vocations, Orem and Ernst were continuously involved on almost a daily basis in the affairs of Sibley. They dominated the Board and its Executive Committee, which routinely accepted their recommendations and ratified their actions. Even more significantly, neither the Finance Committee nor the Investment Committee ever met or conducted business from the date of their creation until 1971, three years after the death of Dr. Orem. As a result, budgetary and investment decisions during this period, like most other management decisions affecting the Hospital's finances, were handled by Orem and Ernst, receiving only cursory supervision from the Executive Committee and the full Board.

[It was only after the deaths of Dr. Orem and Mr. Ernst (in 1968 and 1972, respectively) that other trustees began to assert themselves and exercise supervision over the financial affairs of the hospital. At that point, it became known that over the years "unnecessarily large amounts of [Sibley's] money" had been deposited in accounts bearing little or no interest at banks in which trustees had a financial interest. At the same time, the hospital bought certificates of deposit that paid lower-than-market rates and took out loans with interest rates higher than the interest rates being paid on funds deposited.

Because there was no evidence that the trustees, other than Dr. Orem and Mr. Ernst, had ever actually agreed to engage in or profit from these activities, the court found insufficient evidence to prove a conspiracy among them. The court then proceeds to discuss the allegations of breach of fiduciary duty.]

III. Breach of Duty.
Plaintiffs' second contention is that, even if the facts do not establish a conspiracy, they do reveal serious breaches of duty on

the part of the defendant trustees and the knowing acceptance of benefits from those breaches by the defendant banks and savings and loan associations.

A. The Trustees.
Basically, the trustees are charged with mismanagement, nonmanagement and self-dealing. The applicable law is unsettled. . . . [H]owever, the modern trend is to apply corporate rather than trust principles in determining the liability of the directors of charitable corporations, because their functions are virtually indistinguishable from those of their "pure" corporate counterparts.

1. Mismanagement.
. . . Since the board members of most large charitable corporations fall within the corporate rather than the trust model, being charged with the operation of ongoing businesses, it has been said that they should only be held to the less stringent corporate standard of care. More specifically, directors of charitable corporations are required to exercise ordinary and reasonable care in the performance of their duties, exhibiting honesty and good faith.

2. Nonmanagement.
. . . A corporate director . . . may delegate his investment responsibility to fellow directors, corporate officers, or even outsiders, but he must continue to exercise general supervision over the activities of his delegates. Once again, the rule for charitable corporations is . . . the traditional corporate rule: directors should at least be permitted to delegate investment decisions to a committee of board members, so long as all directors assume the responsibility for supervising such committees by periodically scrutinizing their work.

Total abdication of the supervisory role, however, is improper even under traditional corporate principles. A director who fails to acquire the information necessary to

(continued)

(continued from previous page)

supervise investment policy or consistently fails even to attend the meetings at which such policies are considered has violated his fiduciary duty to the corporation. While a director is, of course, permitted to rely upon the expertise of those to whom he has delegated investment responsibility, such reliance is a tool for interpreting the delegate's reports, not an excuse for dispensing with or ignoring such reports. . . .

3. Self-dealing.
Under District of Columbia Law, neither trustees nor corporate directors are absolutely barred from placing funds under their control into a bank having an interlocking directorship with their own institution. In both cases, however, such transactions will be subjected to the closest scrutiny to determine whether or not the duty of loyalty has been violated. . . .
. . .
  Trustees may be found guilty of a breach of trust even for mere negligence in the maintenance of accounts in banks with which they are associated while corporate directors are generally only required to show "entire fairness" to the corporation and "full disclosure" of the potential conflict of interest to the Board.
  Most courts apply the less stringent corporate rule to charitable corporations in this area as well. It is, however, occasionally added that a director should not only disclose his interlocking responsibilities but also refrain from voting on or otherwise influencing a corporate decision to transact business with a company in which he has a significant interest or control.
  [The court goes on to point out that the hospital board had recently adopted the AHA's policy guidelines that essentially imposed the standards described earlier: (1) a duality or conflict of interest should be disclosed to other members of the board, (2) board members should not vote on such matters, and (3) the disclosure and abstention

from voting should be recorded in the minutes.]
  . . . [T]he Court holds that a director . . . of a charitable hospital . . . is in default of his fiduciary duty to manage the fiscal and investment affairs of the hospital if it has been shown by a preponderance of the evidence that
  (1) . . . he has failed to use due diligence in supervising the actions of those officers, employees or outside experts to whom the responsibility for making day-to-day financial or investment decisions has been delegated; or
  (2) he knowingly permitted the hospital to enter into a business transaction with himself or with any [business entity] in which he then had a substantial interest or held a position as trustee, director, general manager or principal officer [without disclosing that fact]; or
  (3) except [with disclosure], he actively participated in or voted in favor of a decision . . . to transact business with himself or with any [business entity] in which he then had a substantial interest or held a position as trustee, director, general manager or principal officer; or
  (4) he otherwise failed to perform his duties honestly, in good faith, and with a reasonable amount of diligence and care. Applying these standards to the facts in the record, the Court finds that each of the defendant trustees has breached his fiduciary duty to supervise the management of Sibley's investments. . . .
  [In conclusion, the court noted that the plaintiffs pushed for strict sanctions against the various defendants: the removal of certain board members, the cessation of all business transactions with their related firms, an accounting of all hospital funds, and awards of money damages against the individual defendants. But the court declined to adopt these rather severe measures.
  The court points out the factors that it considered significant: (1) the defendant

trustees are a small minority of the board, whereas all board members were in some way guilty of nonmanagement; (2) the defective practices have been corrected, and those who were most responsible for them have either died or been dismissed; (3) the defendants did not profit personally from the transactions; (4) the defendants will soon leave the board because of age, illness, or the completion of a normal term; and (5) this case is essentially the first in the District of Columbia to discuss these issues

comprehensively, and thus no clear legal standards previously existed.

For these reasons, the court declines to remove the defendants from the board, to assess money damages, or to take other more severe actions. Instead, it requires new policies and procedures to make certain that all present and future trustees are aware of the requirements of the law and that they fully disclose all hospital transactions with any financial institutions in which they have an interest or position.]

Discussion Questions

1. If this case were decided today, would the outcome be different? If so, how?
2. As the CEO or board member of a not-for-profit hospital corporation, what measures would you put in place to prevent a repeat of the activities that led to the lawsuit involved here?
3. How would you summarize the duties of board members on the basis of the holding in this case?

The Court Decides

Woodyard, Insurance Commissioner v. Arkansas Diversified Insurance Co.
268 Ark. 94, 594 S.W.2d 13 (1980)

Hickman, J.

The appellant is Arkansas Insurance Commissioner W. H. L. Woodyard, III. The appellee is Arkansas Diversified Insurance Company (ADIC).

ADIC sought a certificate of authority from Woodyard to sell group life insurance to Blue Cross and Blue Shield . . . subscriber groups. Woodyard denied the application. On appeal, his decision was reversed by the Pulaski

County Circuit Court as being arbitrary and not supported by substantial evidence. We find on appeal [that] the circuit court was wrong and [we] reverse the judgment. We affirm the commissioner.

The only evidence before the commissioner was presented by ADIC. The appellee candidly admitted it was a wholly owned subsidiary of a corporation named Arkansas

(continued)

(continued from previous page)

Diversified Services, Inc. (ADS) which is a wholly owned subsidiary of Blue Cross and Blue Shield, Inc.

. . .

ADIC candidly admitted it was created solely to serve Blue Cross customers. It would provide services that could not otherwise be provided by law. . . . ADS wanted its own life [insurance] company to better compete in the market place.

Blue Cross owns all the stock of ADS, which in turn owns all the stock of ADIC. The president of Blue Cross is the president of both ADS and ADIC. Other Blue Cross officials hold positions in ADS and ADIC. The companies use the same location and similar stationery. ADIC will use Blue Cross employees to sell insurance. Underwriting for ADIC will be done by a division of ADS.

There was no real controversy over the commissioner's findings of fact. He concluded that:

(2) That [Arkansas law] would apparently authorize a hospital and medical service corporation [of which Blue Cross is one] to invest in a wholly owned subsidiary insurance corporation with the Commissioner's consent.

(3) That Blue Cross is limited by [law] to transact business as a non-profit hospital and medical service corporation.

(4) That ADIC is not a separate corporate entity from Blue Cross since Blue Cross through ADS owns all the capital stock of ADIC. ADIC has common Officers and Directors with Blue Cross, Blue Cross pays the salary for the Officers and employees of ADIC, ADIC will sell its products only to Blue Cross subscriber groups and the record indicates that ADIC is to be treated as a division of Blue Cross. The evidence indicates that ADIC's management will not act independently but will conduct the affairs of ADIC in a manner calculated primarily to further the interest of Blue Cross.

. . .

The commissioner found that since Blue Cross could not sell life insurance itself, it

should not be able to do so through corporate subsidiaries. We find that decision neither arbitrary nor unsupported by substantial evidence.

. . .

We agree with the commissioner's finding that [Arkansas law] limits the power of medical corporations to providing medical service. If it did not, they could not only sell life insurance, but automobiles or anything else. Clearly, an insurance company organized under a charter or statute empowering it to sell one kind of insurance lacks authority to sell another.

The appellees argue that even if the commissioner was right in ruling Blue Cross could not market its own life insurance policies, Blue Cross could . . . invest in a wholly owned subsidiary which would [have that power]. The statutes, however, provide that such an investment can be made only with the commissioner's consent. . . .

Blue Cross is a tax exempt, non-profit corporation enjoying a financial advantage over conventional insurers. Allowing it to sell, through subsidiaries, its own life insurance policies, could be unfair to competitors. While the commissioner did allow Blue Cross to invest in ADS, we can see why he disapproved of ADIC. ADS, unlike ADIC, could sell only policies written by insurance companies which lacked the competitive advantages of Blue Cross.

The appellee argues the commissioner arbitrarily pierced the corporate veil of these subsidiaries. . . . [C]ourts will ignore the corporate form of a subsidiary where fairness demands it. Usually, this will be where it is necessary to prevent wrongdoing and where the subsidiary is a mere tool of the parent. We believe both criteria were met here. . . .

Blue Cross, through its president and other officials, candidly admitted why they wanted ADIC to sell insurance. Blue Cross can, through its total control of both subsidiaries by stock, officers and directors, direct all efforts and endeavors of ADIC, and collect all profits.

We cannot say the commissioner was wrong in piercing the corporate veil or in denying the application. The facts are clearly there to support his findings. This order is not contrary to law.

Reversed. ■

Discussion Questions

1. How does a Blue Cross health plan fall under the definition of a "hospital and medical service corporation"?
2. What is the function of that type of corporation in the healthcare system? (Other states assign different names to those corporations. Do you know what those names are?)
3. What differences in this situation might have led to a different outcome in the case?

Notes

1. Since 1914, the National Conference of Commissioners on Uniform State Laws has promoted a Uniform Partnership Act (UPA) for adoption by the various states and territories. Louisiana is the only state that has not adopted some version of the UPA. *See* 6 U.L.A. 1 (Supp. 1986) (table of jurisdictions).
2. Trustees of Dartmouth College v. Woodward, 17 U.S. (4 Wheat) 518, 636 (1819).
3. *See, e.g.*, Tovar v. Paxton Memorial Hosp., 29 Ill. App. 3d 218, 330 N.E.2d 247 (1975) (a physician licensed in Kansas but not licensed in Illinois could not maintain an action for an alleged breach of an employment contract with an Illinois hospital because the contract was illegal and thus void).
4. *See generally* Oleksy v. Sisters of Mercy, 92 Mich. App. 770, 285 N.W.2d 455 (1979) (a private charitable hospital has statutory authority to convey its assets to another not-for-profit private hospital; the transaction is not ultra vires).
5. Op. Fla. Att'y Gen. 82-44 (1982).
6. Tift County Hosp. Auth. v. MRS of Tifton, GA, Inc., 255 Ga. 164, 335 S.E.2d 546 (1985).
7. For example, the Michigan statute specifically states that a not-for-profit corporation "may pay compensation in a reasonable amount to shareholders, members, directors, or officers for services rendered to the corporation." Mich. Comp. Laws Ann. § 450.2301(3)(a).
8. *See* 18 C.J.S. *Corporations* § 10 (2009).

9. *See* I.R.C. § 501.

10. *See, e.g.,* Ohio Rev. Code Ann. § 1702.27 (A)(1). The Ohio nonprofit corporation statute states, "The number of directors as fixed by the articles or the regulations shall not be less than three or, if not so fixed, the number shall be three." *See also* Mich. Comp. Laws Ann. § 450.2505 (1) (West Supp. 1986), which states that "the board shall consist of 3 or more directors. The bylaws shall fix the number of directors or establish the manner for fixing the number, unless the articles of incorporation fix the number."

11. For example, a California statute prohibits anyone who owns stock or has any property interest in a private hospital or is a director or officer of a private hospital from serving as a director or officer of a public hospital serving the same area. Cal. Health & Safety Code § 32110 (West 1973 and Supp. 1986). Accordingly, in Franzblau v. Monardo, 108 Cal. App. 3d 522, 166 Cal. Rptr. 610 (1980), the president of a not-for-profit private hospital was prohibited from serving as a director of the public hospital district.

12. W. Va. Code § 16-5B-6a (1985). The law was upheld in the face of a constitutional challenge. Am. Hosp. Ass'n v. Hansbarger, 600 F. Supp. 465 (N.D.W.Va., 1984), *aff'd* Am. Hosp. Ass'n v. Hansbarger, 783 F.2d 1184 (C.A.4 (W.Va.), 1986). In Christie v. Elkins Area Medical Center, 366 S.E.2d 753, 179 W.V. 247 (1988), the court reversed a trial court's finding that a local board was properly constituted and remanded the case for further consideration. The case does not appear in subsequent reports, thus it is surmised that the matter was settled.

13. *See, e.g.,* Mich. Comp. Laws Ann. § 450.2521(3) (West Supp. 1986).

14. With respect to the duty of loyalty, *see* Patient Care Services, S.C. v. Segal, 32 Ill. App. 3d 1021, 337 N.E.2d 471 (1975). A corporate officer and director who actively engaged in a rival and competing business to the detriment of a corporation must answer to the corporation for injury sustained. The defendant physician was an officer and director of the professional service corporation bringing the charge. He had established another professional service corporation to perform identical medical planning services for a hospital client, thereby attempting to seize an opportunity due the plaintiff corporation.

15. In Gilbert v. McLeod Infirmary (219 S.C. 174, 64 S.E.2d 524 [1951]), the sale of hospital property to a corporation controlled by Mr. Aiken, a hospital trustee, was voided even though there was no actual fraud and in spite of the fact that Aiken had refrained from discussing the matter and had not voted on the transaction. However, the attorney for Aiken, who was also a trustee of the board,

had favorably discussed the sale and voted in favor of the proposal. Moreover, Aiken had failed to carry his burden of proof to show fair and adequate consideration for the sale of the property.

16. *See, e.g.*, Wyo. Stat. Ann. § 17-6-104 (1977), *and* Md. Health-General Code Ann. § 19-220 (1982).

17. For example, Michigan's relevant statute provides:

    (1) A director or an officer shall discharge his or her duties ...

    (a) In good faith.

    (b) With the care an ordinarily prudent person would exercise under similar circumstances.

    (c) In a manner he or she reasonably believes is in the best interests of the corporation.

    Mich. Comp. Laws § 450.2451.

18. *See* Reserve Life Ins. Co. v. Salter, 152 F. Supp. 868 (S.D. Miss. 1957).

19. State statutes may specify the items on which directors or trustees may rely in discharging their duties. For example, the Michigan statute (*supra* note 17) does so by saying that a director or officer

    is entitled to rely on information, opinions, reports, or statements, including financial statements and other financial data, if prepared or presented by any of the following:

    (a) One or more directors, officers, or employees of the corporation, or of a domestic or foreign corporation or a business organization under joint control or common control, whom the director or officer reasonably believes to be reliable and competent in the matters presented.

    (b) Legal counsel, public accountants, engineers, or other persons as to matters the director or officer reasonably believes are within the person's professional or expert competence.

    (c) A committee of the board of which he or she is not a member if the director or officer reasonably believes that the committee merits confidence.

20. *See* Epworth Orphanage v. Long, 207 S.C 384, 36 S.E.2d 37 (1945); *see also* Queen of Angels Hosp. v. Younger, 66 Cal. App. 3d 359, 136 Cal. Rptr. 36 (1977) (improper exercise of sound business judgment and breach of fiduciary duty).

21. *See generally* 30 C.J.S., *Employer–Employee Relationships.* Two relevant texts from Health Administration Press are BRUCE FRIED & MYRON FOTTLER, HUMAN RESOURCES IN HEALTHCARE: MANAGING FOR SUCCESS (4th ed., 2015), AND RITA NUMEROF & MICHAEL ABRAMS, EMPLOYEE RETENTION: SOLVING THE HEALTHCARE CRISIS (2003).

22. W. Fletcher, Cyclopedia of the Law of Private Corporations § 41 (perm. ed. 1983).

23. *See, e.g.*, Lowendahl v. Baltimore & Ohio R.R., 247 A.D. 144, 287 N.Y.S. 62, *aff'd*, 272 N.Y. 360, 6 N.E.2d 56 (1936).

24. J. J. McCaskill Co. v. United States, 216 U.S. 504, 515 (1910).

25. "In a sense, faithfulness to these [corporate] formalities is the price paid for the corporate fiction, a relatively small price to pay for limited liability." Labadie Coal Co. v. Black, 672 F.2d 92, 97 (D.C. Cir. 1982).

26. *See* Jabczenski v. Southern Pac. Memorial Hosp., 119 Ariz. 15, 579 P.2d 53 (1978) (mere existence of interlocking directorates between a not-for-profit and a for-profit corporation was insufficient to justify disregarding the corporate identities).

27. 511 F. Supp. 416 (1981), *aff'd*, 685 F.2d 448 (1982).

28. AHA Guide to the Health Care Field at B2 (Health Forum Publishing 2009).

29. *See, e.g.*, Mich. Comp. Laws Ann. §§ 450.1701–.1722, 450.2703–.2722 (West 1973 and Supp. 1986); *see generally* Harry G. Henn & John R. Alexander, Laws of Corporations and Other Business Enterprises at § 346 (West 1983).

30. *See generally* Congressional Budget Office, *Physician Reimbursement Under Medicare: Options for Change* (published April 1986), at http://www.cbo.gov/doc.cfm?index=5967.

31. *Id.* at xviii.

32. *See, e.g.*, Medical Group Management Association, *MGMA Physician Placement Report: 65 Percent of Established Physicians Placed in Hospital-Owned Practices* (published June 3, 2010), at http://www.mgma.com/press/default.aspx?id=33777.

33. Affordable Care Act, Pub. L. No. 111-148, § 3022.

34. *See* Centers for Medicare & Medicaid Services, *Pioneer ACO Model* (updated October 20, 2016), at https://innovation.cms.gov/initiatives/Pioneer-aco-model.

35. ACA § 1899(b)(2).

36. Citizens United v. Federal Election Commission, 558 U.S. 50 (2010).

37. *See* American Hospital Association (AHA), *Mission and Vision* (accessed August 2, 2016), at http://www.aha.org/about/mission.shtml.

LIABILITY OF THE HEALTHCARE INSTITUTION

After reading this chapter, you will

- know that most healthcare institutions began as religious works of mercy, and that as such, they were usually immune from liability for any negligence they might commit;
- understand that the concept of independent contractor is virtually irrelevant today in the world of healthcare malpractice;
- realize that under respondeat superior the corporation is responsible through the acts of an agent, whereas under corporate liability it owes a duty directly to the plaintiff; and
- grasp the complicated liability status of managed care organizations and their financial incentives to minimize the amount of care their enrollees receive.

As discussed in chapter 2, the history of healthcare institutions begins with the almshouses of the Middle Ages. Before the nineteenth century, almshouses had little to do with medical care and more to do with housing unfortunates and keeping them away from "respectable" society. They were religious—mainly Christian—charities and, as the word *almshouses* implies, were supported by donated money and services. A vestige of this history is church groups' (especially Catholic) sponsorship of so many of today's hospitals.

Given their charitable nature, hospitals and many other organizations were held to be immune from tort liability lest their good deeds be diminished by jury awards. Some courts adopted this position because they considered the assets of a charitable corporation to be held in trust for its beneficiaries and feared that the implied trust would be violated by payment of money damages. Others held that the beneficiaries of a charity (including the general public) implicitly waived their rights to sue when accepting the benefits of charitable services. Still others based the rule simply on concepts of public policy, specifying that tort liability should apply only to a profit-making enterprise.[1]

Whatever its rationale, support for the doctrine of **charitable immunity** waned as modern medicine evolved in the twentieth century (see chapter 2),

charitable immunity
the venerable principle (now discredited) that a charitable organization is not to be held liable for the tortious actions of its agents

and the concept had virtually disappeared by the 1970s. The public's perception of hospitals as purely charitable organizations had changed.[2] Health plans and government programs (rather than alms) paid for operational expenses; liability insurance was available to cover defense costs and jury awards; and healthcare more readily adopted the traits of market-driven industries. The courts began to treat not-for-profit enterprises in the same manner as other companies insofar as third party liability claims were concerned, and thus charitable immunity was overturned in a series of state-by-state judicial decisions once the rationale for immunity dissolved. (As discussed in chapter 5, however, government hospitals still enjoy immunity or partial immunity in some jurisdictions, justified as "sovereign immunity" rather than charitable immunity.)

The demise of "charitable immunity" is exemplified by the decisions of two courts. As long ago as 1969—in the state that was the US birthplace of the doctrine—the Massachusetts Supreme Judicial Court decided to abandon it:

> In the past on many occasions we have declined to renounce the defence [sic] of charitable immunity. . . . We took this position because we were of opinion [sic] that any renunciation preferably should be accomplished prospectively and that this should be best done by legislative action. Now it appears that only three or four States still adhere to the doctrine. It seems likely that no legislative action in this Commonwealth is probable in the near future. Accordingly, we take this occasion to give adequate warning that the next time we are squarely confronted by a legal question respecting the charitable immunity doctrine it is our intention to abolish it.[3]

In 2001, Wisconsin's high court, which had never adopted the principle in the first place, declined again to do so, calling this legal fiction "an antiquated doctrine that fails to reflect the emergence of hospitals as modern health care facilities."[4]

With the end of charitable immunity, healthcare became one of the most dramatically changing areas of personal injury law. This chapter reviews evolving legal principles that have affected traditional hospital liability standards since the 1970s:

- Independent contractor status
- Captain-of-the-ship and borrowed-servant doctrines
- Apparent agency or agency by estoppel
- Corporate liability

The chapter begins with a refresher course in the traditional rules of respondeat superior, proceeds to address the principles identified in the previous list, and ends with a section on the liability of managed care and similar organizations.

Respondeat Superior Versus Independent Contractor Status

Respondeat Superior Defined

As noted in chapter 5, *respondeat superior* (vicarious liability) is the principle that an employer is liable for a tort an employee commits within the scope of employment. The idea is based on the principle *qui facit per alium, facit per se* (Latin for "one who acts through another, acts for himself"). Even though the employer is not directly at fault, it controls the means and methods of the employee's work and thus should answer for the employee's negligence. Presumably, the imposition of liability encourages the employer to apply sound procedures for controlling employees' job performance.

Liability asserted on the basis of respondeat superior essentially depends on the answers to three questions:

1. Was a tort committed?
2. Was the person who committed the tort an agent or an employee of the defendant?
3. Was the tort committed within the scope of the agent's or employee's duties?

The duty of a healthcare institution (see Legal Brief) is to have its employees use the same reasonable level of care as that practiced in similar organizations in similar communities.[5] Patients are entitled to the care their medical conditions require.[6] To prove breach of this duty, the plaintiff must usually produce expert testimony about how similar clinicians and hospitals treat his kind of condition.[7] Not surprisingly, the plaintiff's experts will testify that other hospitals or other doctors would have treated the patient differently. The defense will call witnesses who will say, "Oh, no! What the doctor [or nurse, or hospital] did was perfectly reasonable." The battle of the experts is on, and the jury will be asked to decide who is correct.

Sometimes, expert testimony is not necessary—such as when the situation involves routine or nonprofessional care (e.g., helping a patient to the bathroom or out of a wheelchair),[8] when a physician's order is violated,[9] or when common sense makes the breach of duty apparent.[10] Commonsense

Legal Brief

For the sake of simplicity and readability, throughout much of this book the term *hospital* is used as shorthand for *healthcare institution* because the general principles that apply to hospitals also usually apply to other corporate healthcare providers. Discussion that applies solely or primarily to an actual hospital should be apparent from the context.

logic underlies the Department of Health & Human Services' list of adverse events discussed in chapter 5, and expert testimony is not required because lay-persons are capable of determining that reasonable care was not exercised. (See The Court Decides: *Norton v. Argonaut Insurance Co.* at the end of this chapter for a case in which all parties—hospital, physician, and nurse—were held liable for a fatal medication error that common sense indicates was preventable.)

Whether experts testify or not, the principle of vicarious liability is based on public policy considerations. The employer usually has insurance coverage or superior financial means to compensate for the damage caused by the employee's tort. Besides, a corporation can act only through agents and employees. Not holding the organization liable for its employees' actions would mean that the company would not be responsible for decisions made and acts committed in furtherance of institutional aims. The employee who committed the tort can also be held liable for the wrongful act or omission, so the employer and the employee are often sued together; however, the employer is usually the main target because of its "deep pockets."

Independent Contractor Defined

Because respondeat superior is based on employers' right to control the means and methods of employees' work, employers are not liable for the negligence of independent contractors. An independent contractor has sole control over the means and methods of the work to be accomplished, although the person who employs, hires, or appoints a contractor retains the general power of approval over the final work product. For example, if a home owner hires an independent contractor to build a house, provides the plans, and retains the power to approve the final result but does not control the day-to-day activities of the laborers, then the contractor is responsible for the laborers' actions. In effect, the owner is saying, "Here's what I want built. Go do it, and tell me when you're done."

In the context of hospital liability, a physician in private practice who is a member of the medical staff was traditionally considered an independent contractor; the hospital was not liable to the patient for the malpractice or negligence of such a physician (see "The Joint Employer Concept").

Numerous old cases to this effect could be cited.[11] For example, in *Heins v. Synkonis*, the hospital was not held liable for the negligence of a private physician because the hospital merely provided office space for the doctor's outpatient clinic and no actual or apparent employment relationship existed between the hospital and the independent contractor doctor.[12]

Erosion of Physicians' Independent Contractor Status

Heins was decided in 1975, and although old cases are not necessarily bad law, the *Heins* rationale has eroded over the years, making the independent contractor defense less viable today. The following are some of the factors prompting courts to see an employment-like relationship where none would have been found before:

- An increasing number of patients no longer select their own physicians; rather, the hospital, an employer, or some other third party designates the doctor or a panel of doctors.

- Patients use hospitals' emergency services more frequently. Private physicians commonly tell patients to go to the emergency room (ER) (or emergency department [ED]) if they have concerns outside normal office hours. "Meet me at the ER" has morphed into "the ER docs will take care of you."

- Healthcare institutions have increased the number of employed physicians on their staffs and in their clinics.

- Medical practice has become increasingly institutionalized and specialized.

- The number of contracts with hospital-based specialists has increased dramatically.

Employment of Physicians

Because of lifestyle preferences, various economic forces, the effects of the Afford-

The Joint Employer Concept

In some contexts, including healthcare, it is possible for an individual to have more than one employment relationship at the same time for the same job. The situation arises, for example, when a hospital contracts with a staffing agency to provide nurses ("travelers") to augment the regular nursing staff. In the view of the US Equal Employment Opportunity Commission, the National Labor Relations Board, and many state courts, these individuals are employees of *both* the hospital and the staffing agency, thus *both* organizations are liable for the individuals' torts and both may be responsible for ensuring compliance with wage and hour laws, the Family and Medical Leave Act, hiring and termination procedures, labor laws, and other requirements.

A recent decision by the National Labor Relations Board, for example, gave temporary workers at a recycling company the right to be included in the same bargaining unit as the company's full-time employees.[73] Although not yet confirmed by the courts, the decision, if followed to its logical conclusion, would require the employers to bargain jointly with the union and would make them jointly liable for unfair labor practices. The same rationale could be applied to hospitals and the staffing agencies who provide them with "temporary" employees.

Healthcare leaders, especially human resources executives, must take heed when using staffing agencies. They must ensure that both the hospital and the agency are in compliance with all applicable laws and regulations and that "travelers" are accorded the same protections as full-time employees.

able Care Act's (ACA) reforms, and fraud laws that provide "safe harbors" for many transactions with employees (see chapter 15), physicians are increasingly becoming hospital employees. Young physicians coming out of residency often prefer to focus their energies on patient care rather than the business aspects of private practice, for which they may not feel well suited. At the other end of the spectrum, older physicians frequently choose to sell their practices and become employed for many of the same reasons.[13]

According to one report, the number of employed primary care physicians doubled to about 40 per cent between 2000 and 2013, and one-fourth of all specialists who saw patients in hospitals were employees in 2013 compared to only 5 percent in 2000.[14] As the *Atlantic* magazine stated in May 2014, "Hospitals are buying up medical practices at a feverish pace. According to data from the American Hospital Association, the number of physicians employed by hospitals grew by 34 percent between 2000 and 2010, and the pace shows no signs of slackening. [And] a large physician recruiting firm found that in 2004 only 11 percent of physician searches were conducted by hospitals, but by 2013 that figure had risen to 63 percent."[15]

This trend is in sharp contrast to the image of the private practice physician, who was free from external control and whose professional judgment went unquestioned. Such was the autonomy of the medical doctor in the early and mid-twentieth century that "corporate practice of medicine" laws in many states forbade doctors from becoming employees (see Legal Brief in chapter 10, p. 366). Hospitals were, in effect, viewed merely as "doctors' workshops" and thus were not liable for the physicians' medical negligence. Instead, hospitals were responsible for the actions of members of their medical staffs only when those physicians were performing "administrative" rather than "medical" functions.

This understanding began to change in the late 1950s with the landmark case of *Bing v. Thunig.* In that decision the New York Court of Appeals eliminated the distinction between administrative and medical acts and settled the issue of whether the physician's professional status prevented the imposition of vicarious liability on the hospital.[16] A well-known passage from *Bing* reads as follows:

> The conception that the hospital does not undertake to treat the patient, does not undertake to act through its doctors and nurses, but undertakes instead simply to procure them to act upon their own responsibility no longer reflects the fact. Present day hospitals, as their manner of operation plainly demonstrates, do far more than furnish facilities for treatment. They regularly employ on a salary basis a large staff of physicians, nurses and interns, as well as administrative and manual workers, and they charge patients for medical care and treatment, collecting for such services, if necessary, by legal action. Certainly, the person who avails himself of "hospital facilities" expects that the hospital will attempt to cure him, not that its nurses or other employees will act on their own responsibility.[17]

The erosion of the physician's independent contractor status (discussed earlier), coupled with the trend toward employment of physicians and the elimination of any distinction between administrative and medical acts—all these factors combine to make the hospital responsible for the quality of care rendered within its walls (see section titled "Doctrine of Corporate Liability" at p. 226).

Apparent Agency

Even if technically they are not hospital employees, many physicians have contracts with hospitals to provide services to hospital patients. This arrangement is particularly true of anesthesiologists; radiologists; pathologists; and specialists in emergency medicine, nuclear medicine, and other clinical fields. To the average person encountering them in the clinical setting, these physicians appear to be employees even though their contracts state that they are independent contractors.

Depending on the facts, either **apparent agency** (also known as *ostensible agency*) or **agency by estoppel** can counter the independent contractor defense. There is a fine distinction between these concepts, and some courts may note the difference,[18] but as a practical matter they are virtually indistinguishable. The Texas Supreme Court pointed this out in 1998 in *Baptist Memorial Hosp. System v. Sampson*, when it wrote, "Many courts use the terms ostensible agency, apparent agency, apparent authority, and agency by estoppel interchangeably. As a practical matter, there is no distinction among them."[19]

In that case, whether the physician was an independent contractor was a question for the jury, and the court described the gist of the matter as follows: "To establish a hospital's liability for an independent contractor's medical malpractice based on ostensible agency, a plaintiff must show that (1) he or she had a reasonable belief that the physician was the agent or employee of the hospital, (2) such belief was generated by the hospital affirmatively holding out the physician as its agent or employee or knowingly permitting the physician to hold herself out as the hospital's agent or employee, and (3) he or she justifiably relied on the representation of authority."[20]

Two Delaware cases illustrate this principle. In *Vanaman v. Milford Memorial Hospital*, a private physician was on call to provide emergency services.[21] The court held that it was for the jury to decide whether the allegedly negligent doctor treated the patient in a private capacity or while fulfilling the hospital function of providing emergency care. The court said that the hospital could be liable for the doctor's negligence if it held the physician out to be its employee and the patient justifiably relied on that representation. To the same effect is *Schagrin v. Wilmington Medical Center*, in which the court found that a medical partnership staffing an ED may be an agent of the hospital and not an independent contractor—depending on the degree of hospital control, the methods of paying the doctors, and the degree of patients' reliance on the hospital compared with their reliance on the physicians.[22]

Whether a hospital can contractually insulate itself from liability depends on the facts of the particular case, but the courts seem generally inclined to find a hospital liable under principles of vicarious liability—irrespective of a purported independent contractor status—by applying such

apparent agency or **agency by estoppel** closely related doctrines that can be used to counter the independent contractor defense

principles as apparent or ostensible agency or agency by estoppel. These doctrines may be applied even if the allegedly negligent physician is not a medical specialist with an exclusive contract to perform a designated hospital service.

For example, in *Grewe v. Mt. Clemens General Hospital*, the plaintiff was taken to the hospital after suffering a severe electrical shock and shoulder trauma.[23] He was first seen by an internist, who consulted with Dr. Fagen, an orthopedic surgeon. Dr. Fagen diagnosed a dislocated right shoulder and, in turn, designated an orthopedic resident to reduce the dislocation (restore the shoulder to its normal condition), but the reduction was unsuccessful. A specialist in internal medicine, Dr. Katzowitz, was summoned to assist. (The choice of an internist is curious.) According to his own testimony, Dr. Katzowitz did not view the patient's X-rays before attempting to reduce the dislocated shoulder "by placing his foot on the plaintiff's chest and pulling his arm." The plaintiff suffered an injury to a network of nerves in his shoulder (the brachial plexus) and a fracture. Additional surgery was necessary to remove bone fragments and to make other repairs.

The Supreme Court of Michigan held that agency by estoppel is established if the "patient looked to the hospital to provide him with treatment," and it affirmed the jury's verdict against the hospital. The jury had found that the plaintiff had no previous physician–patient relationship with Dr. Katzowitz or the other physicians outside the hospital setting, there was nothing to put the patient on notice that Dr. Katzowitz was an independent contractor, the plaintiff had gone to the hospital expecting to be treated there, and all the physicians were thus ostensible agents of the hospital. Because the patient had not personally selected the physicians, he relied on the institution to provide care. Under the factual circumstances, the hospital was estopped to deny its relationship with the physicians and was held responsible.[24]

We thus see how the doctrines of apparent agency and agency by estoppel have contributed substantially to the demise of the hospital's independent contractor defense. In *Grewe* and similar cases, the doctor was neither an employee of the hospital nor the plaintiff's personal physician. The patients were entitled to jury trials on the issues of whether they had relied on the hospital (rather than on self-selected physicians) to furnish care and whether the hospital had held out the doctors as ostensible employees of the hospital when furnishing emergency services.[25]

Erosion of Captain-of-the-Ship and Borrowed-Servant Doctrines

For many years, two other doctrines helped hospitals escape liability for physicians' acts—the *captain-of-the-ship* and *borrowed-servant* concepts. The first doctrine presumed that a surgeon was the captain of the ship during surgery and, like the captain of a real ship, was responsible for what occurred under her command. Thus, the hospital's argument was that the surgeon, not the hospital, was liable for negligence during surgery. This argument was bolstered by the "borrowed-servant" doctrine, the principle that one who is normally an employee of one person or entity (e.g., an employee of Hospital X) may be borrowed by another—a surgeon, for example—thereby becoming a servant of the surgeon and making the surgeon liable for the "borrowed" employee's negligence.

In any vicarious liability case, the basis for liability is one's right of control over the negligent activities of another. As the number of persons on surgical teams has grown in size and as anesthesiologists, nurses, surgical assistants, and others have been increasingly recognized as performing independent functions pursuant to hospital policies and their own professions' standards of care, the courts have realized that imposing liability on the chief surgeon alone for the negligent acts of all surgical team members is not sound legal doctrine. Whether the surgeon or the hospital was the sole controlling master or whether both had control to justify joint liability is for the jury to decide.

Many cases involving a miscount of instruments or surgical sponges illustrate erosion of the captain-of-the-ship and borrowed-servant doctrines. For example, in *Tonsic v. Wagner*, the trial court applied the captain-of-the-ship doctrine to hold the surgeon liable when neither the scrub nurse, a circulating nurse, nor an intern counted the surgical instruments at the conclusion of a colectomy.[26] As a result, a clamp was not removed from the patient. The trial court did not permit the jury to consider the vicarious liability of the hospital. The Pennsylvania Supreme Court reversed the decision, noting that under the law of agency, a negligent party may be the employee of two masters simultaneously, even though the masters are not joint employers. In such situations both masters may be liable.[27] Accordingly, the plaintiff was entitled to a new trial in her suit against the hospital (see Law in Action).

The trend has been observable for decades.[28] When medical care is provided by highly specialized, sophisticated teams of professionals working in an institutional setting, determining who is exercising what control over whom at any given time is difficult. In such cases, many consider it logical that the corporate institution share the liability.

Law in Action

During a deposition in a case involving a retained sponge, an exchange between the chief operating room nurse and the plaintiff's lawyer went as follows:

ATTORNEY. When the operation was over, did you or anyone else count the sponges that had been used?

NURSE. No, sir.

ATTORNEY. Why not?

NURSE. Well, we didn't count them before the surgery, so it wouldn't have done any good to count them afterward, would it?

The case was settled before trial.

Doctrine of Corporate Liability

Under the doctrine of corporate liability, the hospital itself is negligent. This liability is not "vicarious"—it attaches to the corporation because the hospital owes a legal duty directly to the patient, and this duty is not delegable to the medical staff or other personnel. A Connecticut court defined corporate liability in these words: "Corporate negligence is the failure of those entrusted with the task of providing accommodations and facilities necessary to carry out the charitable purpose of the corporation to follow . . . the established standard of conduct to which the corporation should conform."[29]

What direct duties does the healthcare organization owe the patient or another person? Is a hospital just a space for doctors to practice, where responsibility for patient care is exercised by physicians and clinical personnel under their direction? The hospital does not practice medicine, so how can it be liable? To answer these questions, one must consider the corporate purposes of a hospital or health system. Is its role simply to furnish physical facilities and accommodations wherein private physicians care for and treat their patients? Or is its role broader?

As previously discussed, healthcare systems are more than "doctors' workshops." They arrange, furnish, and provide the community with an entire range of health-related services—preventive, curative, and palliative; outpatient and inpatient; acute and long term. As their vision has expanded, so have their duties.

Before the mid-1960s, courts generally limited hospitals' corporate duties to such issues as selection and retention of employees and maintenance of hospital equipment, buildings, and grounds; these duties remain areas of potential liability today. Negligence regarding equipment is seen when there are unrepaired defects, when equipment is misused,[30] or when it is used for an unintended purpose.[31] The duty of reasonable care regarding the use of equipment and its selection for an intended purpose also includes a duty to inspect the equipment systematically and regularly before use.[32] Rules and regulations of licensing authorities, accreditation standards, and instructional manuals supplied by manufacturers to maintain equipment can be admitted at trial as evidence of expected standards of care. Failure on the part of hospital and medical personnel to comply with such standards constitutes evidence of breach of duty.

Under negligence theories, physicians and institutional providers have a duty to warn a patient of known risks when the patient is furnished with a medical device. Moreover, courts are now extending the duty to include informing patients of risks that become known after the device is furnished. Thus, if a heart pacemaker is implanted and the particular device is later recalled because of a defect, the hospital and the physician have a duty to notify the patient if the physician knows or should know of the recall.

With regard to the availability of equipment and services, one is not required to possess the newest and most modern equipment available on the market, but there is a duty to have available the usual and customary equipment and staff for any service that the hospital renders. (The same applies to physicians' offices, nursing homes, and other facilities.) For example, providers have been found liable for using unsterilized hypodermic needles.[33] In *Garcia v. Memorial Hospital*, a hospital did not have a pediatric endotracheal tube that might have saved a child's life.[34] The hospital operated an ED and held itself out as providing a full range of emergency services, and the court held that availability of a pediatric endotracheal tube is usual and customary in EDs. In another example, a Pennsylvania hospital was found liable when its electrocardiogram machine in the ED broke down and no backup instrument was available.[35] The emergency patient had to be taken to another location for the test, but he died there.

Healthcare organizations also have a corporate responsibility to exercise reasonable care in selecting and retaining employees. In *Wilson N. Jones Memorial Hospital v. Davis*,[36] the hospital had to pay the plaintiff both compensatory and punitive damages for failure to investigate the background and references of an applicant for the position of orderly. The hospital's normal hiring procedure was to obtain four employment references and three personal references. Established policy was to verify at least one of the employment references and one of the personal references before hiring the applicant. In this case, a hospital executive employed the applicant as an orderly without checking *any* of the references. The lame justification, asserted after the fact, was that the hospital had a critical need for personnel.

After the individual began work, an inquiry was sent to one of the references, who verified that the orderly had worked for him for approximately four months but did not answer any of the other questions on the reference form. The hospital failed to follow up. Furthermore, the employee had stated that he received his training as an orderly while in the US Navy, but again the hospital did not inquire, saying the armed services had not been cooperative with it in the past. However, the plaintiff requested information from the Navy and promptly learned that the orderly had been expelled from the Navy's Medical Corps School after a single month's training, that he had been diagnosed as having a serious drug problem, and that he had a criminal record. The orderly also had listed three personal references on his application and included a local telephone number for each. The hospital attempted to contact only one of these references, and that attempt was unsuccessful.

Soon after hire, the orderly attempted to remove a Foley catheter from a patient's bladder without first deflating the bulb; this action seriously injured the patient. The hospital was held liable for both compensatory and punitive damages. The hospital's critical need for orderlies at the time did not justify its failure to exercise reasonable care in the employee selection process. Moreover, the punitive damages awarded in the case were assigned as a result of "such an entire want of care as to indicate that the act ... was the result of conscious indifference to the rights, welfare, and safety of the patients in the hospital."[37]

Failure to Adopt or Follow Rules

Hospital bylaws, rules and regulations, and the accreditation standards of The Joint Commission are admissible as evidence at trial.[38] If violation of a hospital rule is the proximate cause of a plaintiff's injury, liability can be premised on the fact that the rule is the expected standard of care. Violation of a rule or written standard does not automatically amount to negligence, but it is strong evidence. For example, in *Pederson v. Dumouchel*, a hospital was held liable when—in violation of hospital policy—it permitted nonemergency dental surgery to be performed under a general anesthetic without the supervision of a medical doctor.[39]

Typically, the existence of a rule and evidence of its breach are submitted to the jury as a question of fact. As would be expected, evidence that a rule has been violated is often persuasive to jurors. For example, a jury verdict for the plaintiff was affirmed in *Burks v. Christ Hospital*, citing a hospital policy requiring that bedside rails be raised if a patient is restless, obese, or under sedation, unless the attending physician issues an order to the contrary.[40] The plaintiff sustained injuries when he fell from the bed, and the jury was entitled to consider the violation of this written standard as evidence of negligence. In another example, a Michigan case noted that an administrative regulation requiring hospitals to have written policies regarding medical consultations and to record consultations was intended to protect hospitalized patients.[41] Accordingly, the plaintiff was entitled to have the jury instructed on the purpose of this rule.

Another variation of corporate liability is a hospital's failure to have and to implement adequate rules regarding communication of vital information on patient care to others who are or will be responsible for treating the patient. For example, in *Keene v. Methodist Hospital*,[42] an injured patient was seen at about 2 am on December 25 by an on-call physician in a hospital ED. He was sent home after X-rays were taken, and a few hours later a radiologist examined the films and detected a possible skull fracture. The radiologist suggested further X-ray studies and dictated a tentative diagnosis and recommendations into a recorder, but he did not communicate further with the attending physician, the patient, the patient's family, or hospital administration. Because of the Christmas holiday, the dictation was not transcribed for two days. During this period, the patient lost consciousness, was returned to the hospital for emergency surgery, and died as a result of a fractured skull and hemorrhage.

The court stated that the patient "would not have died from his head injuries if he had been treated for a skull fracture during the morning of December 25" and found both the ED physician and the radiologist liable. In addition, the hospital was held liable because "it is the duty of the Hospital to adopt procedures which would ensure that the opinion of a radiologist showing the possibility of a severe injury would be immediately conveyed to the proper persons."[43] Thus, failure to have and to follow proper rules, regulations, or systems when indicated by recognized professional standards can result in liability—whether it is called corporate negligence or vicarious liability.[44]

In any given case, the applicable legal theory—corporate negligence or respondeat superior—is becoming increasingly difficult to determine, but it probably does not matter much. Just as in *Bing v. Thunig*[45]—which in 1957 eliminated any distinction between the administrative and professional acts of nurses for the purposes of respondeat superior—the distinction between hospitals' vicarious liability (respondeat superior) and direct liability (corporate negligence) has nearly disappeared for all practical purposes. In any event, hospital rules, standards of accreditation, and licensure regulations must be realistic, known to all affected persons, implementable, and consistently enforced. Furthermore, the rules must be regularly and systematically reviewed; if they are not realistic and workable, they should be eliminated.

Negligence in Selection and Retention of Medical Staff

The law in most states now recognizes that a corporate healthcare institution owes a duty directly to its patients to exercise reasonable care in the selection and retention of medical staff. The corporation may be liable if it knows or should have known that an individual physician was not competent to perform the permitted clinical procedures. This doctrine emerged from the 1965 landmark case of *Darling v. Charleston Community Memorial Hospital*,[46] in which the Illinois Supreme Court held that a hospital could be liable under either (1) respondeat superior, if nurse employees failed to notify medical and hospital administrators when they knew that a patient was receiving inadequate medical care, or (2) corporate liability, if the hospital failed to review and monitor the quality of care generally rendered to patients by the private physician. The private physician in this case was a general practitioner who had been permitted by the hospital to practice orthopedic medicine and whose clinical competence had not been reviewed in his more than three decades of practice.

Significantly, *Darling* also established that to prove the standard of care, the jury may consider standards set forth in medical staff bylaws as well as those promulgated by The Joint Commission and state licensing authorities. Moreover, the case abolished the "locality rule" in Illinois. In short, the hospital could no longer fully defend itself by asserting that other hospitals in the area also did not enforce their medical staff bylaws or review the performance of their medical staff members.

The Illinois court rejected the view that a hospital simply procures nurses and doctors who then act on their own responsibility. A hospital treats patients and acts through its nurses and doctors, even if the latter are not employees.[47] Following the *Darling* decision, one commentator wrote,

> Even in the absence of an employer–employee . . . relationship . . . there now appears to be some chance . . . to impose liability on the hospital on the theory of independent negligence in failing to review, supervise, or consult about, the treatment given by the physician directly in charge, if the situation indicates that the hospital had the opportunity for such review but failed to exercise it, or that its servants (usually nurses or residents) were negligent in failing to call the attention of the proper hospital authorities to the impropriety or inadequacy of the treatment being given.[48]

Case law has firmly established that hospital administration and medical staff have a joint role with respect to the clinical performance of individual practitioners. The governing body of a hospital has a responsibility to adopt corporate and medical staff bylaws providing for an organized medical staff accountable to the board for quality of care. The governing board grants medical staff appointments, delineates privileges on an individual basis, and reappoints clinicians on the basis of the recommendations of medical staff committees. In ruling on these recommendations, the board must be satisfied that the peer review process is working properly and avoid rubber-stamping recommendations submitted by the medical staff. The responsibility of the governing body is nondelegable; the board does, however, delegate to the medical staff the authority to implement the credentialing process and prepare recommendations for appointments and reappointments (more on this subject in chapter 8).

Other leading cases have recognized the corporate duty of a hospital to exercise reasonable care in the selection and retention of the medical staff. A 1971 Georgia case, *Joiner v. Mitchell County Hospital Authority*, held that members of the medical staff who make physician appointment recommendations to the governing body of a hospital are agents of the hospital.[49] In considering these recommendations, the governing body must act in good faith and with reasonable care.[50] Nevada's Supreme Court recognized a similar institutional duty in *Moore v. Board of Trustees of Carson-Tahoe Hospital*, a case concerning medical staff privileges.[51] The court stated:

> The purpose of the community hospital is to provide patient care of the highest possible quality. To implement this duty of providing competent medical care to the patients, it is the responsibility of the institution to create a workable system

whereby the medical staff of the hospital continually reviews and evaluates the quality of care being rendered within the institution. The staff must be organized with the proper structure to carry out the role delegated to it by the governing body. All powers of the medical staff flow from the board of trustees, and the staff must be held accountable for its control of quality. . . . The role of the hospital vis-à-vis the community is changing rapidly. The hospital's role is no longer limited to the furnishing of physical facilities and equipment where a physician treats his private patients and practices his profession in his own individualized manner.

Licensing [of physicians], per se, furnishes no continuing control with respect to a physician's professional competence and therefore does not assure the public of quality patient care. The protection of the public must come from some other authority, and that in this case is the Hospital Board of Trustees. The Board, of course, may not act arbitrarily or unreasonably in such cases. The Board's actions must be predicated upon a reasonable standard.[52]

In *Gonzales v. Nork*, the defendant performed an unsuccessful and allegedly unnecessary laminectomy and spinal fusion procedure on a 27-year-old man who had been injured in an automobile accident.[53] Various complications developed and substantially reduced the patient's life expectancy. The plaintiff presented evidence showing that the surgeon had performed more than three dozen similar operations negligently or unnecessarily. The trial court issued a lengthy opinion recognizing that the hospital owed a duty of care to the patient with respect to the delineation of surgical privileges extended to private surgeons. The court stated forcefully that this duty included the obligation to protect the patient from acts of malpractice by an independently retained doctor if the hospital knew or should have known that such acts were likely to occur. Even though the hospital had no knowledge of Dr. Nork's propensity to commit malpractice or perform unnecessary surgery, its demonstrated lack of a system for acquiring such knowledge justified a finding of negligence.

A landmark Wisconsin case in 1981 took a particularly enlightened view of the role of a hospital in its relations with the medical staff. In *Johnson v. Misericordia Community Hospital* (see The Court Decides at the end of this chapter), the plaintiff alleged that the hospital was negligent in granting orthopedic surgical privileges to a particular physician.[54] The Wisconsin Supreme Court affirmed a jury verdict for the plaintiff on the following bases:

1. The hospital failed to inquire into the physician's professional background and qualifications prior to granting a staff appointment.
2. The hospital failed to adhere to its own bylaw provisions and to Wisconsin statutes pertaining to medical credentialing.
3. The exercise of ordinary care would have disclosed the physician's lack of qualifications.

4. Had the hospital exercised due diligence, it would not have appointed the physician to the medical staff.

5. By not exercising due diligence, the hospital exposed patients to a "foreseeable risk of unreasonable harm."

Johnson stands for the now well-recognized proposition that, as the Wisconsin court simply phrased it, "a hospital has a duty to exercise due care in the selection of its medical staff."[55]

Only licensed practitioners can practice medicine and exercise clinical judgment for the proper care and treatment of patients, but the governing board and administration are responsible for ensuring that the organized medical staff periodically reviews the clinical behavior of staff physicians. Rather than second-guess medical care, the governing board delegates the review and evaluation functions to the medical staff, which in turn is accountable to the board for its recommendations in a process known as *credentialing* (see a complete discussion in chapter 8).

The medical staff is responsible for developing reasonable criteria and fundamentally fair procedures for evaluation, appointment, and delineation of privileges. The medical staff must gather information and data that support its recommendations and must forward the information to the governing body. The board, in turn, is responsible for approving the criteria and procedures for appointment, the delineation of privileges, and the renewal of appointments. It then acts on the medical staff's recommendations after ensuring that all supporting information is complete.

Hospitals must develop a credentialing process for other professionals—physician's assistants, nurse practitioners, podiatrists, technicians, pharmacists, and other clinicians—who also work in their facilities. Institutions must evaluate the competencies of these individuals just as they do those of the medical staff. Moreover, procedures must be developed to review periodically the performance of each of these professionals. The scope of their clinical activities is a matter for the medical and nursing staffs to develop according to local licensure laws and professional custom and usage.

The cases discussed in this section illustrate significant changes in the theories of hospital liability. The law of agency and respondeat superior no longer suffice to explain corporate duty; rather, in the hospital setting, the rules of respondeat superior and corporate or independent negligence have essentially become one.

Liability of Managed Care Organizations

Managed care organization (MCO) is a general term used to describe any number of health insurance arrangements that are "intended to reduce unnecessary health care costs through a variety of mechanisms, including: economic incentives for physicians and patients to select less costly forms of care; programs for reviewing the medical necessity of specific services; increased beneficiary cost sharing; controls on inpatient admissions and lengths of stay; the establishment of cost-sharing incentives for outpatient surgery; selective contracting with health care providers; and the intensive management of high-cost health care cases."[56]

MCOs take various organizational forms, such as health maintenance organizations (HMOs), preferred provider organizations (PPOs), and independent practice associations. They proliferated in the 1980s, during the frenzy over efficiency and cost savings; as with the first wave of physician–hospital organizations (see chapter 6), whether they have had any significant effect on rising healthcare costs is debatable.

In general, managed care plans tend to emphasize preventive and primary care and to limit access to more costly services. In many MCOs, select primary care physicians act as *gatekeepers* who must be consulted before the patient can see a specialist. Many patients also must obtain MCO authorization for hospitalization or for hospitalization to extend beyond a certain number of days. This process is often referred to as **utilization review (UR)** or **utilization management (UM)**, and the requests for authorization are often handled by nurses specially trained to administer the program. Authorization can be refused for a number of reasons; for example, the proposed treatment may not be a covered benefit, the proposed treatment may not be medically necessary, or the request may not have been made in a timely or procedurally correct manner.

utilization review (UR) systematic (usually retrospective) review of the efficiency and medical necessity of healthcare services on the basis of established guidelines

utilization management (UM) proactive techniques to improve the efficiency and to control the cost of health services by influencing providers' medical decision making; UM typically includes concurrent peer review processes.

Quality Versus Cost Savings

Any of these reasons to deny care can be legitimate, but when UR denials appear to result from financial pressures, aggrieved patients often allege that the health plan neglected quality in favor of economy. They assert that a particular authorization request was denied for other than clinical reasons, that they were refused necessary treatment, or that they were discharged from the hospital prematurely. The aphorism that patients were being sent home "sicker and quicker" arose out of this last claim.

Typical of the cases that first raised these issues were two from California in the late 1980s. In *Wickline v. State,*[57] the plaintiff argued that the decision to admit patients or extend their stay is a medical one that only a physician—and not a health plan—should make; she attempted to assert liability against the state's Medi-Cal program after a UR decision led to her being discharged early, which resulted in complications that caused loss of a leg.

The trial court decided in the patient's favor, but the appellate court reversed the decision while emphasizing the difference between prospective and retrospective UR.

> In . . . prospective utilization review, authority for the rendering of health care ser-
> vices must be obtained before medical care is rendered. Its purpose is to promote
> the well-recognized public interest in controlling health care costs by reducing
> unnecessary services while still intending to assure that appropriate medical and
> hospital services are provided to the patient in need. However, such a cost contain-
> ment strategy creates new and added pressures on the quality assurance portion
> of the utilization review mechanism. The stakes, the risks at issue, are much higher
> when a prospective cost containment review process is utilized than when a retro-
> spective review process is used.
>
> A mistaken conclusion about medical necessity following retrospective
> review will result in the wrongful withholding of payment. An erroneous decision in
> a prospective review process, on the other hand, in practical consequences, results
> in the withholding of necessary care, potentially leading to a patient's permanent
> disability or death.[58]

The court went on to hold that it was ultimately the physician's, not Medi-
Cal's, responsibility to decide when the patient should be discharged. "Third
party payers of health care services can be held legally accountable when
medically inappropriate decisions result from defects in the design or implementation of cost containment mechanisms. . . . However, the physician who
complies without protest with the limitations imposed by a third party payor,
when his medical judgment dictates otherwise, cannot avoid his ultimate
responsibility for his patient's care. He cannot point to the health care payor
as the liability scapegoat when the consequences of his own determinative
medical decisions go sour."[59]

　　　The court concluded that although the physician was "intimidated"
by Medi-Cal's UR decision, he was not "paralyzed" by it and should have
made a greater effort to keep his patient in the hospital. There is irony in this
outcome: the court agreed with the plaintiff's argument that the decision to
discharge is one for physicians to make, and she lost her appeal as a result.

　　　Four years later, the other California case—decided by different judges
on the same appellate court—limited the applicability of *Wickline's* broad
language. In *Wilson v. Blue Cross of Southern California*,[60] a physician had
requested three to four weeks of additional care for a depressed psychiatric
patient. On the basis of a prospective review, the insurance company declined
to pay for any further care. Because nobody else could afford to pay, the
patient was discharged. He committed suicide less than three weeks later.

　　　The *Wilson* court found that there was "substantial evidence that [the deci-
sion] not to approve further hospitalization was a substantial factor in bringing
about the decedent's demise,"[61] and it remanded the case for further proceedings.

　　　In their decision, the justices characterized as **dictum** and overly broad
Wickline's statement that "the decision to discharge is . . . the responsibility
of the patient's own treating doctor." According to the *Wilson* court, "This

dictum (plural,
dicta)
Latin meaning
"remark"—a
comment in a legal
opinion that is not
binding because it
is not required to
reach the decision
but that states
a related legal
principle

broadly stated language was unnecessary to the [earlier] decision and in all contexts does not correctly state the law relative to causation issues in a tort case."[62]

Over the next few years, cases in several other states addressed the issue of MCOs' allegedly wrongful denial of treatment, and the results were mixed. The decisions often depended on interpretation of the Employee Retirement Income Security Act of 1974 (ERISA).[63]

ERISA Preemption Complicates Matters

Congress passed ERISA to protect employer-sponsored pension plans and later expanded the act to cover employee benefit plans, including employer-sponsored health plans. ERISA eliminates conflicting state laws by creating a uniform regulatory structure and preempts (supersedes) "any and all State laws insofar as they may now or hereafter relate to any employee benefit plan."[64]

Because employer-sponsored health plans are ERISA plans, some cases held that this provision bars state tort claims based on MCOs' UR decisions and leaves ERISA as the plaintiffs' only recourse.[65] Unfortunately, from the plaintiffs' standpoint, ERISA has no provisions for compensatory damages—such as would be awarded to make a person whole in a typical negligence case.

As the appeals of these various preemption cases wound their way through the court system, a few states attempted to resolve the problem by passing laws that provide a remedy for claims against MCOs. The Texas statute is typical; it provides, in relevant part, the following:

sec. 88.002

(a) A health insurance carrier, health maintenance organization, or other managed care entity for a health care plan has the duty to exercise ordinary care when making health care treatment decisions and is liable for damages for harm to an insured or enrollee proximately caused by its failure to exercise such ordinary care.

(b) [Any such entity] is also liable for damages for harm to an insured or enrollee proximately caused by the health care treatment decisions made by its:

(1) employees;

(2) agents;

(3) ostensible agents; or

(4) representatives who are acting on its behalf and over whom it has the right to exercise influence or control or has actually exercised influence or control which result in the failure to exercise ordinary care.[66]

The US Court of Appeals for the Fifth Circuit upheld this law in 2000, stating: "Although state efforts to regulate an entity in its capacity as plan administrator are preempted, managed care providers operate in a traditional sphere of state regulation when they wear their hats as medical care providers. . . . We are not persuaded that Congress intended for ERISA to supplant this state regulation of the quality of medical practice."[67]

Similar cases in other states tested similar statutes. Two federal circuits agreed with the Fifth Circuit, but three others did not. By early 2004, the federal circuits were split 3–3 on the question of whether ERISA preempted state law claims against MCOs for their adverse treatment decisions.[68]

The Supreme Court Weighs In (Heavily)

In June 2004, the US Supreme Court handed down a landmark decision in *Aetna Health, Inc. v. Davila*.[69] The facts of the cases—plural, because two lawsuits were consolidated and decided as one—typify many patients' situations. The first patient, Juan Davila, had been prescribed Vioxx for arthritis pain, but his MCO refused to pay for it and approved a less expensive drug instead. According to the decision, Davila "suffered a severe reaction that required extensive treatment and hospitalization."

The second patient had undergone surgery, and her physician felt she needed an extended hospital stay. The MCO's "discharge nurse" denied this request, after which the patient "experienced postsurgery complications forcing her to return to the hospital." She argued in her lawsuit that "these complications would not have occurred had [the MCO] approved coverage for a longer hospital stay."

Both patients sued their health plans on the basis of section 88.002 (the Texas statute quoted earlier), but the US Supreme Court found the Texas law to be invalid per ERISA's preemption language (also quoted earlier). In his opinion for a unanimous Supreme Court, Justice Clarence Thomas wrote, "A benefit determination is part and parcel of the ordinary fiduciary responsibilities connected to the administration of a plan. . . . The fact that a benefits determination is infused with medical judgments does not alter this result."[70] He drew no distinction between medical and nonmedical judgments by benefits plan administrators, and he summed up the Supreme Court's decision as follows: "Respondents bring suit only to rectify a wrongful denial of benefits promised under ERISA-regulated plans, and do not attempt to remedy any violation of a legal duty independent of ERISA. We hold that respondents' state causes of action fall within the scope of [ERISA's preemption language] and are therefore completely pre-empted . . . and removable to federal district court."[71]

ERISA is thus the exclusive remedy for beneficiaries of employer-sponsored health plans when challenging their MCOs' UR decisions. Because it is a federal statute, a state lawsuit alleging an ERISA violation can be "removed" (i.e., transferred) to a federal court for adjudication if the defendant so chooses. The dilemma for plaintiffs is that ERISA allows for no compensatory damages—only contractual damages and equitable relief (such as an injunction); thus, their state court options are precluded and there is no corresponding federal remedy to pursue.

The decision also creates a strange injustice: Tort and bad-faith claims against non-ERISA health plans (i.e., individual insurance policies, government plans, church plans that have elected not to be covered by ERISA) are not affected. Patients who suffer injury as a result of non-ERISA plans' UR decisions are free to pursue traditional remedies in state court, whereas patients with identical injuries resulting from identical decisions made by ERISA plans have no viable claim.

In a strongly worded concurring opinion, joined by Justice Stephen Breyer, Justice Ruth Bader Ginsburg wrote, "I . . . join the Court's opinion. But, with greater enthusiasm . . . I also join 'the rising judicial chorus urging that Congress and [this] Court revisit what is an unjust and increasingly tangled ERISA regime' [quoting a Third Circuit decision in 2003]." She pointed out with favor the suggestion of one court of appeals: "The vital thing . . . is that either Congress or the Court act quickly, because the current situation is plainly untenable."

These exhortations were written in 2004, and the health reform debate of 2009–2010 was a grand opportunity for Congress to address the "tangled ERISA regime," but unfortunately the injustice created by ERISA preemption was not addressed (see Legal Brief).

The court has had at least one other occasion to weigh in recently. In *Gobeille v. Liberty Mutual Ins. Co.*, the justices considered Vermont's "all-payer claims database" system, which required insurers to report data on healthcare costs and treatment outcomes. The question was whether such a system— similar versions of which were in effect in at least 17 other states—impermissibly conflicts with ERISA's dominion over employee benefit plans. By a 6–2 margin, the court held that it does.

Vermont's reporting regime, which compels plans to report detailed information about claims and plan members, both intrudes upon "a central matter of plan administration" and "interferes with nationally uniform plan administration." The State's law and regulation govern plan reporting, disclosure, and— by necessary implication—recordkeeping. These matters are fundamental components of ERISA's regulation of plan administration. Differing, or even parallel, regulations from multiple jurisdictions could create wasteful administrative costs and threaten to subject plans to wide-ranging liability.

Legal Brief

I would like to compliment the House [ACA] bill for one particular achievement. The convoluted language brilliantly upholds the tradition of the original ERISA legislation in defying rational and straightforward analysis. That we're already trying to parse whether ERISA preemption is being relaxed is an indication that Congress isn't sure what to do.

—Peter D. Jacobson, JD, MPH, University of Michigan (personal communication with the author regarding the ACA debates)

> .... ERISA's express pre-emption clause requires invalidation of the Ver-
> mont reporting statute as applied to ERISA plans. The state statute imposes duties
> that are inconsistent with the central design of ERISA, which is to provide a single
> uniform national scheme for the administration of ERISA plans without interfer-
> ence from laws of the several States even when those laws, to a large extent,
> impose parallel requirements.[72]

Thus, it seems ERISA preemption issues will remain a tangled web unless
Congress decides to act. Because the issues pit patient rights against business
interests, and given the discordant political climate in Washington recently,
there is considerable doubt whether that will occur anytime soon.

Summary

This chapter shows that the law has come a long way in recent years as it
relates to healthcare organizations. For more than half of the twentieth century, most hospitals were charitable organizations and thus were immune
from tort liability. After charitable immunity was abolished, courts began
to apply the doctrine of respondeat superior to the healthcare setting, and
a distinction was clearly drawn between an employee and an independent
contractor. But then the concepts of apparent agency and agency by estoppel
emerged, and the captain-of-the-ship and borrowed-servant doctrines fell out
of favor. These new notions have now expanded to the point that the independent contractor defense seems no longer viable in the healthcare field.

More significant, the expanded doctrine of *corporate negligence*—the
nondelegable duty of reviewing and evaluating clinical practices—has virtually obliterated the distinction between hospitals' vicarious liability and direct
liability, at least in the context of medical staff law.

Finally, the rise of managed care in the 1980s and 1990s has prompted
questions about whether efforts to control costs compromise the quality of
care. Because ERISA preempts any state law relating to employee benefit
plans (including employer-based health plans), in many cases MCOs are
immune from liability for coverage decisions that lead to adverse patient
outcomes. Conflicts sometimes arise between advancing patient welfare and
reducing healthcare costs. In the context of ERISA, at least, resolution of the
dilemma may require congressional action.

Discussion Questions

1. Why is the history of healthcare institutions important to understanding
   their legal liability today?

2. Why has the defense of independent contractor status declined in importance in recent years?

3. How is corporate liability different from liability under respondeat superior?

4. What is the liability of an MCO (e.g., HMO, PPO) when it makes decisions about insurance coverage for hospital stays?

5. Why is ERISA preemption an important consideration for MCOs?

6. What is the "tangled ERISA regime," and what are the chances that Congress will unsnarl it? (Students may wish to research any developments on this issue that have occurred since the publication of this book.)

The Court Decides

Norton v. Argonaut Insurance Co.
144 So. 2d 249 (La. Ct. App. 1962)

Landry, J.

[The plaintiffs are the parents of an infant who died after a medication error in a hospital. She was given an injection of a heart drug that should have been administered orally. The trial court found in the plaintiffs' favor, and the defendants appealed.

Shortly after her birth, the Norton baby was diagnosed as having congenital heart disease and was placed on Lanoxin (a form of digitalis) to strengthen her heart and reduce her pulse rate. She was discharged from the hospital at two and a half months, and her mother administered the medication at home by using a medicine dropper. The child was readmitted about two weeks later—on December 29, 1959—by her pediatrician, Dr. Bombet.]

On this occasion [Dr. Bombet] issued admission orders on the infant to be placed in the child's hospital chart or record. Included in his admission orders were instructions regarding medication, diet, etc., and the notation that special medication was being administered by the mother. In this connection it appears that Mrs. Norton preferred to continue administration of the daily maintenance dose of the Lanoxin herself since she had been performing this function since the child's initial admission to the hospital on December 15th. Dr. Bombet noted in the hospital admission orders of December 29, 1959, that special medication was being given by the mother to thusly advise the hospital staff and employees that some medication was being administered the child other than that which he placed on the order sheet and would, therefore, be administered by the hospital nursing staff.

On January 2, 1960 (Saturday) Dr. Stotler examined the Norton baby at approximately noon while in the course of making his rounds in the hospital. As a result of this examination he concluded that the child needed an increase in the daily maintenance dose of Lanoxin and instructed Mrs. Norton, who was present in the room, to increase the daily dose of the Lanoxin for that day only to 3 c.cs. instead of the usual 2.5 c.cs. Following this instruction to Mrs. Norton, Dr. Stotler went to the nurse's station in the hospital pediatric unit floor to check the hospital chart or record on the Norton infant and noted on the Doctor's Order Sheet contained therein certain instructions among which only the following is pertinent to the issues involved herein: "Give 3.0 cc Lanoxin today for 1 dose only."

Dr. Stotler's entry of the foregoing order for medication constitutes the basis of plaintiff's claim against Aetna as the professional liability insurer of Dr. Stotler. It is frankly conceded by Aetna that unless Dr. Stotler indicated on the order sheet that he had instructed the patient's mother to increase the daily maintenance dose of Lanoxin to 3.0 c.cs. and administer the medication, his entry of the aforesaid prescription on the order sheet would indicate that the nursing staff of the hospital was to give the medication prescribed. It is further conceded that under such circumstances the child was subjected to the possibility of being administered a second dose of Lanoxin. The possibility thus presented is exactly what occurred in the instant case. A member of the nursing staff noting Dr. Stotler's orders, administered 3 c.cs. of

Lanoxin in its injectible form instead of the elixir form which Dr. Stotler intended. . . . It is readily conceded by all concerned that the 3 c.cs. of Lanoxin administered the baby by hypodermic was a lethal overdose and was in fact the cause of the infant's demise.

. . . *[The day in question was a Saturday, and the regular staff was not on duty. Mrs. Florence Evans, an RN whose regular duties were administrative in nature, was assisting in the pediatric unit that day. She had not engaged in the actual clinical practice of nursing for some time, and she did not know that Lanoxin was available in oral form; the last she knew, Lanoxin was given only by injection. Noting the doctor's orders for "3 cc of Lanoxin," and seeing no indication that it had been given, she decided to inject the medication herself, even though she sensed that this "appeared to be a rather large dose," according to the court.]*

. . . She discussed the matter very briefly with the student nurse, Miss Meadows, and inquired of the Registered Nurse, Miss Sipes, whether or not the child had previously received Lanoxin. Mrs. Evans then examined the patient's hospital chart and found nothing [to indicate that] the child had been receiving Lanoxin while in the hospital. . . . Considering administration of the drug only by hypodermic needle, Mrs. Evans, accompanied by the Student Nurse, Miss Meadows, went to the medicine room of the pediatric unit and obtained two ampules of Lanoxin each containing 2 c.cs. of the drug in its injectible form. While pondering the advisability of . . . administering what she considered to be a large dose, Mrs. Evans noted that Dr. Beskin, one of the consultants on the child's case, had entered the pediatric ward so Mrs. Evans consulted him about the matter and was advised that if Dr. Stotler prescribed 3 c.cs. he meant 3 c.cs. Still not certain about the matter Mrs. Evans also

discussed the subject with Dr. Ruiz and was informed by him in effect that although the dose was the maximum dose that if the doctor had prescribed that amount she could give it. *[Despite her misgivings, she did give the injection. The baby went into distress, and despite emergency efforts, she died a little more than an hour later.]*

. . . The rule applicable in the instant case is well stated in the following language [of an earlier Louisiana case]: (1) A physician, surgeon or dentist, according to the jurisprudence of this court and of the Louisiana Courts of Appeal, is not required to exercise the highest degree of skill and care possible. As a general rule it is his duty to exercise the degree of skill ordinarily employed, under similar circumstances, by the members of his profession in good standing in the same community or locality, and to use reasonable care and diligence, alone with his best judgment, in the application of his skill to the case.

[I]t is manifest that Dr. Stotler was negligent in failing to denote the intended route of administration and failing to indicate that the medication prescribed had already been given or was to be given by the patient's mother. It is conceded by counsel for Dr. Stotler that the doctor's oversight in this regard exposed the child to the distinct possibility of being given a double oral dose of the medicine. Although it is by no means certain from the evidence that a second dose of oral Lanoxin would have proven fatal, Dr. Stotler's own testimony dose [*sic*] make it clear that in all probability it would have produced nausea. In this regard his testimony is to the effect that even if the strength of two oral doses were sufficient to produce death in all probability death would not result for the reason that nausea produced by overdosing would have most probably induced the child to vomit the second dose thereby saving her life. The contention that

(continued)

(continued from previous page)

Dr. Stotler followed the practice and custom usually engaged in by similar practitioners in the community is clearly refuted and contradicted by the evidence of record herein. Of the four medical experts who testified herein only Dr. Stotler testified in effect that it was the customary and usual practice to write a prescription in the manner shown. The testimony of Drs. Beskin, Bombet and Ruiz falls far short of corroborating Dr. Stotler in this important aspect. The testimony of Dr. Stotler's colleagues was clearly to the effect that the better practice is to specify the route of administration intended. . . . In view of the foregoing, we hold that the act acknowledged by Dr. Stotler does not relieve him from liability to plaintiffs herein on the ground that it accorded with that degree of skill and care employed, under similar circumstances, by other members of his profession in good standing in the community. We find and hold that the record before us fails to establish that physicians in good standing in the community follow the procedure adopted by defendant herein but rather the contrary is shown.

Pretermitting the issue of charitable immunity (with which we are not herein concerned in view of the fact that the suit is against the insurer of the hospital in the instant case) it is the settled jurisprudence of this state that a hospital is responsible for the negligence of its employees including, inter alia, nurses and attendants under the doctrine of respondeat superior.

[I]t is not disputed that Mrs. Evans was not only an employee of the hospital but that on the day in question she was in charge of the entire institution as the senior employee on duty at the time.

Although there have been instances in our jurisprudence wherein the alleged negligence of nurses has been made the basis of an action for damages for personal injuries . . . we are not aware of any prior decision which fixes the responsibility or duty of care owed by nurses to patients under their care or treatment. The general rule, however, seems to be to extend to nurses the same rules which govern the duty and liability of physicians in the performance of professional services. Thus . . . we find the rule stated as follows:

* * * The same rules that govern the duty and liability of physicians and surgeons in the performance of professional services are applicable to practitioners of the kindred branches of the healing profession, such as dentists, and, likewise, are applicable to practitioners such as drugless healers, oculists, and manipulators of X-ray machines and other machines or devices.

The foregoing rule appears to be well-founded and we see no valid reason why it should not be adopted as the law of this state. Tested in the light of [this rule] the negligence of Mrs. Evans is patent upon the face of the record. We readily agree with the statement of Dr. Ruiz that a nurse who is unfamiliar with the fact that the drug in question is prepared in oral form for administration to infants by mouth is not properly and adequately trained for duty in a pediatric ward. As laudable as her intentions are conceded to have been on the occasion in question, her unfamiliarity with the drug was a contributing factor in the child's death. In this regard we are of the opinion that she was negligent in attempting to administer a drug with which she was not familiar. While we concede that a nurse does not have the same degree of knowledge regarding drugs as is possessed by members of the medical profession, nevertheless, common sense dictates that no nurse should attempt to administer a drug under the circumstances shown in [this] case. Not only was Mrs. Evans unfamiliar with the medicine in question but she also violated what has been shown to be the rule generally practiced by the members of the nursing profession in the community and which rule, we might add, strikes us as being most reasonable and prudent, namely, the practice of calling the prescribing physician when in doubt about an order for medication. . . . For obvious reasons we believe it the duty of a nurse when in doubt about an order for medication to make absolutely certain what the doctor intended both as to dosage and route. . . .

. . .

The evidence . . . leaves not the slightest doubt that when Dr. Stotler entered the order for the medication on the chart, it was the duty of the hospital nursing staff to administer it. Dr. Stotler frankly concedes this important fact and for that reason acknowledged that he should have indicated on the chart that the medication had been given or was to be given by the mother, otherwise some nurse on the pediatric unit would give it as was required of the hospital staff. Not only was there a duty on the part of Dr. Stotler to make this clear so as to prevent duplication of the medication but also he was under the obligation of specifying or in some manner indicating the route considering the drug is prepared in two forms in which dosage is measured in cubic centimeters. In dealing with modern drugs, especially of the type with which we are herein concerned, it is the duty of the prescribing physician who knows that the prescribed medication will be administered by a nurse or third party, to make certain as to the lines of communication

between himself and the party whom he knows will ultimately execute his orders. Any failure in such communication which may prove fatal or injurious to the patient must be charged to the prescribing physician who has full knowledge of the drug and its effects upon the human system. The duty of communication between physician and nurse is more important when we consider that the nurse who administers the medication is not held to the same degree of knowledge with respect thereto as the prescribing physician. It, therefore, becomes the duty of the physician to make his intentions clear and unmistakable. If, as the record shows, Dr. Stotler had ordered elixir Lanoxin, or specified the route to be oral, it would have clearly informed all nurses of his intention to administer the medication by mouth. Instead, however, he wrote his order in an uncertain, confusing manner considering that the drug in question comes in oral and injectible form and that in both forms dosage is prescribed in terms of cubic centimeters.

It is settled jurisprudence of this state that where the negligence of two persons combines to produce injury to a third, the parties at fault are [jointly] liable to the injured plaintiff.

[Thus, the court affirms the jury's verdict and holds everybody liable.]■

Discussion Questions

1. How many mistakes can you count in this set of facts? At how many points could the chain of errors have been interrupted?
2. If you were the hospital administrator, the chief of the medical staff, or the chief of nursing, what action would you take to prevent recurrence of this tragedy?
3. This child's death occurred more than 50 years ago, yet a 2007 report by the Institute of Medicine (*Preventing Medication Errors*) states that at least 1.5 million people are injured each year because of medication errors. According to the report, on average at least one medication error is made per hospital per patient per day. What safeguards are in place in hospitals today to prevent these kinds of mistakes?
4. What does *pretermitting* mean?

~ Ⅲ ~

The Court Decides

Johnson v. Misericordia Community Hospital
99 Wis. 2d 708, 301 N.W.2d 156 (1981)

Coffey, J.

[This case involves negligent surgery per-formed on Mr. Johnson by Dr. Salinsky at Misericordia Community Hospital in July 1975. Because of undisputed negligence by the doc-tor, the patient (plaintiff) has "a permanent paralytic condition of his right thigh muscles with resultant atrophy and weakness and loss of function." The doctor settled before trial, but the hospital disputed allegations that it was negligent. A verdict in favor of the plain-tiff was affirmed by the court of appeals.

Misericordia Community Hospital had pre-viously been a religiously affiliated hospital but was sold to a private group of physicians who first operated it as a nursing home but subsequently reinstituted acute care services there. At the time of the incidents in this case, the hospital was not accredited by The Joint Commission.]

On March 5, 1973 . . . Dr. Salinsky applied for orthopedic privileges on the medical staff. In his application, Salinsky stated that he was on the active medical staff of [other hospitals and that] his privileges at other hospitals had never "been suspended, diminished, revoked, or not renewed." In another part of the application form, he failed to answer any of the questions pertaining to his malpractice insurance, i.e., carrier, policy number, amount of coverage, expiration date, [and] agent, and represented that he had requested privileges only for those surgical procedures in which he was qualified by certification.

In addition to requiring the above informa-tion, the application provided that significant misstatements or omissions would be a cause for denial of appointment. Also, in the application, Salinsky authorized Misericordia

to contact his malpractice carriers, past and present, and all the hospitals that he had previously been associated with, for the pur-pose of obtaining any information bearing on his professional competence, as well as his moral and ethical qualifications for staff membership. *[The application also contained language releasing the hospital from any lia-bility as a result of doing a background check on the applicant.]*

Mrs. Jane Bekos, Misericordia's medical staff coordinator (appointed April of 1973) testifying from the hospital records, noted that Salinsky's appointment to the medical staff was recommended by the then hospital administrator, David A. Scott, Sr., on June 22, 1973. Salinsky's appointment and requested orthopedic privileges, according to the hospi-tal records, were not marked approved until August 8, 1973. This approval of his appoint-ment was endorsed by Salinsky himself. Such approval would, according to accepted medical administrative procedure, not be signed by the applicant but by the chief of the respective medical section. Additionally, the record establishes that Salinsky was ele-vated to the position of Chief of Staff shortly after he joined the medical staff. However, the court record and the hospital records are devoid of any information concerning the pro-cedure utilized by the Misericordia authori-ties in approving either Salinsky's appoint-ment to the staff with orthopedic privileges or his elevation to the position of Chief of Staff.

Mrs. Bekos testified that although her hospital administrative duties entailed obtaining all the information available regarding an applicant from the hospitals

and doctors referred to in the application for medical staff privileges, she failed to contact any of the references in Salinsky's case. In her testimony she attempted to justify her failure to investigate Salinsky's application because she believed he had been a member of the medical staff prior to her employment in April of 1973, even though his application was not marked approved until some four months later on August 8, 1973. Further, Mrs. Bekos stated that an examination of the Misericordia records reflected that at no time was an investigation made by anyone of any of the statements recited in his application.
. . .

At trial, the representatives of two Milwaukee hospitals . . . gave testimony concerning the accepted procedure for evaluating applicants for medical staff privileges. Briefly, they stated that the hospital's governing body, i.e., the board of directors or board of trustees, has the ultimate responsibility in granting or denying staff privileges. However, the governing board delegates the responsibility of evaluating the professional qualifications of an applicant for clinical privileges to the medical staff. The credentials committee (or committee of the whole) conducts an investigation of the applying physician's or surgeon's education, training, health, ethics and experience through contacts with his peers in the specialty in which he is seeking privileges, as well as the references listed in his application to determine the veracity of his statements and to solicit comments dealing with the applicant's credentials. Once [this has been done, a recommendation is relayed] to the governing body, which . . . has the final appointing authority.

The record demonstrates that had [such an investigation been conducted, Misericordia] would have found, contrary to [Dr. Salinsky's] representations, that he had in fact experienced denial and restriction of his privileges, as well as never having been granted privileges at the very same hospitals he listed in his application. This information was readily available to Misericordia, and a review of Salinsky's associations with various Milwaukee orthopedic surgeons and hospital personnel would have revealed that they considered Salinsky's competence as an orthopedic surgeon suspect, and viewed it with a great deal of concern.

[The court summarizes some of Dr. Salinsky's professional history. At one hospital, his request for expanded orthopedic privileges was denied after being on the staff for a year and a half. At another, his privileges were temporarily suspended and subsequently limited after a report of "continued flagrant bad practices." At a third, his initial application for privileges was flatly denied. The court adds, "The testimony at trial established many other discrepancies in Salinsky's Misericordia application," and it points out that experts in the field testified that, in their opinion, a prudent hospital would not have granted Salinsky's application under these circumstances.]

The jury found that the hospital was negligent in granting orthopedic surgical privileges to Dr. Salinsky and thus apportioned eighty percent of the causal negligence to Misericordia. Damages were awarded in the sum of $315,000 for past and future personal injuries and $90,000 for past and future impairment of earning capacity. . . .

Issues:

1. Does a hospital owe a duty to its patients to use due care in the selection of its medical staff and the granting of specialized surgical (orthopedic) privileges?

2. What is the standard of care that a hospital must exercise in the discharge of this duty to its patients[,] and did Misericordia fail to exercise that standard of care in this case?

(continued)

(continued from previous page)

At the outset, it must be noted that Dr. Salinsky was an independent contractor, not an employee of Misericordia, and that the plaintiff is not claiming that Misericordia is vicariously liable for the negligence of Dr. Salinsky under the theory of respondeat superior. Rather, Johnson's claim is premised on the alleged duty of care owed by the hospital directly to its patients.

. . . "The concept of duty in Wisconsin, as it relates to negligence cases, is irrevocably interwoven with foreseeability. Foreseeability is a fundamental element of negligence." In [a prior case,] this court set the standard for determining when a duty arises:

> A defendant's duty is established when it can be said that it was foreseeable that his act or omission to act may cause harm to someone. A party is negligent when he commits an act when some harm to someone is foreseeable. Once negligence is established, the defendant is liable for unforeseeable consequences as well as foreseeable ones. In addition, he is liable to unforeseeable plaintiffs.

Further, we defined the term "duty" as it relates to the law of negligence:

> The duty of any person is the obligation of due care to refrain from any act which will cause foreseeable harm to others even though the nature of that harm and the identity of the harmed person or harmed interest is unknown at the time of the act.

. . .

Thus, the issue of whether Misericordia should be held to a duty of due care in the granting of medical staff privileges depends upon whether it is foreseeable that a hospital's failure to properly investigate and verify the accuracy of an applicant's statements dealing with his training, experience and qualifications as well as to weigh and pass judgment on the applicant would present an unreasonable risk of harm to its patients. The failure of a hospital to scrutinize the credentials of its medical staff applicants could foreseeably result in the appointment of unqualified physicians and surgeons to its staff. Thus, the granting of staff privileges to these doctors would undoubtedly create an unreasonable risk of harm or injury to their patients. Therefore, the failure to investigate a medical staff applicant's qualifications for the privileges requested gives rise to a foreseeable risk of unreasonable harm and we hold that a hospital has a duty to exercise due care in the selection of its medical staff.

Our holding herein is in accord with the public's perception of the modern day medical scientific research center with its computed axial tomography (CATscan), radio nucleide imaging thermography, microsurgery, etc., formerly known as a general hospital. The public is indeed entitled to expect quality care and treatment while a patient in our highly technical and medically computed hospital complexes. The concept that a hospital does not undertake to treat patients, does not undertake to act through its doctors and nurses, but only procures them to act solely upon their own responsibility, no longer reflects the fact. . . . [T]he person who avails himself of our modern "hospital facilities" . . . expects that the hospital staff will do all it reasonably can to cure him and does not anticipate that its nurses, doctors and other employees will be acting solely on their own responsibility.

Further, our holding is supported by the decisions of a number of courts from other jurisdictions. These cases hold that a hospital has a direct and independent responsibility to its patients, over and above that of the physicians and surgeons practicing therein, to take reasonable steps to (1) insure that its medical staff is qualified for the privileges granted and/or (2) to evaluate the care provided.

[The court here embarks on a lengthy discussion of similar cases from various other states. It points out the leading case of Darling v. Charleston Community Memorial Hosp., *in which the Supreme Court of Illinois found a direct duty flowing from hospital to patient regarding the qualifications of members of the medical staff. The* Johnson *court favorably quotes from the* Darling *opinion, including the following passage: "The Standards for Hospital Accreditation, the state licensing regulations and the defendant's bylaws demonstrate that the medical profession and other responsible authorities regard it as both desirable and feasible that a hospital assume certain responsibilities for the care of the patient."]*

There was credible evidence to the effect that a hospital, exercising ordinary care, [would have known of the deficiencies in Dr. Salinsky's qualifications and] would not have appointed Salinsky to its medical staff. . . .

This court has held "* * * a jury's finding of negligence * * * will not be set aside when there is any credible evidence that under any reasonable view supports the verdict. * * *" Thus, the jury's finding of negligence on the part of Misericordia must be upheld [because] the testimony of [the expert witnesses] constituted credible evidence which reasonably supports this finding.

In summary, we hold that a hospital owes a duty to its patients to exercise reasonable care in the selection of its medical staff and in granting specialized privileges. The final appointing authority resides in the hospital's governing body, although it must rely on the medical staff and in particular the credentials committee (or committee of the whole) to investigate and evaluate an applicant's qualifications for the requested privileges. However, this delegation of the responsibility to investigate and evaluate the professional competence of applicants for clinical privileges does not relieve the governing body of its duty to appoint only qualified physicians and surgeons to its medical staff and periodically monitor and review their competency. The credentials committee (or committee of the whole) must investigate the qualifications of applicants. *[Paragraph break added.]*

The facts of this case demonstrate that a hospital should, at a minimum, require completion of the application and verify the accuracy of the applicant's statements, especially in regard to his medical education, training and experience. Additionally, it should: (1) solicit information from the applicant's peers, including those not referenced in his application, who are knowledgeable about his education, training, experience, health, competence and ethical character; (2) determine if the applicant is currently licensed to practice in this state and if his licensure or registration has been or is currently being challenged; and (3) inquire whether the applicant has been involved in any adverse malpractice action and whether he has experienced a loss of medical organization membership or medical privileges or membership at any other hospital. The investigating committee must also evaluate the information gained through its inquiries and make a reasonable judgment as to the approval or denial of each application for staff privileges. The hospital will be charged with gaining and evaluating the knowledge that would have been acquired had it exercised ordinary care in investigating its medical staff applicants and the hospital's failure to exercise that degree of care, skill and judgment that is exercised by the average hospital in approving an applicant's request for privileges is negligence. This is not to say that hospitals are insurers of the competence of their medical staff, for a hospital will not be negligent if it exercises the noted standard of care in selecting its staff.

The decision of the Court of Appeals is affirmed. ■

(continued)

(continued from previous page)

Discussion Questions

1. In the opening paragraph of his classic 1881 treatise *The Common Law*, Oliver Wendell Holmes Jr. wrote: "The life of the law has not been logic: it has been experience. The felt necessities of the time, the prevalent moral and political theories, institutions of public policy, avowed or unconscious, even the prejudices which judges share with their fellow-men, have had a good deal more to do than the syllogism in determining the rules by which men should be governed." How is this case an example of the truth of this passage?
2. Do you agree with the court's rationale? What would have been the implications of the opposite result?
3. Do you agree with the court's statement on how the public perceives a modern hospital today? What evidence is there to support this statement?
4. Does this decision mean that a hospital will be liable for every incident of malpractice committed by nonemployee members of its medical staff? Why or why not?

Notes

1. The origin of immunity in the United States is generally attributed to McDonald v. Massachusetts Gen. Hosp., 120 Mass. 432, 21 A.529 (1876). It was a determining factor in the famous case of Schloendorff v. Society of New York Hospital, 211 N.Y. 125, 105 N.E. 92 (1914), which is generally cited today for its dictum on negligence versus battery (see chapter 11).

2. For a landmark case abolishing charitable immunity, *see* President & Directors of Georgetown College v. Hughes, 130 F.2d 810 (D.C. Cir. 1942).

3. Colby v. Carney Hospital, 356 Mass. 527, 254 N.E. 2d 407 (1969).

4. Lewis v. Physicians Ins. Co. of Wisconsin, 627 N.W.2d 484 (Wis. 2001).

5. Foley v. Bishop Clarkson Memorial Hosp., 185 Neb. 89, 173 N.W.2d 881 (1970); Kastler v. Iowa Methodist Hosp., 193 N.W.2d 98 (Iowa 1917); McGillivray v. Rapides Iberia Management Enterprises, 493 So. 2d 819 (La. Ct. App. 1986). Additionally, Lamont v. Brookwood Health Services, Inc., 446 So. 2d 1018 (Ala. 1983), held that the standard of care for hospitals was determined by the national hospital community.

6. Foley v. Bishop Clarkson Memorial Hosp., 185 Neb. at 95, 173 N.W.2d at 885.

7. For example, Reifschneider v. Nebraska Methodist Hosp., 222 Neb. 782, 387 N.W.2d 486 (1986) (when a semiconscious patient was placed on a cart in the hospital emergency department without use of restraints, expert testimony was required to establish expected standard of care); Rosemont, Inc. v. Marshall, 481 So. 2d 1126 (Ala. 1985) (standard of care with respect to observation and supervision of patient's ambulatory status requires expert testimony).

8. For example, Keeton v. Maury County Hosp., 713 S.W.2d 314 (Tenn. App. 1986) (the hospital staff knew or could foresee that the patient would be in danger if moving about unassisted; expert testimony was not necessary to establish breach of duty).

9. Reifschneider v. Nebraska Methodist Hosp., 387 N.W.2d at 489 (violation of a physician's order that patient be attended at all times presented a prima facie case of negligence).

10. Hastings v. Baton Rouge Gen. Hosp., 498 So. 2d 713 (La. 1986) (violation of hospital bylaws constitutes breach of duty and eliminates the need for expert testimony); Therrel v. Fonde, 495 So. 2d 1046 (Ala. 1986) (when facts establish a significant delay in treatment, expert testimony is not necessary to support a jury verdict that the defendant failed to provide adequate security).

11. For example, Mayers v. Litow & Midway Hosp., 154 Cal. App. 2d 413, 316 P.2d 351 (1957); Zelver v. Sequoia Hosp. Dist., 7 Cal. App. 3d 934, 87 Cal. Rptr. 79 (1970); Dickinson v. Mailliard, 175 N.W.2d 588 (Iowa 1970).

12. 58 Mich. App. 119, 227 N.W.2d 247 (1975).

13. Robert Kocher and Nikhil Sahni, *Hospitals' Race to Employ Physicians— The Logic behind a Money-Losing Proposition*, 364 N. ENG. J. MED. 1790 (2011).

14. Bob Herman, *7 Trends in Hospital-Employed Physician Compensation*, BECKER'S HOSP. REV., Jan. 25, 2013.

15. Richard Gunderman, *Should Doctors Work for Hospitals?*, ATLANTIC, May 27, 2014.

16. 2 N.Y.2d 656, 143 N.E.2d 3, 163 N.Y.S.2d 3 (1957).

17. *Id.*, 2 N.Y.2d at 666.

18. *See, e.g.*, Sanchez v. Medicorp Health Sys., 270 Va. 299, 303 (2005).

19. Baptist Memorial Hosp. System v. Sampson, 969 S.W.2d 945 (Tex. 1998).

20. *Id.* at 949.

21. 272 A.2d 718 (Del. 1970).

22. 304 A.2d 61 (Del. Super. Ct. 1973). *See also, e.g.*, Mehlman v. Powell, 281 Md. 269, 378 A.2d 1121 (1977), *and* Paintsville Hosp. Co. v. Rose, 683 S.W.2d 255 (Ky. 1985).

23. 404 Mich. 240, 273 N.W.2d 429 (1978).

24. See also RESTATEMENT (SECOND) OF TORTS § 429 (1965). One who employs an independent contractor to perform services for a client is liable for physical harm caused by negligence of the contractor if that client accepts those services under the reasonable belief that they are being rendered by the employer.

25. A physician who is on call for emergencies in the hospital may be personally liable as the result of a failure to respond. The hospital may also be liable (Hiser v. Randolph, 126 Ariz. 608, 617 P.2d 774 [1980]).

26. 458 Pa. 246, 329 A.2d 497 (1974).

27. *See* RESTATEMENT (SECOND) OF AGENCY § 226 (1958).

28. This trend was anticipated and forecast by Professor Arthur Southwick as early as 1960 when he wrote: "The third trend in the law of hospital liability is the most significant. It is the increasing tendency . . . to impose vicarious liability on facts where none would have been imposed heretofore. By some leading decisions it no longer follows that a professional person using his own skill, judgment and discretion in regard to the means and methods of his work is an independent contractor. . . . Gradually, the test of hospital liability for another's act is becoming simply a question of whether or not the actor causing injury was a part of the medical care organization." Arthur F. Southwick, *Vicarious Liability of Hospitals*, 44 MARQ. L. REV. 151, 182 (1960).

29. Bader v. United Orthodox Synagogue, 148 Conn. 449, 453, 172 A.2d 192, 194 (1961).

30. Shepherd v. McGinnis, 257 Iowa 35, 131 N.W.2d 475 (1964); Ardoin v. Hartford Accident & Indem. Co., 350 So. 2d 205 (La. App. 1977).

31. Phillips v. Powell, 210 Cal. 39, 290 P.2d 441 (1930); Milner v. Huntsville Memorial Hosp., 398 S.W.2d 647 (Tex. App. 1966).

32. South Highlands Infirmary v. Camp, 279 Ala. 1, 180 So. 2d 904 (1965); Nelson v. Swedish Hosp., 241 Minn. 551, 64 N.W.2d 38 (1954).

33. Peck v. Charles B. Towns. Hosp., 275 A.D. 302, 89 N.Y.S.2d 190 (1949).

34. 557 S.W.2d 859 (Tex. 1977).

35. Hamil v. Bashline, 224 Pa. Super. 407, 307 A.2d 57 (1973).

36. 553 S.W.2d 180 (Tex. App. 1977). *See also* Hipp v. Hospital Auth., 104 Ga. App. 174, 121 S.E.2d 273 (1961); Garlington v. Kingsley,

277 So. 2d 183 (La. App. 173), *rev'd on other grounds*, 289 So. 2d 88 (La. 1974).

37. 553 S.W.2d at 181.

38. Darling v. Charleston Community Memorial Hosp., 33 Ill. 2d 326, 211 N.E.2d 253, *cert. denied*, 383 U.S. 946 (1966). There are many other cases in accord, some of which are cited infra.

39. 72 Wash. 2d 73, 431 P.2d 973 (1967).

40. 19 Ohio St. 2d 128, 249 N.E.2d 829 (1969).

41. Kakligian v. Henry Ford Hosp., 48 Mich. App. 325, 210 N.W.2d 463 (1973).

42. 324 F. Supp. 233 (N.D. Ind. 1971).

43. 324 F. Supp. at 235.

44. Hospitals owe a duty to exercise such reasonable care as the patient's known condition requires and to guard against conditions that should have been discovered by the exercise of reasonable care (Foley v. Bishop Clarkson Memorial Hosp., 185 Neb. 89, 173 N.W.2d 881 [1970]). Moreover, hospitals are held to standards and practices prevailing generally, not only in the local community but also in similar or like communities in similar circumstances (Dickinson v. Mailliard, 175 N.W.2d 588 [Iowa 1970]).

45. 2 N.Y.2d 656, 143 N.E.2d 3, 163 N.Y.S.2d 3 (1957).

46. 33 Ill. 2d 326, 211 N.E.2d 253, *cert. denied*, 383 U.S. 946 (1966).

47. In support of its position, the court cited Bing v. Thunig, 2 N.Y.2d 656, 143 N.E.2d 3, 163 N.Y.S.2d 3 (1957).

48. 14 A.L.R.3d 873, 879 (1967).

49. 125 Ga. App. 1, 186 S.E.2d 307, *aff'd*, 229 Ga. 140, 189 S.E.2d 412 (1972).

50. The New York courts have also recognized that hospitals have a duty to patients to select and retain staff physicians with care. *See* Fiorentino v. Wenger, 19 N.Y.2d 407, 227 N.E.2d 296, 299, 280 N.Y.S.2d 373, 378 (1967), in which the court stated: "More particularly, in the context of the present case, a hospital will not be liable for an act of malpractice performed by an independently retained healer, unless it has reason to know that the act of malpractice would take place."

51. 88 Nev. 207, 495 P.2d 605, *cert. denied*, 409 U.S. 879 (1972).

52. *Id.*, 495 P.2d at 608. *See also* Pedroza v. Bryant, 101 Wash. 2d 226, 677 P.2d 166 (1984) (hospitals owe independent duty to patients to use reasonable care in selection and retention of medical staff; duty does not extend to the patient of a physician who allegedly committed malpractice in private office practice).

53. No. 228566 (Super. Ct. Cal., Sacramento County, 1973), *rev'd on other grounds*, 60 Cal. App. 3d 728 (1976).

54. 99 Wis. 2d 708, 301 N.W.2d 156 (1981). The opinion of the intermediate court of appeals is reported at 97 Wis. 2d 521, 294 N.W.2d 501 (1980).

55. 99 Wis. 2d at 723.

56. National Library of Medicine, *Managed Care Programs* (accessed August 8, 2016), at http://www.ncbi.nlm.nih.gov/mesh?term=managed%20care.

57. 192 Cal. App. 3d 1630, 239 Cal. Rptr. 810 (Ct. App. 1986).

58. *Id.* at 811–12.

59. *Id.* at 819.

60. 271 Cal. Rptr. 876 (Ct. App. 1990).

61. *Id.* at 883.

62. *Both quotes id.* at 880.

63. 29 U.S.C. § 1001 et seq.

64. 29 U.S.C. § 1144(a).

65. *See, e.g.*, Corcoran v. United Healthcare, Inc., 965 F.2d 1321 (5th Cir. 1992), *and* Rodriguez v. Pacificare of Tex., Inc., 980 F.2d 1014 (5th Cir. 1993). *But see* Dukes v. U.S. Healthcare, 57 F.3d 350 (3rd Cir. 1995), *and* Pacificare of Oklahoma, Inc. v. Burrage, 59 F.3d 151 (10th Cir. 1995).

66. Tex. Civ. Prac. & Rem. Code Ann. § 88.002.

67. Corporate Health Ins., Inc. v. Texas Dept. of Ins., 215 F.3d 526, 535 (5th Cir. 2000). The case was brought by various health insurers specifically to challenge the statute's validity. The plaintiffs were not ERISA plans.

68. Cases holding that there is no preemption: Cicio v. Does, 321 F.3d 83 (2d Cir. 2003); Roark v. Humana, 307 F.3d 298 (5th Cir. 2002); Land v. CIGNA Healthcare, 339 F.3d 1286 (11th Cir. 2003). Cases holding that ERISA does preempt state claims: Andrews-Clarke v. Travelers Ins. Co., 984 F. Supp. 49 (D. Mass. 1997); DiFelice v. Aetna U.S. Health Care, 346 F.3d 442 (3d Cir. 2003); Marks v. Watters, 322 F.3d 316 (4th Cir. 2003).

69. 542 U.S. 200 (2004).

70. *Id.* at 219.

71. *Id.* at 214.

72. 577 U.S. __ (2016).

73. Browning-Ferris Industries of California, Inc., 362 NLRB No. 186, August 27, 2015.

8

MEDICAL STAFF PRIVILEGES AND PEER REVIEW

After reading this chapter, you will

- know that the hospital board is ultimately responsible for the overall quality of care rendered in the facility,
- understand that medical staff membership is not limited to those with a doctor of medicine (MD) degree,
- recognize the role physicians play in accountable care organizations (ACOs),
- be aware that the courts usually support a hospital's decisions on medical staff privileges if a fundamentally fair process is used,
- appreciate the liability issues inherent in the peer review process under the Health Care Quality Improvement Act (HCQIA), and
- understand the emerging role of complementary and alternative medicine practitioners.

This chapter concentrates on relationships between the general acute care hospital and its organized medical staff, particularly with regard to granting and maintaining medical staff privileges. The chapter also explores differences in the hospital–physician relationship when physicians are employees rather than independent contractors.

With some minor variations, the principles discussed here apply both to hospitals and to other healthcare institutions that grant licensed professionals the privilege to use their facilities to care for patients. Therefore, unless otherwise indicated by the context, in this chapter the word *hospital* usually includes other kinds of healthcare provider organizations. In addition, note that the term *physician* includes not only those with an MD degree but also certain other licensed practitioners as defined by the Medicare statute.

The Medical Staff Organization

A structured medical staff is an essential part of a hospital. It is a miniature version of a corporation, complete with bylaws and rules that regulate the functions delegated to it by the governing board; some medical staffs are, in fact, incorporated, although this is not common. The functions of the medical staff organization include the following:

- Serving as liaison between the board and the medical staff
- Implementing the clinical aspects of corporate policies
- Investigating applicants' backgrounds and recommending applicants for medical staff membership
- Supervising the quality of medical care provided throughout the facility by means of a peer review process
- Providing continuing medical education

The medical staff organization is founded on a set of bylaws approved by the governing board. These bylaws define the structure of the medical staff, its areas of delegated authority, the functions of its committees, and the lines of communication between the staff and the governing board.

If a multihospital system has separate medical staffs for each facility, the corporate (system) governing board must have a mechanism for communicating with each facility's medical staff, and each medical staff must have a means of interacting with the corporate office. Healthcare systems commonly employ a physician liaison—a corporate director of medical affairs—to fulfill this role.

Because peer review and selection of medical staff members are responsibilities of the governing board, physician representation on the board is advisable. Although conflicts between clinical and operational interests can occur, the arguments favoring integration of physicians into hospital governance far outweigh those favoring a board of trustees made up entirely of lay members.

The advent of the Affordable Care Act of 2010 (ACA) raises salient questions about the relationship between the hospital corporation and its medical staff members:

- As hospital–physician integration becomes more prevalent, prompted by arrangements such as ACOs, how will the management and control of operational functions be allocated?
- Will operational functions be shared under these arrangements, or will an "us versus them" attitude persist between the "hospital side" and the "physician side"?

- How can hospital management support physicians in their individual practices in the absence of an ACO or other arrangements?
- How will the ACA affect physicians' right to attain and retain hospital staff appointments?
- Will staff appointments remain traditional, or will they be contractual or take the form of ownership interests or new arrangements?
- Will appointments grant full or only limited privileges?
- How will quality be assessed and controlled?
- As hospital–physician relationships improve or are established, will there be joint liability for decisions about selection of the medical staff?
- If the hospital corporation creates an ACO and the ACO receives a share of Medicare cost savings, how will the revenue be divided among participating physicians and facilities?

Answers to these and similar questions will evolve and become more apparent as the ACA takes hold in the years ahead.

Relationships Among Board, Management, and Medical Staff

For many, many years, hospitals' day-to-day operations have been described as resting on a "three-legged stool" comprising the governing board, medical staff, and executive management. For a hospital to run smoothly and serve its community well, the three legs of that stool must be stable. The Joint Commission puts it this way:

> How well leaders work together and manage conflict affects a hospital's performance. In fulfilling its role, the governing body involves senior managers and leaders of the organized medical staff in governance and management functions.
>
> Good relationships thrive when leaders work together to develop the mission, vision, and goals of the hospital; encourage honest and open communication; and address conflicts of interest.[1]

A breakdown in this tripartite relationship can have serious consequences, as exemplified by a recent case from Minnesota in which a medical staff filed suit against its own hospital. Tension and conflict had begun after a city-owned hospital was acquired by an out-of-state health system in 2009. The hospital board attempted to deal with the situation three years later by unilaterally rescinding and replacing the medical staff organization's bylaws, but disgruntled members of the medical staff commenced litigation. The hospital asked that the case be dismissed on the ground that the medical staff, as such, lacked standing to sue.

At the heart of the case was the issue of who has ultimate control of a hospital: the governing board or the medical staff. The lower courts granted summary judgment in the hospital's favor, and the medical staff appealed. In December 2014, the Minnesota Supreme Court ruled that the medical staff could in fact sue the hospital, and it remanded the case for further proceedings on the merits of the claims.[2]

Thus after more than two years of procedural wrangling and nearly six years of discontent, the ultimate issue remained unsettled, the drama and dysfunction continued, and the scene shifted back to the trial court. The hospital again moved for summary judgment, that motion was again granted, and the medical staff again appealed. In July 2016, the Minnesota Court of Appeals affirmed the trial court's decision.[3] Whether the medical staff will appeal further is unknown, but regardless, one suspects that the friction between the physicians and the governing board will continue for quite some time. This case serves as a reminder of the serious problems that can arise when there are disputes between the medical staff and hospital leadership. Given the ACA's emphasis on hospital–physician integration, maintaining a well-balanced "three-legged stool" is more important than ever (see "The Joint Commission on Discord").

privileging
the process whereby the specific scope and content of patient care (clinical) services are authorized for a healthcare practitioner by a healthcare organization on the basis of evaluation of the individual's credentials and performance[5]

Appointment of the Medical Staff
Duty of Reasonable Care

As discussed in chapter 7, the hospital governing board has ultimate responsibility for the quality of patient care, and members of the governing board have a duty to exercise reasonable care in (1) reviewing the credentials of medical staff applicants and (2) **privileging** them to work in the facility. If the physicians are employees, respondeat superior applies and the hospital may be held liable for negligence in granting medical staff privileges. A hospital also may be held liable for negligence in granting privileges to independent contractors because the hospital's duty to select medical staff physicians carefully and to monitor the quality of care is separate from its responsibility as an employer.[4] This concept is referred to variously as "corporate liability," "institutional liability," or "direct liability."

The governing board may not abdicate its responsibility for quality. The duty cannot be delegated to the medical staff organization, the local medical society, or any other group or individual. Although lay members of the governing board might not be qualified to judge physicians' professional competencies, they must ensure that a reliable review process is in place

The Joint Commission on Discord

The Joint Commission states, "A hospital with an organized medical staff and governing body that cannot agree on amendments to critical documents has evidenced a breakdown in the required collaborative relationship."[87]

so that physicians' peers may do so. The board thus authorizes the medical staff to investigate applicants' backgrounds and quality concerns involving active physician members. The board usually approves the medical staff's recommendations, but the staff's role is advisory only; the board has ultimate decision-making responsibility (see Legal Brief at right).[6]

Due Process and Equal Protection Requirements

As long ago as 1927, the US Supreme Court held that a licensed physician does not have a constitutional right to a medical staff appointment.[7] However, hospitals that are owned by the government are engaged in state action when they make decisions about medical staff privileges. Thus, they must afford medical staff members and applicants the constitutional protections required by the Fourteenth Amendment (see Legal Brief below).

> ### Legal Brief
>
>
>
> A physician friend and I were talking about appointments to the medical staff. He made a comment that led me to ask, "Who makes the decisions about medical staff privileges in your hospital?" His reply was, "The medical staff credentials committee, of course."
>
> I had to disabuse him of this notion. Although the medical staff's recommendations are usually adopted, the board has ultimate responsibility to decide. Board members must therefore ensure that the medical staff committee is following the **credentialing** process properly and must be prepared to ask appropriate questions and exercise independent judgment.

State action is conduct that a person (either an individual or an entity) undertakes on behalf of a governmental body. State actors include government agencies, government-owned corporations, and individuals employed by the state. Others who have only an indirect relationship with the state but whose actions are under some degree of state sanction or control may also be state actors. Clearly, a state-, county-, or city-owned hospital is a state actor, as are its employees and agents. A private corporation that operates a state-owned facility under contract may also be considered to be engaged in state action.

credentialing
a process for establishing the qualifications and competence of medical staff applicants through review of their training, licensure, and practice history

In *Baldetta v. Harborview Medical Center*, the concept of state action was implicated when the plaintiff sued a public hospital where he had been employed.[8] He alleged that his tattoo of the words "HIV-Positive" was protected speech under the First Amendment and that the hospital acted unlawfully when it terminated him for refusing to cover it. The court found in the hospital's favor—the hospital's interests in facilitating its patients' recovery outweighed Baldetta's interest in displaying the tattoo—but the constitutional argument had to be addressed because Harborview is a state-owned facility.

> ### Legal Brief
>
>
>
> No state shall . . . deprive any person of life, liberty, or property, without due process of law; nor deny to any person . . . the equal protection of the laws.
>
> —US Constitution, Fourteenth Amendment

Private hospitals, although highly regulated and funded in large part by government programs (especially Medicare and Medicaid), are not instrumentalities of the state for constitutional purposes.[9] Thus, the government does not aid or approve an activity or cause an injury simply by providing funding to the hospital or by regulating it,[10] and a private hospital is not performing a public function when it appoints physicians to its medical staff.[11] As noted earlier, however, when the government owns the hospital, it must extend due process and equal protection to any physician who applies for a medical staff appointment and to any current staff member who is subject to disciplinary action.[12]

The Fourteenth Amendment refers to two key principles that apply to state actors. The first is *due process*, which concerns the legal relationship between the state and the individual, and it requires essential fairness in the government's handling of that relationship (the Fifth Amendment contains an identical requirement that applies to the federal government). The second is *equal protection of the laws*, which essentially means that a government cannot discriminate on the basis of characteristics such as race, religion, gender, national origin, and socioeconomic status. Both due process and equal protection issues can surface whenever fundamental rights are directly affected by state action, and both require the state actor—a government hospital, for example—to act reasonably, not capriciously or arbitrarily.

In summary, government hospitals are state actors and thus must grant due process and equal protection in their medical staff proceedings and employment policies. Private hospitals are not directly subject to the principles of the Fourteenth Amendment, but (as discussed later in the chapter) they apply essentially the same rights in their medical staff appointment process. Back in the 1980s, the public–private dichotomy was seen as inequitable and anachronistic because public and private hospitals serve the same community. Today, the distinction between the duties of public and private hospitals in matters of medical staff privileges has essentially disappeared.[13] The state action concept remains important, however, in other areas of the law, such as antitrust (see chapter 13).

Standards for Medical Staff Appointments
Fundamental Fairness

Hospitals of all types—whether public or private—must act diligently when considering medical staff appointments and must use fair procedures in applying their bylaws, rules, and regulations. Several statutes and principles mandate this duty, including

- constitutional provisions, when applicable (as explained earlier);
- state nondiscrimination statutes;
- the public policy of fundamental fairness as expressed in judicial decisions;

- state and federal antitrust statutes prohibiting unlawful restraints of trade; and
- tort law precedents prohibiting malicious interference with a physician's right to practice.

Prohibition of Class Discrimination

Constitutional issues aside, hospitals are prohibited by common law from arbitrarily excluding whole classes of practitioners. A seminal case on this point was decided more than 50 years ago in New Jersey. In *Greisman v. Newcomb Hospital*,[14] the plaintiff was a doctor of osteopathy (DO) who had been granted an unrestricted license to practice medicine and surgery in the state of New Jersey. He was the only osteopath in an area of about 100,000 people, and Newcomb Hospital—a private not-for-profit corporation—was the only hospital.

Newcomb Hospital refused to permit Dr. Greisman to apply for admission to its medical staff. Its decision rested on a provision in the hospital's bylaws stating that applicants must be graduates of an American Medical Association (AMA)–approved medical school and must be members of the county medical society. The county had not acted on Dr. Greisman's application to the county medical society, and he was not a graduate of an approved school because the AMA did not approve schools of osteopathy back then.

By the time the case came to the New Jersey Supreme Court, the American Hospital Association and The Joint Commission had changed their policies and had begun to approve of hospitals having DOs on their staffs; following their lead, the AMA adopted a policy statement allowing DOs "where it was determined locally that they practice on the same scientific principles as those adhered to by the American Medical Association."[15] The state medical society in New Jersey had also dropped its opposition. Thus, the Supreme Court of New Jersey—without the benefit of a constitutional or statutory foundation and without relying on tort or antitrust principles— simply held that the hospital could not arbitrarily refuse to consider Dr. Greisman's application. The decision was based on what the court felt was a fundamental public policy: A hospital has a duty to serve the public's best interests, especially when it is the only hospital in town.

In addition to common-law ("judge-made") principles, statutes may prohibit a hospital from summarily dismissing an application solely because the applicant is an osteopath, a podiatrist, or a non-MD practitioner. For example, the relevant Ohio statute reads as follows:

> The governing body of any hospital, in considering and acting upon applications for staff membership or professional privileges within the scope of the applicants' respective licensures, shall not discriminate against a qualified person solely on the basis of whether that person is certified to practice medicine, osteopathic

medicine, or podiatry, or licensed to practice dentistry or psychology. Staff membership or professional privileges shall be considered and acted on in accordance
with standards and procedures established [by the governing body].[16]

The California statute includes an affirmative obligation to allow
podiatrists access to hospital facilities:

The rules of a health facility shall include provisions for use of the facility by, and
staff privileges for, duly licensed podiatrists within the scope of their respective
licensure, subject to rules and regulations governing such use or privileges established by the health facility. Such rules and regulations shall not discriminate on
the basis of whether the staff member holds a[n] MD, DO, or DPM degree.[17]

A similar California provision requiring medical staffs to be open to clinical psychologists includes language that summarizes the general principle at
work: "Competence shall be determined by health facility rules and medical
staff bylaws that are necessary and are applied in good faith, equally and in
a nondiscriminatory manner, to all practitioners, regardless of whether they
hold an MD, DO, DDS, DPM, or doctoral degree in psychology."[18]

The Joint Commission recognizes that the medical staff may include
"any individual permitted by law and by the organization to provide care,
treatment, and services, without direction or supervision."[19] In short, applicants for hospital privileges must be evaluated fairly on the basis of their
professional qualifications and competence. Exclusion of entire classes of
non-MD practitioners is not permitted.

Various state and federal laws also prohibit discrimination on the basis
of race, creed, color, sex, disability, national origin, and other protected categories.[20] Such discrimination violates not only specific statutory prohibitions
but also, in the case of governmental facilities, the equal protection clause of
the Fourteenth Amendment.[21]

General Standards and Judicial Review

If we assume that the hospital does not discriminate against entire classes of
persons, how may it define its qualifications for medical staff privileges? This
question was the focus of *Sosa v. Board of Managers of Val Verde Memorial
Hospital*.[22] Over a number of years, Dr. Sosa had attempted and failed to gain
appointment to the medical staff of Val Verde Memorial Hospital. His application had been denied after the medical staff credentials committee found
his "character, qualifications, and standing in the community" inadequate.
Although the hospital's written criteria were vague, the committee listed nine
specific reasons—each supported by evidence—for denying him privileges
(see Law in Action). The hospital board concurred with the committee's

recommendations, and the US Court of Appeals deemed the hospital's standards sufficiently clear, stating that

staff appointments may be . . . refused if the refusal is based upon any reasonable basis such as the professional and ethical qualifications of the physicians or the common good of the public and the Hospital. *Admittedly, standards such as "character, qualifications, and standing" are very general, but this court recognizes that in the area of personal fitness for medical staff privileges precise standards are difficult if not impossible to articulate.*

The subjectives of selection simply cannot be minutely codified. The governing board of a hospital must therefore be given great latitude in prescribing the necessary qualifications for potential applicants. So long as the hearing process gives notice of the particular charges of incompetency and ethical fallibilities, we need not exact a precis of the standard in codified form.

On the other hand, it is clear that in exercising its broad discretion the board [may] refuse staff applicants only for those matters which are reasonably related to the operation of the hospital. Arbitrariness and false standards are to be eschewed. Moreover, procedural due process must be afforded the applicant so that he may explain or show to be untrue those matters which might lead the board to reject his application.[23] [Emphasis added.]

> ## Law in Action
>
> In Dr. Sosa's case, the evidence showed that the doctor had
>
> - abandoned obstetric patients in active labor because they could not pay his bill;
> - lacked knowledge of basic surgery techniques, operating procedures, and instrument use;
> - demonstrated an unstable physical demeanor and a markedly nervous manner, both of which were likely to jeopardize surgical patients;
> - suffered from an unstable and dangerous mental condition, which manifested in anger and fits of rage;
> - received unsatisfactory reports from references in his application;
> - followed an itinerant medical practice pattern since completing his education;
> - pleaded guilty to two felony charges;
> - had his license to practice suspended in two states; and
> - violated five of the ten principles of medical ethics.

The court concluded with this excellent summary of the principles of judicial review in this area:

It is the [hospital] Board, not the court, which is charged with the responsibility of providing a competent staff of doctors. The Board has chosen to rely on the advice of its Medical Staff, and the court cannot surrogate for the Staff in executing this responsibility. Human lives are at stake, and the governing board must be given discretion in its selection so that it can have confidence in the competence and moral commitment of its staff. The evaluation of professional proficiency of doctors is best left to the specialized expertise of their peers, subject only to limited judicial surveillance. The court is charged with the narrow responsibility of assuring that the qualifications imposed by the Board are reasonably related to the operation of the hospital and fairly administered. *In short, so long as staff selections are administered with fairness, geared by a rationale compatible with hospital responsibility, and unencumbered with irrelevant considerations, a court should not interfere.* Courts must not attempt to take on the escutcheon of Caduceus.[24] [Emphasis added.]

This case demonstrated that due process and fundamental fairness cannot be precisely defined; they are general principles that allow for interpretation based on the time, place, and circumstances of each case. An applicant must be given notice of the charges under consideration and an opportunity to rebut them at a hearing on the matter, but otherwise the standards are, by necessity, loosely defined.

Consistent with this principle, the courts have upheld adverse actions against physicians for the following reasons:

- Lack of surgical judgment, lack of a surgical assistant, and assisting another who had no surgical privileges (all backed by supporting evidence)[25]
- Failure to carry prescribed malpractice insurance coverage[26]
- Failure to comply with rules regarding the maintenance and completion of medical records[27]
- Failure to supply references with the application[28]
- Violation of a rule requiring a full staff member to be in attendance when an associate medical staff member performs major surgery[29]
- Refusal to abide by reasonable medical staff bylaws[30]
- Refusal to serve on a rotating basis in the emergency department[31]
- Failure to consult with other physicians before performing surgery or delivering medical treatment, as defined by medical staff protocols[32]

The circumstances of each case are different, but this list demonstrates that the courts give healthcare institutions considerable leeway to make decisions based on the needs of patients and the quality of care.

Peer Review, Discipline, and the Health Care Quality Improvement Act

The governing board is responsible for monitoring the professional qualifications of the medical staff, but most board directors are not qualified to judge the professional competence of clinicians. For this reason, under the board's supervision the medical staff organization must continually assess the quality of care provided in the facility. (This topic is closely related to the utilization review and case management function discussed in chapter 3.) The following discussion begins with a summary of the common law governing peer review and discipline, proceeds to a lengthy discussion of peer review under the federal Health Care Quality Improvement Act of 1986 (HCQIA), and concludes with a few words about the confidentiality of peer review records and about national fraud data banks.

The Common Law

As noted earlier, the courts generally defer to a hospital's decisions about medical staff discipline if it presents sufficient evidence of incompetence or intolerable behavior. *Moore v. Board of Trustees of Carson-Tahoe Hospital* is a classic example of the hospital's duties under the common law—to wit, to exercise reasonable care in selecting and retaining medical staff and to extend due process to the physician when disciplinary action is undertaken.[33]

Moore involved the termination of a medical staff appointment at a Nevada public hospital. Dr. Moore had been licensed to practice in Nevada and was certified by his professional board in obstetrics and gynecology. The specific acts that led to Dr. Moore's termination were not expressly prohibited in the medical staff bylaws or Carson-Tahoe Hospital's rules and regulations, but the hospital's governing body terminated his privileges on the ground of "unprofessional conduct." The facts showed that he did not exercise proper sterile technique in administering a spinal anesthetic to an obstetrics patient. Specifically, he had not worn sterile gloves while preparing the medication, performing the skin preparation, and handling the spinal needle. Two days later, the chief of the medical staff, with concurrence of another physician, canceled Dr. Moore's scheduled surgery for that day, attesting that he was "in no condition physically or mentally to perform surgery" (see Legal Decision Point).

Dr. Moore brought suit to regain his hospital privileges. He did not allege any deficiency in the procedural aspects of the case because at the hearing he was permitted to have counsel, call witnesses of his own, and cross-examine adverse witnesses. But he claimed that "unprofessional conduct" was too vague a standard on which to revoke his privileges and that he was, therefore, denied *substantive* due process.

The Nevada Supreme Court disagreed, citing this language from a Florida case: "Detailed description of prohibited conduct is concededly impossible, perhaps even undesirable in view of rapidly shifting standards of medical excellence and the fact that a human life may be and quite often is involved in the ultimate decision of the board."[34] The court held that the

Legal Decision Point

Why do you suppose Dr. Moore was in no condition to perform the intended surgery? Should the trial record and appellate decision have described his condition specifically? Why, do you suppose, they did not?

language "unprofessional conduct" was objective enough to justify the board's decision to terminate the doctor's privileges.

In rendering its opinion, the Nevada Supreme Court made these observations about the status of the hospital as an institution, prophetic words that ring even truer more than four decades later:

> Today in response to demands of the public, the hospital is becoming a community health center. The purpose of the community hospital is to provide patient care of the highest possible quality. To implement this duty of providing competent medical care to the patients, it is the responsibility of the institution to create a workable system whereby the medical staff of the hospital continually reviews and evaluates the quality of care being rendered within the institution. The staff must be organized with a proper structure to carry out the role delegated to it by the governing body. All powers of the medical staff flow from the board of trustees, and the staff must be held accountable for its control of quality. The concept of corporate responsibility for the quality of medical care was forcibly advanced in *Darling v. Charleston Community Memorial Hospital*, wherein the Illinois Supreme Court held that hospitals and their governing bodies may be held liable for injuries resulting from imprudent or careless supervision of members of their medical staffs.
>
> *The role of the hospital vis-a-vis the community is changing rapidly. The hospital's role is no longer limited to the furnishing of physical facilities and equipment where a physician treats his private patients and practices his profession in his own individualized manner.*
>
> The right to enjoy medical staff privileges in a community hospital is not an absolute right, but rather is subject to the reasonable rules and regulations of the hospital. Licensing, per se, furnishes no continuing control with respect to a physician's professional competence and therefore does not assure the public of quality patient care. The protection of the public must come from some other authority, and that in this case is the Hospital Board of Trustees. The Board, of course, may not act arbitrarily or unreasonably in such cases. The Board's actions must also be predicated upon a reasonable standard.[35] [Emphasis added.]

Moore stands as an excellent illustration of how (1) the medical staff properly exercises its responsibility for quality-of-care issues, (2) a governing board should act on the medical staff's recommended corrective action before injury to a patient occurs, and (3) courts usually defer to a hospital's decisions if they are based on reasonable criteria related to the quality of care.

Moore and cases like it give healthcare organizations the incentive, authority, and responsibility to focus on quality and to pursue the "triple aim" of better health, better care, and reduced cost (see "The Triple Aim").

Determining practitioners' competency is perhaps the most important function of the organized medical staff and the governing board. Whether for constitutional reasons (in the case of state actors) or because of statutory or common-law principles, decisions about practitioners' privileges must be objective, evidence based, and fundamentally fair. The process should include the practitioner's rights to notice, a timely hearing, an opportunity to produce evidence and cross-examine witnesses, written findings, and an opportunity to appeal. Both Medicare and The Joint Commission confirm these conclusions.[36]

The Joint Commission's accreditation standards for medical staff privileges are based on the following areas of general competency:

- Patient care
- Medical or clinical knowledge
- Practice-based learning and improvement
- Interpersonal and communication skills
- Professionalism
- Systems-based practice[37]

The standards also include the concept of "focused professional practice evaluation" (used when specific questions about competency arise) and "ongoing professional practice evaluation."[38] Together these processes are intended to identify performance issues that affect the quality of care and to resolve them as early as possible, with intervention by the organized medical staff if necessary.

The Triple Aim

According to the Institute for Healthcare Improvement (IHI),

> Focusing on three critical objectives simultaneously can potentially lead us to better models for providing healthcare. We call this approach the "Triple Aim":
>
> - Improve the health of the defined population
> - Enhance the patient care experience (including quality, access and reliability)
> - Reduce, or at least control, the per capita cost of care[88]

In 2007, IHI launched initiatives to translate the Triple Aim concept into specific actions for change. The result was a model and a set of design concepts to fulfill the Triple Aim in practice.

Some components of a system to accomplish the Triple Aim include:

1. A focus on individuals and families
2. Redesign of primary care services and structures
3. Population health management
4. A cost-control platform
5. System integration and execution

Additional information on each component is available at http://www.ihi.org.

Peer Review Under the Health Care Quality Improvement Act

Peer review is meant to be a discreet, retrospective evaluation of physicians' performance to see whether accepted standards of care were met and to suggest quality improvements if they were not. The HCQIA[39] provides a framework for accomplishing peer review and for protecting persons involved in the process.

The courts' deference to hospitals' decisions about staff privileges waned somewhat in the 1970s for two major reasons. The first was the large increase of medical malpractice lawsuits in the 1970s. As the number of suits increased, so did the perception of medical incompetence and a fear that discredited physicians could move across state lines and begin practice again without anyone knowing about their substandard performance. This apprehension prompted the creation of the HCQIA's National Practitioner Data Bank (NPDB).

The second reason for increased scrutiny of hospitals' privileging decisions involved claims of malicious interference with the right to practice and antitrust suits for restraint of trade. The 1988 US Supreme Court case *Patrick v. Burget* is a prime example.[40]

The *Patrick* Case

Dr. Patrick was a general and vascular surgeon in Astoria, Oregon (with an approximate population of 10,000). After practicing with the Astoria Clinic for a year, he started a competing practice and, along with his former colleagues, maintained his surgical privileges at Astoria's only hospital. According to the US Supreme Court's opinion,

> After petitioner established his independent practice, the physicians associated with the Astoria Clinic consistently refused to have professional dealings with him. Petitioner received virtually no referrals from physicians at the Clinic, even though the Clinic at times did not have a general surgeon on its staff. Rather than refer surgery patients to petitioner, Clinic doctors referred them to surgeons located as far as 50 miles from Astoria. In addition, Clinic physicians showed reluctance to assist petitioner with his own patients. Clinic doctors often declined to give consultations, and Clinic surgeons refused to provide backup coverage for patients under petitioner's care. At the same time, Clinic physicians repeatedly criticized petitioner for failing to obtain outside consultations and adequate backup coverage.[41]

Eventually, this "openly hostile" situation (quoting the court of appeals) deteriorated to the point that Astoria Clinic's physicians initiated and participated in peer review actions that terminated Dr. Patrick's medical staff privileges. He then sued under the antitrust laws and won a jury verdict of $650,000, which was tripled to nearly $2 million, as required by antitrust law.

On appeal, the Ninth Circuit found "substantial evidence that [the defendants] had acted in bad faith in the peer review process" and that the process was "shabby, unprincipled and unprofessional."[42] Even so, the appellate court ruled that the clinic's doctors were immune from antitrust liability because of the state action doctrine. (See the section on antitrust law in chapter 13.) The US Supreme Court took the case and reversed the lower court. The high court ruled that Oregon's peer review law did *not* amount to state action and thus did not protect the defendants from liability for their activities on private hospitals' peer review committees (see Law in Action). This decision sent shock waves through the medical community and made physicians and others understandably reluctant to participate in peer review.

As a direct result of the trial court verdict in *Patrick*, and even before the US Supreme Court issued its opinion, Congress passed the HCQIA. The "findings" section of the act summarizes Congress's rationale:

- A rise in the number of malpractice cases
- The potential for incompetent physicians to move from state to state and start practice anew
- The threat of physician liability under the antitrust laws
- The need for improved peer review activities[43]

> ## Law in Action
>
>
>
> In contrast to *Patrick*, and depending on the facts of the situation, the peer review activities of a hospital owned by a government agency—a taxing district or "hospital authority," for example—may amount to state action and thus be exempt from antitrust scrutiny. See, for example, *Crosby v. Hosp. Authority of Valdosta and Lowndes County*, in which the court stated: "Because of the control exercised by the [Hospital] Authority over peer review decisions and the statutory context of peer review in Georgia, we conclude that the actions of individual doctors on peer review committees should be considered [state] actions."[89]

A lengthy excerpt from the HCQIA is reproduced in appendix 8.1 at the end of this chapter.

With these statements as its foundation, the HCQIA grants immunity from most civil money damages to healthcare professionals who engage in peer review (referred to in the act as "professional review activities"; see Legal Brief). The HCQIA also authorized the creation of the NPDB as a reporting system for information on the competence of MDs, DOs, and dentists. Two cases decided by the US Court of Appeals for the Fifth Circuit in 2008 demonstrate the HCQIA's effects.

The *Poliner* Case

In *Poliner v. Texas Health System*, an interventional cardiologist's catheterization lab and echocardiography privileges at Presbyterian Hospital in Dallas were temporarily suspended while his manner of handling certain patients was being investigated.[44] (Today, The Joint Commission would call this type of investigation a "focused professional practice evaluation.") Quality concerns had been reported to the director of the cath lab and

> ## Legal Brief
>
>
>
> The HCQIA was sponsored by Congressman Ron Wyden of Oregon, who specifically referred to the jury verdict in *Patrick* as an example of the need to protect persons who perform peer review.[90]

to the chair of the internal medicine department. The bylaws of this not-for-profit hospital allowed for summary action "when the acts of a practitioner through his lack of competence, impaired status, behavior or failure to care adequately for his patients constitutes a present danger to the health of his patients," so the internal medicine department invoked the suspension after consultations with other physicians and hospital administration.[45] Dr. Poliner agreed, albeit reluctantly, to the temporary suspension of his privilege to use the cath lab.

An ad hoc committee of cardiologists then convened to review a sample of Dr. Poliner's cases. It chose at random the records of 44 patients and found evidence of substandard care in more than half of them. The committee reported its findings to the hospital's internal medicine advisory committee (IMAC). The IMAC's minutes identified the following concerns about Dr. Poliner's competencies:

- Poor clinical judgment
- Inadequate skills, including in angiocardiography and echocardiography
- Unsatisfactory documentation of medical records
- Substandard patient care

On the basis of the evidence before it, the IMAC recommended suspension of Dr. Poliner's cath lab and echocardiography privileges. He requested a hearing, as provided for in the hospital bylaws. The hearing committee (a separate group from the IMAC) upheld the original suspension on the basis of the evidence available at the time but recommended that he be reinstated on the condition that he consult with another cardiologist before performing interventional procedures. After a month, this condition was to be changed to postprocedure review. The hospital's governing board accepted these recommendations and, subject to these conditions, Dr. Poliner was reinstated. Approximately 18 months later, he filed suit against the hospital and the doctors who had been involved in the peer review process.

Dr. Poliner's lawsuit alleged federal and state antitrust violations; violations of the Deceptive Trade Practices Act; and numerous tort claims, including defamation. The case went to a trial by jury on the issue of temporary restrictions of Dr. Poliner's privileges, and the appellate court summarized the outcome as follows:

The jury found for Poliner on his defamation claims. Poliner was able to offer evidence at trial of actual loss of income of about $10,000—but was awarded more than $90 million in defamation damages, nearly all for mental anguish and injury to career. The jury also awarded $110 million in punitive damages. The district court ordered a remittitur of the damages and entered judgment against Defendants.[46]

By its **remittitur**, the trial court reduced the verdict to slightly more than $11 million, still a huge amount considering that the actual damages were only about $10,000. The defendants appealed, arguing that the HCQIA's immunity provisions protect them from liability in any amount. The court of appeals agreed, and in doing so provided a good summary of the HCQIA's history and its immunity provisions:

> Congress passed the Health Care Quality Improvement Act because it was concerned about "[t]he increasing occurrence of medical malpractice and the need to improve the quality of medical care," and because "[t]here is a national need to restrict the ability of incompetent physicians to move from State to State without disclosure or discovery of the physician's previous damaging or incompetent performance." Congress viewed peer review as an important component of remedying these problems, but recognized that lawsuits for money damages dampened the willingness of people to participate in peer review. Accordingly, Congress "grant[ed] limited immunity from suits for money damages to participants in professional peer review actions."
>
> When a "professional review action" as defined by the statute meets certain standards, the HCQIA provides that participants in the peer review "shall not be liable in damages under any law of the United States or of any State (or political subdivision thereof) with respect to the action." The statute establishes four requirements for immunity:
>
> For purposes of the protection set forth in section 11111(a) of this title, a professional review action must be taken—
>
> (1) in the reasonable belief that the action was in the furtherance of quality health care,
>
> (2) after a reasonable effort to obtain the facts of the matter,
>
> (3) after adequate notice and hearing procedures are afforded to the physician involved or after such other procedures as are fair to the physician under the circumstances, and
>
> (4) in the reasonable belief that the action was warranted by the facts known after such reasonable effort to obtain facts and after meeting the requirement of paragraph (3).[47]

The court found that the actions of the ad hoc committee, the IMAC, the Hearing Committee, and the hospital board fit the definition of "professional review actions" (see Legal Brief on p. 270) and that there was a "reasonable belief that the action was in the furtherance of quality health care":

> The ad hoc committee's review, upon which the extension of the abeyance rested, speaks for itself. A group of six cardiologists reviewed 44 of Poliner's cases and concluded that he gave substandard care in more than half of the cases. We

remittitur
a judge's order
reducing an
excessive jury
award

Legal Brief

The HCQIA defines a professional review action in part as "an action or recommendation of a professional review body which is taken or made in the conduct of professional review activity, which is based on the competence or professional conduct of an individual physician (which conduct affects or could affect adversely the health or welfare of a patient or patients), and which affects (or may affect) adversely the clinical privileges, or membership in a professional society, of the physician."[91]

conclude that . . . the belief that temporarily restricting Poliner's cath lab privileges during an investigation would further quality health care was objectively reasonable.[48]

The court added, "No reasonable jury could conclude that Defendants failed to make a 'reasonable effort to obtain the facts.'" The pièce de résistance of the opinion is its closing language:

This case demonstrates how the process provisions of the HCQIA work in tandem: legitimate concerns lead to temporary restrictions and an investigation; an investigation reveals that a doctor may in fact be a danger; and in response, the hospital continues to limit the physician's privileges. The hearing process is allowed to play out unencumbered by the fears and urgency that would necessarily obtain if the physician were midstream returned to full privileges during the few days necessary for a fully informed and considered decision resting on all the facts and a process in which the physician has had an opportunity to confront the facts and give his explanations. The interplay of these provisions may work hardships on individual physicians, but the provisions reflect Congress' balancing of the significant interests of the physician and "the public health ramifications of allowing incompetent physicians to practice while the slow wheels of justice grind."

. . .

The temporary restrictions [of Dr. Poliner's privileges] were "tailored to address the health care concerns" that had been raised—[about] procedures in the cath lab—leaving untouched Poliner's other privileges. Nor was the information relayed to [the chair of the internal medicine department] "so obviously mistaken or inadequate as to make reliance on [it] unreasonable." There was an objectively reasonable basis for concluding that temporarily restricting Poliner's privileges during the course of the investigation was warranted by the facts then known, and for essentially the reasons given above, we hold that Defendants satisfy this prong.

To allow an attack years later upon the ultimate "truth" of judgments made by peer reviewers supported by objective evidence would drain all meaning from the statute. The congressional grant of immunity accepts that few physicians would be willing to serve on peer review committees under such a threat; as our sister circuit explains, "the intent of [the HCQIA] was not to disturb, but to reinforce, the preexisting reluctance of courts to substitute their judgment on the merits for that of health care professionals and of the governing bodies of hospitals in an area within their expertise." At the least, it is not our role to re-weigh this judgment and balancing of interests by Congress.

IV. Conclusion

Not only has Poliner failed to rebut the statutory presumption that the peer review actions were taken in compliance with the statutory standards, the evidence independently demonstrates that the peer review actions met the statutory requirements.

. . .

We REVERSE the judgment of the district court and RENDER judgment for Defendants.[49]

The *Kadlec* Case

In contrast to *Poliner*—in which the HCQIA achieved its purpose of promoting quality care and the defendants were held to be immune from liability—stands *Kadlec Medical Center v. Lakeview Anesthesia Associates*.[50] Although the hospital defendant was not held liable, *Kadlec* demonstrates the difficulties that can be encountered if the HCQIA's provisions are not followed.

When the chain of events leading to this lawsuit began, Dr. Berry was a licensed anesthesiologist. He was a partner in a group medical practice known as Louisiana Anesthesia Associates (LAA) and was under contract with LAA to work at Lakeview Medical Center in southeast Louisiana. He also was a man with a drug problem. When officials at Lakeview and his partners at LAA learned of his substance abuse, Dr. Berry was fired "for cause" by LAA and was not permitted to return to Lakeview. However, no one at LAA or Lakeview reported these facts to the hospital board, the Louisiana Board of Medical Examiners, or the NPDB, as required by the HCQIA.

After leaving LAA and Lakeview, Dr. Berry obtained *locum tenens* (or "traveling physician") privileges in Shreveport, Louisiana, and eventually applied through a staffing firm for a similar position at Kadlec Medical Center in Richland, Washington. On receipt of the application, Kadlec conducted its usual background check, including making inquiries to LAA and Lakeview about Dr. Berry's performance history. LAA's response was false and misleading, and Lakeview's was vague (presumably for fear of a lawsuit for defamation or malicious interference with his professional relations). In the absence of negative background information, Kadlec granted credentials to Dr. Berry. Eventually, his narcotics problem led to the near death of a patient, who was left in a permanent vegetative state.

To defend and settle the resulting lawsuit, Kadlec and its insurance carrier paid more than $8 million in damages. They then sued LAA and Lakeview to recover the money, alleging that Kadlec had been misled and that the defendants had failed to comply with the HCQIA and Louisiana law.

A lengthy excerpt from the court of appeals decision is given at the end of this chapter (see The Court Decides). In the end, the group practice was held liable for fraudulent misrepresentations, but Lakeview was not found liable because it had no duty to respond and the response it sent was so vague that it contained no substantive information. Apparently, in Louisiana, if you don't say anything, you can't misrepresent it.

Lessons from *Poliner* and *Kadlec*

Poliner and *Kadlec* demonstrate the continuing importance of professional review (peer review) activities today. The courts and the public at large want hospitals and physicians to monitor quality and patient safety ever more carefully than they did in the past. Compliance with this expectation seems a reasonable exchange for a grant of immunity from tort liability under the HCQIA and state laws.[51] In addition, various provisions of the ACA mandate that more attention be paid to the quality of healthcare and emphasize the dangers of impaired or incompetent physicians.

One commentator predicts that, despite the hospital's exoneration in *Kadlec*, hospitals generally can "anticipate an expanded obligation to disclose risky physician behavior":

> Just as physicians are not simply service providers, and patients not simply courted consumers, hospitals are not simply doctors' workshops. . . . [They] are increasingly being held liable for the negligent actions of nonemployee physicians. They are increasingly viewed as having a duty to their patients to appropriately monitor the quality of care provided by staff physicians, employed or not, and to credential only those who practice safely and competently. In addition, hospitals face increased obligations to monitor the quality of care provided within their facilities and to report impaired or unsafe physicians. When hospitals can be held responsible under the theories of vicarious liability or negligent credentialing, they have a heightened need for complete credentialing information.[52]

Applying a patient-centric framework to this topic, the commentator sees the healthcare system as a web of relationships, not a series of bilateral transactions: "Although they are likely to be unaffiliated businesses, in the credentialing process hospitals are part of a relational web that aims to ensure high-quality patient care."[53] This vision was what the HCQIA was implicitly promoting, and it would seem to be consistent with the current trend of hospital–physician integration.

Similarly, another commentator argues wants to increase institutions' responsibility for quality and patient safety. He calls this model of fiduciary duty "protective intervention":

> Fiduciary duties are expanding in tandem with expanded tort obligations. . . . The recognition of institutional responsibility to better handle informed consent,

disclosure of data, and revelation of errors turns the hospital finally into a recognizable legal fiduciary with an obligation to protect its patients from harm from third parties.

This duty of "protective intervention" captures the more intense obligations whose shadows we can see cast by regulatory initiatives and institution-assumed obligations. Hospitals now have to collect data on adverse events and report them to the state regulators and to patients in many states. They have to manage and coordinate their care to protect their patients. It is no longer a world in which the hospital is little more than a brick shell for physicians, with a loose contract relationship with patients.

A fiduciary duty provides the building blocks for remedies that strengthen the patient's recovery opportunities. . . . Such an expansion . . . strengthens the hands of internal hospital risk managers and compliance officers, as they advise administrators of the increasing necessity of implementing modern data mining, electronic medical records, reporting of adverse events, and better coordination and management of the institution. And it properly imposes on hospital managers a higher duty to protect their patients, their beneficiaries, from harm to the greatest extent possible. They have become "fiduciaries," stewards of their patients' safety.[54]

As the ACA takes hold, it will be interesting to follow the trend of peer review and HCQIA cases to see whether the courts and legislatures adopt these more intense views on hospitals' obligations.

Confidentiality of Peer Review Records

Additional to the liability and immunity issues raised by *Poliner* and *Kadlec* is the question of the confidentiality of peer review records. Plaintiffs' attorneys often want access to these records to support their clients' cases, and physicians under review often want access to the records to support their claims of bad faith and conspiracy.

To be most effective, the peer review process must be an honest and candid evaluation of a practitioner's activities. Confidentiality of the peer review committee's minutes and deliberations is essential to a full and honest process. As the court in *Bredice v. Doctors Hospital, Inc.* stated in 1973,

There is an overwhelming public interest in having [peer review] meetings held on a confidential basis so that the flow of ideas can continue unimpeded. . . .

Confidentiality is essential to effective functioning of these staff meetings; and these meetings are essential to the continued improvement in the care and treatment of patients. Candid and conscientious evaluation of clinical practices is a sine qua non of adequate hospital care. To subject these discussions and deliberations to the discovery process, without a showing of exceptional necessity, would result in terminating such deliberations. Constructive professional criticism cannot occur in an atmosphere of apprehension that one doctor's suggestion will be used as a denunciation of a colleague's conduct in a malpractice suit.[55]

This view has been reaffirmed over the years. For example, in 1992 a federal court of appeals wrote, "As Congress has recognized, peer review materials are sensitive and inherently confidential, and protecting that confidentiality serves an important public interest. [*Citing the HCQIA.*] . . . The medical peer review process 'is a sine qua non of adequate hospital care.'"[56]

Following the line of reasoning begun in *Bredice*, various state legislatures addressed the confidentiality issue in the early 1970s. Today, all jurisdictions have some form of legislation establishing a degree of peer review privilege. For example, the Georgia statute provides that

the proceedings and records of medical review committees shall not be subject to discovery or introduction into evidence in any civil action against a provider of professional health services arising out of the matters which are the subject of evaluation and review by such committee; and no person who was in attendance at a meeting of such committee shall be permitted or required to testify in any such civil action as to any evidence or other matters produced or presented during the proceedings of such committee or as to any findings, recommendations, evaluations, opinions, or other actions of such committee or any members thereof.[57]

The statutes vary from state to state on such matters as

- the type of legal proceeding to which they apply;
- whether the information is protected from discovery, admission into evidence, or both;
- the type of information and the nature of the committee whose records are confidential; and
- various express exceptions to the protection.

Therefore, the application of the privilege is also likely to vary from state to state and even from court to court, depending on the facts of the case. Furthermore, almost universally the privilege does not apply to records, such as medical records and routine business records, created for purposes other than peer review.

National Fraud Data Banks

As mentioned earlier, one aspect of the HCQIA was the creation of the NPDB to promote patient safety and quality of care. Entities that conduct professional review activities are supposed to report to the NPDB any significant adverse peer review actions taken against physicians and to query the

NPDB during the credentialing process to procure an applicant's disciplinary history. Entities that fail to do so can lose their immunity protections (see HCQIA §§ 11133 and 11135, reproduced in appendix 8.1).

>
>
> ### Law in Action
>
> The National Practitioner Data Bank website is www.npdb.hrsa.gov, and a history of the NPDB can be found at https://www.npdb.hrsa.gov/topNavigation/timeline.jsp.

In addition to the NPDB, in 1996 Congress mandated creation of the Healthcare Integrity and Protection Data Bank (HIPDB) "to combat fraud and abuse in health insurance and health care delivery."[58] The HIPDB was intended to augment other tools, and both it and the NPDB have useful information that can help alleviate the problem of incompetent physicians who cross state lines to begin a new practice. Nevertheless, the two data banks are somewhat redundant, and many were skeptical about them—particularly the NPDB—from the outset. Hospitals and other providers were reluctant to report incidents to the data banks, a good deal of information was out-of-date or inaccurate, and physicians who were wrongly reported had difficulty clearing their names. Even the US Department of Health and Human Services (HHS), the agency that administers the Medicare and Medicaid programs, failed to report all of its adverse actions against providers to the HIPDB as required by law.[59]

Recognizing these deficiencies, HHS strengthened its compliance efforts and improved the NPDB/HIPDB system. Furthermore, the ACA required that the duplication between the data banks be eliminated and the HIPDB be discontinued.[60] This change was implemented in 2013, and there is now a single database for submitting queries and receiving responses (see Law in Action).

Although not perfect, if used correctly, the NPDB can significantly thwart physicians' attempts to move to a new location and receive hospital privileges unencumbered by their past.

Quality Issues and Accountable Care Organizations
Exclusive Contracts with Physicians

For many years, hospitals have entered into exclusive contracts with physicians and physician groups to staff such departments as radiology, emergency, and pathology. These arrangements have withstood legal challenges when they were aimed at improving the quality of patient care.[61]

In *Adler v. Montefiore Hospital Association of Western Pennsylvania*,[62] the plaintiff—Dr. Adler—had been employed by a private hospital for six years as the part-time director of the cardiology laboratory with full medical staff privileges. When Montefiore evolved into a teaching hospital, it hired a full-time director—Dr. Curtiss—to replace Dr. Adler. Dr. Curtiss was then granted exclusive privileges to perform cardiac catheterizations, which significantly limited the number of procedures Dr. Adler was permitted to perform. In Dr. Adler's subsequent lawsuit, the exclusive arrangement was upheld as reasonably related to the hospital's purposes, especially because it was a teaching institution.

Catheterization, the court held, was a laboratory procedure—more like radiology than surgery. The exclusive contract was considered part of the hospital's effort to ensure the quality of care and improve efficiency. Accordingly, the hospital had not violated Dr. Adler's rights to due process and equal protection because he was obliged to yield to reasonable rules intended to benefit the hospital's patients, the physicians, the university's medical students, and the public.

Although decided more than 40 years ago, *Adler* is still cited when courts refuse to intervene in hospitals' decisions to confer exclusive privileges on designated physician groups, even though the contracts have restricted the medical staff privileges of other qualified and competent physicians.[63]

In addition to bringing due process arguments, plaintiffs have challenged exclusive service contracts as violating federal or state antitrust legislation. The underlying purpose of antitrust law is to foster competition in the marketplace, and the argument is that exclusive contracts reduce competition and amount to a "group boycott." For the most part, however, the challenges have not been successful because an exclusive contract is seen as a reasonable restraint of trade that actually promotes competition among hospitals and is consistent with efforts to promote high-quality care.[64] (Antitrust cases are discussed in chapter 13.)

Economic Credentialing

Ideally, decisions on medical staff privileges are based on physician competence and the quality of care. However, the institution's financial stability depends on providing care at a cost that will be reimbursed. When physicians' utilization patterns begin to affect the bottom line negatively, financial considerations may creep into credentialing decisions. This practice is known as *economic credentialing*. Although there is no standard definition of the term, the AMA defines it—disapprovingly—as "the use of economic criteria unrelated to quality of care or professional competence in determining a physician's qualifications for initial or continuing hospital medical staff membership or privileges."[65] Whether economic criteria are permissible is a matter of considerable dispute.

At least two scenarios provide a motive for economic credentialing. The first is admission of patients to an acute care hospital when those patients could be served more economically on an outpatient basis or in another type of inpatient facility (e.g., skilled nursing facility, inpatient hospice, nursing home). The dearth of reported decisions suggests that the utilization review and case management function, rather than the credentialing process, is coping with this situation adequately. Given hospitals' incentive to keep costs as low as possible, this supposition is likely true.

The second scenario involves a kind of *loyalty oath*. Hospitals ask their physicians whether they have any financial interest in a competing facility, such as another hospital, an imaging center, or an ambulatory surgery center. If they do, hospitals condition these physicians' medical staff privileges on their agreement not to use those other facilities (or to use them only a certain percentage of the time) if the same services can be provided at the hospital. This scenario raises issues under both state and federal laws.

A 1978 case upheld this practice. In *Cobb County–Kennestone Hosp. Auth. v. Prince*,[66] a government hospital purchased a whole-body computed tomography (CT) scanner and then resolved that "if a treatment, procedure, diagnostic test or other service is ordered for a patient . . . and that procedure, test or service is routinely offered by the Hospital, then the [hospitalized] patient will receive that service within the confines of the Hospital complex."[67] Some staff physicians—who privately owned and operated a CT scanner outside the hospital complex—challenged this policy as an arbitrary restriction on their medical judgment. In upholding the hospital's policy as reasonable and "strikingly similar" to exclusive service contracts, the Supreme Court of Georgia observed that the hospital's resolution

> is reasonable and reflects a well-intentioned effort by the Authority to deal with the intricate and complex task of providing comprehensive medical services to the citizens of our state. The preeminent consideration in the adoption of such a resolution by the Authority was the health, welfare and safety of the patient. . . . The Authority's resolution is a reasonable and rational administrative decision enacted in order for the Authority to carry out the legislative mandate that it provide adequate medical care in the public interest. The resolution does not invade the physician's province. Although he is required to use the facilities and equipment provided within the hospital complex for testing rather than similar facilities and equipment outside, he is nevertheless free to interpret the results of such tests and free to diagnose and prescribe treatment for all his patients.[68]

A 2006 case, however, did not defer to hospital administration. In *Baptist Health v. Murphy*,[69] the defendant—a multihospital system—adopted a policy to deny staff appointments or clinical privileges "to any practitioner who, directly or indirectly, acquires or holds an ownership or investment interest in a competing hospital."[70] The policy—apparently a revenue-enhancing measure—was challenged by cardiologists who had an ownership interest in another hospital and held medical staff privileges at both Baptist Health and the other facility. The trial court issued a preliminary injunction against enforcement of the policy, and the Supreme Court of Arkansas affirmed that decision, holding that the hospital's actions amounted to an intentional, tortious interference with the physicians' business relationships with their patients:

> Defendant knew that the adoption of the economic credentialing policy would inevitably result in a disruption of the relationship between Plaintiffs and a significant number of their patients. The economic credentialing policy was adopted with the intention of forming a relationship with the Plaintiffs' patients, potential patients, and referring physicians who were required to use its facilities by establishing relationships with cardiologists other than the Plaintiffs. Defendant, by adopting the economic credentialing policy, intended to disrupt the business expectancies arising out of Plaintiffs' relationships with their patients and with referring physicians with whom they have established patterns of referral. Further, by adopting the economic credentialing policy, Defendant intended to disrupt and interfere with the doctor-patient relationship existing between Plaintiffs and their patients and Plaintiffs' ability to provide health care to their patients. Defendant's actions are an attempt to secure treatment of patients at Defendant's facilities and not Plaintiffs' facilities.[71]

After further hearings the Supreme Court of Arkansas again affirmed the decision to enjoin Baptist Health's policy;[72] thus, economic credentialing now appears to be legally objectionable in Arkansas.

As the HHS Office of Inspector General notes, "In addition to the antikickback statute, hospitals should make sure that their credentialing policies comply with all other applicable Federal and State laws and regulations, some of which may prohibit or limit economic credentialing."[73] Thus, hospital administration would be well advised to seek legal counsel when considering adopting a policy that sets economic criteria or establishes a loyalty standard for medical staff appointments and privileges.

Furthermore, note that the ACA amended the physician self-referral (Stark) law and placed severe limitations on physicians' ability to own or invest in hospitals.[74] Physician-owned hospitals that did not have a Medicare provider agreement before December 31, 2010, may not participate in the Medicare program. Those that did have a provider agreement may continue to participate—but only under certain significant conditions that address facility expansion, conflicts of interest, bona fide investments, patient safety issues, and conversion of facilities. If these amendments to the Stark self-referral law remain in place, issues such as those raised in *Baptist Health* may become moot because physician ownership of hospitals will be severely limited. (The Stark law and other fraud statutes are discussed more fully in chapter 15.)

Medical Staff Issues in Accountable Care Organizations

The premise of the ACA was that fundamental change is needed in the US healthcare system. In regard to the medical staff, one of the act's most significant changes was the creation of the Medicare Shared Savings Program under which groups of providers, organized as ACOs, would "work together to manage and coordinate care for Medicare fee-for-service beneficiaries."[75]

In other words, ACOs are meant to improve quality, coordinate care in various settings, and reduce unnecessary costs, and they have the ultimate goals of helping patients get the right care at the right time and avoiding duplication of services. A successful ACO—one that delivers high-quality care and reduces costs—will share in the savings it generates for the Medicare program.

ACOs continue the trend of hospital–physician alignment, which began with physician–hospital organizations in the 1990s. As the economics of physician practice changed and cost-containment pressures increased, employment by a hospital or integrated delivery system became an attractive option for many physicians. Under health reform, hospitals have new reasons to increase the bond with their medical staffs.

Whether as an ACO or otherwise, hospital–physician relationships take various forms: joint ventures; facility leasing; management contracts; and outright employment of the physician by a hospital, clinic, medical foundation, faculty practice plan, or hospital-owned group practice. As ACOs become common and as more physicians become employees, these integrated relationships will add new management challenges and will strain the traditional legal concepts of medical staff privileges.

As a general principle, under a doctrine known as *employment at will*, employees are not entitled to substantive or procedural due process and can be dismissed without a hearing, without prior notice, and without cause—unless their employment contract (if any), the organization's human resources policies, or state laws provide otherwise. Physicians employed by an ACO are covered by the same at-will rule; thus, their legal position is different from that of an independent member of the medical staff. The employed physician's medical staff privileges, however, are a different matter. Unless the employment contract makes employment and staff privileges coterminous, the hospital must take separate action and follow regular medical staff procedures if it wants to revoke the privileges of a physician it has dismissed from employment.

Similarly, a hospital's decision not to renew an exclusive service contract—with a radiology group, for example—usually does not require due process but depends on the term of the contract. For example, in a Minnesota case, a municipal hospital (a state actor) had an unwritten, at-will arrangement with its director of pathology. When the hospital terminated the contract, the physician filed suit, arguing that he should have been afforded formal due process. The court disagreed. Although loss of the directorship position made his medical staff privileges virtually worthless—pathologists do not normally admit and treat patients, after all—that directorship "stemmed solely from his oral contract with the hospital, not [from] his staff membership. Accordingly . . . we must distinguish the termination of a contractually created director's position from the termination or reduction of staff privileges."[76]

These traditional viewpoints may need to be reconsidered and contractual and bylaws provisions reexamined as physicians become more involved in hospital governance under an ACO (see Legal Brief). The concept of economic credentialing discussed earlier may also need to be reviewed. In short, the idea of hospital–physician alignment—being as it is all about money and control—will present myriad new issues in the realm of medical staff privileges, perhaps for the courts but certainly for hospital administration.

Complementary and Alternative Medicine and Integrative Healthcare

In his Pulitzer Prize–winning book *The Social Transformation of American Medicine*, Professor Paul Starr chronicles how physicians gradually assumed a dominant role in the US medical establishment. He notes that a century ago physicians had much less prestige and influence than they have today. They were in competition with faith healers, herbalists (Thomsonians), eclectics (botanics), homeopaths, midwives, naturopaths, hydropathists, osteopaths, chiropractors, and others.

The field changed after the famous *Flexner Report*, issued in 1910, prompted reforms in medical education; when physicians' education caught up with medical science, physicians consolidated their power. By the time of the Great Depression, one survey reported that "all the non-M.D. practitioners combined—osteopaths, chiropractors, Christian Scientists and other faith healers, midwives, and chiropodists—took care of only 5.1 percent of all attended cases of illness [in the study]."[77] Ever since, as one law review article remarked, "Organized medicine . . . has fought to maintain a firm grip on the philosophy of health care generally, as well as on the specific treatments patients should have available to them."[78]

By the 1950s, "mainstream medicine" had essentially suppressed some healers (e.g., homeopaths, eclectics), but it reluctantly acceded to the licensure of others

Legal Brief

Members of a physician group that provides exclusive services for certain hospital departments (e.g., pathology, radiology, anesthesiology) must be members of both the group and the hospital medical staff. Contracts between the hospital and the group should provide that if physicians leave the practice, their medical staff appointments end and they must reapply for privileges to continue practicing in the facility. These contractual arrangements will need to be reviewed if the physician group becomes part of an ACO with the hospital.

(e.g., osteopaths) who had scientific training. By the mid-1960s, the grip that physicians once held had loosened such that Medicare defined *physician* as an individual holding any of these degrees: doctor of medicine (MD), doctor of osteopathic medicine (DO), doctor of dental surgery (DDS), doctor of dental medicine (DMD), doctor of podiatric medicine (DPM), doctor of optometry (OD), and doctor of chiropractic (DC).[79] This definition holds today.

Now the field is changing again. In an ironic twist, some practices that were once disdained are gaining acceptance under the guise of "wellness and prevention." As one court stated in a 2001 case involving a state health plan's insurance coverage,

> there are many medical schools in the United States that are teaching alternative approaches to some traditional practices. As more and more doctors become familiar with alternative practices, we can anticipate the availability and increasing utilization of . . . alternative treatments.
>
> . . .
>
> If a licensed alternative medical provider indicates that the treatment is based on sound medical, biological or scientific principles; widely prescribed and recognized by other alternative medical providers; and considered efficacious and safe, the [state health plan] should not reject the treatment solely because traditional doctors do not yet utilize the treatment or are completely unfamiliar with the practice. In that instance, the new treatment should be carefully evaluated under the other provisions of the plan, and not automatically excluded solely because no traditional physician is as yet prescribing [it].[80]

The treatments to which this court referred are an essential component of *integrative healthcare*—a philosophy that focuses not only on the conventional treatment of a patient's condition but also on the whole person (mind, body, spirit) to promote health and wellness. When used in conjunction with a physician's prescribed therapies, the nontraditional treatments are "complementary"; when used in isolation, they are "alternative." Collectively, the term for such treatments is *complementary and alternative medicine* (CAM) (see Legal Brief). By adopting

Legal Brief

CAM is recognized by the National Institutes of Health and its National Center for Complementary and Alternative Medicine (NCCAM). NCCAM is the federal government's "lead agency for scientific research on the diverse medical and health care systems, practices, and products that are not generally considered part of conventional medicine."[92]

CAM and integrative medicine are mentioned numerous times in the health reform legislation. Such treatments are part of an interdisciplinary, patient-centered "medical home" and are included in a new NIH council on prevention and health promotion. Furthermore, the ACA's definition of *health care workforce* encompasses "all health care providers with direct patient care and support responsibilities, such as . . . licensed complementary and alternative medicine providers [and] integrative health practitioners."[93]

For an example of an integrative healthcare program in a university's physician practice group, see http://fammed.utmb.edu/education/integrative-medicine.

CAM principles, physicians who practice integrative healthcare incorporate some of the very practices the medical establishment scorned two or three generations ago: acupuncture, Eastern medicine, naturopathy, massage therapy, herbal medicine, yoga, meditation, herbalism, Ayurveda, hypnotherapy, and shamanism, to name a few.[81]

CAM principles are seen as entirely consistent with the ACA's emphasis on cost reduction, coordinated care, and chronic disease management, and they are fast becoming part of ACOs' strategies. These practices are also gaining recognition as disciplines worthy of licensure in their own right. For example, at least 17 states, the District of Columbia, and two US territories now have licensing laws for naturopathic doctors.[82]

Legal Issues and Credentialing for Complementary and Alternative Medicine and Integrative Healthcare Providers

Over the years, some CAM and integrative healthcare practitioners have been prosecuted for practicing medicine without a license.[83] Otherwise, research reveals only a few reported cases involving these practitioners, and in those cases CAM was only tangentially related to the issue (e.g., regulatory enforcement for misleading advertising, the revocation of a physician's license because of fraud or gross negligence).[84] In contrast to years ago—when osteopaths, for example, challenged their exclusion from medical staffs— research reveals no recent cases which nonphysician CAM and integrative healthcare practitioners have sought and been denied medical staff privileges.

In independent practice, the liability issues of massage therapists or herbalists, for example, are theirs alone. However, in a hospital setting, the corporation must consider respondeat superior issues and questions about licensure, credentialing, scope of practice, medical supervision, professional liability insurance, and health plan coverage, among others. No single answer can address the myriad questions involved because there is no standard system for credentialing CAM and integrative healthcare providers, and the educational requirements and licensing vary widely from state to state.[85] Organizations will have to address these questions independently as CAM and integrative healthcare become more popular.

Credentialing

Society is more health conscious than ever, and CAM and integrative healthcare have regained credibility. As one article commented, "Legislative recognition trumps medical recognition,"[86] but licensure and scope of practice vary by state. How the issues surrounding hospital credentialing will play out over time remains to be seen, but—as discussed earlier—the general principle remains that decisions should be based on individual merit rather than discrimination against an entire class of providers.

Summary

This chapter focuses on decisions about medical staff privileges. It points out that management and the medical staff are responsible for the credentialing process and may recommend physician applicants. The ultimate responsibility for appointing a competent medical staff, however, lies with the hospital governing board. In recent decades, practitioners other than MDs have been given medical staff privileges, including DOs, DMDs, DPMs, DCs, and other physicians, depending on state law. Decisions on medical staff membership must be based on the individual's qualifications rather than on a bias against a particular school of practice.

The chapter also addresses issues related to the peer review and quality assurance functions, both of which are efforts to monitor the quality of care. It concludes with some thoughts about ACOs and CAM and integrative healthcare.

Discussion Questions

1. Who has ultimate responsibility for decisions about medical staff membership, and why? How should this responsibility be fulfilled?
2. What differences are there, if any, between the due process standards that apply to public hospitals and those that apply to private hospitals?
3. What categories of professionals are permitted membership on the medical staff?
4. What issues of confidentiality and liability does the hospital's peer review function present?
5. Explain how the HCQIA establishes an "objective reasonableness" requirement rather than a subjective "good faith standard" for peer review committees.
6. What are the medical staff privileges of contract physicians and CAM and integrative healthcare providers?
7. Research the status of economic credentialing in your state and the effects of the *Baptist Health* case and similar decisions.
8. Explain the concept of the ACO and its role in the 2010 health reform legislation.

The Court Decides

Kadlec Medical Center v. Lakeview Anesthesia Associates
527 F.3d 412 (5th Cir. 2008)

REAVLEY, Circuit Judge:

Kadlec Medical Center and its insurer, Western Professional Insurance Company, filed this diversity action in Louisiana district court against Louisiana Anesthesia Associates (LAA), its shareholders, and Lakeview Regional Medical Center (Lakeview Medical). The LAA shareholders worked with Dr. Robert Berry—an anesthesiologist and former LAA shareholder—at Lakeview Medical, where the defendants discovered his on-duty use of narcotics. In referral letters written by the defendants and relied on by Kadlec, his future employer, the defendants did not disclose Dr. Berry's drug use.

While under the influence of Demerol at Kadlec, Dr. Berry's negligent performance led to the near-death of a patient, resulting in a lawsuit against Kadlec. Plaintiffs claim here that the defendants' misleading referral letters were a legal cause of plaintiffs' financial injury, i.e., having to pay over $8 million to defend and settle the lawsuit. The jury found in favor of the plaintiffs and judgment followed. We reverse the judgment against Lakeview Medical, vacate the remainder of the judgment, and remand.

I. Factual Background
Dr. Berry was a licensed anesthesiologist in Louisiana and practiced with Drs. William Preau, Mark Dennis, David Baldone, and Allan Parr at LAA. From November 2000 until his termination on March 13, 2001, Dr. Berry was a shareholder of LAA, the exclusive provider of anesthesia services to Lakeview Medical (a Louisiana hospital).

In November 2000, a small management team at Lakeview Medical investigated Dr. Berry after nurses expressed concern about

his undocumented and suspicious withdrawals of Demerol. [The findings were discussed with Dr. Berry's LAA partners, who confronted him with the evidence, but his drug-related problems continued and his performance deteriorated. In March of 2001, Lakeview's CEO Max Lauderdale] . . . decided that it was in the best interest of patient safety that Dr. Berry not practice at the hospital. Dr. Dennis and his three partners at LAA fired Dr. Berry and signed his termination letter on March 27, 2001, which explained that he was fired "for cause":

> [You have been fired for cause because] you have reported to work in an impaired physical, mental, and emotional state. Your impaired condition has prevented you from properly performing your duties and puts our patients at significant risk. . . . [P]lease consider your termination effective March 13, 2001.

At Lakeview Medical, Lauderdale ordered the Chief Nursing Officer to notify the administration if Dr. Berry returned.

Despite recognizing Dr. Berry's drug problem and the danger he posed to patients, neither Dr. Dennis nor Lauderdale reported Dr. Berry's impairment [or discipline] to the hospital's Medical Executive Committee, . . . to Lakeview Medical's Board of Trustees, . . . to the Louisiana Board of Medical Examiners or to the National Practitioner's Data Bank. . . .

After leaving LAA and Lakeview Medical, Dr. Berry briefly obtained work as a *locum tenens* (traveling physician) at a hospital in Shreveport, Louisiana. In October 2001, he applied through Staff Care, a leading *locum tenens* staffing firm, for *locum tenens* privileges at Kadlec Medical Center in Washington State. After receiving his application, Kadlec began its credentialing process. Kadlec examined a variety of materials, including referral letters from LAA and Lakeview Medical.

LAA's Dr. Preau and Dr. Dennis, two months after firing Dr. Berry for his on-the-job drug use, submitted referral letters for Dr. Berry to Staff Care, with the intention that they be provided to future employers. The letter from Dr. Dennis stated that he had worked with Dr. Berry for four years, that he was an excellent clinician, and that he would be an asset to any anesthesia service. Dr. Preau's letter said that he worked with Berry at Lakeview Medical and that he recommended him highly as an anesthesiologist. Dr. Preau's and Dr. Dennis's letters were submitted on June 3, 2001, only sixty-eight days after they fired him for using narcotics while on-duty and stating in his termination letter that Dr. Berry's behavior put "patients at significant risk."

On October 17, 2001, Kadlec sent Lakeview Medical a request for credentialing information about Berry. The request included a detailed confidential questionnaire, a delineation of privileges, and a signed consent for release of information. The interrogatories on the questionnaire asked whether "[Dr. Berry] has been subject to any disciplinary action," if "[Dr. Berry has] the ability (health status) to perform the privileges requested," whether "[Dr. Berry has] shown any signs of behavior/personality problems or impairments," and whether Dr. Berry has satisfactory "judgement" [sic].

Nine days later, Lakeview Medical responded to the requests for credentialing information about fourteen different physicians. In thirteen cases, it responded fully and completely to the request, filling out forms with all the information asked for

by the requesting health care provider. The fourteenth request, from Kadlec concerning Berry, was handled differently. Instead of completing the multi-part forms, Lakeview Medical staff drafted a short letter. In its entirety, it read:

> This letter is written in response to your inquiry regarding [Dr. Berry]. Due to the large volume of inquiries received in this office, the following information is provided.

> Our records indicate that Dr. Robert L. Berry was on the Active Medical Staff of Lakeview Regional Medical Center in the field of Anesthesiology from March 04, 1997 through September 04, 2001.

> If I can be of further assistance, you may contact me at (504) 867-4076.

The letter did not disclose LAA's termination of Dr. Berry; his on-duty drug use; the investigation into Dr. Berry's undocumented and suspicious withdrawals of Demerol that "violated the standard of care"; or any other negative information. The employee who drafted the letter said at trial that she just followed a form letter, which is one of many that Lakeview Medical used.

Kadlec then credentialed Dr. Berry, and he began working there. After working at Kadlec without incident for a number of months, [Dr. Berry's performance began to deteriorate again in November, 2002. He seemed sick on occasion and exhibited mood swings. On November 12 he again appeared sick, several of his surgery patients suffered adverse effects, and he almost passed out during one procedure.]

. . .

Kimberley Jones was Dr. Berry's fifth patient that morning. She was in for what should have been a routine, fifteen minute tubal ligation. When they moved her into the recovery room, one nurse noticed that her fingernails were blue, and she was not

(continued)

(continued from previous page)

breathing. Dr. Berry failed to resuscitate her, and she is now in a permanent vegetative state.

. . .

Jones's family sued Dr. Berry and Kadlec in Washington. Dr. Berry's insurer settled the claim against him. . . . Western, Kadlec's insurer, settled the claim against Kadlec. *[Western's payout was approximately $8.25 million.]*

. . .

III. Discussion
A. The Intentional and Negligent Misrepresentation Claims
The plaintiffs allege that the defendants committed two torts: intentional misrepresentation and negligent misrepresentation. The elements of a claim for *intentional* misrepresentation in Louisiana are: (1) a misrepresentation of a material fact; (2) made with intent to deceive; and (3) causing justifiable reliance with resultant injury. To establish a claim for intentional misrepresentation when it is by silence or inaction, plaintiffs also must show that the defendant owed a duty to the plaintiff to disclose the information. To make out a *negligent* misrepresentation claim in Louisiana: (1) there must be a legal duty on the part of the defendant to supply correct information; (2) there must be a breach of that duty, which can occur by omission as well as by affirmative misrepresentation; and (3) the breach must have caused damages to the plaintiff based on the plaintiff's reasonable reliance on the misrepresentation.

The defendants argue that any representations in, or omissions from, the referral letters cannot establish liability. We begin our analysis below by holding that after choosing to write referral letters, the defendants assumed a duty not to make affirmative misrepresentations in the letters. We next analyze whether the letters were misleading, and we conclude that the LAA defendants' letters were misleading, but the letter from Lakeview

Medical was not. We also examine whether the defendants had an affirmative duty to disclose negative information about Dr. Berry in their referral letters, and we conclude that there was not an affirmative duty to disclose. Based on these holdings, Lakeview Medical did not breach any duty owed to Kadlec, and therefore the judgment against it is reversed. Finally, we examine other challenges to the LAA defendants' liability, and we conclude that they are without merit.

1. The Affirmative Misrepresentations
The defendants owed a duty to Kadlec to avoid affirmative misrepresentations in the referral letters. In Louisiana, "[a]lthough a party may keep absolute silence and violate no rule of law or equity . . . if he volunteers to speak and to convey information which may influence the conduct of the other party, he is bound to [disclose] the whole truth." In negligent misrepresentation cases, Louisiana courts have held that even when there is no initial duty to disclose information, "once [a party] volunteer[s] information, it assume[s] a duty to insure that the information volunteered [is] correct."

Consistent with these cases, the defendants had a legal duty not to make affirmative misrepresentations in their referral letters. . . . Here, defendants were recommending an anesthesiologist, who held the lives of patients in his hands every day. Policy considerations dictate that the defendants had a duty to avoid misrepresentations in their referral letters if they misled plaintiffs into thinking that Dr. Berry was an "excellent" anesthesiologist, when they had information that he was a drug addict. Indeed, if defendants' statements created a misapprehension about Dr. Berry's suitability to work as an anesthesiologist, then by "volunteer[ing] to speak and to convey information which . . . influence[d] the conduct of [Kadlec], [they were] bound to [disclose] the whole truth." In other words, if they created a misapprehension about Dr. Berry due to their own statements, they incurred a duty to disclose information about his drug use and for-cause firing to complete the whole picture.

... The letter from Dr. Preau stated that Dr. Berry was an "excellent anesthesiologist" and that he "recommend[ed] him highly." Dr. Dennis's letter said that Dr. Berry was "an excellent physician" who "he is sure will be an asset to [his future employer's] anesthesia service." These letters are false on their face and materially misleading. ...

The question as to whether Lakeview Medical's letter was misleading is more difficult. The letter does not comment on Dr. Berry's proficiency as an anesthesiologist, and it does not recommend him to Kadlec. ... [W]hatever the real reason that Lakeview Medical did not respond in full to Kadlec's inquiry, Kadlec did not present evidence that this could have affirmatively misled it into thinking that Dr. Berry had an uncheckered history at Lakeview Medical.

Kadlec also says that the letter was misleading because it erroneously reported that Dr. Berry was on Lakeview Medical's active medical staff until September 4, 2001. *[The court finds that although Dr. Berry did not return to work at Lakeview after his March 13 termination, technically he was on the medical staff until he formally resigned on October 1.]*

In sum, we hold that the letters from the LAA defendants were affirmatively misleading, but the letter from Lakeview Medical was not. ... We now examine the theory that, even assuming that there were no misleading statements in the referral letters, the defendants had an affirmative duty to disclose. ...

[The court proceeds to analyze this issue and concludes, despite "compelling policy arguments," that Louisiana courts would not impose on the defendants an affirmative duty to disclose possible impairments. Such a duty would exist, according to the court's reading of Louisiana law, only if there were a "special relationship" between the parties.

That relationship apparently would need to be contractual or fiduciary in nature.]

3. Legal Cause
...

The LAA defendants ... argue that Kadlec had multiple warning signs ... and had it responded with an investigation, plaintiffs' injuries would have been avoided. ... The jury ... concluded that the LAA defendants negligently *and intentionally* misled Kadlec about Dr. Berry's drug addiction. By intentionally covering up Dr. Berry's drug addiction in communications with a future employer, they should have foreseen that the future employer might miss the warning signs of Dr. Berry's addiction. This was within the scope of the risk they took.

Indeed, both plaintiffs' and defendants' witnesses agreed at trial that narcotics addiction is a disease, that addicts try to hide their disease from their co-workers, and that particularly in the case of narcotics-addicted anesthesiologists, for whom livelihood and drug supply are in the same place, colleagues may be the last to know about their addiction and impairment. This is not a case where a future tortious act is so unforeseeable that it should relieve the earlier tortfeasor of liability. ...
...

E. Summary and Remand Instructions
...

The district court entered judgment consistent with how the jury allocated fault among the entities it found to be legally responsible for the plaintiffs' injuries. The jury's allocation was as follows: Dr. Dennis 20%; Dr. Preau 5%; Lakeview Medical 25%; Kadlec 17%; and Dr. Berry 33%. We have affirmed the liability finding of the jury against the LAA defendants. But now that we have reversed the judgment against Lakeview Medical, the question arises whether there must be a reapportionment of fault with a

(continued)

(continued from previous page)

corresponding change to damages assessed against the LAA defendants. It is possible that this is unnecessary, if under Louisiana law we can simply compare the fault percentages of the remaining parties. But Louisiana law might also require a reapportionment of fault and, therefore, a fresh determination of damages. Because there was no briefing on this issue, we vacate the judgment against the LAA defendants and remand the case to the district court to determine what, if anything, needs to be redone on the apportionment and damages issues, and then to enter judgment against the LAA defendants accordingly. ■

Discussion Questions

1. *Kadlec* is a decision by a federal court in a lawsuit brought by a plaintiff located in the state of Washington on a question regarding Louisiana state law. Can you explain why the case was filed in Louisiana and why Louisiana law rather than the law of Washington applies?
2. The US Court of Appeals for the Fifth Circuit is located in New Orleans. Most, if not all, of its judges are likely members of the Louisiana bar. Nevertheless, this *federal* court is presuming to gauge what a *state* court would decide if presented with these issues. What procedural mechanism might the district court or court of appeals have used to dispose of the *Kadlec* case without guessing what the Louisiana courts would do?

~ ~

Notes

1. THE JOINT COMMISSION, 2013 HOSPITAL ACCREDITATION STANDARDS at LD-7.
2. MED. STAFF OF AVERA MARSHALL REG'L MED. CTR. V. AVERA MARSHALL, 857 N.W.2D 695 (Minn., 2014).
3. Meister v. Avera Marshall Reg'l Med. Ctr., No. A15-1982 (Ct. App., July 25, 2016).
4. *See, e.g.*, Johnson v. Misericordia Community Hosp., 99 Wis. 2d 708, 301 N.W.2d 156 (1981), *and* Sophia Elam v. College Park Hosp., 132 Cal. App. 3d 332, 183 Cal. Rptr. 156, *modified*, 133 Cal. App. 3d 94 (1982).
5. THE JOINT COMMISSION, 2013 HOSPITAL ACCREDITATION STANDARDS at GL-9, GL-32.
6. *See generally* Thomas C. Shields, *Guidelines for Reviewing Applications for Privileges*, 9 HOSP. MED. STAFF 11 (September 1980). *See also* Leonard v. Board of Directors, Prower County Hosp. Dist., 673 P.2d 1019 (Colo. App. 1983) (the governing board has the authority to reject a medical staff committee's recommendation and terminate a

physician's privileges), *and* Ad Hoc Executive Comm. of the Medical Staff of Memorial Hosp. v. Runyan, 716 P.2d 465 (Colo. 1986) (the executive committee of the medical staff has no standing to challenge the decision of the board restoring a physician's privileges).

7. Hayman v. Galveston, 273 U.S. 414 (1927).

8. 116 F.3d 482 (1997).

9. *See, e.g.,* Barrett v. United Hosp., 376 F. Supp. 791 (S.D.N.Y. 1974), *aff'd mem.,* 506 F.2d 1395 (2d Cir. 1974), *and* Jackson v. Metropolitan Edison Co., 419 U.S. 345 (1974).

10. Barrett, *supra* note 9, at 800–805.

11. *Id.* at 799; *accord* Lubin v. Crittenden Hosp. Ass'n, 713 F.2d 414 (8th Cir. 1983), *cert. denied,* 465 U.S. 1025 (1984).

12. *See, e.g.,* Sosa v. Board of Managers of Val Verde Memorial Hosp., 437 F.2d 173 (5th Cir. 1971) (notice of charges "reasonably related to operation of hospital" is required for denial of admission to medical staff), *and* Moore v. Board of Trustees of Carson-Tahoe Hosp., 88 Nev. 207, 495 P.2d 605 (1972), *cert. denied,* 409 U.S. 879 (1972).

13. *See, e.g.,* Arthur F. Southwick, *The Physician's Right to Due Process in Public and Private Hospitals: Is There a Difference?* 9:1 MEDICOLEGAL NEWS 4 (1981). First expressed more than three decades ago, these insights have proved true.

14. 40 N.J. 389, 192 A.2d 817 (1963). Some cases are contra; *see, e.g.,* Limmer v. Samaritan Health Serv., 710 P.2d 1077 (Ariz. App. 1985). By statute and accreditation standards, the *Greisman* position has been vindicated.

15. 40 N.J. at 393.

16. Ohio Rev. Code Ann. § 3701.351(B).

17. Cal. Health & Safety Code § 1316.

18. Cal. Health & Safety Code § 1316.5(a)(2).

19. THE JOINT COMMISSION, 2013 HOSPITAL ACCREDITATION STANDARDS at MS-1.

20. *See, e.g.,* Civil Rights Acts of 1964, 42 U.S.C.A. § 2000 (d), *and* 42 U.S.C.A. §§ 1395–1395zz.

21. Foster v. Mobile Hosp. Bd., 398 F.2d 227 (5th Cir. 1968); Meredith v. Allen County War Memorial Hosp., 397 F.2d 33 (6th Cir. 1968); Eaton v. Grubbs, 329 F.2d 710 (4th Cir. 1964); Simkins v. Moses H. Cone Memorial Hosp., 323 F.2d 959 (4th Cir. 1963), *cert. denied,* 376 U.S. 938 (1964) (a private hospital receiving governmental financial support is subject to the Fourteenth Amendment).

22. 437 F.2d 173 (5th Cir. 1971).

23. *Id.* at 176–77 (citations omitted).

24. *Id.* at 177. *See also* Schooler v. Navarro County Memorial Hosp., 375 F. Supp. 841 (N.D. Tex. 1973), *aff'd*, 515 F.2d 509 (5th Cir. 1975) (when procedural due process is followed, a hospital may deny staff appointment if there is evidence that the physician displayed an inability to work harmoniously with other doctors and hospital personnel and charged patients excessive fees).

25. Woodbury v. McKinnon, 447 F.2d 839 (5th Cir. 1971).

26. Pollock v. Methodist Hosp., 392 F. Supp. 393 (E.D. La. 1975). *See also* Jones v. State Bd. of Medicine, 555 P.2d 399 (Idaho 1976) (a statutory requirement that both physicians and hospitals obtain malpractice insurance as a condition of licensure is constitutional); Wilkinson v. Madera Community Hosp., 144 Cal. App. 3d 436, 192 Cal. Rptr. 593 (1983) (a hospital may deny privileges when a doctor's insurance company is not approved by California Department of Insurance); Kling v. St. Paul Fire and Marine Ins. Co., 626 F. Supp. 1285 (C.D. Ill. 1986) (an agreement between hospital and insurance company requiring staff to carry a minimum amount of malpractice insurance is not subject to jurisdiction of Sherman Act).

27. Board of Trustees of the Memorial Hosp. v. Pratt, 72 Wyo. 120, 262 P.2d 682 (1953); Peterson v. Tucson Gen. Hosp., Inc., 559 P.2d 186 (Ariz. Ct. App. 1976).

28. Rao v. Board of County Commiss'rs, 80 Wash. 2d 695, 497 P.2d 591 (1972).

29. Selden v. City of Sterling, 316 Ill. App. 455, 45 N.E.2d 329 (1942).

30. Yeargin v. Hamilton Memorial Hosp., 225 Ga. 661, 171 S.E.2d 136 (1969), *cert. denied*, 397 U.S. 963 (1970).

31. Yeargin v. Hamilton Memorial Hosp., 229 Ga. 870, 195 S.E.2d 8 (1972).

32. Fahey v. Holy Family Hosp., 32 Ill. App. 3d 537, 336 N.E.2d 309 (1975).

33. 88 Nev. 207, 495 P.2d 605 (1972), *cert. denied*, 409 U.S. 879 (1972).

34. North Broward Hosp. Dist. v. Mizell, 148 So. 2d 1, 5 (Fla. 1962).

35. 495 P.2d at 608.

36. *See* Medicare Conditions of Participation, 42 C.F.R. § 482.12, *and* THE JOINT COMMISSION, 2013 HOSPITAL ACCREDITATION STANDARDS at MS-22 et seq. *See also* Darling v. Charleston Community Memorial Hosp., 33 Ill. 2d 326, 211 N.E. 2d 253 (1965), *cert. denied*, 383 U.S. 946 (1966) (Joint Commission standards are admissible in court and failure to adhere to them can constitute evidence of negligence).

37. 2013 HOSPITAL ACCREDITATION STANDARDS at MS-22-23. These competencies were developed jointly by the Accreditation Council for Graduate Medical Education and the American Board of Medical Specialties.

38. *See generally* 2013 Hospital Accreditation Standards MS-34 to MS-39.

39. 42 U.S.C. §§ 11101 et seq.

40. 486 U.S. 94 (1988).

41. 486 U.S. at 96.

42. 486 U.S. at 98 and n. 3.

43. *See generally* Margo Heffernan, *The Health Care Quality Improvement Act of 1986 and the National Practitioner Data Bank: The Controversy Over Practitioner Privacy Versus Public Access*, 84(2) Bull. Med. Libr. Ass'n 263–69 (1996), at http://www.ncbi.nlm.nih.gov/pmc/articles/PMC299426/.

44. 537 F.3d 368 (5th Cir. 2008). Footnotes are omitted from the original passages.

45. 537 F.3d at n. 11.

46. 537 F.3d at 370.

47. 537 F.3d at 376–77.

48. 537 F.3d at 379.

49. 537 F.3d at 384–85.

50. 527 F.3d 412 (5th Cir. 2008).

51. For example, Cal. Bus. & Prof. Code § 805 (Deering 1986); Tex. Rev. Civ. Stat. Ann. art. 4495b, § 4.14 (Vernon 1987); Mich. Comp. Laws Ann. §§ 333.16233, 333.16243, 333.21513 (Supp. 1986).

52. Sallie Thieme Sanford, *Candor after Kadlec: Why, Despite the Fifth Circuit's Decision, Hospitals Should Anticipate an Expanded Obligation to Disclose Risky Physician Behavior*, 1 Drexel L. Rev. 383, 386 (2009).

53. *Id.*

54. *See* Barry R. Furrow, *Patient Safety and the Fiduciary Hospital: Sharpening Judicial Remedies*, 1 Drexel L. Rev. 439, 483 (2009).

55. 50 F.R.D. 249, 250–251 (D.D.C 1970), *aff'd*, 479 F.2d 920 (D.C. Cir. 1973).

56. U.S. v. Harris Methodist Fort Worth, 970 F.2d 94 (5th Cir. 1992). *See also* Laws v. Georgetown University Hospital, 656 F. Supp. 824, 826 (D.D.C.1987), *and* Mewborn v. Heckler, 101 F.R.D. 691 (D.D.C. 1984).

57. O.C.G.A. § 31-7-143 (2010).

58. U.S. Dept. of Health and Human Services, *National Practitioner Data Bank* (accessed August 22, 2016), at https://www.npdb-hipdb.hrsa.gov.

59. OIG Report, *CMS Reporting to the Healthcare Integrity and Protection Internet Bank* (published September 2010), at https://oig.hhs.gov/oei/reports/oei-07-09-00292.asp.

60. Pub. L. No. 111-148, § 6403.

61. *See, e.g.*, Blank v. Palo Alto-Stanford Hosp. Center, 234 Cal. App. 2d 377, 44 Cal. Rptr. 572 (1965), *and* Major v. Memorial Hospitals Ass'n, 84 Cal. Rptr. 2d 510, 71 Cal. App. 4th 1380 (1999).

62. Adler v. Montefiore Hosp. Ass'n of W. Pa., 453 Pa. 60, 311 A.2d 634 (1973), cert. denied, 414 U.S. 1131 (1974); see also Lewin v. St. Joseph Hosp., 82 Cal. App. 3d 368, 146 Cal. Rptr. 892 (1978).

63. Sokol v. University Hosp., Inc., 402 F. Supp. 1029 (Mass. 1975) (a hospital's restriction of cardiac surgery to a single surgeon did not violate either antitrust or civil rights statutes); Moles v. White, 336 So. 2d 427 (Fla. Ct. App. 1976) (an exclusive contract for open-heart surgery did not violate state antitrust statutes, constitutional principles, or common law); Dillard v. Rowland, 520 S.W.2d 81 (Mo. App. 1974) (a private hospital that has an affiliation agreement with a university's medical school may restrict staff appointments to those physicians who also hold a university faculty appointment).

64. *See, e.g.*, Dattilo v. Tucson Gen. Hosp., 23 Ariz. App. 392, 533 P.2d 700 (1975) (an exclusive contract for nuclear medicine did not violate either state or federal antitrust laws); Harron v. United Hosp. Center, Inc., Clarksburg, W. Va., 522 F.2d 1133 (4th Cir. 1975), *cert. denied*, 424 U.S. 916 (1976) (an exclusive radiology contract does not violate the federal Sherman Antitrust Act or the civil rights statutes).

65. Am. Med. Ass'n Policy H-230.976.

66. 242 Ga. 139, 249 S.E.2d 581 (1978).

67. 249 S.E.2d 581, 583.

68. *Id.*

69. 226 S.W.3d 800 (2006).

70. *Id.* at 805.

71. 226 S.W.3d at 808.

72. Baptist Health v. Murphy, 2010 Ark. 358 (2010).

73. HHS Office of Inspector General, Supplemental Compliance Program Guidance for Hospitals, 70 Fed. Reg. 4858, 4870 at note 59, Jan. 31, 2005.

74. 42 U.S.C. § 1395nn, as amended by Pub. L. No. 111-148, § 6001.

75. ACA § 3022.

76. Engelstad v. Virginia Mun. Hosp., 718 F.2d 262 (8th Cir. 1983).

77. PAUL STARR, THE SOCIAL TRANSFORMATION OF AMERICAN MEDICINE 127 (Basic Books 1982).

78. Kathleen M. Boozang, *Western Medicine Opens the Door to Alternative Medicine*, 24 AM. J. L. & MED. 185, 186 (1998), quoted in Murray v. State Health Benefits Comm., 337 N.J. Super. 435, 767 A.2d 509 (N.J. Super. Ch., 2001).

79. 42 U.S.C. § 1395x(r).

80. Murray v. State Health Benefits Comm., 337 N.J. Super. 435, 767 A.2d 509, (N.J. Super. Ch., 2001).

81. *See* National Center for Complementary and Alternative Medicine website at http://nccam.nih.gov/health/whatiscam/#definingcam.

82. *See* North Carolina Association of Naturopathic Physicians, *Licensure of NDs* (accessed August 18, 2016), at http://ncanp.com/about-ncanp/licensure-of-nds/.

83. *See, e.g.*, People v. Cantor, 198 Cal.App.2d Supp. 843, 18 Cal. Rptr. 363 (Cal. Super. 1961) (hypnotist); People v. Amber, 76 Misc.2d 267, 349 N.Y.S.2d 604 (N.Y. Sup. 1973) (naturopathy); Williams v. State ex rel. Medical Licensure Commission, 453 So.2d 1051 (Ala. Civ. App. 1984) (naturopathy and homeopathy); State v. Howard, 337 S.E.2d 598, 78 N.C. App. 262 (N.C. App. 1985) (naturopathy); Sabastier v. State, 504 So.2d 45, 12 Fla. L. Weekly 811 (Fla. App. 4 Dist. 1987) (homeopathy); State Dept. of Health v. Hinze, 441 N.W.2d 593, 232 Neb. 550 (Neb. 1989) (naturopathy); State v. Mountjoy, 891 P.2d 376, 257 Kan. 163 (Kan. 1995) (midwifery).

84. *See, e.g.*, FTC v. Qt, Inc., 448 F. Supp. 2d 908 (N.D. Ill., 2006) (defendants enjoined from falsely advertising their "Q-Ray bracelet" in infomercials as a pain-relieving device), *and* United States v. Lane Labs-USA, Inc., 324 F. Supp. 2d 547 (2004) (defendants enjoined from marketing certain products as treatments for cancer and HIV/AIDS).

85. *See generally* David M. Eisenberg et al., *Credentialing Complementary and Alternative Medical Providers*, 137 ANN. INT. MED. 965 (December 17, 2002). It is noted, by way of comparison, that all states license MDs, DOs, and DCs, but only about half license massage therapists. Only three states license homeopaths who are not also MDs or DOs.

86. *Id.*

87. THE JOINT COMMISSION, 2013 HOSPITAL ACCREDITATION STANDARDS at MS-13.

88. Institute for Healthcare Improvement, *The Triple Aim*, HEALTHCARE EXECUTIVE 64–66 (January/February 2009).

89. 93 F.3d 1515, 1530 (11th Cir., 1996).

90. Am. Bar Ass'n Section of Antitrust Law, PRACTICAL IMPLICATIONS OF THE HEALTH CARE QUALITY IMPROVEMENT ACT at 17 (1994), quoting statement of Rep. Wyden, 89 Cong. Rec. E2366 (daily ed. June 26, 1986).

91. 42 U.S.C. § 11151(9).

92. 42 U.S.C. § 287c-21, *and* http://nccam.nih.gov/about.

93. ACA §§ 3502, 4001, and 5001.

Appendix 8.1: Healthcare Quality Improvement Act of 1986, as Amended

[Note: This lengthy excerpt of the HCQIA is provided for two reasons: first, because of its importance to understanding the related discussion in the body of the chapter; and second, because the act's complex definitions and overall structure make for a good exercise in statutory interpretation. Certain key terms in the definitions section are rendered here in **bold** *font; they are not so in the original.]*

TITLE 42 U.S. Code, CHAPTER 117
ENCOURAGING GOOD FAITH PROFESSIONAL REVIEW ACTIVITIES
SUBCHAPTER I—PROMOTION OF PROFESSIONAL REVIEW ACTIVITIES

§ 11101. Findings
The Congress finds the following:
(1) The increasing occurrence of medical malpractice and the need to improve the quality of medical care have become nationwide problems that warrant greater efforts than those that can be undertaken by any individual State.
(2) There is a national need to restrict the ability of incompetent physicians to move from State to State without disclosure or discovery of the physician's previous damaging or incompetent performance.
(3) This nationwide problem can be remedied through effective professional peer review.
(4) The threat of private money damage liability under Federal laws, including treble damage liability under Federal antitrust law, unreasonably discourages physicians from participating in effective professional peer review.
(5) There is an overriding national need to provide incentive and protection for physicians engaging in effective professional peer review.

§ 11111. Professional review
(a) In general
(1) Limitation on damages for professional review actions

If a professional review action (as defined in section 11151(9) of this title) of a professional review body meets all the standards specified in section 11112(a) of this title, except as provided in subsection (b) of this section—
(A) the professional review body,
(B) any person acting as a member or staff to the body,
(C) any person under a contract or other formal agreement with the body, and
(D) any person who participates with or assists the body with respect to the action,
shall not be liable in damages under any law of the United States or of any State (or political subdivision thereof) with respect to the action. The preceding sentence shall not apply to damages under any law of the United States or any State relating to the civil rights of any person or persons, including the Civil Rights Act of 1964, 42 U.S.C. 2000e, et seq. and the Civil Rights Acts, 42 U.S.C. 1981, et seq. Nothing in this paragraph shall prevent the United States or any Attorney General of a State from bringing an action, including an action under section 15c of title 15, where such an action is otherwise authorized.

(2) Protection for those providing information to professional review bodies

Notwithstanding any other provision of law, no person (whether as a witness or otherwise) providing information to a professional review body regarding the competence or professional conduct of a physician shall be held, by reason of having provided such information, to be liable in damages under any law of the United States or of any State (or political subdivision thereof) unless such information is false and the person providing it knew that such information was false.

(b) Exception

If the Secretary has reason to believe that a health care entity has failed to report information in accordance with section 11133(a) of this title, the Secretary shall conduct an investigation. If, after providing notice of noncompliance, an opportunity to correct the noncompliance, and an opportunity for a hearing, the Secretary determines that a health care entity has failed substantially to report information in accordance with section 11133(a) of this title, the Secretary shall publish the name of the entity in the Federal Register. The protections of subsection (a)(1) of this section shall not apply to an entity the name of which is published in the Federal Register under the previous sentence with respect to professional review actions of the entity commenced during the 3-year period beginning 30 days after the date of publication of the name.

(c) Treatment under State laws *[text omitted]*

§ 11112. Standards for professional review actions

(a) In general

For purposes of the protection set forth in section 11111(a) of this title, a professional review action must be taken—

(1) in the reasonable belief that the action was in the furtherance of quality health care,
(2) after a reasonable effort to obtain the facts of the matter,
(3) after adequate notice and hearing procedures are afforded to the physician involved or after such other procedures as are fair to the physician under the circumstances, and
(4) in the reasonable belief that the action was warranted by the facts known after such reasonable effort to obtain facts and after meeting the requirement of paragraph (3).

A professional review action shall be presumed to have met the preceding standards necessary for the protection set out in section 11111(a) of this title unless the presumption is rebutted by a preponderance of the evidence.

(b) Adequate notice and hearing

A health care entity is deemed to have met the adequate notice and hearing requirement of subsection (a)(3) of this section with respect to a physician if the following conditions are met (or are waived voluntarily by the physician): *[Details omitted regarding the notice of proposed action, notice of hearing, and conduct of the hearing.]*

(c) Adequate procedures in investigations or health emergencies

For purposes of section 11111(a) of this title, nothing in this section shall be construed as—

(1) requiring the procedures referred to in subsection (a)(3) of this section—
   (A) where there is no adverse professional review action taken, or
   (B) in the case of a suspension or restriction of clinical privileges, for a period of not longer than 14 days, during which an investigation is being conducted to determine the need for a professional review action; or

(2) precluding an immediate suspension or restriction of clinical privileges, subject to subsequent notice and hearing or other adequate procedures, where the failure to take such an action may result in an imminent danger to the health of any individual.

§ 11113. Payment of reasonable attorneys' fees and costs *[text omitted]*

§ 11114. Guidelines of Secretary *[text omitted]*

§ 11115. Construction *[text omitted]*

SUBCHAPTER II—REPORTING OF INFORMATION

§ 11131. Requiring reports on medical malpractice payments *[text omitted]*

§ 11132. Reporting of sanctions taken by Boards of Medical Examiners *[text omitted]*

§ 11133. Reporting of certain professional review actions taken by health care entities
(a) Reporting by health care entities
  (1) On physicians
    Each health care entity which—
    (A) takes a professional review action that adversely affects the clinical privileges of a physician for a period longer than 30 days;
    (B) accepts the surrender of clinical privileges of a physician—
      (i) while the physician is under an investigation by the entity relating to possible incompetence or improper professional conduct, or
      (ii) in return for not conducting such an investigation or proceeding; or
    (C) in the case of such an entity which is a professional society, takes a professional review action which adversely affects the membership of a physician in the society,

shall report to the Board of Medical Examiners, in accordance with section 11134(a) of this title, the information described in paragraph (3).
  (2) Permissive reporting on other licensed health care practitioners
    A health care entity may report to the Board of Medical Examiners, in accordance with section 11134(a) of this title, the information described in paragraph (3) in the case of a licensed health care practitioner who is not a physician, if the entity would be required to report such information under paragraph (1) with respect to the practitioner if the practitioner were a physician.
  (3) Information to be reported
  The information to be reported under this subsection is—
    (A) the name of the physician or practitioner involved,
    (B) a description of the acts or omissions or other reasons for the action or, if known, for the surrender, and
    (C) such other information respecting the circumstances of the action or surrender as the Secretary deems appropriate.
(b) Reporting by Board of Medical Examiners
Each Board of Medical Examiners shall report, in accordance with section 11134 of this title, the information reported to it under subsection (a) of this section and known instances of a health care entity's failure to report information under subsection (a)(1) of this section.
(c) Sanctions
  (1) Health care entities
  A health care entity that fails substantially to meet the requirement of subsection (a)(1) of this section shall lose the protections of section 11111(a)(1) of this title if the Secretary publishes the name of the entity under section 11111(b) of this title.

(2) Board of Medical Examiners
If, after notice of noncompliance and providing an opportunity to correct noncompliance, the Secretary determines that a Board of Medical Examiners has failed to report information in accordance with subsection (b) of this section, the Secretary shall designate another qualified entity for the reporting of information under subsection (b) of this section.

(d) References to Board of Medical Examiners
Any reference in this subchapter to a Board of Medical Examiners includes, in the case of a Board in a State that fails to meet the reporting requirements of section 11132(a) of this title or subsection (b) of this section, a reference to such other qualified entity as the Secretary designates.

§ 11134. Form of reporting *[text omitted]*

§ 11135. Duty of hospitals to obtain information
(a) In general
It is the duty of each hospital to request from the Secretary (or the agency designated under section 11134(b) of this title), on and after the date information is first required to be reported under section 11134(a) of this title)
(1) at the time a physician or licensed health care practitioner applies to be on the medical staff (courtesy or otherwise) of, or for clinical privileges at, the hospital, information reported under this subchapter concerning the physician or practitioner, and
(2) once every 2 years information reported under this subchapter concerning any physician or such practitioner who is on the medical staff (courtesy or otherwise) of, or has been granted clinical privileges at, the hospital.
A hospital may request such information at other times.

(b) Failure to obtain information
With respect to a medical malpractice action, a hospital which does not request information respecting a physician or practitioner as required under subsection (a) of this section is presumed to have knowledge of any information reported under this subchapter to the Secretary with respect to the physician or practitioner.
(c) Reliance on information provided
Each hospital may rely upon information provided to the hospital under this chapter and shall not be held liable for such reliance in the absence of the hospital's knowledge that the information provided was false.

§ 11136. Disclosure and correction of information *[text omitted]*

§ 11137. Miscellaneous provisions *[text omitted]*

SUBCHAPTER III—DEFINITIONS AND REPORTS

§ 11151. Definitions
In this chapter:
(1) The term "adversely affecting" includes reducing, restricting, suspending, revoking, denying, or failing to renew clinical privileges or membership in a health care entity.
(2) The term "Board of Medical Examiners" includes a body comparable to such a Board (as determined by the State) with responsibility for the licensing of physicians and also includes a subdivision of such a Board or body.
(3) The term "clinical privileges" includes privileges, membership on the medical staff, and the other circumstances pertaining to the furnishing of medical care under which a physician or other licensed health care practitioner is permitted to furnish such care by a health care entity.
(4) (A) The term **"health care entity" means**—

(i) a hospital that is licensed to provide health care services by the State in which it is located,
(ii) an entity (including a health maintenance organization or group medical practice) that provides health care services and that follows a formal peer review process for the purpose of furthering quality health care (as determined under regulations of the Secretary), and
(iii) subject to subparagraph (B), a professional society (or committee thereof) of physicians or other licensed health care practitioners that follows a formal peer review process for the purpose of furthering quality health care (as determined under regulations of the Secretary).
(B) The term "health care entity" does not include a professional society (or committee thereof) if, within the previous 5 years, the society has been found by the Federal Trade Commission or any court to have engaged in any anti-competitive practice which had the effect of restricting the practice of licensed health care practitioners.
(5) The term "hospital" means an entity described in paragraphs (1) and (7) of section 1395x(e) of this title.
(6) The terms "licensed health care practitioner" and "practitioner" mean, with respect to a State, an individual (other than a physician) who is licensed or otherwise authorized by the State to provide health care services.
(7) The term "medical malpractice action or claim" means a written claim or demand for payment based on a health care provider's furnishing (or failure to furnish) health care services, and includes the filing of a cause of action, based on the law of tort, brought in any court of any State or the United States seeking monetary damages.

(8) The term **"physician" means** a doctor of medicine or osteopathy or a doctor of dental surgery or medical dentistry legally authorized to practice medicine and surgery or dentistry by a State (or any individual who, without authority holds himself or herself out to be so authorized).
(9) The term **"professional review action" means** an action or recommendation of a professional review body which is taken or made in the conduct of professional review activity, which is based on the competence or professional conduct of an individual physician (which conduct affects or could affect adversely the health or welfare of a patient or patients), and which affects (or may affect) adversely the clinical privileges, or membership in a professional society, of the physician. Such term includes a formal decision of a professional review body not to take an action or make a recommendation described in the previous sentence and also includes professional review activities relating to a professional review action. In this chapter, an action is not considered to be based on the competence or professional conduct of a physician if the action is primarily based on—
    (A) the physician's association, or lack of association, with a professional society or association,
    (B) the physician's fees or the physician's advertising or engaging in other competitive acts intended to solicit or retain business,
    (C) the physician's participation in prepaid group health plans, salaried employment, or any other manner of delivering health services whether on a fee-for-service or other basis,
    (D) a physician's association with, supervision of, delegation of authority to, support for, training

of, or participation in a private group practice with, a member or members of a particular class of health care practitioner or professional, or

(E) any other matter that does not relate to the competence or professional conduct of a physician.

(10) The term **"professional review activity" means** an activity of a health care entity with respect to an individual physician—

(A) to determine whether the physician may have clinical privileges with respect to, or membership in, the entity,

(B) to determine the scope or conditions of such privileges or membership, or

(C) to change or modify such privileges or membership.

(11) The term **"professional review body" means** a health care entity and the governing body or any committee of a health care entity which conducts professional review activity, and includes any committee of the medical staff of such an entity when assisting the governing body in a professional review activity.

(12) The term "Secretary" means the Secretary of Health and Human Services.

(13) The term "State" means the 50 States, the District of Columbia, Puerto Rico, the Virgin Islands, Guam, American Samoa, and the Northern Mariana Islands.

(14) The term "State licensing board" means, with respect to a physician or health care provider in a State, the agency of the State which is primarily responsible for the licensing of the physician or provider to furnish health care services.

HEALTH INFORMATION MANAGEMENT

After reading this chapter, you will

- understand that maintaining accurate and complete health records serves many purposes, the most important of which is to aid in clinical decision making;
- know that health information is highly confidential but must be disclosed in many situations;
- appreciate that all healthcare personnel must be familiar with federal and state privacy laws;
- see that the HIPAA privacy standards overlie, but generally do not replace, other confidentiality laws; and
- understand that serious criminal and civil penalties can be assessed for breaches of information security and confidentiality.

Discussions of health information today almost always begin with a mention of the Health Insurance Portability and Accountability Act of 1996 (HIPAA).[1] HIPAA was originally intended to protect health coverage for employees who change or lose their jobs, but despite its name it did not actually provide for "portability" of health insurance. Instead, it prohibited a new employer's health plan from excluding workers or charging them higher premiums because of preexisting conditions, but it did so only under limited circumstances.

> *Quality information is essential to all aspects of today's healthcare system. [Health information management] has the body of knowledge and practice that ensure the availability of health information to facilitate real-time healthcare delivery and critical health-related decision making for multiple purposes across diverse organizations, settings, and disciplines.*
>
> —American Health Information Management Association[93]

There were so many loopholes and exceptions to the law that many consumers received little benefit from it. Thus the lasting legacy of HIPAA does not relate to insurance coverage at all—either portable or otherwise—but to regulations meant to improve the security of electronic health transactions (read: billing) and protect the privacy of health information.[2] These were published by the Department of Health and Human Services after Congress was unable to agree on its own version of federal privacy and security standards.

HIPAA defines *health information* as

> any information, whether oral or recorded *in any form or medium*, that—
> (A) is created or received by a health care provider, health plan, public health authority, employer, life insurer, school or university, or health care clearinghouse; and
> (B) relates to the past, present, or future physical or mental health or condition of an individual; or the past, present, or future payment for the provision of health care to an individual.[3] [Emphasis added.]

This broad definition covers *any* information related to the provision of or payment for healthcare. It includes demographics, insurance coverage, medical history, clinical findings, test results, medical images, procedures performed, and so forth. It also includes information not directly related to health—such as the names of a patient's children, her favorite food, the kind of car she drives, or the high school she attended—if somehow relevant to her healthcare situation in any way.

Health information has been preserved on paper for centuries, but today patient records consist of more than traditional medical charts in color-tabbed folders. For example, they may include photographic and radiographic images (film, digital, or holographic); computer and Internet files (stored in "the cloud" or on hard drives, CDs, flash drives, other media); and sound recordings (e.g., dictation)—all of which may be accessed and perhaps downloaded via a desktop, laptop, or mobile device. In short, the record of care includes all data and information in any format that are "gathered about a patient from the moment he or she enters the hospital [or doctor's office] to the moment of discharge or transfer."[4]

covered entity
a health plan, healthcare clearinghouse, or healthcare provider that transmits any health information in electronic form

Health information is maintained primarily to facilitate continuity of care, but it is also needed for accurate coding and billing, documentation of medical necessity, ethical decision making, protection of patients' and providers' legal interests, public health and research, peer review and quality assurance, medical education, accreditation and licensure, and myriad other purposes. Because health information is used in many ways and by many organizations, HIPAA defines two other terms critical to its application: *covered entity* and *protected health information*.

protected health information (PHI)
any health-related information that identifies or can be used to identify the individual to whom it pertains

Covered Entity, Protected Health Information, and De-identification

A **covered entity** is any healthcare provider, health insurance plan, or billing company. **Protected health information (PHI)** is identifying information (as defined earlier) collected or used by a covered entity. PHI does not include information contained in education or employment records or information that has been "de-identified."[5] Eighteen indicators must be scrubbed from PHI before it can be considered de-identified, including names; small geographic areas; dates related to the individual (e.g., dates of birth and death); phone and fax numbers; mail and e-mail addresses; URLs; identifying numbers (e.g., Social Security and health record numbers); and photographs, fingerprints, and similar images. In short, PHI consists of data containing enough details that would make it easy to track or identify a person, his family and relatives, or his associates; if such identifiers have been removed or the information has been aggregated or encrypted, it does not amount to PHI.

Form and Content of Records

In most states, the form and content of records are dictated by the statutes, rules, and regulations of the licensing agencies. These directives date back to the time records were kept on paper and often merely require that an "adequate" or "complete" record be maintained. A few statutes specify categories of information that must be included but leave other details to the administrative rule. For example, the Florida statute requires that a hospital must use

> a system of problem-oriented medical records for its patients, which system shall include the following elements: basic client data collection; a listing of the patient's problems; the initial plan with diagnostic and therapeutic orders as appropriate for each problem identified; and progress notes, including a discharge summary. The [state licensing] agency shall, by rule, establish criteria for such problem-oriented medical record systems in order to ensure comparability among facilities and to facilitate the compilation of statewide statistics.[6]

The agency's implementing regulation then lists two dozen specific items that must be included in every inpatient record, including, for example, the chief complaint or reason for seeking care, personal and family medical history, reports of physical examinations, lab and imaging reports, consultation reports, specific treatments given, and documentation of informed consent. There are additional requirements for patients undergoing invasive procedures and for ambulatory care patients.[7] In short, the Florida regulatory scheme is detailed about the contents of a medical record, and it must be followed. Health information management (HIM) professionals must ensure that medical records comply with the applicable requirements.

Some states' licensure regulations explicitly authorize an electronic health record (EHR) system, as long as it contains the required content. In theory, a computerized record eliminates handwritten or printed documents, improves accuracy, and saves time and money. The Stimulus Act of 2009,[8]

Legal Brief

In the *2013 Hospital Accreditation Standards* (p. RC-1), The Joint Commission offers the following recommendation.

Whether the hospital keeps paper records, electronic records, or both, the contents of the record remain the same. Special care should be taken, however, by hospitals that are transitioning from paper to electronic systems, as the period of transition can present increased opportunity for errors in record-keeping that can affect the delivery of safe quality care.

This advice should be considered by all providers, not only hospitals.

the Affordable Care Act, and the Health Information Technology for Economic and Clinical Health Act (HITECH, discussed later in this chapter) encourage the widespread adoption of EHRs. The EHR concept raises issues of confidentiality, durability, and compliance with licensure requirements, and as always there is some resistance to change, but healthcare is clearly headed in that direction. Where the law has not kept pace with this technological progress, the advice of legal counsel and state associations should be sought.

The Joint Commission has standards for health records[9] (see Legal Brief) and may revoke an organization's accreditation for failure to comply with its terms. Noncompliance also could be presented as evidence of negligence if such failure was a cause of injury.[10] The federal government set similar standards in its Medicare Conditions of Participation (COP).[11]

In addition to general record-keeping requirements, state laws require hospitals and physicians to maintain certain information and report it to public authorities for statistical purposes. These requirements are discussed later in this chapter.

Record entries must be "authenticated"; that is, they must be dated and signed or otherwise verified by the person making the entry. This notation can be done by electronic signatures, written signatures or initials, rubber stamp signature, or computer key. If rubber stamp or electronic signatures are used, the individual identified by the stamp or electronic authentication must be the only individual who uses it.[12]

A hospital health record is complete when it contains the patient's medical history; admitting diagnosis; consultations and test results; complications; informed consent; physician orders, nursing notes, and medication records; discharge summary (clinical resume) with provisions for follow-up care; and final diagnosis—all within 30 days following discharge. HIM policies must require that attending physicians keep their records current and complete them in a reasonable time (typically, no more than 30 days) after a patient's discharge; disciplinary measures should be prescribed for physicians who do not comply with these requirements.

Failure to maintain complete, accurate, and legible records can have severe adverse effects in civil litigation (see Legal Decision Point). For example, a nurse's failure to record observations of a patient's condition is evidence

Legal Decision Point

Consider the following report:

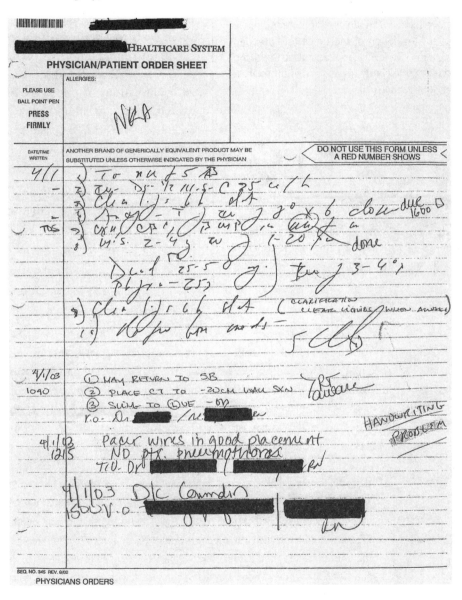

1. What does the first entry dated 4/1 say?
2. A nurse added "clarification: clear liquids when awake" to the report, and an auditor wrote "handwriting problem" in the margin. If an entry is illegible, can the document containing the entry be considered accurate and complete?
3. What are some ways to improve the quality of this physician's records?

Law in Action

A physician left written orders that his patient be given a saline solution of ".3 NS." The attending nurse overlooked the decimal point and gave the patient a solution of ten times the intended concentration. Believing he was not at fault, the physician tried to clarify his original order by tracing over it in pen to read:

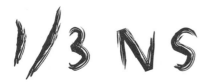

This "clarification" only compounded the problem and looked like a cover-up. The jury returned a verdict in favor of the plaintiffs.

of possible negligence for a jury to consider. Health records are used as evidence in malpractice suits—in fact, they are often the most important "witness" in such cases—so the absence of standard entries or the inclusion of inaccurate information often leads to a verdict for the plaintiff.

Inaccurate information must be corrected as soon as it is discovered. Erasure or obliteration of medical information, even if inaccurate, should not be permitted (see Law in Action). Instead, the person making the change should

- carefully draw a line through the error, leaving the original writing legible;
- describe the reason for the change;
- date the corrected entry; and
- authenticate it in the same manner as any other entry.

The wisdom of following this practice of careful correction is illustrated by a Connecticut case involving a psychiatric patient who had been left unattended in a locked room and was later "found in the room with her head wedged between the side rail and the mattress of her bed, unconscious, with no pulse, blood pressure, or respiratory function." A few days later, on the orders of the director of nursing,

> the original record was surreptitiously removed from the chart and a "revised" record was substituted without the knowledge of the hospital administration and in violation of explicit hospital policy. The substituted record was demonstrably false and conflicted with other records and the testimony of staff members on duty that morning as to their actual observations. The revised record came to light after suit was commenced when a nurse not connected with the psychiatric unit brought to the attention of the hospital administration that she had been forced to rewrite a note on the original record. The trial court instructed the jury without objection that they could consider the substitution of the records as a circumstance indicating the defendant's consciousness of negligence.[13]

A verdict against the hospital in the amount of $3.6 million was upheld on appeal.

The adverse implications of an incomplete health record were demonstrated in *Carr v. St. Paul Fire and Marine Insurance Company*.[14] The patient came to the hospital's emergency department (ED) complaining of severe abdominal pains and vomiting but was examined only by a licensed practical nurse and two orderlies. (The court noted that the nurse and one of the orderlies were "sweethearts" and later married and that all three were "close friends." The relevance of this fact becomes apparent later.) One of the orderlies took the patient's vital signs, but the hospital was unable to contact the patient's doctor, who was out of town. The patient left, saying he would return when his doctor returned. The patient died later that evening after returning to the hospital by ambulance in even greater distress. The death certificate opined that the decedent had suffered a heart attack.

Testimony described the patient's vital signs as "normal" during the first visit, but the three ED personnel "and possibly Dr. Vizant" (who completed the death certificate) were the only ones to view the record of the visit. The friendship among the three ED staff becomes relevant at this point: Someone destroyed the record that night after the patient died.

In the resulting lawsuit, the jury was allowed to infer that the documents probably revealed a medical emergency necessitating attendance by a physician. The court stated:

> No one knows the effect [destruction of the records] had on the jury, but the jury certainly had a right to infer that the record had it been retained would have shown that a medical emergency existed and that a doctor should have been called and that more attention should have been given him than was given.[15]

As this case shows, the best witness in malpractice litigation is often a thorough and complete health record. In many cases, such records are convincing evidence that the patient received reasonable care under all the facts and circumstances. An incomplete or missing record may spell disaster for the defense.

Although clinical records should be comprehensive, *incident reports* are not meant to be part of the health record and should not be included. They are prepared in anticipation of possible litigation and for the hospital's attorneys to use. They often contain information (much of it hearsay) that tends to indicate fault. If they are included in the health record, they will be available as evidence in a lawsuit. In most states, incident reports are considered privileged, not subject to discovery, and not admissible. The incident report process is conducted for educational purposes and to improve general standards of patient care and safety. To serve these ends, incident reports need to be written with candor. Staff cannot be forthright if they are apprehensive that the reports will be available to potential malpractice plaintiffs, so those preparing the documents must be assured of the reports' confidentiality.

Hospital policies regarding retention of health records depend on local law and the standards of professional care appropriate to the type of institution involved. Governing bodies must not only be familiar with applicable legal requirements regarding the length of time that records must be preserved but also analyze their particular medical and administrative needs. For example, to enable epidemiological studies (or for other pedagogic reasons), teaching hospitals and research institutions may wish to retain records longer than typical acute care hospitals do. All institutions need to retain records long enough to facilitate continuing programs of peer review and quality assurance.

The law on record retention varies widely, and from state to state, on such matters as the length of time records must be kept and whether alternative media (e.g., microfilming, electronic formats) may substitute for records that were originally kept on paper. Medicare's COP require that records be maintained for at least five years,[16] but many states specify longer periods. Formats other than paper are permitted unless explicitly proscribed, and some items (e.g., nurses' notes, original X-ray films) may be destroyed sooner than others. To complicate matters, a state's statutes of limitation must be considered. Traditionally, the limitation period for torts did not begin to run against a minor until she reached the age of majority. (If the limitation period were two years and the age of majority were 21, a newborn could file suit a day short of her twenty-third birthday and still have a valid claim.) Many states have changed this common-law rule. Florida, for example, provides:

> In no event shall the action be commenced later than 4 years from the date of the incident or occurrence out of which the cause of action accrued, except that this 4-year period shall not bar an action brought on behalf of a minor on or before the child's eighth birthday.[17]

In summary, the length of time patients' clinical records are retained and those records' format are determined by standards of professional practice, the operational and medical needs of the particular organization, and local law in each state. Institutional policies on these questions must be carefully developed and periodically reviewed with legal counsel. Private organizations such as The Joint Commission and the American Hospital Association (AHA) also have published statements of policy on retention and destruction of records. The current policy statement of the AHA recommends that records be retained for at least ten years. As more and more electronic records are created where paper records would have existed before, storage logistics becomes simpler and retention periods can be extended. Some organizations are now archiving their electronic records permanently.

Access to Health Information
Ownership and Control of Records

State law generally provides that healthcare providers (e.g., physicians, hospitals) own and have physical possession and control of health records.[18] Neither patients nor authorized representatives have a right to physical possession of the original health records, and The Joint Commission flatly states, "Original medical records are not released unless the hospital is responding to law and regulation."[19]

Ownership and the right to control do not prohibit patients and interested third parties from accessing health records. Patients have a right to view and copy their records, have copies sent to any new physician of their choice, and appoint authorized representatives (e.g., their attorneys) to examine the documents. One exception may be cases in which disclosure of information might adversely affect a patient's physical or mental health.[20] In such situations, attending physicians may have the authority to deny patients access to their records.

The estates of deceased physicians and physicians who retire from practice, relocate, or are otherwise unavailable are obligated to notify their former patients and make copies of the records available.[21] Hence, in a New York case, the court invalidated a provision in a deceased physician's will that his executor burn all his professional records.[22] Physicians are also required to transfer a health record (or copies of it) to a former patient's new physician when the patient so requests.

The Patient's Right to Access Under HIPAA

The long-held paternalistic belief that health records are not to be read by the patient is no longer valid. HIPAA and state laws codify patients' right to the information in their health records. HIPAA gives patients the right to examine and obtain copies of their records and request correction of any errors.[23] The request may be denied only for good cause, such as if

- disclosure of the information would be likely to endanger the life or physical safety of the patient or another person;
- the information is contained in psychotherapy notes; or
- it was compiled for use in a civil, criminal, or administrative proceeding.

HIM departments usually have a contract agency whose full-time job it is to copy health records and release the information pursuant to patients' requests. This function is often referred to as *release of information (ROI)*; at most hospitals, the ROI function becomes, in effect, a department of its own within HIM because of the number of subpoenas and other requests for copies.

HIPAA also gives patients greater control over the use of their health information. For example, a signed authorization must be obtained from the patient before health information can be used for marketing or fundraising purposes.

Under HIPAA, patients have a right to obtain a listing (also known as *accounting*) of purposes for which their health information was disclosed other than for treatment, payment, or routine healthcare operations (e.g., peer review, quality assurance) or at their own request. Accordingly, healthcare facilities and physicians must keep account of health information disclosures to the following entities, among others:

- Accrediting agencies, such as The Joint Commission
- State oversight agencies
- Public health organizations
- Law enforcement agencies
- Funeral directors
- Tumor registries

The accounting must indicate the date of the disclosure, the name of the recipient, the information disclosed, and the purpose of the disclosure.[24]

HIPAA does not replace state law protections, and before HIPAA was passed many states already had laws providing for access—but HIPAA does trump any state law that conflicts with its provisions. Thus, for example, HIPAA would nullify a state statute that gave a right of access to a broader class of persons or that would allow records to be released only to other physicians and not to the patients themselves (see The Court Decides: *Opis Management Resources v. Secretary* at the end of this chapter).

Many state statutes do not address the right of minor patients to obtain information from their health records or their parents' right to that information. HIPAA defers to state law regarding parents' right to access their children's records, and it would seem that mature minors who can consent for treatment without parental consent should be permitted to access their own records. Emancipated minors are treated as adults in such matters.

In the past, physicians and hospitals routinely refused to allow patients access to their health records. Three rationales were often asserted: (1) records are technical and not understood by laypersons; (2) revelation of the information might adversely affect the patient's or another's life, health, or physical safety; or (3) the privacy of third parties (by which they usually meant healthcare personnel) should be protected. The first and third reasons are no longer supportable under HIPAA. The second reason remains valid because HIPAA allows physicians to deny patients access to their own records if the information would endanger the life or physical safety of the patient or another person. For example, a person such as a friend or family member who reports domestic violence may fear retaliation by the abuser. In that case, the patient may be denied access if allowing them to see the records would be likely to reveal the source of the information. (Note, however, that a decision to deny access on these grounds may be reviewable, thus expert advice is recommended.)

HIPAA was passed more than 20 years ago, and hospitals and physicians have since reevaluated their policies. Today, health records are available to anyone whom the patient authorizes to receive them. Reasonable safeguards have been instituted to protect healthcare information from unauthorized use and disclosure. Although patients cannot arbitrarily be denied access, hospitals should know by now how to handle such requests. Especially important is the moral and legal duty of the hospital or physician to ensure that patients' authorization of third parties is current and genuine. Healthcare personnel must be sensitive to the validity and authenticity of documents that purport to be a patient's authorization to release information.[25]

Release of Information Without Patient Consent

Confidentiality is governed by both state and federal laws. Accordingly, both HIPAA's privacy regulations and state law must be consulted to determine reliable answers to the questions that continually arise about the release of medical information.

Disclosure of personal information does not offend the US Constitution.[26] Although the US Supreme Court has recognized an individual's constitutional right to make certain personal decisions without interference by the government or other third parties,[27] no federal constitutional provision prohibits the release of health information. As discussed in the next section, in many situations third parties have a legitimate interest in and a legal right to medical information regarding a particular patient. In those cases, release of health information without the patient's consent is permitted and, indeed, sometimes required.

Court Orders and Subpoenas

A valid court order directing that health records be made available to a third party must be honored, and the patient's consent is not required. Generally, the legal process for obtaining health record information is through a *subpoena duces tecum*—a request that a witness bring specified documents to a court or other tribunal that has jurisdiction over pending litigation.

Under most states' procedural rules, during the litigation process attorneys may themselves issue subpoenas for records relating to the other party using blank forms provided by the court. The lawyer for the defendant in a malpractice suit, for example, routinely subpoenas all the plaintiff's health records from other healthcare providers to have the case evaluated by a medical expert. Under HIPAA's privacy standards, if an attorney's subpoena is not accompanied by a court order (i.e., an order signed by a judge or equivalent judicial official) a healthcare provider may release the patient's records only if (1) a patient authorization accompanies the subpoena or (2) the party issuing the subpoena has made a reasonable effort to give the patient notice of the request. If in doubt, the record owner may petition the court for a determination of whether the records must be turned over. (Hospital HIM/ROI departments are usually facile with these requirements and should be consulted. In fact, in most health systems all subpoenas are referred to the HIM department for action.)

Statutory Reports

Certain state and federal statutes require or permit hospitals and medical personnel to report health information to public authorities. These reporting requirements are permissible as a legitimate exercise of the government's power to provide for the general welfare.[28] The disclosures must be "accounted for" (as noted earlier) under HIPAA. Following are some of the kinds of state reporting requirements:

- Vital statistics (deaths, births, fetal deaths)
- Abortions
- Sexually transmitted diseases
- Other communicable diseases
- Injuries that may be the result of criminal acts
- Accidental or self-inflicted wounds
- Drug abuse
- Child or elder abuse or neglect

This list is not exhaustive and the requirements differ somewhat from state to state, so annotating all the requirements here is not possible. Healthcare providers must be familiar with the law of their particular jurisdictions because failure to report to the appropriate public authority may lead to civil liability or criminal penalties.

Duty to Warn Third Parties

In addition to statutory reporting obligations, providers have a common-law duty to warn third parties of foreseeable risks of harm. HIPAA permits such disclosure when the healthcare provider believes it "is necessary to prevent or lessen a serious and imminent threat to the health or safety of a person or the public" and is made to someone who is able to prevent or lessen the threat.[29]

In a California case with a tragic outcome, a male student was receiving voluntary outpatient psychiatric treatment at a university hospital. Several hospital psychotherapists were aware that he had threatened to kill a particular individual. One of the psychologists felt the student should be committed and asked the campus police to detain him, which they did; he was later released, however, when the chief of psychiatry reviewed and reversed the order for detention. Two months later, the student killed his intended victim.

A trial court dismissed the victim's parents' lawsuit, holding that the psychotherapists and the university had no duty to warn the victim. However, the California Supreme Court reversed and remanded the case for trial. The high court felt that, under the circumstances, members of a jury might reasonably conclude that they had a duty to disclose the foreseeable dangers the patient posed (see The Court Decides: *Tarasoff v. Regents of the University of California* at the end of this chapter).

The *Tarasoff* doctrine is limited to situations in which the provider knows the patient is a serious or imminent threat to a readily identifiable victim. One justice noted this limitation in a separate opinion:

> I concur in the result in this instance only because the complaints allege that defendant therapists did in fact predict that [the patient] would kill and were therefore negligent in failing to warn of that danger. Thus the issue here is very narrow: we are not concerned with whether the therapists, pursuant to the standards of their profession, "should have" predicted potential violence; they allegedly did so in actuality. Under these limited circumstances I agree that a cause of action can be stated.[30]

Because the ability to predict dangerousness has been seriously questioned over the years (see Legal Brief), providers are usually held to have no duty to warn of a person's generalized threats to unspecified individuals. For example, in a case interpreting *Tarasoff*, the California Supreme Court held that the government had no duty to warn the community or the police that a juvenile delinquent released from governmental custody to the home of his mother had exhibited violent propensities toward young children. In the absence of an imminent risk to an identifiable victim, the juvenile's criminal act that caused the death of a five-year-old was not foreseeable, and no liability was imposed.[31]

The duty to warn third parties strikes a balance between an individual's right to confidentiality and a third person's

Legal Brief

An Internet search using such key words as *predicting dangerousness* will result in myriad results demonstrating the controversial nature of the assumption that such predictions are reliable. One source flatly states, "In reality, no one can predict future dangerousness precisely and with absolute certainty."[94]

For this reason, trial judges and opposing counsel will likely scrutinize rigorously any opinion of dangerousness so as not to prejudice the individual against whom it is asserted.

right to know that a risk exists. The imminence and probability of the risks and the identification of the probable victim must be carefully considered to justify the conclusion that the third person's interests are paramount to the confidentiality of health information.[32] As a practical matter, the professional who must balance these interests is in the unenviable position of having to predict violent behavior despite medical science's inability to forecast self-injury or injury to others accurately (see discussion of involuntary detention or commitment in chapter 3).

The existence and extent of a defendant's duty is a question of law for the court to determine. If a duty exists, whether it was breached and whether the breach was the proximate cause of injury are questions of fact for a jury. Thus, *foreseeability* is a question for the jury, and reluctance to send this question to the jury may be the reason some jurisdictions have rejected the *Tarasoff* rule in favor of the physician–patient privilege.[33] Even California declined to apply the principle in a case in which a psychiatrist was allegedly aware of a patient's suicidal tendencies and failed to restrain the patient or warn the parents.[34] The court held that *Tarasoff*'s duty to warn applies only when the risk to be prevented is the danger of violent assault, not when the risk is suicide. When the patient is in danger of self-inflicted harm, the proper course would seem to be involuntary commitment.

Peer Review Statutes

As discussed more fully in chapter 8, peer review is a type of quality assurance process. Under federal regulations, peer review organizations have the right to access patient records and other information.[35] The information must be held in confidence and must not be disclosed, except as authorized by law—for example, as aggregate data that do not identify an individual patient or healthcare provider. The HIPAA privacy regulations recognize and permit compliance with these statutes.

Lien Statutes

A third party's legal right to receive medical information regarding a particular patient is further enforced by hospital lien statutes, which exist in approximately one-third of states. The lien laws grant healthcare providers a legal claim under which the cost of hospitalization is paid from damages that a patient recovers from the person or entity whose civil wrong necessitated the patient's treatment. In these cases, the tortfeasor is entitled to access the patient's health information—without patient authorization—to assess the legitimacy of the medical bills.

Liability for Unauthorized Disclosure

The Hippocratic Oath requires physicians to hold inviolate and confidential all information entrusted to them by their patients (see Legal Brief). This ethical obligation may be incorporated in state regulations governing the licensure of physicians and healthcare institutions, and its violation may be a cause for revoking or suspending a license. Whether violation of licensure regulations creates a civil cause of action for damages is a different issue. Clearly, the HIPAA privacy regulations set a standard of care for confidentiality irrespective of other state laws.

No doctrine of confidential or privileged communication between patient and physician or patient and institution existed in early common law. It recognized a doctrine of privileged communication in only three relationships: attorney–client, husband–wife, and clergy–penitent.

> ## Legal Brief
>
>
> What I may see or hear in the course of the treatment or even outside of the treatment in regard to the life of men, which on no account one must spread abroad, I will keep to myself, holding such things shameful to be spoken about.[95]
>
> —The Hippocratic Oath (translation by Ludwig Edelstein)

Most states have now enacted privileged communication statutes to establish a confidential relationship between physicians and patients. Although the details of these statutes differ, they essentially codify the Hippocratic Oath. These statutes do not always apply to out-of-court disclosures; they often apply only to disclosures made in the course of judicial or quasi-judicial proceedings. Furthermore, they may not apply to institutional providers. Thus, a plaintiff often must base cases involving breach of confidence on tort or contract principles.

Action may be brought for at least three types of infringement: defamation of character, invasion of privacy, or breach of an implied contract to respect confidentiality. The first two violations are discussed in the following sections; breach of an implied contract is addressed in chapter 4.

Defamation

As stated in chapter 4, *defamation* is a written or verbal communication to a third party of information that diminishes the esteem, respect, or confidence with which a living person is regarded by exciting adverse or derogatory feelings against that person.[36] Written defamation is *libel*, while spoken defamation is *slander*. In either event, to be considered defamatory the communication must be made (published) to someone other than the aggrieved party. For example, in *Farris v. Tvedten*, a physician's dictated letter addressed personally to a nurse that suggested the nurse may have committed a crime by administering a substitute for a prescribed medicine did not constitute libel because no third party received the communication.[37]

Successful defamation suits for release of information from a health record are uncommon. Even in the absence of a legitimate motive for publishing the information, the truth of a published statement is a complete defense to a defamation charge.[38] Even if the statement is not true, evidence of a proper motive or a reasonable belief that the statement *is* true generally provides a partial defense that may mitigate damages.

In addition, the law has long recognized two privileges that may afford a defense even when a defamatory statement is made. The first is *absolute privilege*, which attaches to judicial and administrative proceedings. In one case, for example, when a hospital honored a court-ordered subpoena and released a health record that indicated the plaintiff was under the influence of alcohol, the release was privileged and defamation was not proved. Whether the record was false had no bearing on the case.[39]

The second is *qualified privilege*, which concerns information reasonably believed to be true and published with a proper motive in mind. Information may be communicated in good faith to protect or advance the legitimate interests of the publisher or to protect someone else's interests. For example, in a New York case, the name of a frequent visitor to a hospital's ED was placed on a list of persons suspected of being drug abusers. The court held that the communications were protected by qualified privilege because hospital personnel had a duty to communicate their opinions to other staff.[40]

Whether the information was reasonably believed to be true and published in good faith is a question of fact for the jury. If the publication was motivated by spite or ill will (*malice in fact*), the publisher may be liable for punitive and compensatory damages. Because most hospitals and physicians do not recklessly disregard the truth or publish information they know to be false, they are unlikely to be held liable for malice in fact.

Examples of qualified privilege predate HIPAA by many years. Even if a disclosure of information could be justified under traditional defamation law, the HIPAA privacy standards may provide other theories on which plaintiffs could premise recovery.

Invasion of Privacy

Invasion of privacy was recognized as a tort following the publication in 1890 of a famous *Harvard Law Review* article coauthored by future US Supreme Court Justice Louis D. Brandeis. Brandeis and his law partner, Samuel Warren, asserted that privacy is a common-law right—"the more general right of the individual to be let alone."[41] More than half a century ago, an Ohio court expounded on this right as follows:

1. The right of privacy is the right of a person to be let alone, to be free from unwarranted publicity, and to live without unwarranted interference by the public in matters with which the public is not necessarily concerned.

2. An actionable invasion of the right of privacy is the unwarranted appropriation or exploitation of one's personality, the publicizing of

one's private affairs with which the public has no legitimate concern, or the wrongful intrusion into one's private activities in such a manner as to outrage or cause mental suffering, shame, or humiliation to a person of ordinary sensibilities.[42]

Most courts recognize the tort, but some have imposed limitations to discourage unwarranted litigation and to strike a proper balance between privacy and free speech. A few states have recognized the right of privacy by enacting statutes that carefully set limitations to the cause of action. In contrast to actions based on the law of defamation, the truth of an unwarranted publication is not necessarily a defense to a suit alleging invasion of privacy. On the other hand, express consent to the publication is a defense.

To succeed in an action for invasion of privacy, the plaintiff does not have to prove monetary loss; damages can be awarded for mental suffering. The right is personal to the individual; the privacy of a deceased person cannot be invaded, so in most cases surviving relatives have no cause of action when the alleged tort occurs after the person's death.[43] Similarly, in contrast to defamation, the "privacy" of a corporation or partnership cannot be invaded; other legal principles, such as copyright and trademark, are used to protect a business entity from unwarranted appropriation of its name.[44]

Cases involving invasion of privacy may include the following:

- Unauthorized commercial appropriation of the plaintiff's name, personality, professional skills, or photograph
- Use of the plaintiff's name or likeness for the defendant's own purposes, even if the use was not commercial and the defendant did not benefit financially from it
- Physical intrusion into someone's private affairs
- Disclosure of private information to those who have no legitimate need to know it

Photography and Observation

The Pennsylvania case of *Clayman v. Bernstein* is an early example of unauthorized use (appropriation) of a patient's likeness for innocent but ulterior purposes.[45] A physician had photographed the plaintiff's facial disfigurement for use in education, but because the patient had not agreed to be photographed, the court found in her favor and prohibited the use of the photos.

More recently, a plastic surgeon was sued for using recognizable before-and-after photos of his patient on television and in a promotion titled "Cream Versus Plastic Surgery" at Garfinckel's department store.[46] Patient consent was an issue in the case; if the patient did give consent, she did not do so in writing. The jury returned sizable verdicts against the surgeon and the department store. Although photos may be taken for inclusion in a patient's health record, these kinds of cases demonstrate that the patient must give written consent. Most healthcare providers have standard consent forms for this purpose.

Providers may be held liable on the basis of any of the principles just discussed for using photography without patient consent or in a manner that does not accord with professional standards of medical practice. Today, the risk is exacerbated by smartphones' photo and video capabilities. Provider organizations need to have clear policies about the use of cell phones and similar devices to photograph patients, and physicians in particular need to be continually reminded that they are subject to HIPAA and other privacy laws.

The issues are similar to those that arise when unauthorized visitors are allowed to observe during surgery or medical examinations; such practices are invasions of the patient's privacy if permitted without consent. Teaching hospitals especially should make clear in the general consent form patients sign at admission that medical students may accompany treating physicians and that the opportunity to observe is an integral part of the students' education.

In cases alleging invasion of privacy, the courts must balance conflicting public policy values: "the right of the individual to be let alone" versus the public's "right to know." The right to be let alone diminishes as one's fame or notoriety increases, as demonstrated by the case about the autopsy photos of NASCAR driver Dale Earnhardt, who was killed in a crash at the Daytona Motor Speedway in 2001.

Like those of any accident victim in Florida, Earnhardt's autopsy records were subject to the state's public records laws, and the autopsy report and certain other items were promptly made available to the public. The autopsy photographs, however, were not. When news organizations tried to obtain copies of the photos, the Earnhardt family objected. The Florida legislature quickly passed an amendment to the public records laws that shielded autopsy photos from disclosure (see Legal Decision Point). The media challenged the law. In ruling that the law is constitutional and that the records (the photographs) must not be released, the court looked into "the seriousness of the intrusion into the family's right to privacy." The opinion states:

> The medical examiner testified that the photographs were "gruesome, grisly and highly disturbing," and the physician attending Mr. Earnhardt after the accident confirmed this. The trial court found that such publication would "be an indecent, outrageous, and intolerable invasion, and would cause deep and serious emotional pain, embarrassment, humiliation and sadness to Dale Earnhardt's surviving family members." It is evident from our review of the record that the publication of the nude and dissected body of Mr. Earnhardt would cause his wife and children pain and sorrow beyond the poor power of our ability to express in words.[47]

Release of medical information to persons who have a legitimate interest in the information does not ordinarily constitute an invasion of the patient's privacy, even absent an explicit consent to do so.[48] Individuals and organizations with a legitimate interest include patients' attorneys, insurance carriers, various government agencies, bona fide research personnel, and family members (in some circumstances, but especially if they are or will be participating in the patient's care and the patient does not object).[49] As mentioned earlier, HIPAA permits release of information for treatment, payment, and healthcare operations (e.g., quality assurance, peer review) and to healthcare oversight agencies. It permits disclosure to a friend or family member if the patient agrees or, if the patient is unable to consent, if disclosure is in the patient's best interests. Persons who consent to publicity or who place themselves in the public eye through their activities and exploits (e.g., musicians, actors, politicians) implicitly waive their rights of privacy to the extent that the public has a legitimate interest in newsworthy events.[50] This principle also applies to persons who are not public figures but who are temporarily in the public eye. Unless news stories and photographs exceed the bounds of ordinary decent conduct, persons cannot complain when, for example, the press reports an accident or a crime they are involved in or when they figure in any other newsworthy event, as long as the publicity is not misleading or the facts are not misrepresented.

Publication of information acknowledging an individual's admission to a hospital, naming the physician, and describing the patient's medical condition in general terms ("good," "fair," "critical," etc.) usually presents no legal risk of liability for invasion of privacy unless the patient objects.[51] If the mere fact of the patient's admission could reveal the presence of a condition thought to be shameful or humiliating, however—as might occur, for example, when the institution in question is known to treat only substance abusers, sex offenders, or those with mental illness—the provider could be held liable for announcing the admission, at least if the patient is not a public figure. Furthermore, irrespective of the kind of facility, HIPAA has provisions allowing the patient to request that no information about his care be released, including the fact that he has been admitted.[52]

Legal Decision Point

In its statute protecting autopsy photographs, the Florida legislature noted

> that the existence of the World Wide Web and the proliferation of personal computers throughout the world encourages and promotes the wide dissemination of photographs and video and audio recordings 24 hours a day and that widespread unauthorized dissemination of autopsy photographs and video and audio recordings would subject the immediate family of the deceased to continuous injury.[96]

Do you think current legal standards regarding these kinds of privacy issues are sufficient?

State and Federal Confidentiality Laws

Physicians and hospital personnel must be familiar with state and federal statutes and regulations that create a positive duty not to release medical information in certain circumstances. HIPAA was mentioned earlier, and state and federal laws provide for "superconfidentiality" of substance abuse, HIV and AIDS, and mental health records. For example, New York's mental hygiene law prohibits state mental institutions from making case records available, except as provided by law; violation of this state statute created civil liability to a patient when a hospital director released the record to an adverse attorney.[53]

Illinois has comprehensive legislation that grants mental health patients or their parents or guardians a right of access to mental health records. It applies principles of confidentiality to all services related to mental health or developmental disability that are furnished by physicians, psychiatrists, psychologists, social workers, and nurses in the community at large.[54] The personal notes of a therapist are part of the accessible record, and no information can be disclosed without written consent of the patient, parent, or guardian except to professional colleagues, peer review committees, and institutions having legal custody of the patient. Furthermore, the statute includes detailed provisions on testimonial disclosures in judicial and quasi-judicial proceedings. Violation of these provisions is a criminal and civil offense; the patient can sue for an injunction and may also seek damages, including recovery of attorneys' fees.

Federal laws such as the Comprehensive Drug Abuse Prevention and Control Act of 1970;[55] the Drug Abuse Office and Treatment Act of 1972;[56] and the Comprehensive Alcohol Abuse and Alcoholism Prevention, Treatment, and Rehabilitation Act Amendments of 1983[57] impose stringent confidentiality of records of patients receiving treatment for drug dependency and alcoholism under programs supported by federal funds. Underlying these rules is the principle that confidentiality encourages patients to seek help for drug and alcohol abuse and psychiatric problems.

The legislation applies to all federally assisted healthcare providers whether the assistance is research on the abuse of drugs or alcohol or through Medicare, Medicaid, or other governmental payment programs. Together, the statutes and attendant regulations provide that medical information is to be disclosed only to those connected with the program.[58] Family members, law enforcement officials, and courts have no access except as specifically provided, unless the patient has given express written consent to the disclosure.

Disclosures without a patient's consent can be made only to personnel in drug or alcohol programs who have a legitimate need to know, to other providers when a medical emergency arises, and to organizations conducting research and evaluations (as long as patients are not identified) and only by special court order based on good cause.[59] These patients may not be identified in any civil, criminal, or administrative procedure, and information cannot be released to law enforcement officials without a court order. Normal civil or criminal proceedings and their usual subpoena processes do not justify breach of a substance abuse or mental health patient's right to confidentiality. Hospital and medical personnel, therefore, must develop policies to prohibit release of all medical information concerning these patients without a court order.

Courts have ordered release of information in proceedings to revoke criminal probation, in cases of child neglect, and for investigation by the Internal Revenue Service (IRS).[60] In one criminal proceeding to determine a person's potential for rehabilitation, good cause for a disclosure was not established when the credibility of a witness was in question.[61] A New York court protected the confidentiality of photographs that had been taken in the waiting room of a methadone treatment clinic and were later sought by law enforcement officials investigating a murder.[62] A judicial **in camera** (Latin phrase meaning "in chamber") review is often necessary to establish good cause and to determine what portion of the record may be released.

in camera
in secret; privately (from Latin: *room, chamber*)

HIPAA Standards, the HITECH Act, and the Red Flags Rule

HIPAA permeates health records law, and no one section of a textbook can do justice to the issues it presents (see Legal Brief). Until this point, therefore, this text has considered HIPAA's effects only as they might illuminate the general privacy concerns that have existed since Hippocrates. The following discussion examines HIPAA standards significant to this chapter, in particular those that

- give patients more control over their PHI than they had previously,
- set limits on the use and disclosure of PHI, and
- hold violators accountable for breaches through enhanced civil and criminal penalties.

Uses and Disclosures of Personal Health Information

HIPAA requires health providers and health plans to provide patients with a notice of privacy practices that explains how patients' PHI will be maintained and used. Patients have the right to prevent

Legal Brief

HIPAA is a massive statute of which only one part addresses the privacy of health information. In this chapter we are concerned primarily with those provisions that deal with privacy issues and their implementing regulations. (As is usually the case, the regulations are more detailed than the law itself.)

The website http://hhs.gov/hipaa/ provides detailed information for individuals and health-care professionals about HIPAA rules, individuals' rights, compliance guidance, FAQs, and more.

some uses of their PHI (e.g., marketing, research, fundraising), but PHI may be used and disclosed for treatment and payment purposes and for routine healthcare operations (e.g., for care management, peer review). If the patient does not object, her name, location, and general condition may be listed in the facility directory. PHI may also be disclosed to friends and family members involved in the patient's care.

Disclosure of PHI is permitted for the following purposes:

- Required by law
- To report abuse, neglect, and domestic violence
- For healthcare oversight activities
- As evidence in judicial and administrative proceedings
- To aid law enforcement investigation
- For coroners, medical examiners, and funeral directors
- For organ, eye, and tissue donation
- For certain research
- To avert a serious threat to health or safety
- For certain governmental functions, such as national security
- For workers' compensation claims

Regardless of whether the disclosure is permitted by law or authorized by the patient, the organization must "limit the protected health information disclosed to the information reasonably necessary to achieve the purpose for which the disclosure is sought."[63] Disclosures that are not permitted by the foregoing cannot be made without the patient's (or legal representative's) written authorization.

HIPAA preempts state laws that provide less protection or grant the patient fewer rights of access. Each state's laws need to be analyzed to determine whether any of its provisions are preempted. In 2002, the Florida Hospital Association convened a committee of attorneys and compliance officers to review more than 200 laws and regulations of that state that affect the privacy of health information. The committee found several provisions that conflict with HIPAA. For example, one section of the Florida mental health law provides that patients have a right to access their records unless the physician determines that release would be "harmful to the patient,"[64] whereas the HIPAA regulations state that access may be denied only if it would endanger the patient's "life or physical safety."[65] As the Florida statute allows a physician to deny access because of potential emotional harm—not only danger to the patient's life or physical safety—the statute is contrary to HIPAA and is preempted.[66]

In the few cases challenging HIPAA's privacy rules, the courts have upheld the regulations. For example, in *South Carolina Medical Association v. Thompson*, a federal court ruled that Congress had not unconstitutionally delegated its legislative power to the executive branch by giving the secretary of the US Department of Health and Human Services (HHS) broad rule-making authority:

> Because Congress laid out an intelligible principle in HIPAA to guide agency action, we reject appellants' claim that the statute impermissibly delegates the legislative function. We also conclude that regulations promulgated pursuant to HIPAA are not beyond the scope of the congressional grant of authority, and that neither the statute nor the regulations are impermissibly vague.[67]

Privacy Breaches and the HITECH Act

Although the HIPAA standards have been part of the regulatory landscape since 1996, privacy breaches continue to occur. Recognizing the need for greater vigilance, in 2009 Congress passed the Health Information Technology for Economic and Clinical Health (HITECH) Act to help clamp down on the problem. The law sharply increased the administrative penalties that can be imposed on violators—to as much as $50,000 per violation—and included criminal penalties of fines and prison time of up to ten years.[68] If a breach of unsecured PHI affects 500 or more individuals, a covered entity must notify the secretary of HHS of the breach no later than 60 calendar days from the discovery of the breach, and the details are posted on the HHS website (see Legal Brief).

In addition to increasing the penalties for HIPAA breaches, the HITECH Act included the following changes (also see The Omnibus Rule, p. 324):

- **Business associates** are also required to notify their affiliated covered entities of breaches of which they become aware.
- Covered entities are required to notify all affected individuals of unauthorized disclosure of their PHI as soon as reasonably possible.
- HIPAA rules extend directly to a covered entity's business associates who have access to PHI.
- An individual's right to obtain an accounting of disclosures is expanded.

business associates outside persons or organizations that use PHI while providing services on behalf of a "covered entity" (a healthcare organization); business associate functions include billing, claims processing, utilization review, and so on.

Legal Brief

The number of privacy breaches has grown steadily, and millions of individuals have been affected. In 2014, for example, the HHS Office for Civil Rights received 277 reports of breaches involving 500 or more individuals, totaling more than 21 million people. That number was up from just over 8 million individuals the year before, and the five-year cumulative total for large breaches alone was more than 41 million. The types of breaches include loss of laptops and other devices, loss of paper records, improper disposal, unauthorized access by healthcare personnel, and hacking of network servers.[97]

The Omnibus Rule

On January 25, 2013, HHS published a massive regulation to implement the HITECH Act, strengthen privacy protections for genetic information, and make certain other modifications to HIPAA rules "to improve their workability and effectiveness and to increase flexibility for and decrease burden on the regulated entities." Known as the *Omnibus Rule*, this regulation comprises 136 pages of the *Federal Register* and affects many portions of Parts 160 and 164 of the Code of Federal Regulations. (*See* 78 Fed. Reg. 5566, Jan. 25, 2013.) Compliance with these provisions was required as of September 23, 2013. Further regulatory "clarification" and judicial interpretation will undoubtedly ensue. Stay tuned.

- The standards for using PHI for marketing and fundraising purposes are different.
- State attorneys general have a new enforcement authority.
- Review of HIPAA-related policies and training programs; business associate agreements; and physical, technical, and administrative safeguards is required.
- Meaningful use objectives for electronic health records are established; the achievement of these objectives qualifies providers for financial bonuses

Medical Identity Theft and the Red Flags Rule

One other significant issue regarding access to health information is identity theft. According to the Federal Trade Commission,

> medical identity theft happens when a person seeks health care using someone else's name or insurance information. A survey conducted by the Federal Trade Commission (FTC) found that close to [450,000 persons each year] have experienced some form of medical identity theft. Victims may find their benefits exhausted or face potentially life-threatening consequences due to inaccuracies in their medical records. The cost to health care providers—left with unpaid bills racked up by scam artists—can be staggering, too.[69]

To address this problem, in 2008 the FTC and a number of other federal agencies published the *Red Flags Rule*, a requirement that certain organizations adopt a written identity theft prevention program.[70] Authority for the rule was grounded in the Fair and Accurate Credit Transactions Act of 2003 (FACTA),[71] which applies to financial institutions and creditors and is aimed primarily at theft of individuals' financial information. However, the agencies interpreted FACTA's term *creditor* to include healthcare providers who allow patients to make installment payments. Following an outcry by the American Medical Association and other provider groups that felt the requirements were burdensome, costly, and unnecessarily complex, Congress amended FACTA and exempted healthcare providers from the identity theft prevention rules.[72]

Notwithstanding this development, hospitals, physicians' offices, and other healthcare providers must be alert for the warning signs of medical identity theft. Given the public's expectation of privacy protections—and bolstered by HIPAA, the HITECH Act, and other privacy and security standards—the spirit of the Red Flags Rule is likely to become the standard of care in identity theft cases.

The following red flags are some of the warning signs of medical identity theft:

- Identification documents appear to have been altered or forged.
- A photograph or the physical description of the patient on file is inconsistent with the appearance of the person presenting for care.
- Identifying information is inconsistent with information already on file (e.g., Social Security number does not match).
- Identifying information is associated with known or suspected fraudulent activity (e.g., address is fictitious or a mail drop; phone number is a pager or an answering service).
- Address or telephone number is the same as that submitted by numerous other patients.
- Mail to the account address is returned despite ongoing patient visits.
- The person fails to provide all requested identifying information.
- When questioned, the person is unable to provide authenticating information beyond that generally available from a wallet or consumer report.[73]

Healthcare providers should adopt some form of identity theft prevention program to address the red flags they might encounter. The program should be tailored to the provider's setting (e.g., physician practice, hospital), and all staff who open patient accounts, handle billing operations, or otherwise deal with patient information must be trained to spot the warning signs (see Legal Brief). Ideally, the program should be approved by the governing board (or at least senior management) and monitored for effectiveness. Identity theft thus becomes another responsibility of the compliance department (see chapter 15).

Confidentiality and Other Issues in Telemedicine

The healthcare field is becoming more comfortable with providing clinical services

Legal Brief

Healthcare organizations' records are subject not only to medical identity theft but to other criminal activity as well. In 2013, the payroll accounts of a public hospital in Leavenworth, Washington, were hacked to the tune of $1.03 million by cyberthieves based in Ukraine and Russia. The thieves used "money mules"—individuals who are duped into being conduits for the transactions—to transfer the money. Once the theft was reported, the unwitting accomplices' personal accounts were frozen, leaving them with nothing but embarrassment and the hassle of explaining their involvement to the authorities. Nearly half a million dollars of the public hospital's money was "gone for good," according to news reports.[98]

Legal Brief

Although some states' definitions vary, Medicare regulations consider telemedicine to involve "multimedia communications equipment that includes, at a minimum, audio and video equipment permitting two-way, real-time interactive communication between the patient and distant site physician or practitioner." The definition excludes telephone calls and use of fax machines or e-mail.[99]

through telemedicine (aka "telehealth" or "e-health"; see Legal Brief). Use of telecommunication technology can improve access to care and clinical outcomes, and thus it presents significant benefit to both the clinician and the patient. However, telemedicine also carries with it certain legal issues and, as is often the case, the legal system lags behind technological developments.

HIPAA's privacy and security standards, including liability for breaches, clearly apply to telemedicine services—thus the security of the online network used for an e-health encounter must be ensured. While providing health services at a distance improves access to care for patients in remote areas or in an emergency, it also raises malpractice issues for the provider and questions about liability insurance coverage. These problems may not be specific to telemedicine, but a heightened regard for thorough documentation is warranted.

Whether a telehealth "visit" is covered by the patient's health insurance may also be an issue. Medicare covers telehealth encounters on a limited basis only, Medicaid reimbursement varies from state to state, and private health plans also vary widely. The practitioner must take these differences into account to avoid possible liability for false claims.

When the clinician and patient are not in the same jurisdiction, questions arise as to which state's medical records and licensure laws apply. Restrictive laws in some states may require a practitioner to obtain a license when delivering care across state lines. If a physician serves patients in several states—or if those patients travel frequently or regularly spend a portion of the year in another location—must the physician be licensed in multiple states, pay multiple licensure fees, and meet the regulatory requirements of each locale? Will a pharmacy in a different state honor a telemedicine physician's prescriptions, especially for controlled substances? May a hospital rely on the credentialing and privileging decisions of the physician's "home" hospital, or must he also obtain privileges and credentials at the distant facility? If the former, is there written documentation of those decisions? How will the distant hospital conduct peer review of the telemedicine practitioner?

Myriad other issues, too numerous to discuss at length here, surround telemedicine technologies. For example, multiple regulatory agencies—the Food and Drug Administration, Federal Communications Commission, Federal Trade Commission, and Office of National Coordinator for Health Information, to name a few—have jurisdiction over some aspect of mobile medical applications and devices that are involved in telemedicine. These agencies' regulations often conflict or overlap with one another.

Telemedicine is a growing field that presents many legal issues but many opportunities as well.

Use of Health Records in Legal Proceedings

As mentioned earlier (under the heading "Liability for Unauthorized Disclosure"), common law formerly did not recognize a *physician–patient* privilege. Today most states have a statute on *testimonial privilege* that prohibits the physician (and perhaps other clinical personnel) from testifying about statements made by the patient in the course of the doctor–patient relationship unless the patient waives the privilege. The purpose of the privilege is to encourage candid communication between doctor and patient and thus promote the quality of care.

A typical privilege statute reads as follows:

> Except as otherwise provided by law, a person duly authorized to practice medicine or surgery shall not disclose any information that the person has acquired in attending a patient in a professional character, if the information was necessary to enable the person to prescribe for the patient as a physician, or to do any act for the patient as a surgeon. If the patient brings an action against any defendant to recover for any personal injuries, or for any malpractice, and the patient produces a physician as a witness in the patient's own behalf who has treated the patient for the injury or for any disease or condition for which the malpractice is alleged, the patient shall be considered to have waived the privilege provided in this section as to another physician who has treated the patient for the injuries, disease, or condition.[74]

As the previously discussed statute recognizes, parties in a lawsuit are deemed to have waived the testimonial privilege by putting their medical conditions at issue. Their records are admissible at trial, and their physicians are allowed to testify. The health information of someone who is not a party to the litigation is not usually admissible in evidence, however. The testimonial privilege protects the confidentiality of those persons and prohibits their physicians from testifying. The privilege statutes also apply to pretrial proceedings and to investigations conducted by state legislative bodies.

When a privilege does not apply, health records are admissible as evidence under one or more of the exceptions to the hearsay rule. The hearsay rule prohibits secondhand evidence, and although health records are technically hearsay, they are considered reliable and are admissible if their authenticity is properly established.[75] Some jurisdictions allow records to be admitted into evidence only when the person who entered the information in the chart is not available to testify in person. In any event, the parties to the litigation often attest to the records' authenticity and agree that they may be used.

The fundamental purpose of litigation is to determine the truth and achieve justice for the parties. Information collected and maintained in the regular course of a patient's care presumably helps establish the truth. Because physicians, nurses, and hospitals do not ordinarily falsify health information, courts can be reasonably confident that the health record accurately reports the facts of the case. In addition, records are usually more reliable than personal recollections. Witnesses are often forgetful or may not be available to testify in person. Furthermore, many people may have made entries on the record. Even in the rare case they are all available, testimony by each person involved would be time-consuming and expensive. To exclude health records from evidence because they are hearsay would defeat the legitimate goals of the judicial process.

Federal Government's Access to Personal Health Information

Under HIPAA, government agencies have access to PHI for healthcare oversight and other legitimate purposes. Even before HIPAA was passed, however, the Federal Rules of Evidence gave the courts broad discretion to determine when to grant access. For example, in one case, the IRS was allowed to obtain the health records of a deceased person to determine whether gifts of property given during the patient's lifetime were made in "contemplation of death" and thus subject to the federal estate tax.[76] In another case, the IRS obtained the surgical records of a physician who had failed to file tax returns.[77] In yet another case, the National Institute of Occupational Safety and Health was allowed to subpoena employees' health records maintained under the Occupational Safety and Health Act.[78] In none of these situations did the respective state's privileged communication statute apply to protect the confidentiality of the records.

In a case widely publicized in 1983, HHS sought the records of a severely disabled newborn (Baby Jane Doe.) The government contended that the parents' refusal to consent to surgery for spina bifida, hydrocephalus, and other severe congenital conditions amounted to unlawful discrimination against a disabled person in violation of federal law. The district court denied the government's request for access to the records, held that Baby Jane Doe's parents had made "a reasonable choice among alternative medical treatments," and found that the parents' refusal to consent to treatment did not violate the Rehabilitation Act of 1973, which prohibits discrimination on the basis of disability.[79] Although access to the records was not granted, the court noted in its opinion that disclosure would not have been barred by a state privilege of confidentiality because no state statutory privilege exists when a federal question is being decided.[80]

State authorities also have obtained information necessary to enforce the law and to protect against fraud and abuse. For example, the US Court of Appeals for the Sixth Circuit held that a psychotherapist was required to disclose the names of patients and the dates of their treatment to a grand jury investigating an alleged scheme to defraud the Michigan Blue Cross Blue Shield plan.[81] In a similar case, a court denied a claim of privilege and permitted the New York Department of Social Services to review a psychiatrist's Medicaid patients' records when investigating the physician's billing practices.[82] In another New York case investigating a death in a hospital's intensive care unit, neither the state's privileged communication statute nor a constitutional right of privacy prohibited a grand jury from accessing patients' medical information.[83] In California and many other jurisdictions, the agency responsible for licensure may review health records when examining the professional conduct of a physician whose hospital privileges have been revoked, although the law may require that the names of patients be deleted.[84]

Law enforcement officials' requests for PHI often present a challenge. Routine requests such as court orders and subpoenas can be handled by a hospital's HIM or ROI department, but many requests are not routine and are made on an emergency basis. For example, law enforcement personnel may request PHI to

- locate a suspect or fugitive,
- retrieve or preserve evidence of a crime,
- deal with imminent threats to public safety, or
- determine the blood alcohol level of a person in custody.

As a general proposition, disclosures of PHI should not be made to law enforcement officials without the patient's consent, explicit statutory authority, or a court order. However, determination of whether disclosure is permitted in a given case involves complicated, fact-dependent legal calculus at which most hospital personnel are not likely to be adept. Institutions should have policies to address these issues, and they must train personnel in the ED, outpatient clinics, and other areas likely to receive the requests.

For its members, the Florida Hospital Association (FHA) published a handbook that compares HIPAA requirements and Florida law and offers general suggestions for dealing with law enforcement personnel:

- Document the law officer's identity (e.g., name, badge number).
- Determine the purpose of the request and whether the officer has legal authority to make it.
- Ask that the request be submitted in writing, preferably in an official document.
- Provide only the minimum amount of information, preferably de-identified.
- Consult the facility's privacy officer, compliance officer, risk manager, or legal counsel if time permits.

In addition to these suggestions, the FHA handbook describes 28 scenarios that hospitals and physicians might encounter. All scenarios are followed by discussion of possible solutions and can be used as an educational resource. Healthcare providers might find it useful to obtain or develop a resource similar to the FHA's handbook and to use it as the basis for their policies and training programs.[85]

State Open Meeting and Public Records Laws

Every state has statutes that determine when government agencies must allow the public to attend meetings and to make minutes and other records available for public inspection.[86] These statutes are often referred to as *sunshine laws*, which connotes that the public is entitled to have light shed on the conduct of governmental affairs. They are also, less colorfully, called *public record laws* or *open meeting laws*.

Therefore, government hospitals and hospital authorities are covered not only by federal statutes and regulations but also by laws at the state, county, and municipal levels, some of which do not apply to other healthcare organizations.[87] For example, a county-owned hospital was subject to the state's sunshine laws and its personnel records were subject to inspection even though they contained information about employees' prior felony convictions, drug and alcohol problems, unlisted phone numbers, physical and mental examinations, and communications from third persons who provided the information believing it was confidential.[88]

Likewise, a county hospital authority in Georgia was subject to that state's similar legislation, and the Supreme Court of Georgia held that a newspaper had the right to access the names, job titles, and salaries of all hospital employees who earned more than $28,000.[89] In Florida, *Gadd v. News-Press Publishing Company, Inc.* held that a newspaper was entitled to view a public hospital's medical staff files and its utilization review documents.[90] Although another Florida statute exempts peer review records and proceedings from use in an action against a provider of health services,[91] the Public Records Act does not do so specifically, so the *Gadd* court held that the apparent inconsistency between the two statutory schemes was a matter for the legislature to resolve. These cases are examples of the typical judicial approach to interpreting the sunshine laws liberally in accordance with legislative intent.

Most of the sunshine statutes contain exceptions to the right of public access. Some of the exceptions are cast in general language, but some are more specific—as is the exception in Florida related to autopsy photos (see the discussion about Dale Earnhardt earlier in the chapter). A court may create an exception when it is presented with a persuasive reason for limiting the applicability of the legislation. Typically, the statutes exclude meetings and records related to pending litigation, negotiations with labor unions, acquisition of capital (e.g., the purchase of real estate), and disciplinary action against governmental personnel.

Questions about public records laws involve balancing various interests. The outcome of each case depends on the language of the relevant statute, judicial understanding of legislative intent, the purposes or motives of those seeking access, and the countervailing interests of the defendant or third parties.

Summary

The title of this chapter reflects a belief that the term *medical records* is passé because information about a person's health (or payment for health-related services) can be maintained in many types of media other than paper. Regardless of the form in which it is maintained, health information must be accurate and its confidentiality must be ensured. This chapter reviews the various ways in which health information is properly used, such as for documentation of treatment, for accurate billing, and as evidence in legal forums. It also discusses HIPAA and other state and federal laws that govern the protection of health information. It outlines circumstances in which third parties may legitimately access individuals' health information with and without patient consent, and it points out the pitfalls that one can encounter when that information is improperly disclosed.

Discussion Questions

1. Describe the nuances of the terms *medical records* and *health information*. Why does HIPAA use the latter term?

2. When might a patient's favorite color or high school alma mater be considered health information?

3. Describe some circumstances in which confidential health information may be disclosed without the patient's consent.

4. Why do you suppose a physician–patient privilege did not exist in common law but had to be created by statute?

5. What is the proper way to make changes to a written health record?

6. Who owns physical health records, X-ray images, and other items containing health information?

7. How can the inability to predict dangerousness be reconciled with the emotional issue of registering convicted sex offenders and preventing them from living in proximity to schools and other places that children frequent?

8. Describe the provisions of the HITECH Act and the Red Flags Rule and how they affect healthcare operations.

The Court Decides

Opis Management Resources, LLC v. Secretary, Fla. Agency for Healthcare Admin.
713 F.3d 1291 (11th Cir., 2013)

BLACK, Circuit Judge:

The issue before us is whether § 400.145 of the Florida Statutes—which provides for the release of medical records of deceased residents of nursing homes to certain specified individuals—is preempted by the federal Health Insurance Portability and Accountability Act of 1996 (HIPAA), 42 U.S.C. § 1320d to d-9, and its implementing regulations. . . .

I. BACKGROUND

The underlying facts are not in dispute. Plaintiffs-Appellees . . . (collectively the Nursing Facilities or the Facilities) are operators and managers of skilled nursing facilities in Florida. In the course of their operations, [they] received requests from spouses and attorneys-in-fact for the medical records of deceased nursing home residents. The Facilities refused to disclose the records because the parties requesting them were not "personal representatives" under the relevant provisions of HIPAA, which regulates the release of protected health information by covered entities. Consequently, the requesting parties filed complaints with the U.S. Department of Health and Human Services Office for Civil Rights, which concluded the Nursing Facilities' actions were consistent with HIPAA.

Defendant-Appellant Florida Agency for Health Care Administration (the State Agency), however, issued citations to the Nursing Facilities for violating Florida law by refusing to release the records. Specifically, the Facilities were cited for violating § 400.145 of the Florida Statutes, which

requires licensed nursing homes to release a former resident's medical records to the spouse, guardian, surrogate, or attorney-in-fact of any such resident.* In written correspondence to individuals who had requested and been denied deceased residents' medical records, the State Agency explained that it interprets § 400.145 in a manner allowing a spouse to qualify as a personal representative such that a deceased spouse's medical records may be disclosed under HIPAA.

Given the dueling interpretations of the relevant statutes, the Nursing Facilities filed a complaint in the district court seeking a declaratory judgment that § 400.145 is preempted by HIPAA. The parties then filed cross-motions for summary judgment. In ruling on the motions, the district court found that § 400.145 was preempted because it impeded the accomplishment and execution of HIPAA's purposes and objectives. The court granted the Nursing Facilities' motion for summary judgment, explaining that the Florida statute affords nursing home residents less protection than is required by the federal law. This appeal followed.

. . .

III. DISCUSSION

[The court begins by reminding readers that the laws of the United States are the supreme law of the land and that where state and federal law directly conflict, "state law must give way." Therefore, HIPAA supersedes any contrary state law. A state law is "contrary" to HIPAA if complying with both the state and

(continued)

(continued from previous page)

federal requirements is impossible or the state law "stands as an obstacle" to achieving HIPAA's objectives. The opinion continues as follows.]

Regarding deceased individuals, the Privacy Rule further specifies that:

If under applicable law an executor, administrator, or other person has authority to act on behalf of a deceased individual or of the individual's estate, a covered entity [such as the plaintiffs] must treat such person as a personal representative under this subchapter, with respect to protected health information relevant to such personal representation.

[Also, if an individual is deceased,] a covered entity may disclose to a family member, or [other relatives, friends or other persons identified by the individual] who were involved in the individual's care or payment for health care prior to the individual's death, protected health information of the individual that is relevant to such person's involvement. . . .

According to the State Agency, § 400.145 enumerates groups of people, including spouses, who may access a deceased resident's medical records "on behalf of" the resident, meaning that they should be treated as personal representatives. Thus, rather than conflicting with HIPAA and the Privacy Rule, § 400.145 supplements and works in tandem with the federal law.

The fatal flaw in the State Agency's argument is that the plain language of § 400.145 does not empower or require an individual to act on behalf of a deceased resident. The unadorned text of the state statute authorizes sweeping disclosures, making a deceased resident's protected health information available to a spouse or other enumerated party upon request, without any need for authorization,

for any conceivable reason, and without regard to the authority of the individual making the request to act in a deceased resident's stead. *See* 45 C.F.R. § 164.502(g)(4) (providing that a person authorized to act on behalf of a deceased individual must be treated as a personal representative "with respect to protected health information *relevant to such personal representation*" (emphasis added)). We therefore agree with the district court that § 400.145 frustrates the federal objective of limiting disclosures of protected health information, and that the statute is thus preempted by the more stringent privacy protections of HIPAA and the Privacy Rule.

. . .

[T]he Florida legislature has not amended or modified § 400.145 to address the impact of HIPAA and its implementing regulations. Section 400.145 does not require a HIPAA-compliant authorization to accompany a request for a deceased individual's medical records, nor can the statute plausibly be read as creating a limited personal representation in the person of a surviving spouse in light of the blanket disclosures that it requires. Given the opportunity, we are confident the Florida legislature could bring § 400.145 into compliance with federal law in any number of ways. Amending the statute, however, is a task for the state legislature, not a panel of federal judges.

. . .

For the foregoing reasons, we agree with the district court that § 400.145 of the Florida Statutes impedes the accomplishment and execution of the full purposes and objectives of HIPAA and the Privacy Rule in keeping an individual's protected health information confidential. Accordingly, the district court's grant of summary judgment is AFFIRMED.

---

*The statute reads, in pertinent part: "400.145: Records of care and treatment of resident; copies to be furnished. — (1) Unless expressly prohibited by a legally competent resident, any nursing home . . . shall furnish to the spouse, guardian, surrogate, proxy, or attorney in fact . . . of a current [or former] resident a copy of that resident's records which are in the possession of the facility." ■

Discussion Questions

1. Summarize in a succinct sentence (or two at the most) why this statute is "contrary" to HIPAA.
2. A similar Florida statute applicable to hospitals reads as follows:

   Any licensed facility shall, upon written request, and only after discharge of the patient, furnish, in a timely manner, without delays for legal review, to any person admitted therein for care and treatment or treated thereat, or to any such person's guardian, curator, or personal representative, or in the absence of one of those persons, to the next of kin of a decedent or the parent of a minor, or to anyone designated by such person in writing, a true and correct copy of all patient records, including X rays, and insurance information concerning such person.[92]

   What HIPAA-related infirmities do you see in this language, and how would the *Opis Management* court decide a claim that this statute is preempted?

The Court Decides

Tarasoff v. Regents of the University of California
17 Cal. 3d 425, 131 Cal. Rptr. 14 (1976)

Tobriner, J.

On October 27, 1969, Prosenjit Poddar killed Tatiana Tarasoff. Plaintiffs, Tatiana's parents, allege that two months earlier Poddar confided his intention to kill Tatiana to Dr. Lawrence Moore, a psychologist employed by the Cowell Memorial Hospital at the University of California at Berkeley. They allege that on Moore's request, the campus police briefly detained Poddar, but released him when he appeared rational. They further claim that Dr. Harvey Powelson, Moore's superior, then directed that no further action be taken to detain Poddar. No one warned plaintiffs of Tatiana's peril.

Concluding that these facts set forth causes of action against neither therapists and policemen involved, nor against the Regents of the University of California as their employer, the superior court sustained defendants' demurrers to plaintiffs' second amended complaints without leave to amend. This appeal ensued.

Plaintiffs' complaints predicate liability on two grounds: defendants' failure to warn plaintiffs of the impending danger and their failure to bring about Poddar's confinement pursuant to the Lanterman-Petris-Short Act

(continued)

(continued from previous page)

[the California law allowing involuntary, psychiatric admission of persons considered dangerous to themselves or others]. Defendants, in turn, assert that they owed no duty of reasonable care to Tatiana and that they are immune from suit under the California Tort Claims Act of 1963.

We shall explain that defendant therapists cannot escape liability merely because Tatiana herself was not their patient. When a therapist determines, or pursuant to the standards of his profession should determine, that his patient presents a serious danger of violence to another, he incurs an obligation to use reasonable care to protect the intended victim against such danger. The discharge of this duty may require the therapist to take one or more of various steps, depending upon the nature of the case. Thus it may call for him to warn the intended victim or others likely to apprise the victim of the danger, to notify the police, or to take whatever other steps are reasonably necessary under the circumstances.

In the case at bar, plaintiffs admit that defendant therapists notified the police, but argue on appeal that the therapists failed to exercise reasonable care to protect Tatiana in that they did not confine Poddar and did not warn Tatiana or others likely to apprise her of the danger. . . .

Plaintiffs . . . can amend their complaints to allege that, regardless of the therapists' unsuccessful attempt to confine Poddar, since they knew that Poddar was at large and dangerous, their failure to warn Tatiana or others likely to apprise her of the danger constituted a breach of the therapists' duty to exercise reasonable care to protect Tatiana. . . .

Plaintiffs' Complaints
. . .

Plaintiffs' first cause of action, [titled] "Failure to Detain a Dangerous Patient," alleges that on August 20, 1969, Poddar was a voluntary outpatient receiving therapy at Cowell Memorial Hospital. Poddar informed Moore, his therapist, that he was going to kill an unnamed girl, readily identifiable as Tatiana, when she returned home from spending the summer in Brazil. Moore, with the concurrence of Dr. Gold, who had initially examined Poddar, and Dr. Yandell, assistant to the director of the department of psychiatry, decided that Poddar should be committed for observation in a mental hospital. Moore orally notified Officers Atkinson and Teel of the campus police that he would request commitment. He then sent a letter to Police Chief William Beall requesting the assistance of the police department in securing Poddar's confinement.

Officers Atkinson, Brownrigg, and Halleran took Poddar into custody, but, satisfied that Poddar was rational, released him on his promise to stay away from Tatiana. Powelson, director of the department of psychiatry at Cowell Memorial Hospital, then asked the police to return Moore's letter, directed that all copies of the letter and notes that Moore had taken as therapist be destroyed, and "ordered no action to place Prosenjit Poddar in 72-hour treatment and evaluation facility."

Plaintiffs' second cause of action, entitled "Failure to Warn on a Dangerous Patient," incorporates the allegations of the first cause of action, but adds the assertion that defendants negligently permitted Poddar to be released from police custody without "notifying the parents of Tatiana Tarasoff that their daughter was in grave danger from Prosenjit Poddar." Poddar persuaded Tatiana's brother to share an apartment with him near Tatiana's residence; shortly after her return from Brazil, Poddar went to her residence and killed her. . . .

[The court holds that the first cause of action is barred by the principle of governmental immunity. The third and fourth— not summarized in this book—were also held to be invalid.] We direct our attention, therefore,

to the issue of whether plaintiffs' second cause of action can be amended to state a basis for recovery.

Plaintiffs can state a cause of action against defendant therapists for negligent failure to protect Tatiana.

The second cause of action can be amended to allege that Tatiana's death proximately resulted from defendants' negligent failure to warn Tatiana or others likely to apprise her of her danger. Plaintiffs contend that as amended, such allegations of negligence and proximate causation, with resulting damages, establish a cause of action. Defendants, however, contend that in the circumstances of the present case they owed no duty of care to Tatiana or her parents and that, in the absence of such duty, they were free to act in careless disregard of Tatiana's life and safety.

. . .

The most important of [various] considerations in establishing duty is foreseeability. As a general principle, a "defendant owes a duty of care to all persons who are foreseeably endangered by his conduct, with respect to all risks which make the conduct unreasonably dangerous." As we shall explain, however, when the avoidance of foreseeable harm requires a defendant to control the conduct of another person, or to warn of such conduct, the common law has traditionally imposed liability only if the defendant bears some special relationship to the dangerous person or to the potential victim. Since the relationship between a therapist and his patient satisfies this requirement, we need not here decide whether foreseeability alone is sufficient to create a duty to exercise reasonable care to protect a potential victim of another's conduct.

Although . . . under the common law, as a general rule, one person owed no duty to control the conduct of another, nor to warn those endangered by such conduct, the courts have carved out an exception to this rule in cases in which the defendant stands in some special relationship to either the person whose conduct needs to be controlled or in a relationship to the foreseeable victim of that conduct. Applying this exception to the present case, we note that a relationship of defendant therapists to either Tatiana or Poddar will suffice to establish a duty of care; as explained in . . . the Restatement Second of Torts, a duty of care may arise from either "(a) a special relation * * * between the actor and the third person which imposes a duty upon the actor to control the third person" conduct, or (b) a special relation * * * between the actor and the other which gives to the other a right of protection."

Although plaintiffs' pleadings assert no special relation between Tatiana and defendant therapists, they establish as between Poddar and defendant therapists the special relation that arises between a patient and his doctor or psychotherapist. Such a relationship may support affirmative duties for the benefit of third persons. Thus, for example, a hospital must exercise reasonable care to control the behavior of a patient which may endanger other persons. A doctor must also warn a patient if the patient's condition or medication renders certain conduct, such as driving a car, dangerous to others.

Although the California decisions that recognize this duty have involved cases in which the defendant stood in a special relationship both to the victim and to the person whose conduct created the danger, we do not think that the duty should logically be constricted to such situations. Decisions of other jurisdictions hold that the single relationship of a doctor to his patient is sufficient to support the duty to exercise reasonable care to protect others against dangers emanating from the patient's illness. The courts hold that a doctor is liable to persons infected by his patient if he negligently fails to diagnose a

(continued)

(continued from previous page)

contagious disease, or, having diagnosed the illness, fails to warn members of the patient's family.

Since it involved a dangerous mental patient, the decision in *Merchants Nat. Bank & Trust Co. of Fargo v. United States* [1967] comes closer to the issue. The Veterans Administration arranged for the patient to work on a local farm, but did not inform the farmer of the man's background. The farmer consequently permitted the patient to come and go freely during nonworking hours; the patient borrowed a car, drove to his wife's residence and killed her. Notwithstanding the lack of any "special relationship" between the Veterans Administration and the wife, the court found the Veterans Administration liable for the wrongful death of the wife.

In their summary of the relevant rulings [two scholars] conclude that the "case law should dispel any notion that to impose on the therapists a duty to take precautions for the safety of persons threatened by a patient, where due care so requires, is in any way opposed to contemporary ground rules on the duty relationship. On the contrary, there now seems to be sufficient authority to support the conclusion that by entering into a doctor–patient relationship the therapist becomes sufficiently involved to assume some responsibility for the safety, not only of the patient himself, but also of any third person whom the doctor knows to be threatened by the patient."

Defendants contend, however, that imposition of a duty to exercise reasonable care to protect third persons is unworkable because therapists cannot accurately predict whether or not a patient will resort to violence. In support of this argument amicus representing the American Psychiatric Association and other professional societies cites numerous articles which indicate that therapists, in the present state of the art, are unable reliably to predict violent acts; their forecasts, amicus claims, tend consistently to overpredict

violence, and indeed are more often wrong than right. Since predictions of violence are often erroneous, amicus concludes, the courts should not render rulings that predicate the liability of therapists upon the validity of such predictions.

. . .

We recognize the difficulty that a therapist encounters in attempting to forecast whether a patient presents a serious danger of violence. Obviously, we do not require that the therapist, in making that determination, render a perfect performance; the therapist need only exercise "that reasonable degree of skill, knowledge, and care ordinarily possessed and exercised by members of [that professional specialty] under similar circumstances." Within the broad range of reasonable practice and treatment in which professional opinion and judgment may differ, the therapist is free to exercise his or her own best judgment without liability; proof, aided by hindsight, that he or she judged wrongly is insufficient to establish negligence.

In the instant case, however, the pleadings do not raise any question as to failure of defendant therapists to predict that Poddar presented a serious danger of violence. On the contrary, the present complaints allege that defendant therapists did in fact predict that Poddar would kill, but were negligent in failing to warn. Amicus contends, however, that even when a therapist does in fact predict that a patient poses a serious danger of violence to others, the therapist should be absolved of any responsibility for failing to act to protect the potential victim. In our view, however, once a therapist does in fact determine, or under applicable professional standards reasonably should have determined, that a patient poses a serious danger of violence to others, he bears a duty to exercise reasonable care to protect the foreseeable victim of that danger. While the discharge of this duty of due care will necessarily vary with the facts of each case, in each instance the adequacy of the therapist's conduct must be measured against the traditional negligence standard of the rendition of reasonable care under the circumstances. As explained in [the same scholars' article]: "* * * the ultimate question of resolving the tension between the conflicting interests of patient and potential victim is one of social policy, not professional expertise. * * * In sum, the therapist owes a legal duty not only to his patient, but also to his patient's would-be victim and is subject in both respects to scrutiny by judge and jury."

. . .

We realize that the open and confidential character of psychotherapeutic dialogue encourages patients to express threats of violence, few of which are ever executed. Certainly a therapist should not be encouraged routinely to reveal such threats; such disclosures could seriously disrupt the patient's relationship with his therapist and with the persons threatened. To the contrary, the therapist's obligations to his patient require that he not disclose a confidence unless such disclosure is necessary to avert danger to others, and even then that he do so discreetly, and in a fashion that would preserve the privacy of his patient to the fullest extent compatible with the prevention of the threatened danger.

The revelation of a communication under the above circumstances is not a breach of trust or a violation of professional ethics;

as stated in the Principles of Medical Ethics of the American Medical Association (1957), section 9: "A physician may not reveal the confidence entrusted to him in the course of medical attendance * * * unless he is required to do so by law or unless it becomes necessary in order to protect the welfare of the individual or of the community." We conclude that the public policy favoring protection of the confidential character of patient–psychotherapist communications must yield to the extent to which disclosure is essential to avert danger to others. The protective privilege ends where the public peril begins.

Our current crowded and computerized society compels the interdependence of its members. In this risk-infested society we can hardly tolerate the further exposure to danger that would result from a concealed knowledge of the therapist that his patient was lethal. If the exercise of reasonable care to protect the threatened victim requires the therapist to warn the endangered party or those who can reasonably be expected to notify him, we see no sufficient societal interest that would protect and justify concealment. The containment of such risks lies in the public interest. For the foregoing reasons, we find that plaintiffs' complaints can be amended to state a cause of action against defendants Moore, Powelson, Gold, and Yandell and against the Regents as their employer, for breach of a duty to exercise reasonable care to protect Tatiana. ■

Discussion Questions

1. This case was brought before the court on this procedural issue: whether the trial court was correct to dismiss the complaint before a trial could be held. What do you suppose happened after the case returned to the trial court?
2. What should the defendants have done differently?
3. Why is the board (the Regents) of the University of California a defendant?

Notes

1. 42 U.S.C. §§ 1320d et seq.
2. 45 C.F.R., Parts 160 and 164.
3. 42 U.S.C. § 1320d(4).
4. THE JOINT COMMISSION, 2013 HOSPITAL ACCREDITATION STANDARDS at RC-1.
5. 45 C.F.R. § 164.514.
6. Fla. Stat. § 395.3015.
7. Fla. Admin. Code R. 59A-3.270, Health Information Management.
8. The American Recovery and Reinvestment Act of 2009, Pub. L. No. 111-5.
9. *See, e.g.*, THE JOINT COMMISSION, 2013 HOSPITAL ACCREDITATION STANDARDS, Standard RC.01.01.01, et seq. The Joint Commission has similar accreditation standards for nonhospital healthcare organizations.
10. Darling v. Charleston Community Memorial Hosp., 33 Ill. 2d 326, 211 N.E.2d 253 (1965), *cert. denied*, 383 U.S. 946 (1966).
11. 42 C.F.R. Part 482.
12. THE JOINT COMMISSION, *supra* note 9, at Standard RC.01.02.01.
13. Pisel v. Stamford Hosp., 430 A.2d 1 (Conn. 1980).
14. 384 F. Supp. 821 (W.D. Ark. 1974).
15. *Id*. at 831.
16. 42 C.F.R. § 482.24.
17. Fla. Stat. § 95.11(4)(b).
18. *See, e.g.*, Fla. Stat. §§ 395.3025 *and* 456.057.
19. THE JOINT COMMISSION, 2013 HOSPITAL ACCREDITATION STANDARDS at RC-5.
20. 21 Fla. Stat. § 395.3025; *see also* Matter of Weiss, 208 Misc. 1010, 147 N.Y.S.2d 455 (Sup. Ct. 1955).
21. Fla. Stat. §§ 456.057 *and* 456.058.
22. In re Culbertson's Will, 57 Misc. 2d 391, 292 N.Y.2d 806 (Sup. Ct. 1968).
23. The regulations implementing the statute are found at 45 C.F.R. Parts 160 and 164. Each specific point made in the text will not be referenced here.
24. 45 C.F.R. § 164.528.
25. Thurman v. Crawford, 652 S.W.2d 240 (Mo. App. 1983) (a hospital may take reasonable precautions to ascertain authenticity of a patient's

consent to release medical information and may refuse to honor consent when the date has been altered).

26. Whalen v. Roe, 429 U.S. 589 (1977).

27. Griswold v. Connecticut, 381 U.S. 479 (1965) (state may not prohibit use of contraceptives or advice or assistance in their use); Roe v. Wade, 410 U.S. 113 (1973), *and* Doe v. Bolton, 410 U.S. 179 (1973) (abortion cases).

28. Robinson v. Hamilton, 60 Iowa 134, 14 N.W. 202 (1882); Planned Parenthood of Central Mo. v. Danforth, 428 U.S. 52 (1976).

29. 45 C.F.R. § 164.512(j).

30. Tarasoff v. Regents of the University of California, 17 Cal. 3d 425, 451 (1976).

31. Thompson v. County of Alameda, 27 Cal. 3d 741, 614 P.2d 728, 167 Cal. Rptr. 70 (1980). *See also* Mangeris v. Gordon, 94 Nev. 400, 580 P.2d 481 (1978); Leedy v. Hartnett, 510 F. Supp. 1125 (M.D. Pa. 1981) (Veterans Administration hospital had no duty to warn of discharged patient's propensity for alcohol-induced violence without a readily identifiable victim), *and* Brady v. Hopper, 570 F. Supp. 1333 (D. Colo. 1983) (the psychiatrist had no duty to warn because the patient, John Hinckley Jr., who attempted to assassinate President Reagan, had not threatened to shoot anyone).

32. Mavroudis v. Superior Court for County of San Mateo, 102 Cal. App. 3d 594, 162 Cal. Rptr. 724 (1980); McIntosh v. Milano, 168 N.J. Super. 466, 403 A.2d 500 (1979).

33. *See, e.g.*, Shaw v. Glickman, 45 Md. App. 718, 415 A.2d 625 (1980); Cole v. Taylor, 301 N.W.2d 766 (Iowa 1981); Case v. United States, 523 F. Supp. 317 (S.D. Ohio 1981); Hawkins v. King County Dep't of Rehabilitative Servs., 602 P.2d 361 (Wash. App. 1979).

34. Bellah v. Greenson, 81 Cal. App. 3d 614, 146 Cal. Rptr. 535 (1978).

35. 42 C.F.R. Parts 462 *and* 476.

36. *See generally* 53 C.J.S., Libel & Slander §§ 1–9 (2009).

37. 623 S.W.2d 205 (Ark. 1981).

38. Koudsi v. Hennepin County Medical Center, 317 N.W.2d 705 (Minn. 1982) (the statement that the plaintiff was a patient in a hospital and had given birth was true and could not be defamation).

39. Gilson v. Knickerbocker Hosp., 280 A.D. 690, 116 N.Y.S.2d 745 (1952).

40. Griffin v. Cortland Memorial Hosp., Inc., 85 A.D.2d 837, 446 N.Y.S.2d 430 (1981) (a notation on a chart that an outpatient was abusing drugs was protected by qualified privilege).

41. Samuel D. Warren and Louis D. Brandeis, *The Right of Privacy*, 4 HARV. L. REV. 193 (1890).

42. Housh v. Peth, 165 Ohio St. 35, 36, 133 N.E.2d 340, 341 (1956).

43. *But cf.* MacDonald v. Time, Inc., 554 F. Supp. 1053 (D. N.J. 1983) (when a living person is libeled, the claim survives death and is saved from abatement by the New Jersey survival statute).

44. *Cf.* Chico Feminist Women's Health Center v. Butte Glenn Medical Soc'y, 557 F. Supp. 1190 (E.D. Cal. 1983) (California constitutional law gave an abortion clinic a cause of action for invasion of privacy—on behalf of women seeking its service—against the hospital, physicians, insurance company, and medical society for statements and activities intended to force the clinic's closure; a corporation did not have cause of action for invasion of privacy in its own right).

45. 38 Pa. D. & C. 543 (1940). *See also* Estate of Berthiaume v. Pratt, 365 A.2d 792 (Me. 1976) (photographing a terminally ill patient for research when the patient objects is an invasion of privacy).

46. *See* Vassiliades v. Garfinckel's, Brooks Bros., 492 A.2d 580 (D.C. App. 1985) (publication of photographs by the physician without the patient's consent may be a tort; this opinion contains an excellent review of the state of the law).

47. Campus Communications, Inc. v. Earnhardt, 821 So. 2d 388, 402 (Fla. App. 2002).

48. Beth Israel Hosp. and Geriatric Center v. District Court in and for the City and County of Denver, 683 P.2d 343 (Colo. 1984) (the physician may have access to health records of his patients especially because case names and not patients' names were requested).

49. Knecht v. Vandalia Medical Center, Inc., 14 Ohio App. 3d 129 (1984) (a qualified privilege based on commonality of interest existed when a woman employed by physicians told her son that his friend was examined for venereal disease).

50. *But see* Sinclair v. Postal Telegraph and Cable Co., 72 N.Y.S.2d 841 (Sup. Ct. 1935) (actors may insist on dignified public presentations of themselves and their work; hence, the defendant's presentation of an actor's picture presenting him in an undignified light, without permission, was wrongful).

51. Koudsi v. Hennepin County Medical Center, 317 N.W.2d 705 (Minn. 1982) (informing a family member that the plaintiff had borne a child in the hospital did not violate any common law or statutory right to confidentiality).

52. 45 C.F.R. § 164.522(b).

53. Munzer v. Blaisdell, 183 Misc. 773, 49 N.Y.S.2d 915 (1944), *aff'd*, 269 A.D. 970, 58 N.Y.S.2d 359 (1945); N.Y. Mental Hyg. Law § 33. 13 (McKinney Supp. 1987).

54. Mental Health and Developmental Disabilities Confidentiality Act, 117, Ill. Ann. Stat. ch. 911–2, §§ 801–17 (Smith-Hurd 1987).

55. 42 U.S.C. § 242(a); 21 U.S.C.S. § 872 (c), (d).

56. 42 U.S.C. § 290ee-3.

57. 42 U.S.C. § 290dd-3.

58. 42 C.F.R. Part 2.

59. 42 U.S.C. § 290ee-30(b)(2)(A-C). Information can also be exchanged between the Armed Forces and the Veterans Administration without violating the statute (42 U.S.C. § 290ee-3(e)).

60. *See* United States v. Hopper, 440 F. Supp. 1208 (N.D. Ill. 1977), Matter of Dwayne G., 97 Misc. 2d 333, 411 N.Y.S.2d 180 (1978), *and* United States v. Providence Hosp., 507 F. Supp. 519 (E.D. Mich. 1981) on these three points, respectively.

61. United States v. Fenyo, 6 M.J. 933 (1979), *and* United States v. Graham, 548 F.2d 1302 (8th Cir. 1977).

62. People v. Newman, 32 N.Y.2d 379, 298 N.E.2d 651, 345 N.Y.S.2d 502 (1973), *cert. denied*, 414 U.S. 1163 (1973).

63. 45 C.F.R. § 164.514(3)(ii).

64. Fla. Stat. § 394.4615(10).

65. 45 C.F.R. § 164.524(a)(3).

66. FLORIDA HOSPITAL ASSOCIATION MANAGEMENT CORP., FLORIDA HIPAA PREEMPTION ANALYSIS (2002).

67. 327 F.3d 346 (4th Cir. 2003). *See also* Citizens for Health v. Leavitt, 428 F.3d. 167 (3d Cir. 2005).

68. 42 U.S.C. §§ 1320d-5 *and* 1320d-6.

69. Federal Trade Comm'n Bureau of Consumer Protection, *Medical Identity Theft: FAQs for Health Care Providers and Health Plans* (published January 2011), at http://www.business.ftc.gov/documents/ bus75-medical-identity-theft-faq-health-care-health-plan.

70. 72 Fed. Reg. 63718 (November 9, 2007), as amended 74 Fed. Reg. 22642 (May 14, 2009), implementing the Fair and Accurate Credit Transactions Act of 2003 (FACT Act), Pub. L. 108-159 and codified at 12 C.F.R. Part 41.

71. 15 U.S.C. §§ 1681 et seq.

72. 15 U.S.C. § 1681m(e)(4)(B).

73. 12 C.F.R. Part 41, Appendix J, Supplement A (2009).

74. Mich. Comp. Laws § 600.2157 (2015).

75. *See, e.g.*, Weis v. Weis, 147 Ohio St. 416, 72 N.E.2d 245 (1947); Sims v. Charlotte Liberty Mutual Ins. Co., 256 N.C. 32, 125 S.E.2d 326 (1962); In re Estate of Searchill, 9 Mich. App. 614, 157 N.W.2d 788 (1968) (the mental competence of the deceased at the time a contested will was executed was at issue; the hospital's health records were admissible on the question of competence); Rivers v. Union Carbide Corp., 426 F.2d 633 (3d Cir. 1970) (hospital records disclosing a history of alcoholism and intoxication at the time of an accident were admissible by virtue of Federal Business Records Act, 28 U.S.C. § 1732).

76. United States v. Kansas City Lutheran Home and Hosp. Ass'n, 297 F. Supp. 239 (W.D. Mo. 1969).

77. United States v. Providence Hosp., 507 F. Supp. 519 (E.D. Mich. 1981).

78. General Motors Corp. v. Director of NIOSH, 636 F.2d 163 (6th Cir. 1980).

79. United States v. University Hosp. of State Univ. of N.Y. at Stony Brook, 575 F. Supp. 607 (E.D.N.Y. 1983). The decision was later affirmed by a federal court of appeals but for different reasons. In the appellate court's view, the factual situation was beyond the contemplation and intent of Congress when it enacted the Rehabilitation Act of 1973— the legislation prohibiting discrimination against disabled persons— and therefore the statute was not relevant. 729 F.2d 144 (2d Cir. 1984).

80. 575 F. Supp. at 611.

81. In re Zuniga, 714 F.2d 632 (6th Cir. 1983).

82. Camperlengo v. Blum, 56 N.Y.2d 251, 436 N.E.2d 1299, 451 N.Y.S.2d 697 (1982).

83. People v. Doe, 116 Misc. 2d 626, 455 N.Y.S.2d 945 (1982).

84. Board of Medical Quality Assurance v. Hazel Hawkins Memorial Hosp., 135 Cal. App. 3d 561, 185 Cal. Rptr. 405 (1982) (a patient's records of disciplinary proceedings, without names, may be subpoenaed).

85. Florida Hosp. Ass'n, HIPAA Requirements and Florida Law: Disclosures of Protected Health Information for Law Enforcement Purposes (May 2006).

86. Reporters Committee for Freedom of the Press, *Open Government Guide* (accessed August 19, 2016), at http://www.rcfp.org/ogg.

87. The Mississippi statute, Section 25-41-3 (1986), however, grants a specific exemption to the boards, committees, and staffs of both "public and private hospitals."

88. Douglas v. Michel, 410 So. 2d 936 (Fla. App. 1982).

89. Richmond County Hosp. Auth. v. Southeastern Newspapers Corp., 311 S.E.2d 806 (Ga. 1984); *see also* Moberly v. Herboldsheimer, 345 A.2d 855 (Md. App. 1975) (a newspaper may compel a municipal hospital to disclose an administrator's salary and fees paid to legal counsel).

90. 412 So. 2d 894 (Fla. App. 1982).

91. Fla. Stat. § 768.40(4) (1985).

92. Fla. Stat. § 395.3025.

93. American Health Information Management Association, 2014 ANNUAL REPORT at 4.

94. R. Phillips, 14 AMA J. ETHICS 472–76 (June 2012).

95. LUDWIG EDELSTEIN, THE HIPPOCRATIC OATH, TEXT, TRANSLATION AND INTERPRETATION (Johns Hopkins Press 1943).

96. Campus Communications, Inc. v. Earnhardt, 821 So. 2d 388, 393 (Fla. App. 2002).

97. HHS Office for Civil Rights, 2013–2014 Report to Congress on the Breach Notification Program, http://www.hhs.gov/hipaa/for-professionals/breach-notification/reports-congress/index.html.

98. Jefferson Robbins, *At Least 46 Percent of Hospital's Hacked Money Gone for Good* (published June 19, 2013), at http://www.wenatcheeworld.com/news/2013/jun/03/at-least-40-percent-ofhospitals-hacked-money/.

99. 42 C.F.R. § 410.78(a)(3).

10

EMERGENCY CARE

A s noted in chapter 3, under common law a hospital has no duty to admit or serve all who present for treatment. Similarly, individuals have no common-law duty to aid another person, even in an emergency. As with most generalizations, there are exceptions to the rule. One relates to the duty to evaluate all patients who present for service and to render emergency care to those who need it. The courts began to recognize this duty in the late 1960s, and federal law later codified it in the Emergency Medical Treatment and Labor Act (EMTALA).[1] The law is consistent with the philosophy that healthcare at the time of an emergency is a moral right and must be provided regardless of the patient's ability to pay.

Accordingly, hospitals and their staffs must be organized and prepared to meet this duty—if they are equipped to do so. This caveat raises the question of whether a hospital must maintain a facility for emergency care. If it offers such services, the extent of the institution's duty to the patient becomes the question.

The Need for Emergency Care Facilities

The American Hospital Association reports that the number of hospitals with emergency departments (EDs) is dropping steadily, while the number of ED visits is on the rise.[2] Given the need for these services, and despite the fact that common law does not generally impose a duty on hospitals to treat emergency patients, many states have some form of emergency medical services act.[3] Some of these laws specifically require hospitals to maintain emergency facilities. The Tennessee statute, for example, states that

> every hospital, either public or private, that does business within this state and provides general medical and surgical services shall provide a hospital emergency service . . . and shall furnish such hospital emergency services to [anyone who seeks them] in case of injury or acute medical condition where the injury or condition is liable to cause death or severe injury or illness.[4]

New York's statute is less explicit but provides that the operating certificates (licenses) of any general hospital can be revoked for refusing to provide emergency care.[5] As a practical matter, these statutes require that some level of emergency services be provided; thus, most general hospitals today offer at least some type of urgent care, if not a fully operational ED.

While these laws and the EMTALA statute mirror the public's expectation to receive emergency care, not all hospitals are capable of providing it. First, there are various kinds of emergency services; examples include basic life support, intermediate life support, interhospital (transfer) care, and several levels of trauma care. Second, small and specialty hospitals are typically not staffed or equipped to provide any but the most basic services. In larger hospitals and major trauma centers, the chronic overcrowding of EDs complicates matters significantly.

To address these issues, for some years now the American College of Emergency Physicians (ACEP) has pushed for passage of a bill intended to improve access to emergency services and the quality of care furnished in EDs. If passed, the so-called Access to Emergency Medical Services Act would establish a bipartisan commission "to examine the factors that affect the effective delivery of such services" and to provide "additional payments for certain physician services furnished in such EDs."[6] ACEP's bill has not been enacted, but the Affordable Care Act provides for the Department of Health and Human Services (HHS) to award multiyear contracts and grants "to support pilot projects that design, implement, and evaluate innovative models of regionalized, comprehensive, and accountable emergency care and trauma systems."[7] Whether these projects will mitigate the problem of access to emergency services remains to be seen.

Duty to Treat and Aid
Under Early Common Law
Although contrary to human instinct, the adage "no one has a duty to stop a blind man from walking off a cliff" applies to physicians and hospitals as

well as laypersons. Hence, a physician has no common-law responsibility to respond to a call for help when he has no preexisting relationship with the patient (see Legal Decision Point).

Childs v. Weis[8] clearly illustrates the application of this common-law rule. At about 2:00 am on November 27, 1966, Daisy Childs arrived at a hospital emergency room in rural Greenville, Texas, some 45 miles northeast of Dallas. She had been visiting the nearby town of Lone Oak when she started bleeding and suffering labor pains. She went to the Greenville hospital because her home and obstetrician were an hour or more away and she felt she could not make it there in time for the delivery.

Legal Decision Point

A physician declines to put a special tag on her license plate that would identify her as a medical doctor (MD). She fears that police would stop her at the scene of an accident and require her to render aid, thus exposing her to lawsuits.

This scenario presents interesting legal and ethical questions. What is a physician's legal and moral obligation to provide care at the scene of an accident? Do random members of the public have such obligations? How real is the risk of liability under such circumstances? What would you do in this situation? (See also the discussion of Good Samaritan statutes later in this chapter.)

Mrs. Childs was examined by Nurse Beckham, who telephoned the physician on call, Dr. Weis, at his home. (The hospital did not require physicians on call to see and examine all emergency patients.) According to Dr. Weis's affidavit, Nurse Beckham told him "that there was a negro girl in the emergency room having a 'bloody show' and some 'labor pains.'" He stated that he told her "to have the girl call her doctor in Garland and see what he wanted her to do." There was some dispute regarding Nurse Beckham's comprehension and communication of the doctor's message. Mrs. Childs testified that according to the nurse, "The doctor said that I would have to go to my doctor in Dallas."[9] When the patient objected that it was too far, the nurse assured her she would make it in time. The premature baby was born in Mrs. Childs's car about an hour later en route to another facility. The child lived only 12 hours.

In the lawsuit that followed, the case against the physician was dismissed at the trial court, and the appellate court affirmed that decision. It held that a doctor's duty depended on the existence of a contract with the patient, and because the doctor and Mrs. Childs had no such contract, he had no duty to treat her. In other words, no doctor–patient relationship had been established, so the physician was not liable. The hospital, being government owned, enjoyed sovereign immunity, and thus the case against it was dismissed. Whether Nurse Beckham was liable for possibly miscommunicating Dr. Weis's instructions was a question for the jury to decide, and that aspect of the case was sent back to the trial court for further proceedings.[10] The case reports say nothing further about Mrs. Childs and her baby, so we do not know the final outcome of the trial court proceedings.

The *Childs* case is recounted here in some detail as a blunt reminder of the insensitivity of the traditional common-law rule. Fortunately, application of this rule has changed since the 1960s. Just as *Hill v. Ohio County* in chapter 3 would have been decided differently today, so too would *Childs* have been. (Arguably, these cases may have been decided incorrectly even then.)

Enlightened Judicial Decisions

At about the time of the *Childs* case, various courts gradually and without the benefit of statutes began to establish a duty to render emergency care. In *Williams v. Hospital Authority of Hall County*, for example, a Georgia appellate court held that a government hospital with an ED was obligated to extend aid to an accident victim who had presented for treatment of a fracture.[11] The court stressed that the defendant hospital was a public, tax-supported institution and expressly rejected the hospital's argument that it had an absolute right to refuse to provide emergency services. The judge described the refusal to serve when emergency care was needed and available as "repugnant."

The Missouri Supreme Court extended the same philosophy to a private hospital in *Stanturf v. Sipes*.[12] A private hospital refused to treat a patient with frozen feet because he could not make a cash deposit, and it persisted in its refusal even after friends tendered the money. The hospital apparently doubted that it would collect further payment. The delay necessitated the amputation of both feet. In the high court's opinion, the trial court committed reversible error by applying the traditional rule and granting summary judgment for the hospital. Rather, the plaintiff was entitled to a trial on the factual issues of whether an emergency existed, whether aid had been provided, and whether reasonable care had been exercised. (Because the case does not appear again in judicial reports, it likely was settled.)

In an Arizona case, *Guerrero v. Copper Queen Hospital*, the judge ruled that a licensed private hospital with an ED must provide care regardless of the patient's ability to pay.[13] A subsequent case—*Thompson v. Sun City Community Hospital, Inc.*[14]—extended the principle of Guerrero. *Thompson* involved a youngster who had suffered a severe injury to his thigh and a transected femoral artery. He was first treated in the defendant hospital's ED but then transferred to a public hospital even though additional treatment was needed immediately. He survived, but his leg was permanently impaired. The court found that the patient was transferred for financial reasons and that "as a matter of law this was a breach of the hospital's duty."[15] Because the permanent impairment might have been inevitable, the jury was left to decide whether the inappropriate transfer increased the harm to the patient.

In contrast to the common-law rule, police officers, fire department personnel, emergency medical technicians, and similar public employees have a duty to aid victims of accidents or other emergencies. Legislation normally specifies their responsibilities and the geographic boundaries of their departmental operations. Few, if any, actions alleging negligence in administering first aid in a medical emergency have been brought against police and fire department personnel (or physician bystanders, for that matter). More common are lawsuits contending that injuries were aggravated or harm was done while transporting patients to hospitals for treatment. Depending on evolving local law, individuals who serve in a public capacity may be immune from personal liability simply because in rendering care they are performing a discretionary act that requires personal decision and judgment.

Statutory Requirements

Statutes in some states have for years required certain hospitals to provide emergency care, and discrimination on the basis of race, color, creed, national origin, or other prohibited category violates various federal and state civil rights statutes and regulations governing Medicare and Medicaid programs. In 1985, however, concerns about reports of alleged *patient dumping*—the practice of refusing to treat or transferring uninsured patients unable to pay for medical care—prompted Congress to pass EMTALA (see Law in Action).

In part, EMTALA provides the following:

§ 1395dd. examination and treatment for emergency medical conditions and women in labor.

(a) medical screening requirement. In the case of a hospital that has a hospital emergency department, if any individual (whether or not eligible for benefits under this subchapter [Medicare]) comes to the emergency department and a request is made on the individual's behalf for examination or treatment for a medical condition, the hospital must provide for an appropriate medical screening examination within the capability of the hospital's emergency department, including ancillary services routinely available to the emergency department, to determine whether or not an emergency medical condition (within the meaning of subsection (e)(1)) exists.

(b) necessary stabilizing treatment for emergency medical conditions and labor

(1) In general If any individual (whether or not eligible for benefits under this subchapter) comes to a hospital and the hospital determines that the individual has an emergency medical condition, the hospital must provide either—

(A) within the staff and facilities available at the hospital, for such further medical examination and such treatment as may be required to stabilize the medical condition, or

Law in Action

Part of the Consolidated Omnibus Budget Reconciliation Act (COBRA) of 1985, EMTALA is also known as the "antidumping act" or (sometimes) "medical COBRA." Its purpose was to provide an "adequate first response to a medical crisis" for all patients and "send a clear signal to the hospital community . . . that all Americans, regardless of wealth or status, should know that a hospital will provide what services it can when they are truly in physical distress."[66]

(B) for transfer of the individual to another medical facility in accordance with subsection (c) of this section.

. . .

(e) Definitions

In this section:

(1) The term "emergency medical condition" means—

(A) a medical condition manifesting itself by acute symptoms of sufficient severity (including severe pain) such that the absence of immediate medical attention could reasonably be expected to result in

(i) placing the health of the individual (or, with respect to a pregnant woman, the health of the woman or her unborn child) in serious jeopardy,

(ii) serious impairment to bodily functions, or

(iii) serious dysfunction of any bodily organ or part; or

(B) with respect to a pregnant woman who is having contractions—

(i) that there is inadequate time to effect a safe transfer to another hospital before delivery, or

(ii) that transfer may pose a threat to the health or safety of the woman or the unborn child.

The statute and its regulations—42 C.F.R. § 489.24—apply to all patients, not merely those who are uninsured and unable to pay for care,[16] and to any hospital that participates in Medicare, which of course is virtually all hospitals in the United States. Violations can result in large civil fines and exclusion from the Medicare program, and individuals who suffer personal harm can recover damages from the hospital.

EMTALA requires that the patient be given an "appropriate medical screening examination," but that term is not defined; included services can vary from case to case. For instance, a quick history and physical may be enough for a child with a fever and a cold, but another child with a fever might require extensive diagnostic services if he exhibits symptoms of meningitis. Thus, EMTALA does not simply require a physical examination; it requires the exercise of good clinical judgment and the use of all indicated ancillary diagnostic techniques to determine whether an emergency, in fact, exists.

If the screening examination reveals that an emergency exists, the condition must be treated until it has been stabilized, unless the patient requests a transfer or the medical benefits of transfer outweigh the risk. When a transfer is appropriate, it must be in the patient's best interests and meet certain standards of care, including the following:

- The hospital must provide what treatment it can to minimize the risks involved.

- The facility must locate a capable hospital willing to accept the patient.
- Medical records—original or copied—must accompany the patient to the second facility.
- Qualified staff and proper equipment must be used to complete the transfer.

Essentially, unless a transfer is in the patient's best interests, EMTALA requires that all patients known to have emergency conditions be given medically proper care until their condition is stable. This care need not result in eventual admission to the hospital, and (once the condition is stable) discharge or transfer does not violate EMTALA. However, the statute specifically states that stabilizing care may not be delayed for the purpose of determining the patient's "method of payment or insurance status."[17]

Ambiguities in Applying the Statute

EMTALA's statutory requirements may seem straightforward, but they carry considerable ambiguity when applied to real-life situations. For example, when does the duty to stabilize begin? What is an "appropriate medical screening examination"? When has the patient come to the hospital? Does the hospital's motive for denying treatment matter? These questions are discussed in the following sections.

Appropriate Medical Screening

The first ambiguity concerns the point at which the duty to stabilize begins. According to the statute, it arises when "the hospital determines that the individual has an emergency medical condition."[18] If the patient is in the ED, the hospital must conduct an appropriate medical screening examination to make this determination. Because EMTALA does not define the services included in an appropriate screening, the distinction between an appropriate examination and an inappropriate examination has been the subject of considerable litigation and commentary.

Consider *Summers v. Baptist Medical Center Arkadelphia*,[19] which involved a man (Summers) who fell from a platform in a tree while deer hunting. Complaining of popping sounds when he breathed and pains in his chest, he was taken to the ED of Baptist Medical Center. There, a physician examined him and ordered X-rays of his spine, which supposedly showed only an old fracture. No full X-rays of the chest were taken. Believing that the man was suffering muscle spasms, the doctor gave him injections of pain medication. Summers then rode five hours home in a pickup truck. Two days later, when his pain became unbearable, he went to another hospital and was diagnosed with a broken thoracic vertebra, a broken sternum, and a broken rib. According to the trial record, the examining physician classified these injuries as life threatening.

To summarize, the ED physician at Baptist Medical Center performed a medical screening examination and determined in good faith—albeit perhaps negligently—that Summers's condition was not a medical emergency. The physician therefore did not admit him to the hospital and, unwittingly, did not stabilize his condition. The physician at the second hospital also performed a medical screening examination, but this physician perceived the emergency and treated Summers for his injuries. Clearly, the examination at the second hospital was appropriate and triggered the obligation to stabilize the patient. But was the presumably negligent examination at Baptist Medical Center also an "appropriate" one under EMTALA?

If an appropriate *transfer* is one that is medically proper and serves the patient's best interests, we might conclude that a *screening examination* is appropriate if it meets the same criteria. If so, the negligent examination at Baptist Medical Center should have been deemed an EMTALA violation. Some commentators strongly support this view. They lament that *appropriate transfer* is defined in terms of medical standards of care but *appropriate medical screening* is said to mean only that all similarly situated patients receive the same examination, whether it be negligent or not.[20] They assert that if *appropriate* means "not negligent" in one part of the statute, it should mean the same in another.

The *Summers* court acknowledged that this interpretation has some superficial appeal:

> One possible meaning, perhaps the most natural one, would be that medical screening examinations must be correct, properly done, [and] if not perfect, at least not negligent. It would be easy to say, for example, simply as a matter of the English language, that a negligently performed screening examination is not an appropriate one.[21]

Nevertheless, the court rejected this interpretation and held that the screening examination at Baptist Medical Center was appropriate in the context of the statute. It may have been negligent, but the physician acted in good faith and did not detect the patient's emergency condition. Because the duty to stabilize does not arise until "the hospital [or physician] determines that the individual has an emergency medical condition,"[22] the hospital and the physician were not charged with having constructive knowledge of a condition they should have diagnosed but did not.

In rejecting the argument that a negligent examination is per se inappropriate, the court pointed out that the purpose of the statute was to prevent patient dumping—not to create "a general federal cause of action for medical malpractice in emergency rooms."[23] Indeed, Mr. Summers's position, if adopted, would require the parties to conduct a miniature medical malpractice trial on the issue of appropriateness for every case in which no emergency medical condition was diagnosed. The *Summers* court was not about to assume that by enacting EMTALA, Congress intended this result. Instead, the court held that

> an inappropriate screening examination is one that has a disparate impact on the plaintiff. Patients are entitled under EMTALA, not to correct or non-negligent treatment in all circumstances, but to be treated as other similarly situated patients are treated, within the hospital's capabilities. Determining what its screening procedures will be is up to the hospital. Having done so, it must apply them alike to all patients.[24]

The *Summers* decision is consistent with the majority view that a negligent screening exam, in and of itself, is not an EMTALA violation. For example, in *Gatewood v. Washington Healthcare Corp.*, a US Court of Appeals held that EMTALA "is not intended to duplicate preexisting legal protections, but rather to create a new cause of action, generally unavailable under state tort law, for what amounts to failure to treat."[25]

The commentators quoted earlier in connection with the *Summers* case argued that EMTALA should be viewed as "a statute designed to protect the health of the consumers of emergency room services rather than an emergency room civil rights statute." They feel that, unless this view prevails, "the effect will be to render EMTALA a serpent without fangs" (an allusion to EMTALA being part of the COBRA of 1985).[26] Given our federal system of government, however, arguably this "cobra" has venom enough for its intended prey (see Law in Action, p. 351). The *Summers* court made this point when it wrote:

> Congress can of course, within constitutional limits, federalize anything it wants to. Whether it chooses to do so is a matter of policy for it to decide, not us. But in construing statutes that are less than explicit, the courts will not assume a purpose to create a vast new realm of federal law, creating a federal remedy for injuries that state tort law already addresses. If Congress wishes to take such a far-reaching step, we expect it to say so clearly.[27]

Other decisions addressing the medical screening issue seem to agree that EMTALA is essentially a civil rights statute.[28] It imposes on a hospital the duty to treat all individuals alike, triage them consistently, and stabilize those with emergency conditions. Undiagnosed emergencies that go untreated are matters for state medical malpractice law, not EMTALA.[29]

Behavioral Health Patients

As discussed in chapter 3 (under the heading "Admission and Treatment of Mentally Ill Patients") predictions of dangerousness in the case of behavioral health patients are inherently unreliable. This fact makes application of EMTALA's "appropriate medical screening" requirement even more problematic when such patients are involved.

What is an "appropriate" screening for a psychiatric patient? How would that screening differ from one involving a patient who presents with an injury or medical condition but who has underlying mental health or substance abuse issues? What persons are qualified to perform such screenings? Who is competent to consent to or refuse transfer of such a patient? What are the risks involved in sending a behavioral health patient home?

Moses v. Providence Hospital and Medical Centers, a case presenting these very kinds of issues, is set forth in The Court Decides at the end of this chapter.

Coming to the Hospital

The next ambiguity concerns the scope of EMTALA. Does it apply only to persons in the ED? Or does it apply also to those with emergency conditions elsewhere on or near hospital property? According to § 1395dd(a), the statute applies when "any individual . . . *comes to the emergency department* and a request is made . . . for examination or treatment." Subparagraph (b), however, states, "If any individual . . . *comes to the hospital* and the hospital determines that the individual has an emergency medical condition, the hospital must provide [stabilization or appropriate transfer]" (italics added).

The problems with these provisions came into sharp focus in 1998 when a teenage gunshot victim in Chicago died after he was left a few yards from a hospital ED entrance. Although they had been alerted to the situation, hospital staff refused to render aid because they were under instructions not to treat anyone off the hospital's property. Police officers eventually moved the victim into the hospital, but he died shortly thereafter.[30]

As a result of this case, HHS amended its regulations to extend the responsibility of the ED to anyone who presents on the hospital's campus, which it defines as

> the physical area immediately adjacent to the provider's main buildings, other areas and structures that are not strictly contiguous to the main buildings but are located within 250 yards of the main buildings, and any other areas determined on an individual case basis, by the [Medicare] regional office, to be part of the provider's campus.[31]

This definition raises its own set of questions and ambiguities. What are the main buildings? Is a hospital-owned but mostly physician-occupied medical office building a main building of the hospital? Where does one begin to measure the 250 yards? What if, for example, there is a small public park between two "main buildings" that are already 200 yards apart? If someone's emergency occurs in the park, is it considered to have happened on the hospital's campus?

Choosing to **pretermit** these questions, we proceed to other issues concerning the point at which the screening requirement is triggered. For example, a court found that an EMTALA violation had occurred when a patient with unstable depression committed suicide the day after he was discharged from a psychiatric unit. Another court found a violation in the case of a patient in labor who was transferred to the defendant hospital's labor room from another hospital.[32] Both cases involved emergency conditions that presumably were known *in the hospital* but occurred outside the ED.

pretermit
to disregard, overlook, or intentionally omit

At least one court has found potential liability for the discharge of a psychiatric patient who murdered his wife ten days later.[33] At issue was not only whether the psychiatric emergency was known in the hospital but also whether injury to someone other than the patient can support an EMTALA claim. The US Court of Appeals answered the latter question in the affirmative and remanded the case for a jury to decide: "We believe that whether [the patient] had an emergency medical condition that the hospital recognized upon screening him is an issue of fact that the court should have left for a jury to decide."[34]

Baber v. Hospital Corporation of America[35] involved more complicated facts but no EMTALA liability. Baber had been taken by her brother to the ED of Raleigh General Hospital (RGH) near Beckley, West Virginia, at 10:40 one evening. She was agitated, had disorderly thought patterns, and had been drinking heavily. It was determined that she had stopped taking the antipsychotic medications prescribed by her private psychiatrist. She was uncooperative, paced continually throughout the ED, and could not be calmed by verbal orders. The administration of two medications (Thorazine and Haldol) did not alleviate her hyperactivity and agitation.

While roaming the ED, Baber had a seizure, fell, and sustained a laceration to her scalp but suffered no other apparent injury. The laceration was sutured, and the patient became calmer. She was observed carefully for more than an hour. Noticing no neurological symptoms, the ED physician at RGH consulted Baber's psychiatrist. Both doctors agreed that her behavior was consistent with her chronic mental illness and that she should receive inpatient psychiatric care.

At 1:35 am, Baber was transferred directly to the psychiatric department of Beckley Appalachian Regional Hospital (BARH). She did not go through the BARH ED, but because she was under restraints, the nursing staff in the psychiatric ward checked on her every 15 minutes. At 3:45 am, Baber had a grand mal seizure and was taken to the ED, where her pupils were found to be unresponsive and CPR was performed. A CT (computed tomography) scan revealed a fractured skull and a subdural hematoma, both apparently caused by the fall suffered hours earlier at RGH. She was transferred back to RGH because it had a neurosurgeon on staff, but Baber became comatose and died later that day.

Baber's estate brought suit against the physicians, RGH, BARH, and the parent companies of the two hospitals. The suits against the physicians were dismissed because EMTALA does not provide for private causes of action. The ruling on the two hospitals is more interesting.

Baber was in RGH's ED for approximately three hours, and staff were aware of her psychiatric condition. Both the ED physician at RGH and the private psychiatrist felt that Baber's transfer to BARH was appropriate and in her best interests. They did not suspect that she had incurred a significant physical injury from the fall. Even though her brother asked that she be x-rayed, per standard practice no X-ray or CT scan was ordered because the patient's signs and symptoms did not warrant it. The court held that RGH satisfied its EMTALA obligations; it applied to Baber the same standard screening procedure it applied to all patients in similar circumstances. By itself, the failure to diagnose the physical injury did not violate the EMTALA statute.

At BARH, the situation was even less favorable for the plaintiff's case because the patient was not seen in the ED and BARH had no reason to suspect an emergency condition—the skull fracture and subdural hematoma—until her fatal symptoms developed. On behalf of the estate, the patient's brother argued that an appropriate medical screening examination should be given to all patients wherever in the hospital they may be located, but the court dismissed this position summarily:

> Despite the clear language of the statute . . . Mr. Baber asks us to require that hospitals provide an appropriate medical screening to all patients seeking treatment from any section or department of a hospital. We decline to accept Mr. Baber's invitation to change the plain language of the statute because . . . to do so would "transcend our judicial function."[36]

Although Baber undeniably had an emergency medical condition—one that ultimately took her life—EMTALA simply does not address the peculiar circumstances of the case.

The EMTALA regulations do not define "comes to the hospital," but they define "comes to the emergency department" as requesting examination or treatment on hospital property.[37] As discussed earlier, hospital property means the main hospital buildings and surrounding areas within 250 yards. According to the regulations, ambulances owned or operated by the hospital, wherever they are located, are also considered hospital property.[38] Persons in non-hospital-owned ambulances on hospital property are also considered to have come to the ED.[39] Finally, the regulations define "hospital with an emergency department" to mean one that offers emergency services, irrespective of whether it has a defined emergency department. Virtually every US hospital today that accepts Medicare patients fits this description.[40]

With the exception of situations similar to those in *Baber* (i.e., the patient is in the hospital but not in the ED, is not requesting examination or treatment, and has an undiagnosed emergency condition), EMTALA's territorial swath is wide. In at least two cases, it was widened beyond owned and proximate property to include non-owned ambulances off hospital property.

Patients in Ambulances

In the 2001 case *Arrington v. Wong*,[41] a patient who had suffered an apparent heart attack was being taken by ambulance to Queens Hospital in Honolulu, the closest medical facility in the area. The emergency medical services (EMS) personnel called ahead to announce their estimated time of arrival and to describe the patient's condition. After learning that the patient's doctor practiced at Tripler Army Medical Center a few miles away, the Queens Hospital physician responded, "I think it would be okay to go to Tripler." The ambulance diverted, and the patient died about 40 minutes after arriving at the army facility. The EMS personnel were not Queens Hospital employees, and the hospital did not own the ambulance.

The US Court of Appeals for the Ninth Circuit held that because the hospital was not on *diversionary status* (i.e., unable to accept patients because of heavy volume), then—quoting HHS regulation—"it would defeat the purpose of EMTALA if we were to allow hospitals to rely on narrow, legalistic definitions of 'comes to the emergency department' or of 'emergency department' to escape their EMTALA obligations."[42] Relying heavily on the government's regulations to interpret an ambiguous provision, the court wrote:

> The "overarching purpose of [EMTALA is to ensure] that patients, particularly the indigent and underinsured, receive adequate emergency medical care." [Quoting another case.] The agency's interpretation achieves this purpose, ensuring that emergency patients may be diverted to other hospitals only when the diverting hospital has a valid, treatment-related reason for doing so. The agency's interpretation works no hardship on the hospital, as the [EMTALA regulation] "only requires hospitals that offer emergency services to provide screening and stabilizing treatment within the scope of their capabilities." Furthermore, a failure to treat an emergency patient, by diverting him to another hospital, may have lethal consequences. Finally, when a hospital is unable to handle the case load and is in diversionary status, it may divert emergency patients even if they are in the process of being transported to that hospital because it is the closest. Because

Legal Brief

According to these decisions, a patient who *is in the process of coming* to the hospital *has come* to the hospital.

What?! Doesn't the plain wording "comes to the emergency department" mean that the patient is already there?

Ah, but just a minute! In *Macbeth* one of the witches utters the famous line, "By the pricking of my thumbs, something wicked this way comes." The wicked something is Macbeth himself, who clearly has not yet arrived physically on the scene but whom the witch already senses. If only some congressional bard had written, "when someone to the ED comes."

the agency's regulation is consistent with the purposes and language of the statute, we find that interpretation reasonable (and certainly not arbitrary or capricious).[43]

This language formed the basis for the First Circuit's decision eight years later in *Morales v. Sociedad Española de Auxilio Mutua y Beneficencia*. On facts similar to those of *Arrington* (see Legal Brief), the court overturned a summary judgment in the hospital's favor and remanded the case for trial. It held as follows:

We think it is appropriate to resolve the ambiguous "comes to" language in accordance with statutory intent. First and foremost, that intent dictates that the statute and its implementing regulations must be interpreted in a way that prevents hospitals from "dumping" patients.

An interpretation of the statute concluding that an individual en route to the hospital, under the plaintiff's version of the facts, has "come[ ] to" the emergency department fits most squarely with this intent. This reading comports with EMTALA's primary goal and hinders efforts to turn away prospective patients because of their economic status. In that way, it enhances the ability of indigent individuals to receive timely first-response care.[44]

Beller v. Health and Hospital Corp. of Marion County, in The Court Decides at the end of this chapter, is another illustration of the ambiguities involved in the "comes to the hospital" language of the statute.

Motive

The final vexing ambiguity concerns motive: For there to be an EMTALA violation, should the defendant's decision have been motivated by the patient's inability to pay? Despite some early district court cases holding that such an allegation is necessary,[45] the appellate courts seem to agree that no particular motive need be alleged or proven. They reason that EMTALA achieves its purpose (to discourage the practice of dumping indigent patients) by requiring that all patients (insured, uninsured, and self-pay alike) receive uniform treatment. If one does not receive uniform treatment, the reason for the lack of uniformity is immaterial.

The Sixth Circuit raised this issue in *Cleland v. Bronson Health Care Group, Inc.*:[46]

We can think of many reasons other than indigency that might lead a hospital to give less than standard attention to a person who arrives at the emergency room. These might include: prejudice against the race, sex, or ethnic group of the patient; distaste for the patient's condition (e.g., AIDS); personal dislike or antagonism between the medical personnel and the patient; disapproval of the patient's occupation; or political or cultural opposition. If a hospital refused treatment to persons for any of these reasons, or gave cursory treatment, the evil inflicted would be quite akin to that discussed by Congress in the legislative history and the patient would fall squarely within the statutory language.[47]

Some legal experts have interpreted this passage to mean that liability can be found only if the hospital had an improper motive. However, the *Cleland* court implicitly recognized that a bad motive of some kind is inherent in all treatment that is less than standard and therefore need not be a specific element of an EMTALA offense. Plaintiffs' lawyers would prefer to have evidence of an ulterior motive because a bad motive can help the case survive a motion for summary judgment and would make a significant impression on the jury, but the lack of such evidence is not necessarily fatal.

Congress chose to address the issue of patient dumping by creating a kind of "emergency room civil rights statute" that requires equal treatment for all. If inequality is found, a violation has occurred and proving the motivation for the less-than-standard treatment is not necessary.

The US Supreme Court agrees with this interpretation. *Roberts v. Galen of Virginia* concerned an uninsured patient (Johnson) who had suffered massive head, neck, and spinal injuries in a vehicle crash. She spent six weeks in a hospital in Louisville, Kentucky, and then was transferred to an Indiana hospital and eventually to a third hospital (also in Indiana), where she remained for "many months." Medical bills mounted to nearly $400,000, and she applied for financial assistance under Indiana's Medicaid program. Her application was denied for failure to meet state residency requirements.

Johnson's guardian (Roberts) filed suit against the Kentucky hospital, alleging that Johnson's transfer to Indiana violated EMTALA. The trial court granted the hospital's motion for summary judgment on the ground that Roberts had not proven that an improper motive was involved in the decision to transfer the patient. Citing *Cleland*, the court of appeals affirmed, but the Supreme Court reversed. In a **per curiam** decision, the court held,

per curiam
literally, "by the court"; a decision issued by all or a majority of the judges deciding a case and for which individual authorship is not given

There is no question that the text of §1395dd(b) does not require an "appropriate" stabilization, nor can it reasonably be read to require an improper motive. This fact is conceded by the [defendant], which notes in its brief that "the 'motive' test adopted by the court below lacks support in any of the traditional sources of statutory construction." Although the concession of a point on appeal by the

respondent is by no means dispositive of a legal issue, we take it as further indication of the correctness of our decision today, and hold that §1395dd(b) contains no
express or implied "improper motive" requirement.[48]

EMTALA has been a significant issue for years, made especially
troublesome because of its ambiguities and the fact that a violation can subject the offender to civil fines and possible exclusion from federal healthcare
programs. For these reasons, healthcare executives must ensure that their
ED policies are clearly understood by all personnel involved in rendering
emergency care.

Duty to Exercise Reasonable Care
Liability and Negligence

EMTALA considerations aside, there is long-standing precedent that once
care has begun, it must be exercised with due care. The rule clearly applies to
both physicians and hospitals. The slightest act of aid to the patient may trigger the application of this judicial doctrine. Illustrative of this rule in action is
Bourgeois v. Dade County, in which the police brought an unconscious man
to a county hospital. The physician on emergency call examined him cursorily
and did not order X-rays. The doctor decided that the patient was intoxicated,
and with the doctor's approval the patient was removed to jail, where he died.
It was later established that the patient had been suffering from broken ribs
and a punctured lung. The issue of negligence was one for the jury to decide.[49]

Many other cases have found providers liable for negligence on these
principles. Prominent among them are *Jones v. City of New York*,[50] *New Biloxi
Hospital, Inc. v. Frazier*,[51] and *Methodist Hospital v. Ball*.[52] In all three cases,
the facts were fundamentally the same: Victims of violence or accident were
accepted into the ED, and the hospital staff failed to exercise reasonable care
in diagnosing and treating them.

In *Jones*, an intern of a voluntary hospital did no more than clean and
dress a patient's stab wounds before ordering a transfer to a city hospital.
The delay caused the patient's death. In *Frazier* and *Ball*, the patients were
unattended for 45 minutes and 1 hour, respectively; were given minimal
attention and diagnosis by hospital nursing and medical staffs; and then were
transferred to other institutions, with adverse results. These cases are more
than 50 years old, but they still underscore the legal and moral necessity of
exercising reasonable care in making emergency diagnoses and deciding the
course and place of treatment.[53] They also show that careful triage is essential.
Attention to other patients is no excuse for delay.[54]

A healthcare provider can be liable for reasons other than the negligence of hospital physicians. This fundamental principle is illustrated by a
South Dakota case, *Fjerstad v. Knutson*.[55] An intern (who was not a licensed

physician) was on duty in Sioux Valley Hospital's ED. He examined the patient, ordered a blood test and throat culture, and gave him a prescription for an antibiotic. Unable to reach the physician on call, the intern released the patient, who died the following morning from asphyxia caused by a blocked trachea. In the case against the intern and the hospital, the trial court instructed the jury that the hospital could not be held liable unless the intern was found negligent. The jury's verdicts were for both defendants, but the plaintiff's appeal succeeded at obtaining a new trial against the hospital.

The judge's instruction to the jury was wrong. The appellate court observed that the jury would have been justified in finding the hospital negligent, even if the intern had not been negligent, because of its failure to have a physician available for consultation with the ED staff. The failure was a violation of the institution's own standards, which required interns to contact the physician on call before treating emergency patients and before prescribing drugs. Such alleged breaches were sufficient to create an issue for a jury (see Law in Action). Further, on the question of proximate cause, the plaintiff had presented expert testimony at trial establishing that a person with the decedent's symptoms should have been hospitalized and that his life probably could have been saved.

Hospital Admissions and Transfers

Obviously, not all ED patients can or need to be admitted to the hospital. Transfer to another hospital is justified when the patient's condition has been stabilized or otherwise meets EMTALA standards. Indeed, a hospital is under a positive duty to transfer a patient to another institution if it does not have the appropriate facilities and staff to care for the patient properly.[56] The transferring institution also has a duty to forward the patient's diagnosis and other appropriate medical information, and the receiving hospital has a duty to obtain this information.[57]

As these cases demonstrate, patients who present at a hospital's ED should never be turned away until they have been seen and examined by qualified healthcare personnel, who should determine the seriousness of the illness or injury and then order admission, a return home, or a transfer to another facility, depending on the circumstances.

Law in Action

It was the policy of the hospital not to release emergency room patients until the on-call physician or the patient's local doctor had been contacted. Interns were to initiate a course of treatment only in emergencies, and they were not to prescribe drugs without consulting a licensed physician.

. . . [T]he separate liability of Sioux Valley Hospital was not properly submitted to the jury.

. . . The evidence of the hospital's breach of its own standards is sufficient to create a jury issue.

The failure to have an emergency room doctor available and failing to consult with him violated the hospital's own standard for treatment.

—*Fjerstad v. Knutson,*
271 N.W.2d 8 (S.D. 1978)

Legal Brief

Governmental regulations, the standards of professional associations, and a hospital's own policies and medical staff bylaws can be evidence for a jury to consider in a lawsuit.[67]

Undue delays should not be tolerated. These policies should be stated clearly in written rules that hospital and ED personnel can readily carry out. Because ignoring or violating written rules can be evidence of negligence, written hospital policies must be followed meticulously.

Full staff compliance with the standards of emergency care promulgated by public and private agencies and professional groups is also important. Among the standards issued by public agencies are the rules and regulations of state licensing agencies. Standards published by private agencies such as The Joint Commission have the same legal implications (see Legal Brief). For example, Joint Commission standards stress ongoing assessment of patients' needs throughout their anticipated course of treatment, especially at the patient's first point of contact, which is often the ED. Qualified practitioners must assess all aspects of the patient's condition, including physical, functional, and psychosocial status, and consider such additional factors as physical disabilities, language barriers, and vision or hearing impairments.[58]

Law in Action

In a case I handled as a lawyer in the Navy, a military physician saw a patient in the ED and sent him home, where he died. At issue in the case was what discharge instructions, if any, the doctor gave the patient and family when the patient was released. Discharge instructions include signs and symptoms to watch for if the patient's condition does not improve. They were to be written in the medical record and explained to the patient or family members on his release from the ED.

In this case the doctor had not provided discharge instructions at the time of the patient's release; in an apparent attempt to escape liability, he retrieved the original record from the ED and added directions to be alert for exactly the types of symptoms the patient later developed. The doctor forgot, however, that the record was written on self-duplicating ("NCR paper") forms and that a duplicate was filed in the patient's Navy medical record and kept in a separate department. The discrepancy was discovered when the fraudulently altered original record was compared to the duplicate. As a result, the physician was disciplined and the malpractice case had to be settled.

A medical record must be maintained for every emergency patient, and a copy must accompany the patient in the case of transfer. Such records are necessary for provision of adequate medical care and are vital evidence in the event of any subsequent legal dispute. Records should include the instructions for continuing care given to the patient at discharge and the information furnished to the institution or physician to whom the patient is referred (see Law in Action).

Staffing the Emergency Department

All of the foregoing suggests that the duty of reasonable care owed to emergency patients mandates a well-organized department staffed with qualified personnel and equipped with the physical means necessary to ensure prompt diagnosis, stabilization, treatment, and referral. Persons in charge of the ED must be an integral part of the organization and must be accountable for the quality of care. Ultimately, the governing body of the hospital is responsible for the professional standards of the ED, just as it is responsible for other clinical standards of the institution. Medical staff privileges must be delineated for each ED physician as they are for physicians in other departments.

For hospitals of significant size, ED coverage by physicians on call alone is asking for trouble. This situation presents too much opportunity for incorrect diagnoses to be made and treatment delays to occur, both of which lead to unfortunate situations and increase liability problems.

Ironically, specialized medical practice is in some respects more subject to liability. Emergency medicine has become a branch of its own, and many physicians in other disciplines are not competent to deal with emergency cases. Such physicians should not be on ED duty; neither should unsupervised first-year residents, physicians' assistants, and others who lack training in emergency medicine. Hospitals that wish to offer full-scale emergency services should staff the department with full-time licensed and certified physicians, nurses, and other personnel trained to handle emergency cases (see Law in Action).

Hospitals have several alternatives for staffing the ED. In most states, the *corporate practice of medicine* rule has been abolished (see Legal Brief on the next page) and not-for-profit institutions may employ doctors directly. More typical than direct employment of ED physicians is a contractual arrangement in which a physician corporation or partnership provides full-time ED coverage. When entering into such an arrangement, the hospital must not abdicate its ultimate responsibility for the quality of healthcare. The contract must provide guidelines for full-time coverage, supervision of hospital nurses and house staff, maintenance of equipment and facilities, billing, and referral of patients. The document must also specify the duration of the arrangement and provisions for renewal. Above all, the medical staff of the hospital must be involved in monitoring the standards of practice in the ED and delineating clinical privileges, even when service is contracted to an independent group of physicians. This medical staff function must be clearly articulated in the contract, and the ED physicians should be required to carry adequate malpractice insurance and agree to indemnify the hospital if malpractice judgments arise from their negligence.

Law in Action

In one hospital, all physicians rotated through the ED. A psychiatrist was staffing the ED one night when an obviously intoxicated woman was brought in complaining of headaches and neck pain after a fall at home. The psychiatrist dismissed her story as the ramblings of a besotted crock and sent her home. As a result of an undiagnosed neck fracture, the patient suffered permanent paralysis. When asked why he did not order cervical X-rays, the doctor—unhappy to have been put on ED call in the first place—replied, "I'm a psychiatrist. I don't look for anything below here," pointing to his eyebrows. The lawsuit was settled, of course.

Although psychiatrists are MDs, this anecdote from my experience is a reminder that not all MDs are qualified to serve in the ED.

Legal Brief

The prohibition on the corporate practice of medicine (CPM) was announced many years ago as a means of discouraging commercialization and exploitation of the medical profession and to emphasize that the physician's individual loyalties belong solely to the patient. It was developed, however, in the context of for-profit corporations that wished to hire physicians to care for their employees, and thus CPM is believed to have little or no relevance to modern not-for-profit hospitals.

In those few states where these laws remain on the books, creative contractual arrangements or even statutory exemptions are often available to bypass their effect. For example, California—which continues the CPM prohibition more stringently than most states do—allows exceptions for professional medical corporations and foundations, teaching hospitals, some community clinics, substance abuse programs, and some not-for-profit organizations. See, for example, *Cal. Med. Ass'n v. Regents, Univ. of Cal.*, 79 Cal. App. 4th 542 (2000), in which the court wrote, "Concerns about for-profit corporations have nothing to do with non-profit teaching hospitals."

The financial arrangements between the hospital and the contracting group may legally allow two charges to the patient: one for hospital services and another for the physician's service. The group may bill the patient directly or assign the account to the hospital for collection.

Good Samaritan Statutes

Most states have statutes—commonly called *Good Samaritan laws*—that encourage physicians and other professionals to extend aid to strangers at the scene of an emergency. The essence of the legislation provides that physicians, registered nurses, or other healthcare professionals—or "any person" in some statutes—cannot be held liable for ordinary negligence when extending aid at an emergency scene, as long as the aid is extended in good faith and without gross negligence.[59] The statutes vary greatly from state to state with regard to persons covered, the protections they receive, and the circumstances under which the statutes apply.

The need for these statutes is questionable. Few Good Samaritan, "accident by the side of the road" situations have come to trial, but the laws were passed anyway at the behest of medical lobbying groups. Furthermore, many states' Good Samaritan statutes apply only to certain people. Professionals or laypersons not specifically designated in the relevant local statute are not protected by the legislation; they are held to the well-recognized common-law rule that once assistance has started, they have a duty to exercise care that is reasonable under the circumstances.

Some of the statutes grant immunity to professionals licensed to practice in other jurisdictions, but others do not. Thus, states that do not grant immunity consider such individuals to be laypersons when they render aid outside the state of their licensure. Most early Good Samaritan laws applied only to physicians and did not cover ambulance attendants or other emergency services personnel. Many jurisdictions now have an entirely separate statute granting immunity to such persons, and many states adopted special legislation for emergency medical care in response to a 1973 federal law that offered financial incentives and otherwise encouraged the development of local and regional emergency services by professional paramedics working outside a healthcare institution.[60] The federal statute has since been repealed, but the state Good Samaritan laws remain.

Few lawsuits are on record against allegedly negligent Good Samaritans. Moreover, the refusal of a physician or another professional to assist at the scene of an emergency has never posed a serious threat of legal liability as long as the person did not already have an established duty to act. (The ethical implications of refusing assistance are beyond the scope of this text.) In short, the fear of lawsuits that prompted the enactment of the Good Samaritan legislation was unfounded. Moreover, *reasonable care* in an emergency outside of a hospital would be a rather low standard because the common law would not expect a physician, for instance, to have lifesaving equipment or drugs at the scene of a highway accident or when treating a victim of sudden illness on an airplane.

Some of the statutes do not specify where the emergency care must take place for the assister to qualify for immunity. In some cases, the applicability of certain states' statutes to emergencies that arise in hospitals has been uncertain. In some jurisdictions either the Good Samaritan statute or a statute covering emergency medical services specifically extends immunity during an in-hospital emergency as long as the person had no preexisting duty to respond. Hence, in a Michigan case, a hospital staff surgeon who was not on call was allowed to claim immunity after he was paged to attend to a motor vehicle accident victim who was already in the hospital.[61] Similarly, courts have interpreted California's statute as granting immunity to physicians who voluntarily provide services to hospitalized patients in an emergency.[62]

Finally, the Good Samaritan legislation often does not apply to people who have a preexisting duty to respond. In litigation involving the Michigan statute, a hospital was not granted immunity when a code-blue team transporting an unconscious person allegedly permitted the patient's unsupported head to strike a guardrail.[63] Because the hospital and patient had a preexisting relationship, the statute did not abrogate the usual common law with respect to hospital liability. Furthermore, a California case, *Colby v. Schwartz*, held that two surgeons on a hospital's emergency call panel could not claim immunity under the statute because they had a duty to respond and thus were not "volunteers."[64]

Extending immunity to those who render in-hospital emergency treatment was one of several malpractice reforms enacted a few years ago, but neither this nor similar ideas have had a significant effect on reducing the costs of litigation. It is not clear from a public policy standpoint whether Good Samaritan statutes have had any effect (either positive or negative) on bystanders' willingness to assist at the scene of an accident. The limited applicability of the statutes, their wide variation from state to state, and their many ambiguities have made the legislation arguably more counterproductive than productive. An alternative approach would be to enact legislation requiring all persons—professional and lay—to render aid to any stranger in peril, as has been done in some states and in countries that operate under the Napoleonic Code (the system based on French law). A grant of immunity from tort liability, in the absence of gross negligence or wanton misconduct, would then be justified.

Summary

This chapter reviews the common-law rule that individuals have no duty to provide emergency care and its numerous exceptions, both judicial and statutory. It provides considerable detail on the federal statute EMTALA, which currently sets the standard for ED personnel's review of patients' conditions, and presents examples of liability for failure to meet those standards. The chapter concludes with a brief discussion of Good Samaritan statutes, which are probably unnecessary but have afforded some medical personnel a measure of emotional comfort.

Discussion Questions

1. What is the common law's traditional viewpoint concerning a bystander's duty to come to the aid of a person in need? How, if at all, is that duty different today? How might it differ depending on who the bystander is?
2. Discuss the *Childs* case with your classmates. Why do you suppose the hospital did not have a physician present or immediately available to assist in its ED? Why would a physician not come to the hospital and personally examine a woman in labor? What were the motives of the parties involved?
3. Describe a hospital's duty to a person who comes to the ED requesting treatment. Is this duty the same if the person is indigent?
4. In the *Arrington* opinion regarding what it means when someone "comes to the hospital," the US Court of Appeals for the Ninth District wrote approvingly of HHS's position that "it would defeat the purpose of EMTALA if we were to allow hospitals to rely on narrow, legalistic definitions of 'comes to the emergency department' or of 'emergency department' to escape their EMTALA obligations."[65]

Which is the more "legalistic" interpretation—that of HHS and the court or that of the person who reads nuances into the plain words of the statute? The case is an excellent example of how seemingly simple language can create serious problems of interpretation. How might you have written the statute to avoid the kinds of ambiguities seen in these cases?

5. Is *Arrington* the work of "activist judges" who are "making law," as some critics claim about decisions they do not agree with?

6. What are the liability hazards of requiring all members of the medical staff to take ED duty?

7. What effects have Good Samaritan statutes had on the duty to render aid in an emergency?

The Court Decides

Moses v. Providence Hospital and Medical Centers, Inc.
561 F.3d 573 (6th Cir. 2009)

Clay, Circuit Judge

[The plaintiff is the representative of the estate of Marie Moses-Irons. She alleges that the defendants violated EMTALA by releasing Moses-Irons's husband, Howard, from the hospital ten days before he murdered her. The trial court granted summary judgment in favor of the defendants, and the plaintiff appeals.

The opinion notes that Howard was taken to the emergency room of Providence Hospital with physical symptoms that included severe headaches, muscle soreness, high blood pressure, and vomiting. He was also experiencing slurred speech, disorientation, hallucinations, and delusions. Moses-Irons reported these symptoms to the emergency room staff and also informed them that Howard had "demonstrated threatening behavior, which made her fearful for her safety." Howard was then admitted and examined numerous times over the next few days by a neurologist, an internist, and a psychiatrist, among other clinical personnel. His physical symptoms apparently improved, but the psychiatrist determined on day 5 that he was still not "medically stable from a psychiatric standpoint" and decided that he should be transferred to the hospital's psychiatric unit, known as 4 East. For reasons that are unclear from the opinion, this transfer did not occur; instead, the patient was released on day 6. A hospital clinical progress report signed by the internist that day stated, "(Patient) declines 4 East, wants to go home. His affect is brighter. No physical symptoms now. (Patient) wishes to go home, wife fears him. Denies any suicidality." Ten days following his release, he murdered his wife. The opinion continues, as follows.]

Defendants argue that, if Howard did have an emergency medical condition when he came to the hospital, the hospital's decision to admit him for six days and perform further testing satisfied its obligations under EMTALA to treat so as to stabilize the patient. We disagree.

Contrary to Defendants' interpretation, EMTALA imposes an obligation on a hospital beyond simply admitting a patient. . . . The statute requires "such treatment as may be required to stabilize the medical condition," and forbids the patient's release unless his condition has "been stabilized." A patient with an emergency medical condition is "stabilized" when "no material deterioration of the condition is likely . . . to result from or occur during" the patient's release from the hospital. Thus, EMTALA requires a hospital to treat a patient with an emergency condition in such a way that, on the patient's release, no further deterioration of the condition is likely. In the case of most emergency conditions, it is unreasonable to believe that such treatment could be provided by admitting the patient and then discharging him. . . .

In short, the hospital was required under EMTALA not just to admit Howard into the inpatient care unit, but to *treat* him in order to stabilize him. Accordingly, Defendants are not entitled to summary judgment simply on the ground that the hospital admitted Howard as an inpatient and subjected him to several days of testing.

The district court's reasoning in granting summary judgment was partially predicated on its finding that the hospital conducted an appropriate screening, and that "no emergency medical condition was recognized on the screening." We believe that whether Howard had an emergency medical condition that the hospital recognized upon screening him is an issue of fact that the court should have left for a jury to decide.

. . . .

At the time he came to the hospital, Howard was experiencing slurred speech, disorientation, hallucinations and delusions, and was making threatening statements, including telling his wife that he had "bought caskets." Howard's condition included physical symptoms such as severe headaches, muscle soreness, high blood pressure and vomiting. Moreover [a psychiatric expert's] report, based on a review of Howard's hospital records, concluded that Howard had an emergency medical condition upon arriving at the hospital. Thus, there is plenty of evidence in the record to create an issue of fact with respect to whether Howard's condition was a mental health emergency.

. . . On the first day of testing, [the neurologist's] note that "an acute psychotic episode must be ruled out" indicated both the possible seriousness of Howard's condition and the need for further testing. . . . [And the psychiatrist who] diagnosed Howard . . . as having "atypical psychosis," determined that Howard should be transferred to 4 East, and instructed 4 East doctors to take "suicide precautions." A legitimate possibility that the patient might commit suicide would appear to "place the health of the individual . . . in serious jeopardy," and could thus fall under the category of "emergency medical condition." It is noteworthy that [the psychiatrist] recommended Howard be transferred to 4 East, the unit for patients "who are acutely mentally ill." This evidence supports Plaintiff's claim that the hospital physicians believed Howard had an emergency medical condition upon his admission.

[To counter some defense evidence that tended to show the patient had stabilized by the time he was discharged, the plaintiff made the following points.] First, the "final diagnosis" of . . . "atypical psychosis [with] delusional disorder" was substantially the same as [the] diagnosis [the day before], which included "atypical psychosis." Moreover, [the expert's] report concludes that "the symptoms and mental state described [earlier] could not be resolved in one to two days, yet the decision to discharge Mr. Howard was made one day later." The doctors were aware on the day they released Howard that Howard's wife did not think he had improved, and in fact still "fear[ed] him." Finally, [a note written the day before discharge read] "will accept [Howard] to 4 east if [his] insurance will accept criteria" [and this] creates at the very least a credibility issue with respect to whether the hospital physicians actually believed that no emergency condition existed upon Howard's release.

. . . Because issues of fact exist relating to Howard's medical condition—upon his initial screening as well as prior to his release—the district court erred in granting summary judgment on this ground.

For the reasons set forth above, with respect to Plaintiff's claims against the hospital, the judgment of the district court is REVERSED and REMANDED for further proceedings consistent with this opinion. ■

Discussion Questions

1. What additional information would you like to have about the facts of this situation?
2. What is the EMTALA standard by which the decision to release this type of patient should be made?
3. According to the opinion of the court, was that standard met in this case?

The Court Decides

Beller v. Health and Hospital Corp. of Marion County
703 F.3d 388 (7th Cir. 2012)

Rovner, Circuit Judge

The plaintiffs brought suit alleging that the defendant, Health and Hospital Corporation of Marion County, Indiana d/b/a Wishard Memorial Hospital . . . violated [EMTALA] by failing to stabilize Melissa Welch and her minor son, Joshua Beller, during an emergency medical situation. The district court granted summary judgment for Wishard, and the plaintiffs appeal.

On June 14, 2001, Melissa Welch called 911 and a Wishard ambulance was dispatched to her home. Welch was 34 weeks pregnant, and the paramedics ascertained that her water broke and she had a prolapsed umbilical cord. The paramedics tried to relieve pressure on the cord, and after consulting with the nurse at Welch's obstetrician's office, agreed that Welch needed to be transported to the nearest hospital. They then contacted the St. Francis Beech Grove ("Beech Grove") emergency room and transported her there. Beech Grove did not have an obstetrics facility. Rather than delivering the baby there, the physician at Beech Grove examined Welch and then sent her in the Wishard ambulance to St. Francis Hospital South. There, Joshua Beller was delivered by Caesarean section, but he had suffered hypoxia resulting in severe brain damage. The plaintiffs allege that Wishard violated the EMTALA by transferring Joshua to Beech Grove instead of stabilizing him by delivering him, and that the failure resulted in his permanent injuries.
. . .

The issue in this case is whether the plaintiffs had "come to the emergency room" of Wishard Memorial Hospital when they were transported in the Wishard ambulance. The

regulations to the EMTALA, promulgated by the Department of Health and Human Services' Center for Medicare and Medicaid Services ("DHHS"), provide a definition of when a person is deemed to have "come to the emergency room," but the 2001 definition in effect at the time of the incident was subsequently amended. Both parties agree that under the 2003 definition, the plaintiffs would not have "come to the emergency room" of Wishard, and therefore the claim could not proceed. The core issue, then, is which definition applies.

The 2001 regulation provides that:

Comes to the emergency department means . . . that the individual is on the hospital property. For purposes of this section . . . [p]roperty . . . includes ambulances owned and operated by the hospital even if the ambulance is not on hospital grounds. 42 C.F.R. § 489.24(b) (2001). That regulation was later amended in 2003, and although it still provided that an individual in an ambulance owned and operated by the hospital is deemed to have come to the emergency room, it also stated that such person is not considered to have come to the emergency room of that hospital if

(i) (t)he ambulance is operated under communitywide emergency medical service (EMS) protocols that direct it to transport the individual to a hospital other than the hospital that owns the ambulance. . . .

The Wishard ambulance was operating under EMS protocols at the time it transported the plaintiffs to Beech Grove . . . [but because] the 2003 amendment occurred after the incident, the question is whether it can be applied retroactively. . . . [In a 1988 case] the Supreme Court held that an administrative agency may not promulgate retroactive rules unless Congress has provided the agency with express authority to do so and, even if such authority is given, an agency rule will not be accorded retroactive effect unless the agency uses language in the rule expressly requiring that result. [However,] not all rules create substantive changes. Some rules simply clarify unsettled or confusing areas of law and rather than changing the law, those rules merely restate what the law has always been according to the agency. . . . Therefore, the dispositive question is whether the 2003 amendment of the definition of "comes to the emergency department" was merely a clarification of the meaning of that phrase, or whether it presented a substantive change in the definition.

The district court held that the amended definition of "comes to the emergency department" was a clarification . . . and granted summary judgment in favor of the defendant. In so holding, the court gave deference to the DHHS' characterization of the 2003 amendment as a clarification, and concluded that the amendment was intended to alleviate confusion surrounding hospital-owned ambulances operating under the EMS protocols. On appeal, the plaintiffs challenge both of those bases. They argue that it is not clear that the DHHS in fact considered the 2003 amendment to be a clarification. Moreover, they assert that even if the DHHS did characterize it as a clarification, the district court gave undue deference to that determination and erred in failing to conduct its own analysis to ascertain whether the amendment was a substantive change or a clarification.

In determining whether a rule constitutes a change in law or a clarification of existing law, the intent of the promulgating agency must be accorded great weight. We therefore will defer to an agency's expressed intent that a regulation be deemed a clarification unless the prior interpretation of the regulation is "patently inconsistent" with the later one.

We agree with the district court's conclusion that the DHHS considered the 2003 regulation to be a clarification of the definition of "comes to the emergency department." In its Final Rule implementing the 2003 amendment, the DHHS repeatedly stated that the changes were clarifications in order to address confusion as to the scope of the 2001 definition. In fact, the title states "Clarifying Policies Related to the Responsibilities of Medicare–Participating Hospitals in Treating Individuals With Emergency Medical Conditions." The Final Rule . . . indicated that the "reiterations and clarifying changes are needed to ensure uniform and consistent application of policy and to avoid any misunderstanding of EMTALA requirements by individuals, physicians, or hospital employees." Moreover . . . DHHS stated "we proposed to clarify . . . an exception to our existing rule requiring EMTALA applicability to hospitals that own and operate ambulances. We proposed to account for hospital-owned ambulances operating under communitywide EMS protocols." The DHHS then proceeded again to refer to its rule as a "proposal to clarify that EMTALA does not apply to a hospital-owned ambulance when the ambulance is operating under communitywide protocols that require it to transport an individual to a hospital other than the hospital that owns the ambulance."

Those statements are unambiguous, and we agree with the district court. . . . [The] characterization of the 2001 definition by the plaintiffs ignores its plain language. The 2001 definition stated that a person "comes to the emergency department" if the person is on

(continued)

(continued from previous page)

hospital property, and [that] hospital property includes "ambulances owned and operated by the hospital even if the ambulance is not on hospital grounds." The plaintiffs' statement that a person therefore had come to the emergency department if she was in a "hospital-owned ambulance" ignores the second qualifier, which is that the ambulance must be owned "and operated by" a hospital. The 2003 definition clarified what it meant for an ambulance to be "operated by" a hospital.... That is a classic situation of a clarifying regulation. The plaintiffs' exclusive focus on the ownership of the ambulance, and their failure to recognize the 2001 requirement that the ambulance must also be operated by the hospital, misses the critical point. The advent of the EMS protocols caused confusion in that an ambulance could be owned by a hospital but not operated under its direction. The 2003 regulation clarified with respect to that and another recurring situation, that the individuals would not be deemed to have come to the emergency room of the hospital because the ambulance was under the operation of others.

There is nothing inconsistent in the 2003 and 2001 definitions. The two are consistent in holding that an individual will be deemed to have come to the emergency department if that person is in an ambulance owned and operated by the hospital.... Because the Wishard ambulance was operating under the EMS protocol at the time the plaintiffs were in it, the plaintiffs had not come to the Wishard emergency department under the EMTALA, and the plaintiffs' claim cannot succeed. The decision of the district court granting summary judgment in favor of the defendant is Affirmed. ∎

Discussion Questions

1. Do you agree that the 2003 amendment was a "clarification" and not a substantive change to the EMTALA regulation?
2. Should the HHS denomination of the amendment be determinative?
3. Why is the named defendant the "Health and Hospital Corporation of Marion County" and not Wishard Hospital?
4. Had the outcome here favored the plaintiffs, what would the next procedural steps have been and what would the likely outcome of the case be on its merits?

Notes

1. 42 U.S.C. § 1395dd.
2. *See* the AHA's annual research and trends *Chartbook*, at http://www.aha.org/research/ reports/tw/chartbook/index.shtml. In 1991, more than 5,100 EDs reported 88.5 million visits. In 2011, there were nearly 130 million visits to fewer than 4,500 EDs. (*Id.* at table 3.3.)
3. *See, e.g.*, 210 Ill. Comp. Stat. 50/1 et seq.
4. Tenn. Code Ann. § 68-140-301.
5. N.Y. Pub. Health Law § 2806.1.

6. *See* Govtrack.us, *S. 1003 (110th): Access to Emergency Medical Services Act of 2007* (updated March 28, 2007), at http://www.govtrack.us/congress/bill.xpd?bill=s110-1003.

7. ACA § 3504, amending 42 U.S.C. § 300d et seq.

8. 440 S.W.2d 104 (Tex. Ct. Civ. App. 1969).

9. *Id*. at 106–8.

10. Childs v. Greenville Hosp. Auth., 479 S.W.2d 399 (Tex. Ct. Civ. App. 1972).

11. 119 Ga. App. 626, 168 S.E.2d 336 (1969).

12. 447 S.W.2d 558, 35 A.L.R.3d 834 (Mo. Sup. Ct. 1969).

13. 22 Ariz. App. 611, 529 P.2d 1205 (1974), *aff'd*, 537 P.2d 1329 (1975).

14. Thompson v. Sun City Community Hosp., Inc., 141 Ariz. 597, 688 P.2d 605 (1984).

15. 688 P.2d at 612.

16. *See, e.g.*, Cleland v. Bronson Health Care Group, Inc., 917 F.2d 266 (6th Cir. 1990); Gatewood v. Washington Healthcare Corp., 933 F.2d 1037 (D.C. Cir. 1991); Brooker v. Desert Hosp. Corp., 947 F.2d 412 (9th Cir. 1991); Collins v. DePaul Hosp., 963 F.2d 303 (10th Cir. 1992); Summers v. Baptist Medical Ctr. Arkadelphia, 91 F.3d 1132 (8th Cir., 1996).

17. 42 U.S.C. § 1395dd(h).

18. 42 U.S.C. § 1395dd(b)(1).

19. *Supra* note 16.

20. Timothy H. Bosler & Patrick M. Davis, *Is EMTALA a Defanged Cobra?* 51 J. Mo. Bar. 165, 167–168 (May/June 1995).

21. 91 F.3d at 1138.

22. 42 U.S.C. § 1395dd(b)(1).

23. Summers v. Baptist Medical Ctr. Arkadelphia, *supra* note 16 at 1137.

24. *Id*. at 1138.

25. 933 F.2d 1037, 1041 (D.C. Cir. 1991).

26. Bosler & Davis, *supra* note 20 at 168. The authors also argued that, because of EMTALA, hospitals should adopt "standardized treatment protocols" for use in EDs. They cite as support for this proposition a 1990 standard of The Joint Commission, which indeed called for written emergency procedures. The Joint Commission's hospital accreditation standards are revised periodically, and although written policies and protocols are favored and are something an accreditation team will look for, they no longer are an absolute Joint Commission requirement.

27. 91 F.3d at 1140–41.

28. *See, e.g.*, Bryant v. Adventist Health Sys., 289 F.3d 1162 (9th Cir. 2002); Phillips v. Hillcrest Med. Ctr., 244 F.3d 790 (10th Cir. 2001); Del Carmen Guadalupe v. Agosto, 299 F.3d 15 (1st Cir. 2002).

29. "EMTALA is implicated only when individuals who are perceived to have the same medical condition receive disparate treatment; it is not implicated whenever individuals who turn out in fact to have had the same condition receive disparate treatment. The Act would otherwise become indistinguishable from state malpractice law." Summers v. Baptist Medical Ctr. Arkadelphia, 91 F.3d 1132, 1147 (1996).

30. *See* New York Times, *Family Agrees on $12 Million in Hospital Suit* (published May 2, 2003), at http://www.nytimes.com/2003/05/02/us/family-agrees-on-12-million-inhospital-suit.html. The hospital was fined $40,000, and it settled with the family for $12 million.

31. 42 C.F.R. § 413.65.

32. Respectively, these two cases are Helton v. Phelps County Regional Medical Ctr., 794 F. Supp. 332 (E.D. Mo. 1992), *and* Smith v. Richmond Memorial Hosp., 416 S.E.2d 689 (Va. 1992).

33. Moses v. Providence Hosp. and Medical Centers, 561 F.3d 573 (6th Cir. 2009).

34. *Id.* at 584.

35. 977 F.2d 872 (4th Cir. 1992).

36. *Id.* at 884.

37. 42 C.F.R. § 489.24(b) (1995).

38. *Id.*

39. *Id.* In Johnson v. University of Chicago Hosps., 982 F.2d 230 (1992), an infant was being transferred to a hospital by a Chicago Fire Department ambulance. When the ambulance was only five blocks away, the hospital advised the ambulance by radio that its ED was overcrowded and that it should go instead to a certain other hospital. The Seventh Circuit held that the patient had not come to the ED within the meaning of EMTALA.

40. 42 C.F.R. § 489.24(b).

41. 237 F.3d 1066 (9th Cir. 2001).

42. *Id.* at 1072.

43. Id. at 1074–75.

44. 524 F.3d 54, 60 (1st Cir. 2008).

45. *See, e.g.*, Evitt v. University Heights Hosp., 727 F. Supp. 495 (S.D. Ind. 1989), *and* Steward v. Myrick, 731 F. Supp. 433 (D. Kan. 1990).

46. 917 F.2d 266 (6th Cir. 1990).

47. 917 F.2d at 272.

48. 525 U.S. 249 (1999).

49. 99 So. 2d 575, 72 A.L.R.2d 391 (Fla. 1957).

50. 134 N.Y.S.2d 779 (Sup. Ct. 1954), *modified*, 286 A.D. 825, 143 N.Y.S.2d 628 (1955).

51. 245 Miss. 185, 146 So. 2d 882 (1962).

52. 50 Tenn. App. 460, 362 S.W.2d 475 (1961).

53. *See also* Barcia v. Society of N.Y. Hosp., 39 Misc. 2d 526, 241 N.Y.S. 2d 373 (Sup. Ct. 1963) (inadequate examination and a decision by a hospital intern in the ED to send the patient home before results of the patient's throat culture were known); Heddinger v. Ashford Memorial Community Hosp., 734 F.2d 81 (1st Cir. 1984) (had medical standards been followed, the patient's finger would not have required amputation; the jury verdict awarding $175,000 was justified); Tatrai v. Presbyterian Univ. Hosp., 439 A.2d 1162 (Pa. 1982) (a hospital employee treated in her employer's ED had cause of action in negligence; workers' compensation was not her exclusive remedy).

54. To collect damages, the plaintiff must prove—usually by expert testimony—that delayed diagnosis and treatment, or a delay occasioned by transfer to another institution, was the proximate cause of death or a worsened condition. *See, e.g.*, Ruvio v. North Broward Hosp. Dist., 186 So. 2d 45 (Fla Dist. Ct. App. 1966), *cert. denied*, 195 So. 2d 567 (Fla. 1966), *and* Cooper v. Sisters of Charity of Cincinnati, Inc., 27 Ohio St. 2d 242, 272 N.E.2d 97 (1971) (although a physician was negligent in not adequately examining a minor struck by a truck, no proof was shown that an appropriate examination would have saved the patient; hence, neither the physician nor the hospital was liable). *Accord* Rosen v. Parkway Hosp., 265 So. 2d 93 (Fla. Dist. Ct. App. 1972). *Cf.* Martin v. Washington Hosp. Center, 423 A.2d 913 (D.C. App. 1980) (expert testimony is not required on issue of proximate cause when jury has enough information to enable factual inferences; the jury's verdict for plaintiff was justified when hospital emergency personnel released a patient, suffering anxiety caused by drug abuse, died in an automobile accident 12 hours later); Valdez v. Lyman-Roberts Hosp., Inc., 638 S.W.2d 111 (Tex. Ct. App. 1982) (when evidence creates a reasonable inference that a patient's condition could have been stabilized with proper care, a jury question is presented on the issue of proximate cause).

55. 271 N.W.2d 8 (S.D. 1978).

56. Carrasco v. Bankoff, 220 Cal. App. 2d 230, 33 Cal. Rptr. 673, 97 A.L.R.2d 464 (1963).

57. Mulligan v. Wetchler, 39 A.D.2d 102, 332 N.Y.S.2d 68 (1972).

58. *See generally* THE JOINT COMMISSION, 2013 HOSPITAL ACCREDITATION STANDARDS, at PC-1 et seq.

59. For example, Michigan's statute protects a "physician, physician's assistant, registered professional nurse, or licensed practical nurse who in good faith renders emergency care without compensation at the scene of an emergency" if no gross negligence or willful and wanton misconduct occurred and no previous patient relationship existed. Mich. Comp. Laws Ann. § 691.1501. Another section provides protection for those who respond to in-hospital emergencies. Mich. Comp. Laws Ann. § 691.1502.

60. Emergency Medical Services Systems Act of 1973, Pub. L. No. 93-145, codified as 42 U.S.C. § 300d-d-3 (repealed October 1, 1981).

61. Matts v. Homsi, 106 Mich. App. 563, 308 N.W.2d 284 (1981).

62. McKenna v. Cedars of Lebanon Hosp., 93 Cal. App. 3d 282, 155 Cal. Rptr. 631 (1979) (a resident physician is not on call and not a member of the hospital rescue team); Burciaga v. St. John's Hosp., 232 Cal Rptr. 75 (1986) (a staff pediatrician responded to a medical emergency by treating a newborn infant at the request of the obstetrician attending the mother); *see also* Markman v. Kotler, 52 A.D.2d 579, 382 N.Y.S.2d 522 (1976) (the Good Samaritan statute applied even though a previous doctor–patient relationship existed).

63. Hamburger v. Henry Ford Hosp., 91 Mich. App. 580, 284 N.W.2d 155 (1979).

64. 78 Cal. App. 3d 885, 144 Cal. Rptr. 624 (1978); *see also* Gragg v. Neurological Assocs., 152 Ga. App. 586, 263 S.E.2d 496 (1979) (a surgeon who responded to an emergency in the hospital's operating room is not protected by the Good Samaritan statute), *and* Guerrero v. Copper Queen Hosp., 112 Ariz. 104, 537 P.2d 1329 (1975) (the Good Samaritan law does not apply to hospital staff).

65. 237 F.3d at 1072.

66. *Baber v. Hospital Corp. of Am.*, 977 F.2d 872 (4th Cir. 1992), quoting Sen. David Durenberger, 131 Cong. Rec. S. 13904 (October 23, 1985).

67. Darling v. Charleston Community Memorial Hosp., 33 Ill. 2d 326, 211 N.E.2d 253, 14 A.L.R.3d 860 (1965).

CONSENT FOR TREATMENT AND WITHHOLDING CONSENT

After reading this chapter, you will

- understand the two basic types of consent for medical treatment and when each is used,
- recognize situations to which the concept of implied consent applies,
- know what information must be given to a patient (or legal surrogate) for a consent to qualify as informed consent,
- be able to distinguish between the physician's role and the hospital's role in obtaining informed consent,
- be aware of the difficulties inherent in decisions to forgo life-sustaining treatment for minors and incompetent adults,
- have greater empathy for those involved in decisions to withdraw artificial nutrition and hydration from a person in a persistent vegetative state, and
- have a greater appreciation for the importance of advance directives and healthcare powers of attorney.

The United States has always been enthralled with the concept of individual rights: the right to free speech, a fair trial, privacy, freedom of religion, due process, equal protection of law, and so forth. Public policy issues are frequently argued in terms of rights—"I/we have a right to/not to [insert your cause here]." Rights language has strong, popular appeal. It harks back to colonial times, when heroes such as Washington, Jefferson, and Adams founded this country on the "self-evident truths" enumerated in the Declaration of Independence.

Aside from the emotional appeal of rights language, there is a practical advantage to using it: Convince someone that what you want is a right—especially a constitutional right—and you have essentially won the argument. Rights language is absolute; it is not concerned with such niceties as cost, practicality, the common good, or the reasonableness of others' viewpoints.

The subject of this chapter is strongly affected by rights language. The patient (or the patient's surrogate) has a fundamental right to decide whether to permit nonemergency medical or surgical treatment, and any unauthorized, intentional touching of the patient's person is battery, even if the patient is not harmed (see the discussion of assault and battery in chapter 4). The classic judicial statement of this general principle was written a century ago by Justice Benjamin Cardozo in *Schloendorff v. Society of New York Hospital*:

> Every human being of adult years and sound mind has a right to determine what shall be done with his own body; and a surgeon who performs an operation without his patient's consent commits an assault for which he is liable in damages. This is true except in cases of emergency, where the patient is unconscious and where it is necessary to operate before consent can be obtained.[1]

Building on Justice Cardozo's idea, for more than 40 years the courts have recognized that an effective consent must be an *informed consent*[2] (see Law in Action). In other words, consent is more than a patient's signature on a form; it must be based on reasonably complete and understandable information about the

- diagnosis (or suspected diagnosis),
- proposed treatment,
- risks and benefits of treatment,
- alternative treatments and their risks and benefits,
- prognosis with and without treatment,
- probable course of recovery or recuperation, and
- consequences of not consenting.

This information must be provided by the physician, and the patient must be given an adequate opportunity to reflect on it and ask questions. Consent given in the absence of this essential information is not informed and is invalid. A physician who fails to provide this information is likely to be held liable if an untoward outcome results from any treatment provided.

Law in Action

Although *Schloendorff* is a century old, its language is timeless. Less so is the main holding of the case: "It is the settled rule that [a charitable] hospital is not liable for the negligence of its physicians and nurses in the treatment of patients."[84]

As we learned in chapter 7, charitable immunity is no longer a viable concept. It was alive and well in 1914, however, and for that reason Schloendorff's lawsuit against the hospital was unsuccessful.

Types of Consent and Recommended Procedures

Legally sufficient consent can be express or implied. The difference between express consent and implied consent is the method by which the patient or the one authorized to consent manifests agreement. Express consent is given in words—whether spoken or written—while implied consent is manifested by action that shows the patient agrees to the treatment. To be sufficient, either type of consent requires that the person be legally competent and possess a reasonable amount of knowledge and understanding about the proposed medical or surgical treatment.

Express consent need not be given in writing; spoken consent is adequate if proven, but it is rare today because of liability concerns. Even written consent may be negated if the patient presents evidence that he lacked a basic understanding of the elements listed earlier. For example, in *Rogers v. Lumbermens Mutual Casualty Company*,[3] the patient signed a general consent form. The defendant surgeon successfully performed a hysterectomy, but the patient subsequently showed that she had thought she was consenting to an appendectomy and had not understood the true nature of the operation. The defendant had no evidence that the situation was an emergency, so the generalized consent (although written) was deemed worthless. The fact that the hysterectomy was medically advisable was immaterial; it did not justify proceeding without consent. The surgeon's skillful performance was also immaterial. Similarly, surgery performed by a person other than the surgeon named by the patient constitutes battery by the "ghost" surgeon, and the surgeon who failed to perform the operation could be charged with malpractice.[4]

To prevent these legal problems, physicians and hospitals use two types of consent forms. The first is the *general consent form*, which a patient (or legal surrogate) is asked to sign as part of the registration process to grant the hospital permission to provide routine care and nursing services (e.g., to take the patient's vital signs, weight, and medical history). Among other things, this form documents that various people (e.g., nurses, laboratory technicians) will be closely involved in the patient's treatment, the patient understands the nature of the basic care he is to receive, and the hospital does not guarantee a cure.

The second is a *special consent form*, which a patient (or legal surrogate) is asked to sign whenever surgery or special diagnostic procedures are indicated. This form must be obtained from the consenting individual *after* the physician has clearly explained all the necessary information and has answered all of the patient's questions. In addition, this informed consent conversation must be held in a language the individual can understand. If the patient or surrogate has limited proficiency in English or uses sign language, an interpreter must be employed (see Law in Action at the top of p. 382).

Nonphysicians must not conduct the informed consent session. Because the patient must fully understand the nature and extent of the proposed procedure, only a physician can properly communicate the information

Law in Action

An interpreter does not merely restate the spoken word from one language to another. She must also understand and convey the full meaning of both sides of the conversation, including medical terminology, idioms, slang, body language, and the culture of both parties.

In one encounter, an obstetrician was explaining to a non-English-speaking woman how to administer medication to her newborn after they left the hospital. This first-time mother was from a culture that taught women always to be respectful of authority figures (in this case, a male physician—in a white coat, no less). Each time the doctor asked her (through the interpreter) whether she understood, the mother nodded obligingly and said "yes." However, it was obvious to the interpreter—who was from the same culture as the mother—that she did not understand.

The interpreter stopped the conversation and said, "Doctor, she's saying 'yes,' but she doesn't really have a clue what you mean." The interpreter recommended that they bring in the doctor's female colleague to explain the instructions to the new mother. Somewhat abashed, the male doctor agreed, and the colleague—sans white coat—was able to conduct this important patient education discussion successfully, thus preventing a potential disaster for all concerned.

and answer the patient's questions. The physician must note the conversation in the medical record and describe the patient's level of understanding.

After the physician has discussed the matter, the consent form must be signed and witnessed. At a minimum, the form should

- name the physician;
- point out that others will be involved in the patient's care;
- list in lay terms the procedure(s) to be undertaken (see Law in Action, below left);
- recite that the patient understands;
- recite consent to the administration of anesthesia, if any, under the supervision of a named physician or nurse; and
- state that the patient has received an explanation of the contemplated procedures.

In addition, the consent form should explain that unforeseen conditions sometimes arise and that additional or different procedures may be necessary. It should state that the patient is aware of this possibility and consents to such additional or different procedures as may be advisable in the physician's judgment if the situation prevents the medical personnel from obtaining a new consent.

A consent obtained by misrepresentation is no consent at all. Moreover, signatures obtained while the patient is under the influence of drugs (e.g., preoperative anesthesia) may be worthless if the patient is able to show that he was unable to understand the consequences of the purported consent.[5]

Hospitals and physician practices generally have consent forms available for

Law in Action

A hospital's preprinted form said a patient was consenting to a "bilateral salpingo-oophorectomy." How many laypeople would know what this term means? How should the form be revised, and how should the physician approach the informed consent discussion with the patient?

their most common procedures and medical treatments. These forms should be reviewed for clinical accuracy, legal sufficiency, and reading level. They should also be translated into the most common non-English languages spoken in the service area (e.g., Spanish, Creole, Russian, Mandarin). Experience shows that physicians' use of consent forms has beneficial effects on the physician–patient relationship. It improves rapport, gives the physician a checklist to discuss with the patient, ensures that the patient understands the content of the form, and offers some measure of protection from claims that the patient did not truly consent. Tactful application of any technique that enhances communication between doctor and patient is always encouraged. Proper consent procedures are recommended primarily for this reason, not just as a matter of legal formality.

Consent in Medical Emergencies

No consent is required in a medical emergency; in the absence of a competent refusal, the law presumes that consent would be given. This rule applies to all patients, regardless of age, and is sometimes called *implied consent* (although grammatically it should be "inferred" or "presumed" consent).

What constitutes a medical emergency is not always easy to define. To justify medical treatment without consent, the provider must show that the urgency of the situation precluded it from obtaining consent in a timely manner. A conscious, competent adult is entitled to refuse even lifesaving care; therefore, treatment without consent is permitted only if patients or those authorized to act for them are unable—as a result of the emergency situation—to express approval or disapproval of the proposed treatment. Also, *emergency* means a situation that presents an immediate danger of death or permanent impairment of health. A mere desire to treat quickly is not the same as an emergency. If delaying treatment to obtain consent would not increase the hazards to the patient, the circumstances would not be considered an emergency, so treatment without consent would not be justified.[6] The description of an emergency provided in the Emergency Medical Treatment and Labor Act is the established minimum definition of the term (see chapter 10).[7]

Extending Surgery

When a surgeon encounters unanticipated conditions during surgery, whether the situation amounts to an emergency that justifies treatment beyond the scope of the patient's consent becomes a legal issue. The traditional rule is that unless a true emergency exists, the original surgery should be completed and the new condition should be addressed at a later time. As a result, however, the patient is subjected to a second procedure along with the risks inherent in the additional surgery.

Most of the cases that have dealt with this issue are decades old[8]—probably because today's consents typically include language permitting the surgeon (in the exercise of professional judgment) to extend the planned procedure and treat unexpected conditions discovered during the course of the operation. For example, the consent might be worded as follows:

> I understand that during the course of the operation/procedure, unforeseen conditions may be discovered which require an extension of the original procedure or a different procedure from that described above. I REQUEST AND AUTHORIZE my physician or other physicians who may be assisting to perform such additional surgical procedures as are indicated by good medical practice which they deem to be in my best interest by exercise of their medical judgment.[9]

In one Georgia case,[10] a patient had signed this type of consent prior to delivery of her baby by cesarean section. During the course of the successful birth, the obstetrician "discovered a grapefruit-sized tumor covering [the patient's] right ovary and adher[ing] to the uterus."[11] Doctors removed the tumor, but the operation caused uterine bleeding that the doctors felt might be life-threatening. The patient's husband was informed of the situation and was told that a hysterectomy was necessary; he was not asked to consent. The doctors then performed the surgery.

When the patient sued, the trial court found no evidence of negligence, treated the case as an allegation of battery—to which consent is a defense—and found in favor of the defendants. The court of appeals agreed, stating that "based on the validity of the consent form executed by [the patient], summary judgment was proper and the judgment is therefore affirmed."

Physicians must explain to patients all aspects of any surgery, including the possible need to extend the procedure if unforeseen circumstances arise. With proper counseling, the risks inherent in extending surgery can be minimized, as this case indicates.

The Healthcare Institution's Role in Consent Cases

To assist in the consent process, hospital risk management departments typically maintain several hundred detailed consent forms—one for each of the many procedures regularly performed in the facility. These forms are made available for physicians' use in counseling their patients about the risks and alternatives of proposed treatments. The risk management department should have protocols and procedures concerning who is authorized to consent on a patient's behalf when the patient is unable to do so. For example, in the Georgia case, a risk management counselor could have been consulted to assist in discussing the hysterectomy intervention with the patient's husband. (Whether the husband's consent was required and whether his consent would have been effectual had it been obtained are separate issues.)

How far must a hospital go to ensure that its medical staff physicians are obtaining informed consent from their patients? In essence, the physician's duty is to obtain consent; the hospital's duty is to determine whether the doctor has fulfilled that responsibility.[12] The hospital should not be held liable for an inadequate informed consent discussion by a physician who is not its employee, but it needs to have a mechanism in place to verify that documentation of consent is present.[13] Specifically, the hospital must have policies and procedures pertaining to documentation of consent, and it must have protocols to ensure that those rules are followed. Someone on the hospital staff (e.g., an operating room supervisor) should be assigned responsibility for checking the patient's identity and making certain that no procedure is performed without documentation of consent in the medical record.

The hospital discharges its duty properly by making physicians aware of their responsibility to inform patients, by making tools such as standard consent forms available, and by insisting that adequate written documentation of patients' consent be placed in the medical record. The hospital need not be a party to or participate in a physician's consent discussions, but if nursing or administrative staff of the hospital know that sufficient consent was not given, the hospital should prevent the unauthorized treatment from occurring.

How "Informed" Must Informed Consent Be?

How far must a physician go in the informed consent discussion to ensure that the patient understands the terms of the proposed treatment?

How Much Information Should Be Given to a Patient?

Patients should be reasonably well informed and have trust and confidence in those caring for them. The patient's welfare and individual needs are the foremost considerations. Physicians should review the following questions when deciding how much to tell patients:

- Is the patient likely to be unaware of a known hazard or risk?
- Would a reasonably prudent patient be likely to withhold consent if she were aware of the risk?
- Is there any acceptable justification for failing to disclose the risk or hazard?
- Is the risk or hazard, however remote, likely to be significant to this patient's decision to grant consent?
- Would I (the physician) disclose the information if the patient were one of my family members?

Court cases centering on questions of informed consent usually result from misrepresentation of the facts, lack of information about consequences, or lack of information about risks.

Misrepresentation of the Facts

Physicians have been charged with misleading their patients—intentionally or otherwise—by misrepresenting the proposed treatment, the basis for the first type of case. *Rogers v. Lumbermens Mutual Casualty Company*,[14] discussed earlier, is one example: The doctor did not reveal the true nature of the proposed surgery (hysterectomy), and the patient thought she was consenting to another procedure (appendectomy).

Apparent misrepresentation was also at issue in *Corn v. French*.[15] After examining the patient, the physician recommended that she submit to a "test" for a possible malignancy. When the patient asked the doctor if he intended to remove her breast, he said, "I have no intentions of removing your breast. I wouldn't think of doing so without first making a test." The patient, however, was given a written consent form indicating that a mastectomy was to be performed. Although she did not know what the term "mastectomy" meant, she signed the form, and her breast was removed. Later, pathology results showed no malignancy. The appellate court held that there was sufficient evidence for the case to proceed to trial. The outcome of the case is unknown—it was likely settled—but it seems there was a high possibility of liability for battery, even without proof of negligence.

In summary, the doctor–patient relationship dictates, at a minimum, full disclosure of the nature of the diagnosed condition, all significant facts concerning the proposed surgery, and an explanation of the probable risks involved.

Lack of Information About Consequences

The second type of case is based on the concept that the patient is entitled to know the inevitable consequences of the contemplated surgery. For example, in *Bang v. Charles T. Miller Hospital*,[16] the patient expressly consented to a transurethral resection of the prostate, but he was not told that because of the particular circumstances—including his age and the possibility of infection—this professionally acceptable surgical technique would likely render him sterile. It did, and the surgeon was held liable for lack of informed consent. This case also stands for the proposition that a patient is entitled to an explanation of the alternatives to a proposed course of treatment. In this situation, the surgeon should have explained to the patient that other treatments were available that might prevent sterility but might also entail a substantial risk of infection.

Lack of Information About Risks

Perhaps the most difficult type of case calls into question the extent of the physician's duty to disclose the risks of the proposed treatment. One approach to this question is illustrated by *Natanson v. Kline*[17] and *Mitchell v. Robinson*.[18] These cases were decided on the basis of what has come to be known as the *reasonable-doctor rule*—the physician must disclose all risks that a reasonable doctor would disclose under the circumstances.

In *Natanson*, the physician recommended cobalt radiation therapy following removal of the patient's cancerous breast. The therapy was skillfully performed, but the patient was not informed that the therapy involved substantial risk of tissue damage. The Kansas Supreme Court held that the patient was entitled to be informed in advance of the hazards known to the doctor and that the physician was obligated to make such "reasonable disclosures" as other medical practitioners would make under the circumstances.

In *Mitchell*, the Missouri Supreme Court held that the plaintiff—who was given electroshock and insulin therapy for "serious depression and rather severe anxiety, complicated by alcoholism"—had the right to be informed that 18–25 percent of patients who underwent such treatment suffered convulsions as a result. In this particular case, a convulsion fractured some of the patient's vertebrae. Although there was no allegation or evidence of negligence in the diagnosis or treatment, the court held that it was for the jury to decide what amounted to reasonable disclosure and whether the doctor was negligent in failing to apprise the patient of the risks.

The reasonable-doctor rule is highly favorable to physicians. Many cases reject the idea that the duty depends on what other doctors do; instead, they hold that the physician should disclose the facts and risks that are likely to be relevant *to the patient*. This standard—characterized as the *reasonable-patient* or *right-to-know* rule—eliminates the need for expert testimony on what other physicians do. The issue will still be for the jury to decide, but it will turn on lay testimony rather than expert evidence.

One of the cases that rejected the reasonable-doctor rule was *Wilkinson v. Vesey*.[19] A diagnosis of malignancy was made without benefit of a biopsy. Radiation treatments caused severe burns that required eight subsequent operations, after which the patient discovered that she had never suffered from cancer in the first place. The Rhode Island Supreme Court ruled that the patient was entitled to know all "material" (important) information, regardless of how much other physicians usually tell their patients. In effect, the court held that expert testimony would be required to determine the medical profession's knowledge of the risks involved but that the information the patient needed to make an intelligent choice would be a question for laypeople (the jury) to decide. The materiality of the information depends on both the inherent danger of the treatment and any other factors that would be significant to a reasonable person. The statistical remoteness of a risk does not determine its materiality because even a small chance of serious consequences may be significant to a reasonable person.

Legal Brief

The reasonable-patient test is based on one question: What would a prudent person in the patient's position have decided if adequately informed of all significant perils?

The reasonable-patient concept (see Legal Brief) was perhaps best summarized in the landmark 1972 California Supreme Court case of *Cobbs v. Grant*:

A physician's duty to disclose is not governed by the standard practice in the community; rather it is a duty imposed by law. A physician violates his duty to his patient and subjects himself to liability if he withholds any facts [that] are necessary to form the basis of an intelligent consent by the patient to the proposed treatment.[20]

See The Court Decides: *Cobbs v. Grant* at the end of this chapter.

Informed Refusal

The reasonable-patient concept has been extended beyond informed consent to include *informed refusal*. In *Truman v. Thomas*, a young woman (the patient) refused to have a recommended Pap test—a test for cervical cancer—apparently because she was unable to afford it.[21] The physician had treated the patient over a six-year period for several routine conditions, rendered advice on family matters, and cared for her during her second pregnancy, but he did not specifically advise her of the risks involved in forgoing the Pap test (see Legal Decision Point). When a specialist eventually discovered a tumor, it was far too advanced for surgical removal and alternative forms of treatment proved unsuccessful. The patient died at age 30. The California Supreme Court held that the trial court erred by not instructing the jury that the physician had a duty to disclose all relevant and material information, including the risks of refusing recommended care.

As these cases show, physicians must exercise "reasonable care under the circumstances." Unless physicians know that a patient is already aware of the risk or that a given risk would not have any apparent significance to the patient's decision—or unless they can establish that disclosure would

Legal Decision Point

One can perhaps sympathize with both the patient and the physician in the *Truman v. Thomas* case. To prepare for class discussions, try to articulate the rationale for each side's actions (or inactions) during the course of the doctor–patient relationship.

adversely affect the rationality of a patient's decision—they must provide the patient with all significant information needed to give an informed consent. All such matters are to be submitted to the jury for decision without requiring the plaintiff to present expert testimony showing the materiality of the nondisclosure, although experts must be used to establish medical facts, such as the risks of a given procedure.

In a few old cases,[22] the courts held that the physician may limit or withhold information from the patient for sound therapeutic reasons—for example, if full disclosure would complicate or hinder treatment because of a patient's emotional state. This paternalistic viewpoint is disfavored today, and occasions justifying this "therapeutic privilege" are extremely rare. The privilege is unlikely to stand if the facts indicate that a competent and rational patient would have declined treatment had there been full disclosure. If such an occasion arises, the physician must document it fully in the medical record, and consultation with a colleague is advisable.

Innovative Therapy Versus Clinical Research

From our discussion thus far, you can deduce that informed consent for any innovative therapy would be especially important to obtain. Because the treatment has not yet been recognized as standard practice, and because the potential risks and benefits of the therapy are uncertain, such consent must be evidenced by a specially drafted form. In a malpractice case involving a well-known cardiologist and surgeon, the estate of a deceased patient alleged that the surgeon and his physician team failed to obtain informed consent for ventriculoplasty surgery (a then-innovative procedure to repair a certain kind of heart defect). The court rendered a direct verdict for the physicians after they presented a carefully prepared consent form and gave a clear testimony of the events.[23]

A difference exists between innovative therapy and clinical research, however. Like standard medical practice, *innovative therapy* is designed to enhance the well-being of the patient and is reasonably expected to be successful. In contrast, *clinical research* is a departure from standard practice that is intended to test a hypothesis or develop new knowledge.[24] Research is conducted to prove or disprove a hypothesis about a new course of treatment of potential benefit to a large number of patients; whether it may benefit the individual patient is not the primary consideration.

Because the risks and benefits of innovative therapy and clinical research are uncertain, the patient must be fully informed, and a signed, specially drafted form must serve as evidence of written consent. Legal advice is strongly recommended. The duty of physicians recommending innovative therapy is determined by the general principles of tort law and malpractice liability on a state-by-state basis, but certain federal regulations—such as those regarding new drugs and medical devices—may impose standards in addition to those of tort law.

When clinical research involves human subjects, a complex regulatory scheme governs the selection of subjects, documentation of informed consent, review by an institutional review board, and processes for ensuring human subjects' safety and privacy (see Legal Brief). Each institution

that conducts research involving human
subjects must seek competent legal advice
and adhere to special laws and regulations,
which are beyond the scope of this text.[25]

Consent of a Spouse or Relative

Marriage or blood relationship alone does
not entitle someone to consent to treatment on the patient's behalf.[26]
Although information may be shared with family members in many cases,
a spouse's or relative's consent to treat the patient is rarely sought. (The
sharing of protected health information with persons involved in a patient's
care raises numerous legal issues. See the section on the Health Insurance
Portability and Accountability Act in chapter 9 for a detailed discussion of
this topic.)

In a few special circumstances, however, a spouse's consent may be
required, even if the patient is competent. Artificial insemination and surrogate motherhood are two such cases. The state statutes regulating these
procedures often require that both the husband and wife consent voluntarily
to artificial insemination involving a third party donor. Similarly, if a married
woman agrees to be a surrogate mother, her husband must consent that he
acknowledges he is not the father of the child to countermand the usual presumption that a married man is the father of a child born to his wife.

On the other hand, if the patient's health and welfare are at risk, the
spouse's consent need not be obtained, even if reproductive capacity will
be affected adversely. An Oklahoma case held that the husband, who had
not consented to his wife's hysterectomy, had no cause of action for loss of
consortium.[27] The wife's right to health is supreme, and her decision alone—
based on the professional advice of her physician—overrules her husband's
wishes.

If the patient is not competent to consent and has not appointed an
agent to act on his behalf, state law usually provides for a hierarchy of individuals who may make healthcare decisions
for him (see Legal Decision Point). Florida
law, for example, provides that the following persons in the patient's life—and in
this order of priority—may consent for the
incompetent patient:

1.   Judicially appointed guardian
2.   Spouse

Legal Decision Point

What are your home state's standards for the
hierarchy of individuals who may consent for an
incompetent patient? Perform some research in
advance of class discussion.

3. Adult child or, if more than one, a majority of the adult children
4. Parent
5. Adult sibling or, if more than one, a majority of the adult siblings
6. Adult relative who has care and concern for the patient
7. Close friend[28]

Withholding and discontinuing lifesaving treatment are discussed later in this chapter.

Life-or-Death Decisions
A Competent Adult's Refusal to Consent

Recall that an emergency normally eliminates the need to obtain consent. Because preservation of life and prevention of permanent impairment are basic values in our society, when a patient is incapable of expressing consent and the healthcare surrogate is unavailable, the law presumes that consent would be given.

The legal situation is different when a competent adult patient refuses to consent to medical or surgical treatment. A patient's refusal to consent must be honored, even if death will likely result, unless a compelling state interest (such as when minor children would suffer as a result) overrides the patient's refusal. In other words, the personal right of self-determination normally trumps society's interest in preserving life. A provider would incur civil and possibly criminal liability for rendering treatment in the face of a competent patient's refusal. There are several leading cases to this effect.[29]

Moreover, the common-law right to refuse medical care—expressed while competent and proven by clear and convincing evidence—must be honored even if the patient later becomes incompetent. On such facts, a court should not order continuation of treatment, and the substituted judgment doctrine (discussed later) would not apply.[30]

"Assisted Death" Statutes

The right to die does not normally encompass affirmative steps to end the patient's life. "Active euthanasia" (aka "assisted suicide" or "assisted death") is considered homicide in most states, but there has long been pressure to change the traditional rule.

For more than a century there has been debate about whether to allow physicians to assist terminally ill persons in ending their lives.[31] The debate is complicated by various moral and ethical considerations, by the fact that physicians have surreptitiously assisted with euthanasia on occasion over the years, by recollections of the eugenics movement of the early 20th century (see discussion of *Buck v. Bell* in chapter 14), and by the public notoriety of

Legal Brief

Dr. Kevorkian was convicted of murder after recording himself actively killing a patient via lethal injection and allowing the recording to be shown on *60 Minutes*. Excerpts of the *60 Minutes* interview and related videos can be found on YouTube.

Doctor Jack Kevorkian in the 1990s (see Legal Brief).

Notwithstanding the highly intense emotions that surround the issue, laws enabling physicians to assist patients hastening their own deaths were passed by voters in Oregon and Washington in 2004 and 2008, respectively. The California legislature passed a similar bill in 2015, and it was signed into law by the governor.[32] Assisted suicide is legal in Montana per a court ruling, and legislation is being considered in several other states.

The legality of aiding a person to die has reached the US Supreme Court on at least three occasions. In two 1997 cases the court ruled unanimously that there is no constitutional right to have assistance in carrying out suicide and, therefore, that the states have the right to prohibit it if they wish.[33] In 2006 the Court ruled that the federal government could not enforce the Controlled Substances Act against physicians who prescribe drugs for assisted suicide if the physician's actions comply with state law, thus implicitly ruling that states may also permit the practice if they choose to do so.[34]

Legal Brief

At least four states—California, Montana, Oregon, and Vermont—allow physician-assisted suicide under certain limited conditions. For example, the Washington statute requires, among other things, that the patient

- be a competent adult;
- be terminally ill with less than six months' time to live;
- make a voluntary request;
- be informed of all other options, including palliative and hospice care;
- obtain two independent persons to witness the request; and
- wait a certain period to receive lethal medications.

In Montana, a state supreme court decision held that assisted suicide is not against public policy and that physicians may be shielded from prosecution if they indirectly aid in the deaths of "terminally ill, mentally competent adult patients" by prescribing a lethal dose of medication which the patients then self-administer. The decision falls short of establishing physician-assisted suicide as a right, and it seems to turn on the question of how direct the physician's participation is beyond merely prescribing the medication.[85]

The existing assisted death statutes are intended only for competent, terminally ill adults who are expected to have less than six months to live. Procedural safeguards are written into the laws—for example, requiring a second physician to concur in the opinion that the patient is competent—and patients are allowed to change their minds (see Legal Brief).

Nevertheless, many commentators express concerns about the laws. They raise questions about unscrupulous relatives who wish to hasten the patient's demise, about the specter of "doctor shopping" to find physicians who will agree with the patient's decision, and about the vulnerability of poor people and undocumented immigrants. There are even questions about what to list as the immediate cause of death on death certificates and whether life insurance policies with suicide exclusion clauses would be payable. (The California law specifically states that insurance coverage may not be denied because of the individual's decision to end his own life.)

Disability rights organizations and some religious groups have mounted strong opposition, but opinion polls tend to show that a majority of voters favor such laws. As one might imagine, this decades-old debate is likely to continue for years to come.

Incompetence

Incompetence (non compos mentis) is a legal status, not a medical diagnosis, but this determination is best made on the basis of a physician's professional judgment. The test is whether patients are capable of understanding their condition, the medical advice they have been given, and the consequences of refusing to consent.

Irrationality does not necessarily indicate incompetence. In one famous case, a 72-year-old man with extensive gangrene in both legs faced death within three weeks unless he agreed to have them amputated; with surgery, his chances of recovery were good. When he decided against surgery, the hospital petitioned the court for a determination of incompetence, appointment of a guardian, and permission to amputate and give other necessary treatment. The hospital argued that the man's refusal was "an aberration from normal behavior" and that the refusal amounted to suicide. However, the court decided that even though the decision might seem irrational, the man was competent. The extensive surgery was unacceptable to him, and his right to privacy outweighed the state's interest in preserving his life.[35]

A patient's right to choose or to refuse treatment is based on common law, the right of self-determination on which the doctrine of informed consent is grounded, and the right to privacy first enunciated in abortion decisions. (Statutory provisions are discussed later in this chapter.) This right is not unfettered, and the state is said to have four interests that may override the individual's freedom to decide:

1. Preservation of life
2. Protection of innocent third parties
3. Preservation of the ethical integrity of the medical profession
4. Prevention of suicide

The interest most often asserted in overriding a patient's objections and ordering treatment is the protection of third parties—usually minor children or a fetus. For example, in *In re Application of the President and Directors of Georgetown College, Inc.*, despite a woman's refusal on religious grounds, the court ordered her to receive a blood transfusion for the sake of her seven-month-old child.[36] The survival of dependent children, however, is not always sufficient to override the patient's right of refusal. In another case, the court did not order a transfusion to save the life of a 34-year-old Jehovah's Witness, even though he had two young children. The judge was convinced that adequate provision had been made for the children's welfare.[37]

The state has sometimes been said to have an interest in "maintaining the ethical integrity of the medical profession."[38] This argument asserts that physicians should not be forced to give (or withhold) treatment against their medical judgment or to assist in suicide because doing so will expose them to possible criminal charges or malpractice suits. This alleged state interest, however, is no longer persuasive.[39] Instead, the courts and legislatures have attempted to provide legal protection for physicians who agree to carry out their patients' wishes. For example, according to the Natural Death Act (passed by a number of states), healthcare providers who comply with the law are immune from criminal prosecution or civil liability.

Courts have recognized that in some instances, withholding or withdrawing life-sustaining treatment is consistent with medical ethics:

> It is perfectly apparent . . . that humane decisions against resuscitative or mainte-nance therapy are frequently a recognized de facto response in the medical world to the irreversible, terminal, pain-ridden patient, especially with familial consent. . . . Physicians distinguish between curing the ill and comforting and easing the dying. . . . Many of them have refused to inflict an undesired prolongation of the process of dying on a patient in irreversible condition when it is clear that such "therapy" offers neither human nor humane benefit.[40]

Many courts have held that, in itself, society's interest in preserving life is not sufficient to prevent a competent adult from making her own decisions about treatment—at least if no third persons might be affected.[41] The less hopeful the patient's condition and the more intrusive the therapy, the weaker the state's interest in preserving life. Even when the prognosis for recovery is good, the patient's right is usually upheld.[42]

Because most courts have determined that forgoing medical treatment is not the equivalent of suicide but rather a decision to permit nature to take its course, the fourth interest of the state—prevention of suicide—is usually not persuasive in cases involving termination of treatment. However, the line between actively taking life—suicide or euthanasia—and letting nature take its course is not always clear. For example, an 85-year-old resident of a nursing home was suffering from multiple ailments and deteriorating health. Although the resident (a former college president) did not have a terminal illness, he was discouraged about his future and decided to hasten his death by fasting. A court found that the man was competent and had the right to refuse food and that the nursing home was neither obligated nor authorized to force-feed him. The man was permitted to die of starvation.[43]

By contrast, a 26-year-old woman who had been severely disabled by cerebral palsy since birth checked herself into the psychiatric unit of a hospital and demanded that she not be fed but given only medication to relieve her pain. Her intent was to starve herself to death. When the hospital sought to force-feed her, she petitioned the court for an injunction to prevent the hospital from doing so, asserting her constitutional right to privacy. The court refused to issue an injunction, finding that the patient was not terminally ill and that society had no duty to help her end her life. The court found that the state's interests in preserving life, maintaining the integrity of the medical profession, and protecting third parties outweighed her right of self-determination because other patients might be adversely affected if they knew the hospital was helping a patient to die.[44]

Three years later, this woman's health had so deteriorated that she was in constant pain and was hospitalized because she was unable to care for herself. After her physicians determined that she was not obtaining sufficient nutrition through spoon-feeding, a nasogastric tube was inserted despite her objections. A trial court denied the patient's request to have the tube removed but was overruled by the appellate court, which held that the patient, who was still mentally competent, had a constitutional right of privacy that included the right to refuse medical treatment. The court further ruled that the decision to refuse the tube feedings was not equivalent to suicide and that the patient's motives were irrelevant.[45]

Consent Issues for Incompetent Adults

A patient may be unable to grant consent by reason of incompetence or other disability. A duly appointed guardian or healthcare surrogate can give valid consent based on the patient's known wishes. This concept is relatively simple, but its application becomes complicated when the individual has never been competent to express his intent.[46] Treatment decisions for these patients involve three questions that have troubled the courts and caregivers for decades:

1. Who should make the decision?
2. What standards should apply?
3. What procedures should be followed?

The first landmark case dealing with these types of consent issues was *In re Quinlan*.[47] In 1975, 22-year-old Karen Quinlan sustained severe brain

Legal Brief

Persistent vegetative state (PVS) is a condition in which the patient is alive and appears to be awake but has no detectable awareness. It is a permanent organic brain syndrome resulting from prolonged anoxia (lack of oxygen to the brain) and character- ized by the absence of higher mental functions such as thought, reason, and emotion. The PVS patient is incapable of performing voluntary acts and responds only reflexively to external stimuli. There is some controversy about whether the con- dition is reversible, but no case of recovery from PVS has been documented.

damage, perhaps as a result of consuming alcohol or drugs. She was comatose and on a respirator and remained for several months in a persistent vegetative state (see Legal Brief). When the hopelessness of the situation eventually became apparent, Karen's parents asked that her life support system be disconnected. Her physicians and the hospital refused, and her father filed suit to be appointed his daughter's guardian and to have the court authorize the withdrawal of the respirator. (The expression "pull the plug" is sometimes used in these cases, but it hardly does jus- tice to the legal, medical, and emotional issues involved.)

All parties stipulated that Karen was incompetent and that she was not dead by either the classical medical definition of *death* (cessation of circula- tion and respiration) or the definition of *brain death* (permanent cessation of all brain functions, including those of the brain stem; see Legal Brief). At the time, New Jersey did not have a statutory definition of death, and there were no judicial decisions on the concept of brain death, although Karen would not have met the criteria for death—no matter how it would have been measured.

The trial court denied Mr. Quinlan's requests for guardianship and

Legal Brief

Physicians have no legal or ethical duty to treat a dead body. Seemingly obvious, this rule becomes relevant when determining the point at which a person is dead and life support systems may be disconnected. The common law defined *death* as the "cessation of life," which is not a particularly helpful standard. Until the 1970s, death meant the cessation of respiration and circulation. With the use of mechanical respirators and other devices, however, respiration and circulation can often be continued indefinitely. For this reason, most states have adopted *brain death*—the complete cessa- tion of all functions of the entire brain, including the brain stem—as the legal standard for diagnos- ing death.

termination of the respirator.[48] On appeal, the New Jersey Supreme Court held that Mr. Quinlan was entitled to be appointed guardian of his daughter, could select a physician of his choice to care for her, and could participate with this physician and the hospital's medical ethics committee in a decision to withdraw the respirator. The legal basis for the decision was the patient's right of privacy, which gave her (through her guardian) the right to decline treatment.

The court went on to rule that when a patient is incompetent and cannot express her wishes, the guardian may use the *substituted judgment* doctrine—that is, the guardian must determine *what the patient herself would decide* under the circumstances, not necessarily what the guardian thinks is in the patient's best interests or what the guardian would want for himself. To guard against possible abuse, the court required the guardian and the attending physicians to consult with a hospital ethics committee, which would review the medical evidence and render an opinion about the probability that the patient would emerge from her chronic vegetative state.

In summary, the court held that if Mr. Quinlan, the attending physicians, and the hospital's ethics committee concurred, Karen's life support system could be withdrawn without incurring civil or criminal liability, the fear of which was the reason for the physicians' refusal. Having received the judicial imprimatur they were seeking and the ethics committee's approval, the physicians weaned Karen from the respirator; however, she unexpectedly continued to breathe on her own. For the next nine years, she received antibiotics to ward off infection and was fed a high-calorie diet through a nasogastric tube. She died in 1985.

Other courts have followed *Quinlan* and adopted the substituted judgment standard. *Superintendent of Belchertown State School v. Saikewicz* applied it in the case of a 67-year-old man (Saikewicz) who had always been profoundly mentally retarded (he had an IQ of 10 and a mental age of less than 3). He was suffering from an acute form of leukemia for which chemotherapy was the indicated treatment. The state institution where he lived petitioned the court for appointment of a personal guardian and of a guardian ad litem (for the litigation) to decide what treatment he should receive.

His illness was incurable, and without chemotherapy he would die a relatively painless death within weeks or months. With chemotherapy, he had a 30 to 40 percent chance of remission (abatement of symptoms), but if remission occurred it would last for only 2–13 months. The chemotherapy would not cure the illness and was expected to cause serious and painful side effects. The guardian ad litem thought that withholding treatment would be in the patient's best interests; he stated:

> If [Saikewicz] is treated with toxic drugs he will be involuntarily immersed in a state of painful suffering, the reason for which he will never understand. Patients who request treatment know the risks involved and can appreciate the painful side effects when [those side effects] arrive. They know the reason for the pain and their hope makes it tolerable.[49]

The probate judge weighed the factors for and against chemotherapy and concluded that treatment should be withheld. Weighing in favor of treatment were the facts that most people would elect chemotherapy and that chemotherapy would offer the patient a chance for a longer life. Weighing against treatment were the patient's age, the probable side effects, the slim chance of remission versus the certainty that the treatment would cause suffering, the patient's inability to cooperate with those administering the treatment, and the patient's quality of life if the treatment was successful.

Adopting the *Quinlan* standard, the appellate court approved of the probate judge's decision, convinced that it "was based on a regard for [Saikewicz's] actual interests and preferences" and was supported by the facts of the case. However, the court rejected any analysis that would equate *quality* of life with the *value* of a life. It interpreted the judge's reference to "quality of life" "as a reference to the continuing state of pain and disorientation precipitated by the chemotherapy treatment."[50]

Cases involving people who, like Saikewicz, have never been competent and have never been able to express their intentions demonstrate that the substituted judgment doctrine is pure fiction. Surrogate decision makers cannot possibly know what such a patient's "actual interests and preferences" would be. The guardians may be well intentioned and may actually make decisions in the patient's best interests, but any such decisions are subjective and—consciously or not—are based on the values, biases, and experiences of the proxy decision makers (see Legal Brief).

In the years immediately following *Quinlan*, numerous cases addressed the questions of who could make decisions for incompetent patients and whether the courts must be involved in all cases. The *Quinlan* court believed that routine involvement by the courts would be "impossibly cumbersome," and most other courts have agreed. Of course, when the patient has no family or guardian, or when family members disagree about what action to take, the courts are proper forums for resolving the matter. The courts have also become involved when the views of the family members conflict with those of the healthcare providers. One such case, *Cruzan v. Director, Missouri Department of Health*,[51] was the occasion for the US Supreme Court's first—and, to date, only—decision regarding termination of medical treatment for incompetent patients.

The case revolves around Nancy Cruzan, a young woman who lay in PVS at a state hospital as a result of the injuries she suffered in an automobile accident. Although she could breathe without assistance, she had to receive nutrition and hydration through artificial means. Realizing over time that she would never regain her mental faculties, her parents asked officials at the hospital to remove her feeding tube and allow her to die. When the hospital refused, the parents filed suit to compel termination of the treatment. At trial, evidence was presented that Nancy

Legal Brief

The viewpoint that guardians' decisions are influenced by their own beliefs was recognized in another New Jersey case, *Matter of Conroy*, decided the year Karen Quinlan died (1985). The court stated that determining the patients' wishes is impossible and that it is "naïve to pretend that the right to self-determination serves as the basis for substituted decision-making."[86]

had "expressed thoughts at age twenty-five in somewhat serious conversations with a housemate friend that if sick or injured she would not wish to continue her life unless she could live at least 'half-way normally.'"[52] On the basis of this evidence, the trial court ordered in favor of the parents.

The state appealed, and the Missouri Supreme Court reversed the trial court's findings. Although it recognized the right to refuse treatment on the basis of the common-law doctrine of informed consent, the Missouri Supreme Court held that the state had a strong public policy favoring life over death and that evidence of an individual's wishes regarding termination of treatment must be "clear and convincing." The court found that Nancy's "somewhat serious conversation" was not sufficient to meet this standard. On certiorari, the Missouri Supreme Court's decision was affirmed on narrow grounds, with the US Supreme Court holding that nothing in the US Constitution "prohibits Missouri from choosing the rule of decision which it did." The opinion reads, in part, as follows:

> The choice between life and death is a deeply personal decision of obvious and overwhelming finality. We believe Missouri may legitimately seek to safeguard the personal element of this choice through the imposition of heightened evidentiary requirements. It cannot be disputed that the Due Process Clause protects an interest in life as well as interest in refusing life-sustaining medical treatment. Not all incompetent patients will have loved ones available to serve as surrogate decision makers. And even where family members are present, "[t]here will, of course, be some unfortunate situations in which family members will not act to protect a patient." A State is entitled to guard against potential abuses in such situations. Similarly, a State is entitled to consider that a judicial proceeding to make a determination regarding an incompetent's wishes may very well not be an adversarial one, with the added guarantee of accurate fact finding that the adversary process brings with it. Finally, we think a State may properly decline to make judgments about the "quality" of life that a particular individual may enjoy, and simply assert an unqualified interest in the preservation of human life to be weighed against the constitutionally protected interests of the individual.
>
> In our view, Missouri has permissibly sought to advance these interests through the adoption of a "clear and convincing" standard of proof to govern such proceedings.[53]

Following this decision, *Cruzan* returned to the trial court, where the judge—after hearing additional testimony—ruled that the evidence was clear and convincing and thus Nancy's artificial nutrition and hydration could be withdrawn. The state's attorney general declined to appeal, the treatment was terminated, and Nancy died in a matter of days (see Law in Action on next page).

No other state has a clear-and-convincing standard of proof, and thankfully most of these difficult, heartrending decisions today are made by

Law in Action

Nancy Cruzan's artificial feeding was discontinued in mid-December 1990. Fifteen members of Operation Rescue (an antieuthanasia group), including a nurse, appeared at the hospital to reinsert the feeding tube, but they were arrested. Nancy died on December 26, 1990, more than seven years after her auto accident.

The Cruzan family's chief antagonist throughout the ordeal was Missouri Attorney General William L. Webster. He was nominated to run for governor in 1992, but his campaign was marked by allegations of corruption and he lost the election. The following year, Webster pleaded guilty to embezzlement charges stemming from his handling of a workers' compensation fund while he was attorney general. He was sentenced to two years in prison.

Nancy's father, depressed and apparently overwhelmed by grief, took his own life in 1996.

physicians and family members without judicial intervention. One notable exception is the tragic, much publicized, and highly politicized case of Terri Schiavo.

Terri, a 26-year-old woman from St. Petersburg, Florida, suffered a cardiac arrest of undetermined cause on February 25, 1990. Emergency personnel took her to a local hospital, where she was ventilated and given a tracheotomy but never regained consciousness. A PVS patient, she survived on nutrition provided through a feeding tube, received continuous nursing home care, and had no reasonable likelihood of recovery.

In 1998, Terri's husband and guardian Michael petitioned to be allowed to terminate her life support procedures, but her parents opposed this decision. Years of contentious litigation followed, including 13 Florida appellate court decisions and five orders by the US Supreme Court (each of which denied certiorari). On October 15, 2003, the feeding tube was removed, but six days later the Florida legislature passed what came to be known as "Terri's Law"—a single-purpose, politically motivated statute intended to permit Governor Jeb Bush to order reinsertion of the feeding tube. Amid considerable media and public interest, the tube was subsequently reinserted. After more legal maneuvering (Terri's parents opposed her husband's decisions at every turn), the Florida Supreme Court unanimously held Terri's Law to be unconstitutional.

The case returned to the lower courts for more procedural squabbling, more efforts by conservative Republicans and others to overturn the judicial decision, and even an attempt by Congress to hold hearings and thus delay the outcome (see Legal Brief). In the end, the trial court's order to discontinue artificial nutrition and hydration stood, and on March 31, 2005—more than 15 years after she collapsed into unconsciousness—Terri died. Thus concluded one of the longest, saddest, and most contentious right-to-die cases ever.

Legal Brief

The Florida Supreme Court's decision is provided at some length in The Court Decides: *Bush v. Schiavo* at the end of this chapter, not only because it ended the legal phase of this family's long misfortune but also because of the insights it offers on the separation of powers in the US system of government.

Consent Issues for Minors

As previously noted, an emergency involves an immediate threat to life or health that would cause permanent injury or death if treatment were delayed, so express consent is not necessary. The medical advisability of treatment in itself does not create an emergency if a delay to obtain consent would not permanently harm the patient. When the patient is a minor, physicians and hospital staff should normally make a reasonable effort to reach the parents (or the person standing in a parental relationship) if they have an opportunity to do so. If they decide to treat the minor without the parents' consent, the medical emergency should be documented and supported by professional consultation.

Though more than a century old, the case of *Luka v. Lowrie* is most illustrative of a situation involving consent for treatment of a minor.[54] A 15-year-old Michigan boy was hit by a train, and his left foot was "mangled and crushed." He was taken to a hospital and within a few minutes lapsed into unconsciousness. Five physicians examined him and decided that to save his life they would have to amputate his foot. Dr. Lowrie, one of the defendants, inquired about the parents' or other relatives' whereabouts. On learning that no one was available, and seeing the emergent nature of the situation, "the foot was amputated and the patient recovered."

In the subsequent malpractice suit, the patient claimed "that his foot should not have been amputated at all, and particularly that it should not have been amputated without first obtaining his consent or the consent of his parents, who went to the hospital as soon as possible after learning of the accident."[55]

The trial court heard testimony from the plaintiff's experts, who testified that it was possible the foot might have been saved without amputation. On cross-examination, however, they all agreed "that the proper course for a surgeon to pursue . . . is to consult with another or others, and then exercise the best judgment and skill of which he is capable."[56] Because Dr. Lowrie had consulted amid the emergency with four "house surgeons"—all of whom agreed with his opinion that immediate amputation was necessary—the trial court directed a verdict for the defendants, and the Supreme Court of Michigan affirmed:

> The fact that surgeons are called upon daily, in all our large cities, to operate instantly in emergency cases in order that life may be preserved, should be considered. Many small children are injured upon the streets in large cities. To hold that a surgeon must wait until perhaps he may be able to secure the consent of the parents before giving to the injured one the benefit of his skill and learning, to the end that life may be preserved, would, we believe, result in the loss of many

lives which might otherwise be saved. It is not to be presumed that competent surgeons will wantonly operate, nor that they will fail to obtain the consent of parents to operations where such consent may be reasonably obtained in view of the exigency. Their work, however, is highly humane and very largely charitable in character, and no rule should be announced which would tend in the slightest degree to deprive sufferers of the benefit of their services.[57]

Age of Majority

Proper consent for the treatment of minors in cases of nonemergency requires that physicians and hospital personnel first determine the age of majority in their jurisdiction. Under early common law, the age of majority was 21 years but in most states is now 18. (Majority is reached the day before the patient's birthday.) In many jurisdictions, married persons are considered adults—regardless of age—and parents who are minors may consent to the treatment of their children. The statutory and case law of each jurisdiction must be consulted to determine the age and circumstances necessary to have legal permission to consent. Hospitals should have clear policies outlining the age of majority for their states.

Emancipated Minors

Most states have statutes that provide for the emancipation of minors from the "disability of age." California, for example, provides the following:

A person under the age of 18 years is an emancipated minor if any of the following conditions is satisfied:

(a) The person has entered into a valid marriage, whether or not the marriage has been dissolved.

(b) The person is on active duty with the armed forces of the United States.

(c) The person has received a declaration of emancipation pursuant to [another provision of the California Family Code].[58]

California also has a provision specifically allowing minors to consent to their own medical or dental care if they are aged 15 or older, are living apart from their parents, and are managing their own financial affairs.[59]

Mature Minors

A common-law doctrine at work in a few states allows mature minors to consent to medical procedures on their own initiative. For example, the Supreme Court of Tennessee adopted the "mature minor exception" to the parental consent requirement in the case of a patient who was nearly 18 years old at the time she sought treatment. The court wrote as follows:

Whether a minor has the capacity to consent to medical treatment depends upon the age, ability, experience, education, training, and degree of maturity or judgment obtained by the minor, as well as upon the conduct and demeanor of the minor at the time of the incident involved. Moreover, the totality of the circumstances, the nature of the treatment and its risks or probable consequences, and the minor's ability to appreciate the risks and consequences are to be considered. Guided by the presumptions in the Rule of Sevens, these are questions of fact for the jury to decide.

In our opinion, adoption of the mature minor exception to the general common law rule [requiring parental consent] would be wholly consistent with the existing statutory and tort law in this State as part of "the normal course of the growth and development of the law." Accordingly, we hold that the mature minor exception is part of the common law of Tennessee. Its application is a question of fact for the jury to determine whether the minor has the capacity to consent to and appreciate the nature, the risks, and the consequences of the medical treatment involved.[60]

The basis for the common-law rule that a parent's consent is necessary is the belief that minors are incapable, by reason of their youth, of understanding the nature and consequences of their own acts and must therefore be protected from the folly of their decisions. In terms of intelligence and insight, however, there is nothing magical about age 18 or 21—or 57, for that matter. Research reveals no judicial decisions that hold a physician or a hospital liable for treatment of a mature minor without the parents' consent when the treatment was beneficial. Thus, public policy and common sense permit mature minors—depending on the circumstances—to consent to some health services.

Physicians and hospitals should encourage minors to involve their parents in medical decision making, but necessary medical treatment should never be withheld from a mature and knowledgeable minor solely because parental consent has not been obtained. Damages for failure to treat might be far greater than damages for treatment without consent. Accordingly, providers of medical care should develop guidelines for the treatment of minors based on local law, recognized standards of clinical care, and common sense. Statements of professional associations may be helpful in drafting these policy guidelines (see Legal Brief).

Infants and Young Minors

In situations involving young minors, parental consent is clearly necessary (except in emergencies), and occasionally the question arises whether both parents must

Legal Brief

The American Medical Association's Code of Medical Ethics, Opinion 5.055, "Confidential Care for Minors," states in part that "where the law does not require otherwise, physicians should permit a competent minor to consent to medical care and should not notify parents without the patient's consent. Depending on the seriousness of the decision, competence may be evaluated by physicians for most minors."

consent. Normally, the consent of either parent is sufficient, but if the parents are divorced or voluntarily separated, the consent of the custodial parent is preferred. Individuals who have temporary custody of a minor child, whether a relative or not, are not by that fact alone authorized to give consent. Baby-sitters, therefore, have no authority to consent unless given specific authority by the minor's parent. When they are to be away from their children for a significant length of time, prudent parents notify their regular caregivers and give the temporary custodians written authorization. Some states have statutes addressing this situation.

Refusal of Consent for Treatment of Minors

If the parent or guardian consents to treatment but a mature minor refuses, the physician and the hospital should not proceed; if mature minors are capable of giving consent, they are also capable of refusing and should be treated as adults. If the tables are turned—the mature minor consents, but the parents refuse—the minor's wishes should still trump the parents'. In both situations, an effort should first be made to resolve the conflict. (Disregarding the interests of a nonpatient involves less legal risk than disregarding the interests of a patient, especially if the treatment is relatively routine.)

If the parent refuses to consent to treatment of a minor who is incapable of expressing consent, the situation poses greater practical, ethical, and legal difficulties, especially when serious consequences attend the decision. If the patient's condition is too serious to delay treatment until a court order is obtained, the physician and the hospital should proceed with treatment despite parental objections. In situations in which life or health is at stake, humanitarian action to save life is preferable to inaction that may cause death (even if technically the parents may have a viable cause of action). In most of these situations, parents filing suit would be able to receive only small damages, if any. Defense attorneys have a stronger argument if their client tried to save a life rather than stood by passively and watched a child suffer and die.

If clinical judgment favors treatment but the patient's condition will not be seriously harmed by a delay, and if no parental consent is forthcoming, the physician or the hospital should seek a court order. The delay may not be long; it will depend on local procedure and on the working relations that the medical personnel and attorneys have developed with the court. Judges have been known to act quickly and at all hours when necessary.

Under the early common law, parents' refusal to consent was not considered neglect and courts had little power to order medical care for a minor over the parents' objections. All states now have statutes granting the appropriate court jurisdiction to protect the interests of dependent and neglected children. These protective statutes differ, but in general the state, a social agency, a hospital, a physician, and even relatives of a neglected child may petition the court for an order to remove the child from the parents' custody and assign a court-appointed guardian. Most of these statutes also require that suspected child neglect or abuse be reported to the appropriate authorities. Thus, the physician and hospital have an affirmative duty toward a child who needs medical care.

These statutes are a valid exercise of the state's power to protect the general health and welfare of society. Hence, they are constitutional, even when their application conflicts with or violates the parents' religious beliefs. In *State v. Perricone*,[61] the New Jersey Supreme Court affirmed a trial court's order that a blood transfusion be performed on an infant child whose parents were Jehovah's Witnesses. With respect to the constitutional issue of the parents' religious freedom, the court said that

> the [First] Amendment embraces two concepts—freedom to believe and freedom to act. The first is absolute, but, in the nature of things, the second cannot be. The right to practice religion freely does not include the liberty to expose . . . a child . . . to ill health or death. Parents may be free to become martyrs themselves. But it does not follow they are free, in identical circumstances, to make martyrs of their children before they have reached the age of full and legal discretion when they can make that choice for themselves.[62]

Decisions in these types of cases turn on whether parental refusal to consent to medical care for a child fits the state's definition of child neglect. Other factors include the medical condition of the child, whether an emergency is present, the probable outcome if treatment is withheld, the child's age, whether the child's wishes have been considered (even though he is a minor), and the basis for parental refusal. Even in states whose statutes do not explicitly consider refusal to consent as child neglect, most courts have readily found it to be so and have upheld orders for treatment. In *Jefferson v. Griffin Spalding County Hospital Authority*, statutory protection was even extended to an *unborn* child; overriding the religious objections of the pregnant woman, the court transferred custody to the state, and a cesarean section was ordered to save the child's life.[63]

Disabled Newborns

Infants are in the same legal position as other immature minors: The parents are authorized to consent or withhold consent to treatment as long as they are competent to do so and their actions do not constitute neglect of their child. However, modern technology is keeping alive newborn infants who, just a few years ago, would not have survived because of low birth weight or severe birth defects. Decisions to administer or withhold treatment for these newborns can be extremely difficult. Whether a decision to withhold or withdraw treatment constitutes neglect or is medically, ethically, and legally sound is not always clear. Furthermore, the same questions that arise for incompetent adults arise for infants: Who should make such decisions, and what standards should prevail?

If treatment is available that would clearly benefit an ill newborn—particularly if such treatment is necessary to save the child's life or prevent serious, permanent consequences—those providing medical care should respond to the parents' refusal in the manner suggested in the previous section. If time permits, a court order should be sought; if it does not, the child should be treated despite the parents' objections. A third alternative is to render sufficient treatment to keep the child alive, pending judicial decisions about future treatment.

Infants with terminal illnesses or those in PVS have the same rights as incompetent adults with such conditions. Ordinarily, the parents or guardians may have treatment withheld or discontinued if further treatment would be clearly futile or inhumane. *In re L.H.R.* involved a terminally ill infant who was in PVS, and the court found that a life support system was prolonging the dying process rather than the infant's life.[64] The court ruled that the right of a terminally ill person to refuse treatment was not lost because of incompetence or youth. The parent or legal guardian could exercise the right on the child's behalf after the attending physician's diagnosis and prognosis were confirmed by two other physicians who had no interest in the outcome. The court did not require review by either an ethics committee or a court.[65]

Newborns with serious birth defects or extremely low birth weight raise more difficult issues. For example, the proposed treatment may be beneficial, even lifesaving, but will leave the infant with a disability. The disability might be caused by the treatment itself (e.g., blindness from the administration of oxygen), or it might result from an existing condition, such as Down syndrome or spina bifida. In other cases, the proposed therapy might be neither clearly beneficial nor clearly futile: The child might survive with therapy but has only a dim chance of living a long life and likely will suffer. In making these difficult decisions, parents or other surrogates must be fully informed of the medical alternatives and the prognosis, and all means must be used to ensure that such children are protected from decisions that are clearly contrary to their best interests.

The well-publicized case of Baby Doe focused national attention on the manner of deciding whether to treat seriously ill newborns.[66] In 1982, a boy was born in Indiana with Down syndrome and a surgically correctable condition that prevented him from eating normally. His parents discussed his care with attending physicians and decided not to consent to the corrective surgery. Food and water were also to be withheld. Following a petition alleging neglect, a hearing was held within days. The probate court found that his parents were not neglectful but had made a reasonable choice among acceptable medical alternatives. Before an attempted appeal could be processed, Baby Doe died. Thereafter, the parents' decision was widely criticized as being against the best interests of the child.

Another notorious case involved Baby Jane Doe (see chapter 9).[67] The infant was born in 1983 with spina bifida and other serious disorders. Surgery is the usual corrective treatment in such cases, but her parents—after lengthy consultation with neurological experts, nurses, religious counselors, and a social worker—chose to forgo surgery and adopt a more conservative course of treatment. When this decision was challenged in court, physicians testified during the hearing that the parents' choice was "well within accepted medical standards." The trial court opined that the child was being deprived of adequate medical care and that her life was in "imminent danger," but an appellate court reversed the decision. According to the higher court, the record contained no evidence supporting the lower court's finding; instead, the two physicians who testified had agreed "that the parents' choice of a course of conservative treatment, instead of surgery, was well within accepted medical standards and that there was no medical reason to disturb the parents' decision." The appellate court concluded, "This not a case where an infant is being deprived of medical treatment to achieve a quick and supposedly merciful death. Rather, it is a situation where the parents have chosen one course of appropriate medical treatment over another" (see Legal Decision Point).[68]

Cases such as these created a great deal of discussion and legislative activity for a number of years. For example, the federal Child Abuse Treatment and Prevention Act now provides that a state may receive federal grant money only after it establishes procedures and programs for responding to reports of medical neglect, including reports of withholding medically indicated treatment for disabled infants with life-threatening illnesses. The act defines *withholding* as "the failure to respond to the infant's life-threatening conditions by providing treatment (including appropriate nutrition, hydration, and medication) which, in the treating physician's (or physicians') reasonable medical judgment, will be most likely to be effective in ameliorating or correcting all such conditions."[69] Exceptions are allowed if the infant is irreversibly comatose and if the treatment would merely delay death; would not correct all of the life-threatening conditions or would otherwise do nothing to help save the child's life; or would be futile and, under the circumstances, inhumane.[70] Various states have also passed laws covering medical treatment for newborns and other children.

Decisions concerning treatment for seriously ill newborns are clearly no longer

---

Legal Decision Point

The Baby Jane Doe case was decided in large part on the basis of medical opinion that the parents' decision to refuse treatment was medically acceptable. Are such decisions ones for medical experts to make? What other disciplines are relevant? What makes a decision "medically acceptable"? Is a medically acceptable decision necessarily a morally acceptable one?

immune from public scrutiny. Hospitals, physicians, and parents have positive duties to act in a child's best interests. In the past, hospitals or physicians could look the other way if a parent refused consent for necessary care; today, the law imposes a duty to act. As in the case of incompetent adults, hospitals must consult with their attorneys to ascertain the applicable state and federal laws and develop procedures for complying with those laws.

Legislation and Protocols on End-of-Life Issues
Brain Death

As medical science advanced in the 1960s and 1970s, decisions at the end of life presented some vexing legal and ethical questions. One of the first was how to define death, given that respirators are able to keep a body "alive" even after the brain ceases to function. Legislatures responded by adopting some version of the Uniform Determination of Death Act (UDDA), which provides that "an individual who has sustained either (1) irreversible cessation of circulatory and respiratory functions, or (2) irreversible cessation of all functions of the entire brain, including the brain stem, is dead. A determination of death must be made in accordance with accepted medical standards."[71]

"Uniform" laws are model statutes proposed by the Uniform Law Commission for adoption by state legislatures. The UDDA definition has now been adopted in one form or another in virtually every state, either by statute, regulation, or judicial decision.

Advance Directives

Next came cases such as *Quinlan* and *Cruzan,* in which the patient was clearly alive but was in a persistent coma (or even a state of seeming wakefulness) but subsisted on artificial means of life support. Legislatures enacted "natural death" acts and "living will" statutes aimed at allowing terminally ill patients to die with dignity. These laws' approaches to the issue and the types of cases they cover vary from state to state, but they offer guidance and some measure of protection to those who face troubling end-of-life situations.

California was the first to pass such a statute. It provided that competent adults could execute a directive—commonly called a *living will*—to instruct their physician to withhold or withdraw certain life-sustaining procedures in the event of a terminal illness. The law was intended to be a model on which other states could base their own statutes, but soon the courts discovered that the lawmakers had not anticipated the many difficult situations that the living will documents did not address. For example, because the California statute contemplated only terminal illness, living wills provided no succor for individuals such as Karen Quinlan or Nancy Cruzan, whose conditions were not terminal but for whom medical technology was not therapeutic. Living wills also did not assist persons who failed to sign them.

To remedy some of the shortcomings of the living will laws, many states developed durable power of attorney (DPOA) statutes allowing individuals to designate a proxy who will make healthcare decisions for them if they become incompetent (see Legal Brief). The proxy's decisions are as valid as the decisions the patient would have made had she been competent. On behalf of the patient, and applying the substituted judgment doctrine discussed earlier, a proxy can consent to or refuse treatments as though the patient were doing so herself. Physicians who rely in good faith on the decisions of the proxy are provided immunity from civil and criminal liability and professional disciplinary action.[72]

The DPOA laws resolved some of the shortcomings of living wills, but they still required people to take affirmative action to sign the DPOA document and varied from state to state. In the early 1990s, a statutory framework called the Uniform Health-Care Decisions Act (UHCDA) was proposed by the National Conference of Commissioners on Uniform State Laws and backed by the American Bar Association. Adopted by a number of states, this model statute

- affirms an individual's right to decline life-sustaining treatment;
- lets the principal designate an agent to make decisions the principal would make if he were competent;
- is flexible enough to allow the principal to give instructions as broadly or as narrowly as she may choose;
- permits designated surrogates, family members, or close friends to make decisions if no agent or guardian has been appointed;
- allows states to replace their various pieces of legislation with one statute;
- provides an easily understood model form to simplify the directive process;
- requires healthcare providers to comply with the patient's or agent's instructions; and
- lays out a dispute resolution process to be used in the event of disagreements.

A sample UHCDA-model advance directive form is shown in appendix 11.1.

Death with Dignity Laws

In addition to living wills and durable powers of attorney as tools to assist in end-of-life situations, six states now allow

Legal Brief

A regular power of attorney gives an agent the authority to act on behalf of a principal, but it ceases to be effective in the event of the principal's death or disability. A durable power of attorney (either for financial or healthcare affairs) is effective as long as the principal is alive, even if she is incapacitated.

Legal Brief

At the time of publication, physician-assisted dying laws were in effect in Oregon (permitted since late 1997), Washington (2009), Vermont (2013), California (June 2016), and Colorado (by referendum, November 2016). In Montana, physician assistance in dying has been legal since 2009 under a ruling of the state supreme court.

physicians to aid competent, terminally ill patients to end their own lives (see Legal Brief). Oregon's statute was the first of such laws, and it serves as a model for others.[73]

Under the Oregon law, a competent adult resident of the state who has been diagnosed with a terminal illness that will lead to death within six months may request a licensed physician (doctor of medicine or doctor of osteopathy) to prescribe medications to end life. If certain procedural safeguards are met—such as a second physician confirming that the patient meets statutory criteria—the individual may self-administer the medications (usually barbiturates). According to the state's department of health, in the 17 years since the law was enacted, 1,545 people have been provided with prescriptions written for life-ending medications and 991 patients have died from ingesting them.[74]

The Oregon law was opposed by "right to life" groups, conservative members of Congress, and the George W. Bush administration. The issue went to court in 2001 after Attorney General John Ashcroft attempted to investigate and prosecute physicians who prescribed controlled drugs to help terminally ill patients die. The statute was upheld by the trial court, which ruled that the US Department of Justice lacked authority to overturn a state law. The Ninth Circuit agreed, and the case then headed to the US Supreme Court.

On January 17, 2006, Justice Anthony Kennedy delivered the Supreme Court's decision affirming the lower courts.[75] In his opinion, Kennedy ruled that although the attorney general has rulemaking power under the Controlled Substances Act (CSA), "he is not authorized to make a rule declaring illegitimate a medical standard for care and treatment of patients that is specifically authorized under state law."[76] Kennedy added, "The authority claimed by the Attorney General is both beyond his expertise and incongruous with the statutory purposes and design [of the CSA]."[77] Thus the court deferred to the state's determination that use of controlled substances to end life can be considered a legitimate medical purpose.

Despite other attempts in Congress to derail it, the Oregon Death with Dignity Act has been a stable part of Oregon law ever since the Supreme Court ruling. A study conducted in 2013 showed that is the act is supported by about 80 percent of Oregon voters.[78]

The California law, known as the End of Life Option Act,[79] took effect on June 9, 2016. Like the Oregon law, the California statute was quickly challenged in court. The plaintiffs in the case—a number of physicians, the American Academy of Medical Ethics (doing business as the Christian Medical and Dental Society), and Life Legal Defense Foundation—sought an injunction against the law on various grounds, most especially because of a provision stating that actions taken under the law *do not* "constitute suicide, assisted suicide, homicide, or elder abuse."[80] At time of writing (September 2016), the case is pending but the motion for preliminary injunction has been denied. Irrespective of the ultimate outcome in the trial court, an appeal will certainly ensue. Stay tuned.

The National POLST Paradigm

Another important development is a movement to adopt forms that convert patients' preferences for end-of-life care into enforceable medical orders. Issued by a physician or other licensed practitioner, these portable orders are valid in multiple care settings, including acute care hospitals, long-term care facilities, and hospices. The Physician Orders for Life-Sustaining Treatment (POLST), called by various other names in different states, is an effort by the medical and legal communities to overcome the limitations of legal documents such as living wills and advance directives.

Begun in Oregon and now used or being developed in a number of states,[81] POLST is described on the National POLST Paradigm Task Force (NPPTF) website in these terms:

1. The POLST Form is a set of medical orders, similar to the do not resuscitate (allow natural death) order. POLST is not an advance directive. POLST does not substitute for naming a health care agent or durable power of attorney for health care.

2. A POLST Paradigm Form is not for everyone. Only those who are seriously ill or frail, or for whom their physicians would not be surprised if they died in the next year, should have one.

3. The POLST Form is completed as a result of the process of informed, shared decision-making. During the conversation, the patient discusses his or her values, beliefs, and goals for care, and the health care professional presents the patient's diagnosis, prognosis, and treatment alternatives, including the benefits and burdens of life-sustaining treatment. Together they reach an informed decision about desired treatment, based on the person's values, beliefs and goals for care.

4. The POLST Form allows patients to have their religious values respected. For example, the POLST Form allows Catholics to make decisions consistent with the United States Conference of Catholic Bishops Ethical and Religious Directives for Catholic Health Care Services, 5th ed. (2009) and ensures that those decisions will be honored in an emergency and across care transitions.

5. The POLST Form enables physicians to order treatments patients would want and to direct that treatment that patients would not want, those they consider "extraordinary" and excessively burdensome, shall not be provided.

6. The POLST Form requires that "ordinary" measures to improve the patient's comfort and food and fluid by mouth, as tolerated, are always provided.

7. The POLST Form is actionable and prevents initiation of unwanted, disproportionately burdensome extraordinary treatment.

8. State law authorizes certain health care professionals to sign medical orders; the POLST Form is signed by those health care professionals who are accountable for the medical orders.

9. The POLST Paradigm requires health care professionals be trained to conduct shared decision-making discussions with patients and families so that POLST Forms are completed properly.

10. The POLST Form may be signed by the patient or designated decision-maker . . . but it is not required in all states. The NPPTF encourages patient or designated decision-maker signatures for all states seeking endorsement. Informed, shared decision making is a key component of the POLST Paradigm process.

11. The POLST Paradigm recognizes that allowing natural death to occur is not the same as killing. POLST does not allow for active euthanasia or physician assisted suicide.[82]

A sample POLST paradigm form is shown in appendix 11.2. Forms in other states are virtually identical. Depending on the wording of existing legislation, questions about the use of POLST forms may be encountered in some jurisdictions, but most states have either endorsed or are developing a POLST program and would be unlikely to prohibit use of the forms.

All healthcare providers should have procedures for handling end-of-life decisions for patients in accordance with the laws of their state and the patients' or surrogates' instructions. Licensed practitioners should discuss treatment options while the patient has capacity, especially if the illness is considered terminal. The practitioner can call the patient's attention to options for end-of-life care, advance directives, and designation of a surrogate and can then issue enforceable medical orders consistent with the patient's wishes. These orders, the relevant discussions and decisions, and copies of an advance directive, DPOA, POLST, or other such document must be included in the medical record.

Patient Self-Determination Act

The Patient Self-Determination Act of 1991 (PSDA)[83] is a federal law that requires facilities that receive federal funding to summarize the facility's policies regarding advance directives, advise patients of their right to make medical decisions, and obtain and include in the medical record any such documents the patient might have executed. The PSDA also requires that facility staff be educated about these issues and never discriminate against patients on the basis of whether they do or do not have advance directives. These procedures are now a routine part of the patient registration process.

Summary

This chapter explores the difference between *consent* (a concept that arose from the law of battery) and *informed consent* (a concept that relates to the standards of medical practice). If a patient's consent to a medical procedure is not well informed, it is not consent at all. For consent to be informed, the patient or legal surrogate must have a basic understanding of the patient's diagnosis and prognosis, the nature of the proposed treatment, the inherent risks, any possible alternative treatments, and the risks of refusing treatment. The chapter also considers consent issues in emergencies and such thorny issues as the right to die (i.e., refusal to consent to life-sustaining treatment) and consent for patients who are not competent to make choices for themselves (including infants and young children). The chapter ends with discussion of various methods of documenting and enforcing patients' end-of-life preferences: living wills, DPOA, advance directive, POLST, and PSDA.

Discussion Questions

1. What are the two types of consent for medical treatment? When does each apply?
2. What is the standard for consent in an emergency?
3. What is the hospital's role in obtaining informed consent?
4. What is required for informed consent to be valid?
5. What is the parallel between *Helling v. Carey* in chapter 5 and the cases in this chapter that disapprove of the reasonable-doctor rule for informed consent?
6. How does the principle of informed consent apply to competent patients who refuse lifesaving treatment? How does it apply to incompetent patients who have signed an advance directive?
7. How does informed consent apply to someone who had not signed an advance directive? To a newborn? To a mature minor?
8. Under what circumstances may consent be refused for the artificial administration of nutrition and hydration?

9. What are the advantages and disadvantages of living wills, DPOA for healthcare, statutory advance directives, and POLST?

10. What are the requirements of the PSDA?

11. What is the status of the "assisted death" issue in your state, and how do you feel about it?

The Court Decides

Cobbs v. Grant
8 Cal. 3d 229, 502 P.2d 1, 104 Cal. Rptr. 505 (1972)

Mosk, J.

This medical malpractice case involves two issues: first, whether there was sufficient evidence of negligence in the performing of surgery to sustain a jury verdict for plaintiff; second, whether, under plaintiff's alternative theory, the instructions to the jury adequately set forth the nature of a medical doctor's duty to obtain the informed consent of a patient before undertaking treatment. We conclude there was insufficient evidence to support the jury's verdict under the theory that the defendant was negligent during the operation. Since there was a general verdict and we are unable to ascertain upon which of the two concepts the jury relied, we must reverse the judgment and remand for a new trial. To assist the trial court upon remand we analyze the doctor's duty to obtain the patient's informed consent and suggest principles for guidance in drafting new instructions on this question.

Plaintiff was admitted to the hospital in August 1964 for treatment of a duodenal ulcer. He was given a series of tests to ascertain the severity of his condition and, though administered medication to ease his discomfort, he continued to complain of lower abdominal pain and nausea. His family physician, Dr. Jerome Sands, concluding that surgery was indicated, discussed prospective surgery with plaintiff and advised him in general terms of the risks of undergoing a general anesthetic. Dr. Sands called in defendant, Dr. Dudley F. P. Grant, a surgeon, who after examining plaintiff, agreed with Dr. Sands that plaintiff had an intractable peptic duodenal ulcer and that surgery was indicated.

Although Dr. Grant explained the nature of the operation to plaintiff, he did not discuss any of the inherent risks of the surgery.

A two-hour operation was performed the next day, in the course of which the presence of a small ulcer was confirmed. Following the surgery the ulcer disappeared. Plaintiff's recovery appeared to be uneventful, and he was permitted to go home eight days later. However, the day after he returned home, plaintiff began to experience intense pain in his abdomen. He immediately called Dr. Sands who advised him to return to the hospital. Two hours after his readmission plaintiff went into shock and emergency surgery was performed. It was discovered plaintiff was bleeding internally as a result of a severed artery at the hilum of his spleen. Because of the seriousness of the hemorrhaging and since the spleen of an adult may be removed without adverse effects, defendant decided to remove the spleen. Injuries to the spleen that compel a subsequent operation are a risk inherent in the type of surgery performed on plaintiff and occur in approximately 5 percent of such operations.

After removal of his spleen, plaintiff recuperated for two weeks in the hospital. A month after discharge he was readmitted because of sharp pains in his stomach. X-rays disclosed plaintiff was developing a gastric ulcer. The evolution of a new ulcer is another risk inherent in surgery performed to relieve a duodenal ulcer. Dr. Sands initially decided to attempt to treat this nascent gastric ulcer with antacids and a strict diet. However, some four months later plaintiff was again

(continued)

(continued from previous page)

hospitalized when the gastric ulcer continued to deteriorate and he experienced severe pain. When plaintiff began to vomit blood the defendant and Dr. Sands concluded that a third operation was indicated: a gastrectomy with removal of 50 percent of plaintiff's stomach to reduce its acid-producing capacity. Some time after the surgery, plaintiff was discharged, but subsequently had to be hospitalized yet again when he began to bleed internally due to the premature absorption of a suture, another inherent risk of surgery. After plaintiff was hospitalized, the bleeding began to abate and a week later he was finally discharged.

Plaintiff brought this malpractice suit against his surgeon, Dr. Grant. The action was consolidated for trial with a similar action against the hospital. The jury returned a general verdict against the hospital in the amount of $45,000. This judgment has been satisfied. The jury also returned a general verdict against defendant Grant in the amount of $23,800.

He appeals.

The jury could have found for plaintiff either by determining that defendant negligently performed the operation, or on the theory that defendant's failure to disclose the inherent risks of the initial surgery vitiated plaintiff's consent to operate. Defendant attacks both possible grounds of the verdict. He contends, first, [that] there was insufficient evidence to sustain a verdict of negligence, and, second, [that] the [trial] court committed prejudicial error in its instruction to the jury on the issue of informed consent.

[In the first section of the opinion, the court agrees with the defendant's argument that the evidence did not justify a verdict of negligence. Because of the general verdict, the court could not determine on which basis the jury found for the plaintiff. Accordingly, the court reverses the judgment and orders a retrial. In the second section, the court finds that the failure to provide information

on which to make an informed consent decision—although technically a battery—is really a case of professional malpractice (i.e., negligence). The opinion then segues into a discussion of the standard of care in these kinds of cases.]

Since this is an appropriate case for the application of a negligence theory, it remains for us to determine [whether] the standard of care described in the jury instruction on this subject properly delineates defendant's duty to inform plaintiff of the inherent risks of the surgery. In pertinent part, the court gave the following instruction: "A physician's duty to disclose is not governed by the standard practice in the community; rather it is a duty imposed by law. A physician violates his duty to his patient and subjects himself to liability if he withholds any facts which are necessary to form the basis of an intelligent consent by the patient to the proposed treatment."

Defendant raises two objections to the foregoing instruction. First, he points out that the majority of the California cases have measured the duty to disclose not in terms of an absolute, but as a duty to reveal such information as would be disclosed by a doctor in good standing within the medical community. . . . One commentator has imperiously declared that "good medical practice is good law." Moreover, with one state and one federal exception every jurisdiction that has considered this question has adopted the community standard as the applicable test. Defendant's second contention is that this near unanimity reflects strong policy reasons for vesting in the medical community the unquestioned discretion to determine [whether] the withholding of information by a doctor from his patient is justified at the time the patient weighs the risks of the treatment against the risks of refusing treatment.

The thesis that medical doctors are invested with discretion to withhold information from their patients has been frequently ventilated in both legal and medical literature. . . . Despite what defendant characterizes as the prevailing rule, it has never been unequivocally adopted by an authoritative source. Therefore we probe anew into the rationale which purportedly justifies, in accordance with medical rather than legal standards, the withholding of information from a patient.

Preliminarily we employ several postulates. The first is that patients are generally persons unlearned in the medical sciences and therefore, except in rare cases, courts may safely assume the knowledge of patient and physician are not in parity. The second is that a person of adult years and in sound mind has the right, in the exercise of control over his own body, to determine whether or not to submit to lawful medical treatment. The third is that the patient's consent to treatment, to be effective, must be an informed consent. And the fourth is that the patient, being unlearned in medical sciences, has an abject dependence upon and trust in his physician for the information upon which he relies during the decisional process, thus raising an obligation in the physician that transcends arms-length transactions.

From the foregoing axiomatic ingredients emerges a necessity, and a resultant requirement, for divulgence by the physician to his patient of all information relevant to a meaningful decisional process. In many instances, to the physician, whose training and experience enable a self-satisfying evaluation, the particular treatment which should be undertaken may seem evident, but it is the prerogative of the patient, not the physician, to determine for himself the direction in which he believes his interests lie. To enable the patient to chart his course knowledgeably, reasonable familiarity with the therapeutic alternatives and their hazards becomes essential.

Therefore, we hold, as an integral part of the physician's overall obligation to the patient there is a duty of reasonable disclosure of the available choices with respect to proposed therapy and of the dangers inherently and potentially involved in each.

A concomitant issue is the yardstick to be applied in determining reasonableness of disclosure. This defendant and the majority of courts have related the duty to the custom of physicians practicing in the community. The majority rule is needlessly overbroad. Even if there can be said to be a medical community standard as to the disclosure requirement for any prescribed treatment, it appears so nebulous that doctors become, in effect, vested with virtual absolute discretion. Unlimited discretion in the physician is irreconcilable with the basic right of the patient to make the ultimate informed decision regarding the course of treatment to which he knowledgeably consents to be subjected.

A medical doctor, being the expert, appreciates the risks inherent in the procedure he is prescribing, the risks of a decision not to undergo the treatment, and the probability of a successful outcome of the treatment. But once this information has been disclosed, that aspect of the doctor's expert function has been performed. The weighing of these risks against the individual subjective fears and hopes of the patient is not an expert skill. Such evaluation and decision is a nonmedical judgment reserved to the patient alone. A patient should be denied the opportunity to weigh the risks only where it is evident he cannot evaluate the data, as for example, where there is an emergency or the patient is a child or incompetent. For this reason, the law provides that in an emergency consent is implied, and if the patient is a minor or incompetent, the authority to consent is transferred to the patient's legal guardian or closest available relative. In all cases other than the foregoing, the decision whether or not to undertake treatment is

(continued)

(continued from previous page)

vested in the party most directly affected: the patient.

The scope of the disclosure required of physicians defies simple definition. Some courts have spoken of "full disclosure" and others refer to "full and complete" disclosure, but such facile expressions obscure common practicalities. Two qualifications to a requirement of "full disclosure" need little explication. First, the patient's interest in information does not extend to a lengthy polysyllabic discourse on all possible complications. A mini-course in medical science is not required; the patient is concerned with the risk of death or bodily harm, and problems of recuperation. Second, there is no physician's duty to discuss the relatively minor risks inherent in common procedures, when it is common knowledge that such risks inherent in the procedure are of very low incidence. When there is a common procedure a doctor must, of course, make such inquiries as are required to determine if for the particular patient the treatment under consideration is contraindicated—for example, to determine if the patient has had adverse reactions to antibiotics; but no warning beyond such inquiries is required as to the remote possibility of death or serious bodily harm.

However, when there is a more complicated procedure, as the surgery in the case before us, the jury should be instructed that when a given procedure inherently involves a known risk of death or serious bodily harm, a medical doctor has a duty to disclose to his patient the potential of death or serious harm, and to explain in lay terms the complications that might possibly occur. Beyond the foregoing minimal disclosure, a doctor must also reveal to his patient such additional information as a skilled practitioner of good standing would provide under similar circumstances.

In sum, the patient's right of self-decision is the measure of the physician's duty to reveal. That right can be effectively exercised only if the patient possesses adequate information to enable an intelligent choice. The scope of the physician's communications to the patient, then, must be measured by the patient's need, and that need is whatever information is material to the decision. Thus the test for determining whether a potential peril must be divulged is its materiality to the patient's decision.

We point out, for guidance on retrial, an additional problem which suggests itself. There must be a causal relationship between the physician's failure to inform and the injury to the plaintiff. Such causal connection arises only if it is established that had revelation been made consent to treatment would not have been given. Here the record discloses no testimony that had plaintiff been informed of the risks of surgery he would not have consented to the operation.

The patient-plaintiff may testify on this subject but the issue extends beyond his credibility. Since at the time of trial the uncommunicated hazard has materialized, it would be surprising if the patient-plaintiff did not claim that had he been informed of the dangers he would have declined treatment. Subjectively he may believe so, with the 20/20 vision of hindsight, but we doubt that justice will be served by placing the physician in jeopardy of the patient's bitterness and disillusionment. Thus an objective test is preferable: i.e., what would a prudent person in the patient's position have decided if adequately informed of all significant perils. . . .

Whenever appropriate, the court should instruct the jury on the defenses available to a doctor who has failed to make the disclosure required by law. Thus, a medical doctor need not make disclosure of risks when the patient requests that he not be so informed. Such a disclosure need not be made if the procedure is simple and the danger remote and commonly appreciated to be remote. A disclosure need not be made beyond that required within the medical community when a doctor can prove . . . [that] he relied upon facts which would demonstrate to a reasonable man the disclosure would have so seriously upset the patient that the patient would not have been able to dispassionately weigh the risks of refusing to undergo the recommended treatment. Any defense, of course, must be consistent with what has been termed the "fiducial qualities" of the physician-patient relationship.

The judgment is reversed.

Discussion Questions

1. How do you suppose the physician community reacted to this decision?
2. How would you explain the decision to someone who disagrees with it?
3. Is it fair for Dr. Grant to be held to a standard of care that did not exist at the time of Cobbs's treatment?
4. Can you explain why the reasonable-patient test is called "objective" while testimony from the patient on the question of causation is considered unreliable?
5. The court said there was not enough evidence to support a verdict of negligence, yet the original gastrectomy led to multiple hospital stays and two follow-up surgeries. These complications were known risks that can occur even if the surgeon performs the operation flawlessly. If you were the patient and knew about these risks, would you decide to consent to the first surgery? What factors would you consider?

~ ~

The Court Decides

Bush v. Schiavo
885 So. 2d. 321 (2004)

Pariente, C.J.

[The facts of the case are summarized in the text on p. 400. In addressing the constitutionality of Terri's Law, the Florida Supreme Court provides insights into the separation of powers between branches of government and the legislature's attempt to interfere in the judicial process.]

The narrow issue in this case requires this Court to decide the constitutionality of a law passed by the Legislature that directly affected Theresa Schiavo, who has been in a persistent vegetative state since 1990. This Court, after careful consideration of the arguments of the parties and amici, the constitutional issues raised, the precise wording of the challenged law, and the underlying procedural history of this case, concludes that the law violates the fundamental constitutional tenet of separation of powers and is therefore unconstitutional both on its face and as applied to Theresa Schiavo. Accordingly, we affirm the trial court's order declaring the law unconstitutional.

(continued)

(continued from previous page)

ANALYSIS

We begin our discussion by emphasizing that our task in this case is to review the constitutionality of chapter 2003-418 [Terri's Law], not to reexamine the guardianship court's orders directing the removal of Theresa's nutrition and hydration tube, or to review the Second District's numerous decisions in the guardianship case. Although we recognize that the parties continue to dispute the findings made in the prior proceedings, these proceedings are relevant to our decision only to the extent that they occurred and resulted in a final judgment directing the withdrawal of life-prolonging procedures.

The language of [the statute] is clear. It states in full:

> Section 1. (1) The Governor shall have the authority to issue a one-time stay to prevent the withholding of nutrition and hydration from a patient if, as of October 15, 2003:
>
> > (a) That patient has no written advance directive;
> > (b) The court has found that patient to be in a persistent vegetative state;
> > (c) That patient has had nutrition and hydration withheld; and
> > (d) A member of that patient's family has challenged the withholding of nutrition and hydration.
>
> (2) The Governor's authority to issue the stay expires 15 days after the effective date of this act, and the expiration of the authority does not impact the validity or the effect of any stay issued pursuant to this act. The Governor may lift the stay authorized under this act at any time. A person may not be held civilly liable and is not subject to regulatory or disciplinary sanctions for taking any action to comply with a stay issued by the Governor pursuant to this act.
>
> (3) Upon issuance of a stay, the chief judge of the circuit court shall appoint a guardian ad litem for the patient to make recommendations to the Governor and the court.
>
> Section 2. This act shall take effect upon becoming a law.

Thus, chapter 2003-418 allowed the Governor to issue a stay to prevent the withholding of nutrition and hydration from a patient under the circumstances provided for in subsections (1)(a)-(d). Under the fifteen-day sunset provision, the Governor's authority to issue the stay expired on November 5, 2003. The Governor's authority to lift the stay continues indefinitely.

. . .

SEPARATION OF POWERS

The cornerstone of American democracy known as separation of powers recognizes three separate branches of government—the executive, the legislative, and the judicial—each with its own powers and responsibilities. In Florida, the constitutional doctrine has been expressly codified in article II, section 3 of the Florida Constitution, which not only divides state government into three branches but also expressly prohibits one branch from exercising the powers of the other two branches:

> Branches of Government.—The powers of the state government shall be divided into legislative, executive and judicial branches. No person belonging to one branch shall exercise any powers appertaining to either of the other branches unless expressly provided herein.

. . .

Encroachment on the Judicial Branch

In this case, the undisputed facts show that the guardianship court authorized Michael to proceed with the discontinuance of Theresa's life support after the issue was fully litigated in a proceeding in which the Schindlers were afforded the opportunity to present evidence on all issues. This order as well as the order denying the Schindlers' motion for relief from judgment were affirmed on direct appeal. The Schindlers sought review in this Court, which was denied. Thereafter, the tube was removed. Subsequently, pursuant to the Governor's executive order, the nutrition and hydration tube was reinserted. Thus, the Act, as applied in this case, resulted in an executive order that effectively reversed a properly rendered final judgment and thereby constituted an unconstitutional encroachment on the power that has been reserved for the independent judiciary.

. . .

Under procedures enacted by the Legislature . . . circuit courts are charged with adjudicating issues regarding incompetent individuals. The trial courts of this State are called upon to make many of the most difficult decisions facing society. [T]hese decisions literally affect the lives or deaths of patients. The trial courts also handle other weighty decisions affecting the welfare of children such as termination of parental rights and child custody. When the prescribed procedures are followed according to our rules of court and the governing statutes, a final judgment is issued, and all post-judgment procedures are followed, it is without question an invasion of the authority of the judicial branch for the Legislature to pass a law that allows the executive branch to interfere with the final judicial determination in a case. That is precisely what occurred here and for that reason the Act is unconstitutional as applied to Theresa Schiavo.

Delegation of Legislative Authority

In addition to concluding that the Act is unconstitutional as applied in this case

because it encroaches on the power of the judicial branch, we further conclude that the Act is unconstitutional on its face because it delegates legislative power to the Governor. The Legislature is permitted to transfer subordinate functions "to permit administration of legislative policy by an agency with the expertise and flexibility to deal with complex and fluid conditions." However, under article II, section 3 of the constitution the Legislature "may not delegate the power to enact a law or the right to exercise unrestricted discretion in applying the law." This prohibition, known as the nondelegation doctrine, requires that "fundamental and primary policy decisions . . . be made by members of the legislature who are elected to perform those tasks, and [that the] administration of legislative programs must be pursuant to some minimal standards and guidelines ascertainable by reference to the enactment establishing the program." In other words, statutes granting power to the executive branch "must clearly announce adequate standards to guide . . . in the execution of the powers delegated. The statute must so clearly define the power delegated that the [executive] is precluded from acting through whim, showing favoritism, or exercising unbridled discretion."

. . .

In this case, the circuit court found that chapter 2003-418 contains no guidelines or standards that "would serve to limit the Governor from exercising completely unrestricted discretion in applying the law to" those who fall within its terms. The circuit court explained:

> The terms of the Act affirmatively confirm the discretionary power conferred upon the Governor. He is given the "authority to issue a one-time stay to prevent the withholding of nutrition and hydration from a patient" under

(continued)

(continued from previous page)

certain circumstances but, he is not required to do so. Likewise, the act provides that the Governor "*may* lift the stay authorized under this act at any time. The Governor *may* revoke the stay upon a finding that a change in the condition of the patient warrants revocation." (Emphasis added). In both instances there is nothing to provide the Governor with any direction or guidelines for the exercise of this delegated authority. The Act does not suggest what constitutes "a change in condition of the patient" that could "warrant revocation." Even when such an undefined "change" occurs, the Governor is not compelled to act. The Act confers upon the Governor the unfettered discretion to determine what the terms of the Act mean and when, or if, he may act under it.

We agree with this analysis. [T]he Legislature failed to provide any standards by which the Governor should determine whether, in any given case, a stay should be issued and how long a stay should remain in effect. Further, the Legislature has failed to provide any criteria for lifting the stay. This absolute, unfettered discretion to decide whether to issue and then when to lift a stay makes the Governor's decision virtually unreviewable. . . .

CONCLUSION
We recognize that the tragic circumstances underlying this case make it difficult to put emotions aside and focus solely on the legal issue presented. We are not insensitive to the struggle that all members of Theresa's family have endured since she fell unconscious in 1990. However, we are a nation of laws and we must govern our decisions by the rule of law and not by our own emotions. Our hearts can fully comprehend the grief so fully demonstrated by Theresa's family members on

this record. But our hearts are not the law. What is in the Constitution always must prevail over emotion. Our oaths as judges require that this principle is our polestar, and it alone.

As the Second District noted in one of the multiple appeals in this case, we "are called upon to make a collective, objective decision concerning a question of law. Each of us, however, has our own family, our own loved ones, our own children. . . . But in the end, this case is not about the aspirations that loving parents have for their children." Rather, as our decision today makes clear, this case is about maintaining the integrity of a constitutional system of government with three independent and coequal branches, none of which can either encroach upon the powers of another branch or improperly delegate its own responsibilities.

The continuing vitality of our system of separation of powers precludes the other two branches from nullifying the judicial branch's final orders. If the Legislature with the assent of the Governor can do what was attempted here, the judicial branch would be subordinated to the final directive of the other branches. Also subordinated would be the rights of individuals, including the well-established privacy right to self-determination. No court judgment could ever be considered truly final and no constitutional right truly secure, because the precedent of this case would hold to the contrary. Vested rights could be stripped away based on popular clamor. The essential core of what the Founding Fathers sought to change from their experience with English rule would be lost, especially their belief that our courts exist precisely to preserve the rights of individuals, even when doing so is contrary to popular will.

The trial court's decision regarding Theresa Schiavo was made in accordance with the procedures and protections set forth by the judicial branch and in accordance with the statutes passed by the Legislature in effect at that time. That decision is final and the Legislature's attempt to alter that final adjudication is unconstitutional as applied to Theresa Schiavo. Further, even if there had been no final judgment in this case, the Legislature provided the Governor constitutionally inadequate standards for the application of the legislative authority delegated in [the statute]. Because chapter 2003-418 runs afoul of article II, section 3 of the Florida Constitution in both respects, we affirm the circuit court's final summary judgment.

It is so ordered. ◼

Discussion Questions

1. Be prepared to describe the religious, political, and sociological factors that may have influenced this drama.
2. On what grounds, if any, might Congress have jurisdiction over these types of issues?
3. If this kind of case were to arise at your healthcare facility, how might you attempt to avoid this lengthy, contentious, and expensive conflict?

Notes

1. 211 N.Y. 125, 129, 105 N.E. 92, 93 (1914).
2. *See, e.g.*, Canterbury v. Spence, 464 F.2d 772 (D.C. Cir. 1972), *and* Cobbs v. Grant, 8 Cal. 3d 229, 104 Cal. Rptr. 505 (1972).
3. 119 So. 2d 649 (La. Ct. App. 1960); *see also* Pegram v. Sisco, 406 F. Supp. 776 (D. Ark. 1976) (a signed consent form in generalized language does not relieve a surgeon from explaining the nature of diagnosis, material elements, and risks of recommended treatment using radium implants as well as alternative methods of treatment).
4. Perna v. Pirozzi, 92 N.J. 446, 457 A.2d 431 (1983).
5. *See, e.g.*, Demers v. Gerety, 85 N.M. 641, 515 P.2d 645 (Ct. App. 1973) (a consent form signed when a patient was under the influence of Nembutal was not effective); *rev'd and remanded on procedural grounds*, 86 N.M. 141, 520 P.2d 869 (1974).
6. *See* Zoski v. Gaines, 271 Mich. 1, 260 N.W. 99 (1935), in which a surgeon was held liable for removal of a minor's tonsils without parental consent. For a contrasting situation involving an immediate threat to life or health, see Luka v. Lowrie, 171 Mich. 122, 136 N.W. 1106 (1912), discussed in this chapter under the section "Consent Issues for Minors."
7. 42 U.S.C. § 1395dd(e).

8. *See, e.g.*, Mohr v. Williams, 95 Minn. 261, 104 N.W. 12 (1905); Wells v. Van Nort, 100 Ohio St. 101 (1919); Tabor v. Scobee, 254 S.W.2d 474 (Ky. Ct. App. 1951).

9. Smith v. Portera, No. E2004-02960-COA-R3-CV (TN 5/27/2005).

10. Davidson v. Shirley, 616 F.2d 224 (5th Cir. 1980).

11. *Id.* at 226.

12. Cooper v. Curry, 92 N.M. 417, 589 P.2d 201 (N.M. App., 1978); *see also* Magana v. Elie, 108 Ill. App. 3d 1028, 439 N.E.2d 1319 (1982).

13. Fiorentino v. Wenger, 19 N.Y.2d 407, 227 N.E.2d 296, 280 N.Y.S.2d 373 (1967). *See also* Cross v. Trapp, 294 S.E.2d 446 (W. Va. 1982) (as a matter of law, a hospital is not liable for a physician's alleged inadequate explanation of risks of surgery).

14. *Supra* note 3.

15. 71 Nev. 280, 289 P.2d 173 (1955).

16. 251 Minn. 427, 88 N.W.2d 186 (1958).

17. 186 Kan. 393, 350 P.2d 1093 (1960), *second opinion*, 187 Kan. 186, 354 P.2d 670 (1960).

18. 334 S.W.2d 11 (Mo. 1960), 79 A.L.R.2d 1017; 360 S.W.2d 673 (Mo. 1962) (retrial in this litigation resulted in a verdict for defendants as they satisfactorily proved that they had adequately informed the patient). *See also* Shack v. Holland, 389 N.Y.S.2d 988 (Sup. Ct. 1976) (the absence of informed consent from a mother with respect to risks, hazards, and alternative delivery procedures is malpractice and gives the child born permanently deformed a derivative cause of action; the statute of limitations begins to run when the child is 21 years old).

19. 110 R.I. 606, 295 A.2d 676 (1972).

20. 8 Cal. 3d 229, 104 Cal. Rptr. 505 (1972).

21. Truman v. Thomas, 27 Cal. 3d 285, 165 Cal. Rptr. 308, 611 P.2d 902 (1980).

22. Lester v. Aetna Casualty Co., 240 F.2d 676 (5th Cir. 1957); Roberts v. Woods, 206 F. Supp. 579 (S.D. Ala. 1962); Nishi v. Hartwell, 52 Haw. 188, 473 P.2d 116, *reh'g denied*, 52 Haw. 296 (1970); Harnish v. Children's Hosp. Medical Center, 387 Mass. 152, 439 N.E.2d 240 (1982); Starnes v. Taylor, 272 N.C. 386, 158 S.E.2d 339 (1968).

23. Karp v. Cooley, 349 F. Supp. 827 (S.D. Tex. 1972), *aff'd*, 493 F.2d 408 (5th Cir.), *cert. denied*, 419 U.S. 845 (1974); *see also* Schwartz v. Boston Hosp. for Women, 422 F. Supp. 53 (S.D.N.Y. 1976) (a hospital has a responsibility to obtain informed consent when the patient is a participant in a surgical research program).

24. US Dep't of HEW, *Part A, Boundaries Between Practice & Research*, ETHICAL PRINCIPLES AND GUIDELINES FOR THE PROTECTION OF HUMAN

SUBJECTS OF RESEARCH ("The Belmont Report") (originally published April 18, 1979; online version reviewed March 15, 2016), at http://www.hhs.gov/ohrp/regulations-and-policy/belmont-report/.

25. National Research Act, Pub. L. No. 93-348, 88 Stat. 342 (codified in various sections of Title 42, U.S.C.), *and* 45 C.F.R., Part 46.

26. Jeffcoat v. Phillips, 417 S.W.2d 903 (Tex. Civ. App. 1967) (a husband's consent was not necessary for surgery on his wife; jury found as fact that the patient had given effective consent); Rytkonen v. Lojacono, 269 Mich. 270, 257 N.W. 703 (1934) (a wife's consent was not necessary for operation on her husband; he had consented); Janney v. Housekeeper, 70 Md. 162, 16 A. 382 (1889) (a husband's consent was not necessary for surgical procedure on his wife); Gravis v. Physician's and Surgeon's Hosp. of Alice, 427 S.W.2d 310 (Tex. 1968) ("the relationship of husband and wife does not in itself make one spouse the agent of the other").

27. Murray v. Vandevander, 522 P.2d 302 (Okla. Ct. App. 1974).

28. Fla. Stat. § 765.401.

29. *See, e.g.*, Satz v. Perlmutter, 362 So. 2d 160 (Fla. Dist. Ct. 1978), *approved*, 379 So. 2d 359 (Fla. 1980) (a 73-year-old man with Lou Gehrig's disease had a right to have his mechanical respirator disconnected); In re Quackenbush, 156 N.J. Super. 282, 383 A.2d 785 (Morris County Ct. 1978) (a competent patient with a gangrenous condition in both legs could refuse consent to amputation even though it was necessary to save his life); Kirby v. Spivey, 167 Ga. App. 751, 307 S.E.2d 538 (1983) (it is not malpractice for a physician to respect the refusal of a competent patient to seek recommended treatment); Erickson v. Dilgard, 44 Misc. 2d 27, 252 N.Y.S.2d 705 (Sup. Ct. 1962) (the court refused to order a blood transfusion for a competent adult); Winters v. Miller, 446 F.2d 65 (2d Cir.), *cert. denied*, 404 U.S.985 (1971) (medication may not be administered to a mentally ill patient contrary to her wishes when she has not been declared legally incompetent); In re Estate of Brooks, 32 Ill. 2d 361, 205 N.E.2d 435 (1965) (a court may not order administration of blood contrary to a patient's wishes based on religious convictions); Palm Springs Gen. Hosp. v. Martinez, No. 71–12687 (Cir. Ct. Fla. 1971) (physicians and hospital were not civilly liable for complying with a competent, terminally ill patient's wishes to withdraw treatment).

30. Eichner v. Dillon, 73 A.D.2d 431, 426 N.Y.S.2d 517 (1980).

31. *See, e.g.,* Appel, "A Duty to Kill? A Duty to Die? Rethinking the Euthanasia Controversy of 1906," 78 BULL. HIST. MED. 610 (2004), *and* Emanuel, "The History of Euthanasia Debates in the United States and Britain," 121 ANN. INT. MED. 793 (1994).

32. "End of Life Option Act," Cal. Health & Safety Code Part 1.85.

33. *See* Washington v. Glucksberg, 521 U.S. 702 (1997) *and* Vacco v. Quill, 521 U.S. 793 (1997).

34. Gonzales v. Oregon, 546 U.S. 243 (2006).

35. In re Quackenbush, 156 N.J. Super. at 290, 383 A.2d at 789.

36. 331 F.2d 1000, 118 App. D.C. 80 (1964); *see also* Raleigh Fitkin-Paul Morgan Memorial Hosp. v. Anderson, 42 N.J. 421, 201 A.2d 537, *cert. denied*, 337 U.S. 985 (1964) (a blood transfusion was ordered to preserve the life of an unborn child; courts also order treatment to protect the public's health). *See also* Jacobson v. Massachusetts, 197 U.S. 11 (1905) (compulsory vaccination).

37. In re Osborne, 294 A.2d 372 (D.C. Cir. 1972).

38. In re Eichner, 73 A.D.2d at 456, 426 N.Y.S.2d at 537.

39. In John F. Kennedy Memorial Hosp. v. Heston, 58 N.J. 576, 279 A.2d 670 (1971), the court—in ruling that the state had a compelling interest to preserve the life of a 22-year-old competent adult—ordered blood transfusions despite her refusal on religious grounds, giving great weight to the interests of the hospital, nurses, and physicians in carrying out their professional duties. *Heston* was expressly overruled in In re Conroy, 98 N.J. 321, 486 A.2d 1209 (1985).

40. In re Quinlan, 70 N.J. 10, 355 A.2d 647, 667, *cert. denied*, 429 U.S. 922 (1976); *see also* Leach v. Akron Gen. Medical Center, 68 Ohio Misc. 1, 426 N.E.2d 809 (1980).

41. Bartling v. Superior Court, 163 Cal. App. 3d 186, 209 Cal. Rptr. 220 (1984) (a competent adult with serious illnesses that were incurable but not diagnosed as terminal had a right to have life support equipment disconnected); Tune v. Walter Reed Army Medical Center, 602 F. Supp. 1452 (D.C.D.C. 1985) (a 71-year-old woman with terminal adenocarcinoma had a right to have the respirator that sustained her life disconnected in spite of US Army policy precluding the withdrawal of life support systems); Satz v. Perlmutter, 379 So. 2d 359 (Fla. 1980) (a 73-year-old competent patient had a right to have a respirator removed when all affected family members consented).

42. *See, e.g.*, In re Melideo, 88 Misc. 2d 974, 390 N.Y.S.2d 523 (Sup. Ct. 1976) (a Jehovah's Witness was permitted to refuse blood transfusion, even though death was likely to result); Lane v. Candura, 6 Mass. App. 377, 376 N.E.2d 1232 (1978) (the court would not order amputation of the gangrenous leg of a 77-year-old competent woman over her objection).

43. In re Plaza Health & Rehabilitation Center (Sup. Ct., Onandaga County, N.Y., February 2, 1984).

44. Bouvia v. Riverside County Gen. Hosp., No. 159780 (Super. Ct., Riverside City, Cal., December 16, 1983).

45. Bouvia v. Superior Court (Glenchur), 179 Cal. App. 3d 1127, 225 Cal. Rptr. 297 (1986).

46. *See, e.g.*, In re Torres, 357 N.W.2d 332 (Minn. 1984); Severns v. Wilmington Medical Center, Inc., 421 A.2d 1334 (Del. 1980); John F. Kennedy Memorial Hosp., Inc. v. Bludworth, 452 So. 2d 921 (Fla. 1984), *aff'g* 432 So. 2d 611 (Fla. Dist. Ct. App. 1983); Superintendent of Belchertown State School v. Saikewicz, 373 Mass. 728, 370 N.E.2d 417 (1977); In re Quinlan, 70 N.J. 10, 355 A.2d 647, *cert. denied*, 429 U.S. 922 (1976); Eichner v. Dillon, 73 A.D.2d 431, 426 N.Y.S.2d 517 (1980); In re Storar, 52 N.Y.2d 363, 420 N.E.2d 64, 438 N.Y.S.2d 266, *cert. denied*, 454 U.S. 858 (1981); Leach v. Akron Gen. Medical Center, 68 Ohio Misc. 1, 426 N.E.2d 809 (1980); In re Colyer, 99 Wash. 2d 114, 660 P.2d 738 (1983).

47. 70 N.J. 10, 355 A.2d 647 (1976).

48. In re Quinlan, 137 N.J. Super. 227, 348 A.2d 801 (Ch. Div. 1975), *modified*, 70 N.J. 10 (1976).

49. 373 Mass. 728, 370 N.E.2d 417 (1977).

50. 373 Mass. at 754–5. Other cases applying the substituted judgment doctrine include In re Hier, 18 Mass. App. 200, 464 N.E.2d 959 (1984); John F. Kennedy Memorial Hosp., Inc. v. Bludworth, 452 So. 2d 921 (Fla. 1984), *aff'd* 432 So. 2d 611 (Fla. Dist. Ct. App. 1983); In re Storar, 52 N.Y.2d 363, 420 N.E.2d 64, 438 N.Y.S.2d 266, *cert. denied*, 454 U.S. 858 (1981).

51. 497 U.S. 261 (1990).

52. *Id.* at 268.

53. *Id.* at 281–82.

54. 171 Mich. 122, 136 N.W. 1106 (1912).

55. 136 N.W. at 1106.

56. *Id.* at 1109.

57. *Id.* at 1110–11.

58. Cal. Fam. Code § 7002.

59. Cal. Fam. Code § 6922.

60. Cardwell v. Bechtol, 724 S.W.2d 739 (Tenn. 1987).

61. 37 N.J. 463, 181 A.2d 751 (1962), *cert. denied*, 371 U.S. 890 (1962).

62. 37 N.J. at 472, 474.

63. 247 Ga. 86, 274 S.E.2d 457 (1981).

64. 253 Ga. 439, 321 S.E.2d 716 (1984).

65. *See also* In re Guardianship of Barry, 445 So. 2d 365 (Fla. App. 2d Dist. 1984) (the court authorized parents to consent to withdrawal of life support systems for a terminally ill, comatose 10-month-old child on the basis of the child's right to privacy); In re Benjamin C. (Sup. Ct. Cal., February 15, 1979) (consistent with generally accepted medical standards, parents could rely on the physician's judgment in authorizing disconnection of life support systems for a 3-year-old auto accident victim who was comatose); Custody of a Minor, 385 Mass. 697, 434 N.E.2d 601 (1982) (the court applied the substituted judgment doctrine and authorized a "do not resuscitate" order for an abandoned, terminally ill newborn; the medical testimony was that heroic efforts to resuscitate the infant would not be in the child's best interests and would "offend medical ethics").

66. In re Infant Doe, No. 1-782A157 (Ind. App., April 14, 1982). The medical circumstances of Baby Doe are described in a letter from John E. Pless, MD, to the editor of the *New England Journal of Medicine*, titled "The Story of Baby Doe," 309 New Eng. J. of Med. 664 (1983).

67. Weber v. Stony Brook Hosp., 467 N.Y.S.2d 685, 95 A.D.2d 587 (1983), *aff'd*, 469 N.Y.S.2d 63, 60 N.Y.2d 208 (1983).

68. *Id.* at 467 N.Y.S.2d 687, 95 A.D. 589.

69. 42 U.S.C. § 501(g)(5).

70. *See* 42 U.S.C. §§ 5106a and 5106g.

71. *See*, Uniform Law Commission, *Determination of Death Act* (accessed September 9, 2016), at http://www.uniformlaws.org/Act.aspx?title=Determination%20of%20Death%20Act.

72. *See, e.g.*, Cal. Civ. Code §§ 2430/2443 (West Supp. 1985).

73. Or. Rev. Stat. §§ 127.800 to 127.897 (2015).

74. Oregon Public Health Division, *Oregon Death with Dignity Act: 2015 Data Summary* (published February 4, 2016), at https://public.health.oregon.gov/ProviderPartnerResources/EvaluationResearch/DeathwithDignityAct/Documents/year18.pdf.

75. Gonzales v. Oregon, 546 U.S. 243 (2006).

76. *Id.* at 258.

77. *Id.* at 267.

78. Peggy Jo Ann Sandeen, *Public Opinion and the Oregon Death with Dignity Act* (published June 2013), at http://pdxscholar.library.pdx.edu/cgi/viewcontent.cgi?article=2014&context=open_access_etds.

79. Cal. Health & Safety Code §§ 443 to 443.22 (2015).

80. *Id.* at § 443.18.

81. For the status in a specific state, *see* National POLST Paradigm Task Force, *Programs in Your State* (accessed September 9, 2016), at http://polst.org/programs-in-your-state/.

82. *See generally* http://polst.org/about-the-national-polst-paradigm/what-is-polst/ (accessed Dec. 28, 2016).

83. 42 U.S.C. §1395cc.

84. 105 N.E. at 93.

85. Baxter v. State, 354 Mont. 234, 224 P.3d 1211 (2009).

86. 98 N.J. 321, 486 A.2d 1209 (1985).

Appendix 11.1: Sample Advance Directive Form

GEORGIA ADVANCE DIRECTIVE FOR HEALTH CARE

By:_____ Date of Birth:_____ (Print Name)

(Month/Day/Year)

This advance directive for health care has four parts:

PART ONE: HEALTH CARE AGENT. *This part allows you to choose someone to make health care decisions for you when you cannot (or do not want to) make health care decisions for yourself. The person you choose is called a health care agent. You may also have your health care agent make decisions for you after your death with respect to an autopsy, organ donation, body donation, and final disposition of your body. You should talk to your health care agent about this important role.*

PART TWO: TREATMENT PREFERENCES. *This part allows you to state your treatment preferences if you have a terminal condition or if you are in a state of permanent unconsciousness. PART TWO will become effective only if you are unable to communicate your treatment preferences. Reasonable and appropriate efforts will be made to communicate with you about your treatment preferences before PART TWO becomes effective. You should talk to your family and others close to you about your treatment preferences.*

PART THREE: GUARDIANSHIP. *This part allows you to nominate a person to be your guardian should one ever be needed.*

PART FOUR:
EFFECTIVENESS AND SIGNATURES. *This part requires your signature and the signatures of two witnesses. You must complete PART FOUR if you have filled out any other part of this form.*

You may fill out any or all of the first three parts listed above. You must fill out PART FOUR of this form in order for this form to be effective.

You should give a copy of this completed form to people who might need it, such as your health care agent, your family, and your physician. Keep a copy of this completed form at home in a place where it can easily be found if it is needed. Review this completed form periodically to make sure it still reflects your preferences. If your preferences change, complete a new advance directive for health care.

Using this form of advance directive for health care is completely optional. Other forms of advance directives for health care may be used in Georgia.

You may revoke this completed form at any time. This completed form will replace any advance directive for health care, durable power of attorney for health care, health care proxy, or living will that you have completed before completing this form.

PART ONE: HEALTH CARE AGENT

[PART ONE will be effective even if PART TWO is not completed. A physician or health care provider who is directly involved in your health care may not serve as your health care agent. If you are married, a future divorce or annulment of your marriage will revoke the selection of your current spouse as your health care agent. If you are not married, a future marriage will revoke the selection of your health care agent unless the person you selected as your health care agent is your new spouse.]

Sample Advance Directive Form, page 1

(1) Health Care Agent

I select the following person as my health care agent to make health care decisions for me:

Name:
Address: _____
Telephone Numbers: _____
                    (Home, Work, and Mobile)

(2) Back-up Health Care Agent
[This section is optional. PART ONE will be effective even if this section is left blank.]

If my health care agent cannot be contacted in a reasonable time period and cannot be located with reasonable efforts or for any reason my health care agent is unavailable or unable or unwilling to act as my health care agent, then I select the following, each to act successively in the order named, as my back-up health care agent(s):

Name:
Address: _____
Telephone Numbers: _____
                    (Home, Work, and Mobile)

Name:
Address: _____
Telephone Numbers: _____
                    (Home, Work, and Mobile)

(3) General Powers of Health Care Agent

My health care agent will make health care decisions for me when I am unable to communicate my health care decisions or I choose to have my health care agent communicate my health care decisions.

My health care agent will have the same authority to make any health care decision that I could make. My health care agent's authority includes, for example, the power to:

- Admit me to or discharge me from any hospital, skilled nursing facility, hospice, or other health care facility or service;
- Request, consent to, withhold, or withdraw any type of health care; and
- Contract for any health care facility or service for me, and to obligate me to pay for these services (and my health care agent will not be financially liable for any services or care contracted for me or on my behalf).

My health care agent will be my personal representative for all purposes of federal or state law related to privacy of medical records (including the Health Insurance Portability and Accountability Act of 1996) and will have the same access to my medical records that I have and can disclose the contents of my medical records to others for my ongoing health care.

Sample Advance Directive Form, page 2

My health care agent may accompany me in an ambulance or air ambulance if in the opinion of the ambulance personnel protocol permits a passenger, and my health care agent may visit or consult with me in person while I am in a hospital, skilled nursing facility, hospice, or other health care facility or service if its protocol permits visitation.

My health care agent may present a copy of this advance directive for health care in lieu of the original and the copy will have the same meaning and effect as the original.

I understand that under Georgia law:
- My health care agent may refuse to act as my health care agent;
- A court can take away the powers of my health care agent if it finds that my health care agent is not acting properly; and
- My health care agent does not have the power to make health care decisions for me regarding psychosurgery, sterilization, or treatment or involuntary hospitalization for mental or emotional illness, developmental disability, or addictive disease.

(4) Guidance for Health Care Agent
When making health care decisions for me, my health care agent should think about what action would be consistent with past conversations we have had, my treatment preferences as expressed in PART TWO (if I have filled out PART TWO), my religious and other beliefs and values, and how I have handled medical and other important issues in the past. If what I would decide is still unclear, then my health care agent should make decisions for me that my health care agent believes are in my best interest, considering the benefits, burdens, and risks of my current circumstances and treatment options.

(5) Powers of Health Care Agent After Death
(A) Autopsy
My health care agent will have the power to authorize an autopsy of my body unless I have limited my health care agent's power by initialing below.

_____(Initials) My health care agent will not have the power to authorize an autopsy of my body (unless an autopsy is required by law).

(B) Organ Donation and Donation of Body
My health care agent will have the power to make a disposition of any part or all of my body for medical purposes pursuant to the Georgia Revised Uniform Anatomical Gift Act, unless I have limited my health care agent's power by initialing below.

[Initial each statement that you want to apply.]

_____(Initials) My health care agent will not have the power to make a disposition of my body for use in a medical study program.
_____(Initials) My health care agent will not have the power to donate any of my organs.

(C) Final Disposition of Body
My health care agent will have the power to make decisions about the final disposition of my body unless I have initialed below.

Sample Advance Directive Form, page 3

_____(Initials) I want the following person to make decisions about the final disposition of my body:

Name:
Address: _____
Telephone Numbers: _____
(Home, Work, and Mobile)

I wish for my body to be:
_____(Initials) Buried

OR

_____(Initials) Cremated

PART TWO: TREATMENT PREFERENCES

[PART TWO will be effective only if you are unable to communicate your treatment preferences after reasonable and appropriate efforts have been made to communicate with you about your treatment preferences. PART TWO will be effective even if PART ONE is not completed. If you have not selected a health care agent in PART ONE, or if your health care agent is not available, then PART TWO will provide your physician and other health care providers with your treatment preferences. If you have selected a health care agent in PART ONE, then your health care agent will have the authority to make all health care decisions for you regarding matters covered by PART TWO. Your health care agent will be guided by your treatment preferences and other factors described in Section (4) of PART ONE.]

(6) Conditions

PART TWO will be effective if I am in any of the following conditions:

[Initial each condition in which you want PART TWO to be effective.]

_____(Initials) A terminal condition, which means I have an incurable or irreversible condition that will result in my death in a relatively short period of time.
_____(Initials) A state of permanent unconsciousness, which means I am in an incurable or irreversible condition in which I am not aware of myself or my environment and I show no behavioral response to my environment.

My condition will be determined in writing after personal examination by my attending physician and a second physician in accordance with currently accepted medical standards.

(7) Treatment Preferences

[State your treatment preference by initialing (A), (B), or (C). If you choose (C), state your additional treatment preferences by initialing one or more of the statements following (C). You may provide additional instructions about your treatment preferences in the next section. You will be provided with comfort care, including pain relief, but you may also want to state your specific preferences regarding pain relief in the next section.]

If I am in any condition that I initialed in Section (6) above and I can no longer communicate my treatment preferences after reasonable and appropriate efforts have been made to communicate with me about my treatment preferences, then:

(A) _____(Initials) Try to extend my life for as long as possible, using all medications, machines, or other medical procedures that in reasonable medical judgment could keep me alive. If I am unable to take nutrition or fluids by mouth, then I want to receive nutrition or fluids by tube or other medical means.

OR

(B) _____(Initials) Allow my natural death to occur. I do not want any medications, machines, or other medical procedures that in reasonable medical judgment could keep me alive but cannot cure me. I do not want to receive nutrition or fluids by tube or other medical means except as needed to provide pain medication.

OR

(C)_____(Initials) I do not want any medications, machines, or other medical procedures that in reasonable medical judgment could keep me alive but cannot cure me, except as follows:

[Initial each statement that you want to apply to option (C).]

_____(Initials) If I am unable to take nutrition by mouth, I want to receive nutrition by tube or other medical means.
_____(Initials) If I am unable to take fluids by mouth, I want to receive fluids by tube or other medical means.
_____(Initials) If I need assistance to breathe, I want to have a ventilator used.
_____(Initials) If my heart or pulse has stopped, I want to have cardiopulmonary resuscitation (CPR) used.

(8) Additional Statements

[This section is optional. PART TWO will be effective even if this section is left blank. This section allows you to state additional treatment preferences, to provide additional guidance to your health care agent (if you have selected a health care agent in PART ONE), or to provide information about your personal and religious values about your medical treatment. For example, you may want to state your treatment preferences regarding medications to fight infection, surgery, amputation, blood transfusion, or kidney dialysis. Understanding that you cannot foresee everything that could happen to you after you can no longer communicate your treatment preferences, you may want to provide guidance to your health care agent (if you have selected a health care agent in PART ONE) about following your treatment preferences. You may want to state your specific preferences regarding pain relief.]

_____

_____

_____

_____

_____

Sample Advance Directive Form, page 5

(9) In Case of Pregnancy

[PART TWO will be effective even if this section is left blank.]

I understand that under Georgia law, PART TWO generally will have no force and effect if I am pregnant unless the fetus is not viable and I indicate by initialing below that I want PART TWO to be carried out.

_____(Initials) I want PART TWO to be carried out if my fetus is not viable.

PART THREE: GUARDIANSHIP

(10) Guardianship

[PART THREE is optional. This advance directive for health care will be effective even if PART THREE is left blank. If you wish to nominate a person to be your guardian in the event a court decides that a guardian should be appointed, complete PART THREE. A court will appoint a guardian for you if the court finds that you are not able to make significant responsible decisions for yourself regarding your personal support, safety, or welfare. A court will appoint the person nominated by you if the court finds that the appointment will serve your best interest and welfare. If you have selected a health care agent in PART ONE, you may (but are not required to) nominate the same person to be your guardian. If your health care agent and guardian are not the same person, your health care agent will have priority over your guardian in making your health care decisions, unless a court determines otherwise.]

[State your preference by initialing (A) or (B). Choose (A) only if you have also completed PART ONE.]

(A)_____ (Initials) I nominate the person serving as my health care agent under PART ONE to serve as my guardian.

OR

(B)_____ (Initials) I nominate the following person to serve as my guardian:

Name:
Address: _____
Telephone Numbers: _____
(Home, Work, and Mobile)

PART FOUR: EFFECTIVENESS AND SIGNATURES

This advance directive for health care will become effective only if I am unable or choose not to make or communicate my own health care decisions.

This form revokes any advance directive for health care, durable power of attorney for health care, health care proxy, or living will that I have completed before this date.

Unless I have initialed below and have provided alternative future dates or events, this advance directive for health care will become effective at the time I sign it and will remain effective until my death (and after my death to the extent authorized in Section (5) of PART ONE).

_____(Initials) This advance directive for health care will become effective on or upon _____ and will terminate on or upon _____.

[You must sign and date or acknowledge signing and dating this form in the presence of two witnesses. Both witnesses must be of sound mind and must be at least 18 years of age, but the witnesses do not have to be together or present with you when you sign this form.

A witness:
- *Cannot be a person who was selected to be your health care agent or back-up health care agent in PART ONE;*
- *Cannot be a person who will knowingly inherit anything from you or otherwise knowingly gain a financial benefit from your death; or*
- *Cannot be a person who is directly involved in your health care.*

Only one of the witnesses may be an employee, agent, or medical staff member of the hospital, skilled nursing facility, hospice, or other health care facility in which you are receiving health care (but this witness cannot be directly involved in your health care).]

By signing below, I state that I am emotionally and mentally capable of making this advance directive for healthcare and that I understand its purpose and effect.

_____
(Signature of Declarant)   (Date)

The declarant signed this form in my presence or acknowledged signing this form to me. Based upon my personal observation, the declarant appeared to be emotionally and mentally capable of making this advance directive for health care and signed this form willingly and voluntarily.

_____
(Signature of First Witness)   (Date)

Print Name: _____

Address: _____

_____
(Signature of Second Witness)   (Date)

Print Name:_____

Address: _____

[This form does not need to be notarized.]

Sample Advance Directive Form, page 7

Appendix 11.2: Sample POLST Form

Physician Orders for Life-Sustaining Treatment (POLST)

Follow these medical orders until orders change. Any section not completed implies full treatment for that section.

Patient Last Name:	Patient First Name:	Patient Middle Name:	Last 4 SSN: ☐ ☐ ☐ ☐

Address: (street / city / state / zip):	Date of Birth: (mm/dd/yyyy) _____ / _____ / _____	Gender: ☐ **M** ☐ **F**

A *Check One*	**CARDIOPULMONARY RESUSCITATION (CPR):** *Unresponsive, pulseless, & not breathing.*
	☐ **Attempt Resuscitation/CPR** ☐ **Do Not Attempt Resuscitation/DNR**
	If patient is not in cardiopulmonary arrest, follow orders in **B** and **C**.

B *Check One*	**MEDICAL INTERVENTIONS:** *If patient has pulse and is breathing.*
	☐ **Comfort Measures Only**. Provide treatments to relieve pain and suffering through the use of any medication by any route, positioning, wound care and other measures. Use oxygen, suction and manual treatment of airway obstruction as needed for comfort. *Patient prefers no transfer to hospital* for life-sustaining treatments. *Transfer if comfort needs cannot be met in current location.* <u>Treatment Plan</u>: **Provide treatments for comfort through symptom management.**
	☐ **Limited Treatment**. In addition to care described in Comfort Measures Only, use medical treatment, antibiotics, IV fluids and cardiac monitor as indicated. No intubation, advanced airway interventions, or mechanical ventilation. May consider less invasive airway support (e.g. CPAP, BiPAP). *Transfer to hospital if indicated. Generally avoid the intensive care unit.* <u>Treatment Plan</u>: **Provide basic medical treatments.**
	☐ **Full Treatment**. In addition to care described in Comfort Measures Only and Limited Treatment, use intubation, advanced airway interventions, and mechanical ventilation as indicated. *Transfer to hospital and/or intensive care unit if indicated.* <u>Treatment Plan</u>: **All treatments including breathing machine.**
	Additional Orders: _____

C *Check One*	**ARTIFICIALLY ADMINISTERED NUTRITION:** *Offer food by mouth if feasible.*
	☐ Long-term artificial nutrition by tube. ☐ Defined trial period of artificial nutrition by tube. ☐ No artificial nutrition by tube.	*Additional Orders (e.g., defining the length of a trial period):* _____

D *Must Fill Out*	**DOCUMENTATION OF DISCUSSION: (REQUIRED)** *See reverse side for add'l info.*
	☐ Patient (If patient lacks capacity, must check a box below) _____
	☐ Health Care Representative (legally appointed by advance directive or court)
	☐ Surrogate defined by facility policy or Surrogate for patient with developmental disabilities or significant mental health condition (Note: Special requirements for completion- see reverse side)
	Representative/Surrogate Name: _____ Relationship: _____

E	**PATIENT OR SURROGATE SIGNATURE AND OREGON POLST REGISTRY OPT OUT**
	Signature: *recommended*	This form will be sent to the POLST Registry unless the patient wishes to opt out, if so check opt out box: ☐

F *Must Print Name, Sign & Date*	**ATTESTATION OF MD / DO / NP / PA (REQUIRED)**
	By signing below, I attest that these medical orders are, to the best of my knowledge, consistent with the patient's **current** medical condition and preferences.
	Print Signing MD / DO / NP / PA Name: *required*	Signer Phone Number:	Signer License Number: *(optional)*
	MD / DO / NP / PA Signature: *required*	Date: *required*	Office Use Only

SEND FORM WITH PATIENT WHENEVER TRANSFERRED OR DISCHARGED
SUBMIT COPY OF BOTH SIDES OF FORM TO REGISTRY IF PATIENT DID NOT OPT OUT IN SECTION E

Sample POLST Form, page 1

HIPAA PERMITS DISCLOSURE TO HEALTH CARE PROFESSIONALS & ELECTRONIC REGISTRY AS NECESSARY FOR TREATMENT

Information for patient named on this form   PATIENT'S NAME: _____

The POLST form is **always voluntary** and is usually for persons with serious illness or frailty. POLST records your wishes for medical treatment in your current state of health (states your treatment wishes if something happened tonight). Once initial medical treatment is begun and the risks and benefits of further therapy are clear, your treatment wishes may change. Your medical care and this form can be changed to reflect your new wishes at any time. No form, however, can address all the medical treatment decisions that may need to be made. An Advance Directive is recommended for all capable adults and allows you to document in detail your future health care instructions and/or name a Health Care Representative to speak for you if you are unable to speak for yourself. Consider reviewing your Advance Directive and giving a copy of it to your health care professional.

Contact Information (Optional)

Health Care Representative or Surrogate:	Relationship:	Phone Number:	Address:

Health Care Professional Information

Preparer Name:	Preparer Title:	Phone Number:	Date Prepared:

PA's Supervising Physician: Phone Number:

Primary Care Professional:

Directions for Health Care Professionals

Completing POLST

- Completing a POLST is always voluntary and cannot be mandated for a patient.
- An order of CPR in Section A is incompatible with an order for Comfort Measures Only in Section B (will not be accepted in Registry).
- For information on legally appointed health care representatives and their authority, refer to ORS 127.505 - 127.660.
- Should reflect current preferences of persons with serious illness or frailty. Also, encourage completion of an Advance Directive.
- Verbal / phone orders are acceptable with follow-up signature by MD/DO/NP/PA in accordance with facility/community policy.
- Use of original form is encouraged. Photocopies, faxes, and electronic registry forms are also legal and valid.
- A person with developmental disabilities or significant mental health condition requires additional consideration before completing the POLST form; refer to *Guidance for Health Care Professionals* at www.or.polst.org.

Oregon POLST Registry Information

Health Care Professionals:
(1) You are **required** to send a copy of both sides of this POLST form to the Oregon POLST Registry unless the patient opts out.
(2) The following sections must be completed:
- Patient's full name
- Date of birth
- MD / DO / NP / PA signature
- Date signed

Registry Contact Information:
Phone: 503-418-4083
Fax or eFAX: 503-418-2161
www.orpolstregistry.org
polstreg@ohsu.edu

Oregon POLST Registry
3181 SW Sam Jackson Park Rd.
Mail Code: CDW-EM
Portland, OR 97239

Patients:
Mailed confirmation packets from Registry may take four weeks for delivery.

MAY PUT REGISTRY ID STICKER HERE:

Updating POLST: A POLST Form only needs to be revised if patient treatment preferences have changed.

This POLST should be reviewed periodically, including when:
- The patient is transferred from one care setting or care level to another (including upon admission or at discharge), or
- There is a substantial change in the patient's health status.
If patient wishes haven't changed, the POLST Form does not need to be revised, updated, rewritten or resent to the Registry.

Voiding POLST: A copy of the voided POLST **must** be sent to the Registry unless patient has opted-out.

- A person with capacity, or the valid surrogate of a person without capacity, can void the form and request alternative treatment.
- Draw line through sections A through E and write "VOID" in large letters if POLST is replaced or becomes invalid.
- Send a copy of the voided form to the POLST Registry (**required** unless patient has opted out).
- If included in an electronic medical record, follow voiding procedures of facility/community.

For permission to use the copyrighted form contact the OHSU Center for Ethics in Health Care at orpolst@ohsu.edu or (503) 494-3965. Information on the Oregon POLST Program is available online at **www.or.polst.org** or at **orpolst@ohsu.edu**

SEND FORM WITH PATIENT WHENEVER TRANSFERRED OR DISCHARGED, SUBMIT COPY TO REGISTRY

© CENTER FOR ETHICS IN HEALTH CARE, Oregon Health & Science University.   2014

Sample POLST Form, page 2

TAXATION OF HEALTHCARE INSTITUTIONS 12

After reading this chapter, you will

- know the difference between tax-exempt and not-for-profit status,
- recognize the differences between standards for exemption from federal income taxation and standards for exemption from state ad valorem (property) taxation,
- be familiar with an important state supreme court decision denying property tax exemption to a church-affiliated health system,
- appreciate the federal rules regarding lobbying and political campaign activity and how they apply to 501(c)(3) organizations,
- understand the meaning of "used for charitable purposes," and
- know how the Affordable Care Act may affect the tax status of not-for-profit healthcare organizations.

Introduction

To be exempt from taxation, an organization must meet the criteria of the tax law in question. Not-for-profit status is a prerequisite to tax-exempt status, but the two concepts are not the same. The former is based on state corporation law, while the latter depends on the federal or state tax law from which the organization wishes to be excused. The various tax law criteria must be examined carefully because an organization can be exempt under one statute (e.g., federal income, excise tax) but taxable under another (e.g., state property tax).

Nature of a Charitable Corporation

Among the organizations exempt from federal income taxation are those described in Internal Revenue Code (IRC) section 501(c)(3):

Section 501(c)(3)

Corporations, and any community chest, fund, or foundation, [that is] *organized and operated exclusively for religious, charitable, scientific, testing for public safety, literary, or educational purposes* . . . no part of the net earnings of which inures to the benefit of any private shareholder or individual, no substantial part of the activities of which is carrying on propaganda, or otherwise attempting, to influence legislation [with one exception], and which does not participate in, or intervene in . . . any political campaign on behalf of (or in opposition to) any candidate for public office.[1] [Emphasis added.]

Most healthcare institutions that claim tax-exempt status rely on section 501(c)(3). In particular, they claim to be organized for "charitable purposes"—which raises two legitimate questions: What is a charity? What is a charitable purpose?

What Is a Charity?

charity
an organization that exists to help those in need or to provide religious, educational, scientific, or similar aid to the public

Somewhat surprisingly, the IRC does not define either **charity** or *charitable purpose*. Even though the terms have lain encysted in the tax code for many decades and are used in various state constitutions and statutes, only since the mid-1980s have they been subjected to any critical analysis. A passage from the famous *Dartmouth College* case of 1819 is one example of language in which the meaning of these terms is assumed to be self-evident. In the opinion, while quoting from *Blackstone's Commentaries*, Chief Justice John Marshall wrote:

[Dartmouth College] is an eleemosynary corporation. It is a private charity, originally founded and endowed by an individual, with a charter obtained for it at his [the King's] request, for the better administration of his charity. "The eleemosynary sort of corporations are such as are constituted for the perpetual distributions of the free-alms or bounty of the founder of them, to such persons as he has directed. Of this are all hospitals for the maintenance of the poor, sick and impotent; and all colleges both in our universities and out of them." 1 Bl. Com. 471.[2]

The chief justice then proceeded to discuss eleemosynary (philanthropic) corporations and their legal history as they were viewed about 200 years ago:

Eleemosynary corporations are for the management of private property, according to the will of the donors; they are private corporations. A college is as much a private corporation as [a] hospital; especially, a college founded as this was, by private bounty. *A college is a charity.* "The establishment of learning," says Lord HARDWICKE, "is a charity, and so considered in the statute of Elizabeth. A devise [a testamentary gift] to a college, for their benefit, is a laudable charity, and deserves encouragement." 1 Ves. 537. The legal signification of a charity is derived chiefly from the statute 43 Eliz., c. 4. "Those purposes," says Sir. W. GRANT, "are considered charitable, which that statute enumerates." 9 Ves. 405. Colleges are enumerated as charities in that statute. The government, in these cases, lends its aid to perpetuate the beneficent [*sic*] intention of the donor, by granting a charter, under which his private charity shall continue to be dispensed, after his death. This is done, either by incorporating the objects of the charity, as, for instance, the scholars in a college, or *the poor in a hospital*; or by incorporating those who are to be governors or trustees of the charity.[3] [Emphasis added.]

These passages have some notable aspects. The first concerns the use of the word *hospital* itself. According to the Oxford English Dictionary, it comes from the Latin *hospitalis*—the root of our English words "hospitality" and "hospitable"—and originally referred to an institution for welcoming and housing travelers and persons who were needy, infirm, or aged. For example, London's Foundling Hospital was established in 1739 for the "education and maintenance of exposed and deserted young children," not for the purpose of providing medical care.[4] Today we might call such an institution a "home" or an "orphanage" rather than a "hospital." The sense of *hospital* as an establishment providing medical or surgical treatment developed only gradually with the advancement of modern medicine (see chapter 2).

The second salient point in Marshall's opinion is the reference to "Bl. Com."—Blackstone's *Commentaries on the Laws of England*, the leading eighteenth-century treatise on English law—and to various statutes dating back to the reign of Queen Elizabeth I. The Statute of Elizabeth (43 Eliz., c. 4), also known as the Charitable Uses Act, was passed in 1601. Thus, the *Dartmouth College* case is both a good example of how English common law carried over to the United States and evidence that courts and legislatures have struggled with the concept of charity for more than four centuries.

Third, Chief Justice Marshall equated hospitals and colleges, assumed without discussion that they are charities, and cited them both as examples of organizations "constituted for the perpetual distributions of . . . free-alms or bounty." Is his description characteristic of today's healthcare institutions— or today's colleges, for that matter?

Fourth, the chief justice assumed that the beneficiaries of hospitals were poor in addition to being "sick and impotent" (by which he meant "infirm"). His concept of a hospital echoes the description in chapter 2 of the almshouses in the Middle Ages—pits of misery and horror—and is consistent with the meaning of the word in Marshall's time.

Fifth, research reveals that hospitals per se were not among the enumerated charities in the Statute of Elizabeth; the sole reference to healthcare in that law was "maintenance of sick and maimed soldiers and mariners."[5]

The final notable point, which confirms the premise of our current discussion, is Chief Justice Marshall's failure to provide a clear definition of the very term that is at the heart of the case. Apparently, *charity* could only be described, not defined, in 1819.

Two centuries later, a clear definition of the word remains elusive. For example, in *Provena Covenant Medical Center v. Department of Revenue*,[6] the Supreme Court of Illinois quoted with approval an 1893 case that had quoted an 1867 case from Massachusetts:

> A charity, in a legal sense, may be more fully defined as a gift, to be applied consistently with existing laws, for the benefit of an indefinite number of persons, either by bringing their hearts under the influence of education or religion, by relieving their bodies from disease, suffering or constraint, by assisting them to establish themselves for life, or by erecting or maintaining public buildings or works, or otherwise lessening the burthens of government.[7]

This ancient description has been repeated, rephrased, reinterpreted, and regurgitated many times, but as venerable as it is, its clarity has not improved and it is little help in deciding real-life cases. As demonstrated later in this chapter, antediluvian language can be problematic when applied to twenty-first century circumstances.

At the least, it seems that a charity must benefit a large segment of the public ("an indefinite number of persons") and not restrict its offerings to a privileged few. Thus, charities are distinguished from the broader category of not-for-profit organizations; that is, charitable corporations are not-for-profit, but not all not-for-profit organizations are charities. Countless not-for-profits—for example, social clubs, fraternal organizations, and labor unions—may extend a significant degree of social service and community benefit without operating for purposes that would exempt them from taxation.

suspect class
a group of people often subjected to discrimination because of stereotyping; criteria for suspect classification and thus careful judicial review include race, religion, national origin, gender, and so on.

A charity's benefits can be restricted to a particular type of beneficiary. In healthcare, prominent examples are children's hospitals and women's hospitals. In other words, organizations do not jeopardize their charitable status by confining their activities to a particular purpose and restricting benefits to a particular category of people (as long as the restriction does not discriminate against a **suspect class** of people) or by restricting their activities because they lack particular types of staff and facilities. Whether the benefits of a charity may be restricted to the members of a particular church, lodge, or labor union or to the employees of a particular company depends on the issue involved in the particular case.

If state law requires tax-exempt organizations to be "purely public charities," their beneficiaries usually may not be restricted to the members of a specific church denomination, fraternal order, or similar group. An old but still respected case is *City of Philadelphia v. Masonic Home of Pennsylvania* (1894), which denied real estate tax exemption to a home for aged Masons because it served only them, not the general public, and therefore was not "purely public."[8] Nine decades later, the court in the 1982 case *West Allegheny Hospital v. Board of Property Assessment, Appeals and Review* relied on *Masonic Home* when it decided that a community hospital was tax exempt because it was open to all without regard to "race, color, creed, national origin or sex" and was not restricted to members of a particular social organization.[9]

By way of comparison, Kansas does not require a charity to be "public" in the same sense that Pennsylvania does. Therefore, in Kansas, a hospital may be considered tax exempt even if it serves only specific groups—for example, Masons, Methodist clergy, or members of Roman Catholic religious orders.[10] The definition of and limitations on the class of persons to be served by a "charity" thus depend on local law and are open questions in many jurisdictions. The point comes into focus with respect to specialized institutions, such as hospitals that care only for patients with a particular disease or disability. Discrimination on the basis of indigence or suspect classification is still prohibited, but an institution does not forfeit its charitable status by restricting benefits on the basis of its purpose, facilities, staff, or ability to serve particular conditions.

As discussed in chapter 10, a hospital may not restrict its provision of emergency care to those able to pay. A related question concerns whether the organization must render some amount of free care to maintain its charity status. This issue has become contentious in recent years, particularly in the context of whether the hospital must pay ad valorem taxes on the property it owns. This question will be revisited later in this chapter.

Pretermitting property tax issues for the moment, the question becomes: Is the provision of medical care in itself a charitable purpose? For many years, the answer was beyond **peradventure**, as reflected in the following language from a 1944 New York decision:

peradventure
chance or
uncertainty;
doubt; question

> Hospitals which are devoted to the care of the sick and injured, which aid in maintaining public health and which make valuable contributions to the advancement of medical science are rightly regarded as benevolent and charitable. A hospital. . . which devotes all of its funds exclusively to the maintenance of the institution is a public charity and this is so irrespective of whether patients are required to pay for the services rendered.[11]

However that case was decided during World War II, and a lot has changed in three-quarters of a century. The assumption that a hospital is a charity has come into question lately, as litigants and policymakers challenge whether not-for-profit hospitals are in any significant way different from their for-profit counterparts. This question is a serious public policy issue given the fiscal pressures facing state and local governments and the potential property tax revenues that could be generated by placing hospital property on the tax assessor's rolls.

Federal Tax Issues

Healthcare organizations' exemption from federal income tax is based on IRC section 501(c)(3). The following explores some significant questions regarding exemption from federal income tax.

Basic Requirements for Federal Exemption
Charitable Purpose
Is the provision of healthcare a *charitable* purpose? Section 501(c)(3) does not define the term "charitable." The regulations contain the following relevant but less than enlightening language:

> **Charitable defined.** The term charitable is used in its generally accepted legal sense and is, therefore, not to be construed as limited by the separate enumeration in section 501(c)(3) of other tax-exempt purposes which may fall within the broad outlines of *charity* as developed by judicial decisions. Such term includes: Relief of the poor and distressed or of the underprivileged; advancement of religion; advancement of education or science; erection or maintenance of public buildings, monuments, or works; lessening of the burdens of Government; and promotion of social welfare by organizations designed to accomplish any of the above purposes, or (i) to lessen neighborhood tensions; (ii) to eliminate prejudice and discrimination; (iii) to defend human and civil rights secured by law; or (iv) to combat community deterioration and juvenile delinquency.[12]

One thing is clear: healthcare is not listed among these activities. So where does it fit? Does it lessen the burdens of the government? Would the government necessarily need to provide healthcare as a social service if community hospitals did not exist? Does providing care amount to relief of the poor? Are "the poor" only the indigent, or does the term include those poor in health or spirit? *Should* it be interpreted that way?

We sense that charity involves benevolence—assisting the less fortunate, doing good works, and promoting the general welfare—but an instinctive response does little to resolve the legal issues, and the answers remain unclear. Apparently, charity—like pornography, famously—is hard to define, but you know it when you see it.

No Private Inurement

In addition to being organized and operated for charitable purposes (whatever that means), a tax-exempt organization's net earnings may not **inure** to the benefit of any private individual or corporation. The statute and regulations do not define *inure* for these purposes, and the dictionary definition—"to make accustomed"—is ill fitting. Nevertheless, the regulations' intent is relatively clear: A charity's net earnings must be permanently dedicated to exempt purposes and may not be distributed to private interests.

This requirement goes hand in hand with the concept of public benefit, and it raises many questions. Each case must be decided on its own merits, and no single factor or set of factors is conclusive in determining whether a corporation claiming tax-exempt status is truly providing a community benefit or is merely a shield for conferring a financial gain on proprietary interests. The courts consider several factors, most of which flow from or relate directly to corporate control.

When control of a corporation rests exclusively with a small group of individuals, the parties' motives should be subject to close scrutiny. Private gain is indicated by such factors as (1) division of income among trustees, members, or officers of the corporation; (2) private use of corporate funds or facilities; (3) in the case of a hospital, exclusive privileges to admit or treat patients; and (4) failure to provide services to those unable to pay.[13] Even if tax-exempt status is granted without requiring the hospital to provide free care, its charity record is evidence of a willingness to serve the public. In other words, the absence or rarity of charity work may be evidence of private gain.

Because of changes in healthcare financing in the last quarter of the twentieth century, hospitals developed various economic incentive plans to attract physicians to the medical staff, encourage the economical use of hospital facilities, and (one hopes) reduce overall costs. The theory is that if physicians share in net revenues, they will have a financial incentive to be efficient and all parties will benefit. As long as the doctors' compensation is reasonable and furthers the charitable purpose of the institution, its tax-exempt status is not jeopardized.[14] Of course, the institution must receive and should document services of value in return for the incentives it grants the doctors. (Note that such arrangements implicate state or federal antikickback and self-referral laws, as discussed in chapter 15.)

In addition, federal law imposes sizable financial penalties on persons who receive "excess benefits" and on the organizational managers who approve the transactions.[15] Tax-exempt organizations are advised to develop compensation and conflict-of-interest policies to ensure the propriety of transactions with corporate insiders, including physicians. Failure to abide by such policies puts the insiders and corporate managers at substantial monetary risk.

inure
a term used but not defined in IRC section 501(c)(3); in context, it means a charity's income or assets may not benefit, accrue to, or be distributed to private interests.

No Lobbying or Political Activity

Not only does section 501(c)(3) bar private inurement; it also prohibits exempt organizations from campaigning and electioneering on behalf of or in opposition to candidates for political office. However, they may engage in **lobbying** as long as that activity does not amount to a "substantial part" of their overall operations. What amounts to a substantial part is a matter of some dispute, so public charities (except certain religious organizations) are permitted to file an election with the Internal Revenue Service (IRS) indicating their intent to engage in lobbying. If they do so, they are subject to defined limitations on their lobbying expenditures. The following are not considered lobbying expenses:

lobbying
activity intended to influence the outcome of pending legislation

- Publishing nonpartisan research data
- Providing testimony to a legislative body
- Sending communications to a governmental official outside the legislative branch

Health Reform Adds New Requirements

The preceding discussion concerns the effect of excess benefits transactions, lobbying, and political campaign activity on an organization's tax status, not the fraud laws or recent "transparency and program integrity" provisions of the health reform statutes. The Affordable Care Act adds a number of new requirements to the tax code and imposes additional standards regarding care of the poor.[16] To qualify for the federal exemption, charitable hospitals now must

- conduct a community health needs assessment (CHNA) at least once every three years,
- adopt an implementation strategy to meet the health needs identified in the assessment,
- publicize and implement a written financial assistance policy— essentially a charity care policy for services to indigent patients,
- adopt a written policy on nondiscrimination in emergency services,
- limit the amounts charged for care to indigent patients, and
- not attempt "extraordinary collection actions" without first determining whether the patient meets financial assistance criteria.

The CHNA must include "input from persons who represent the broad interests of the community served by the hospital facility, including those with special knowledge of or expertise in public health" and must be made "widely available to the public."[17] Failure to comply subjects hospitals to a penalty tax.

The Affordable Care Act also adds new review and reporting requirements. IRC section 501(r) requires hospitals to be audited at least once every three years for compliance with the CHNA requirement, and organizations will need to file their audited financial statements and report annually to the IRS how they are meeting community needs. Finally, the Affordable Care Act requires the secretaries of the departments of Treasury and Health and Human Services to report annually to Congress the levels of charity care hospitals are providing, hospitals' bad debt expenses, unreimbursed services, and similar items.

In a nutshell, a healthcare organization seeking to maintain federal tax exemption needs to meet these new charity care and community benefit requirements in addition to meeting the traditional charitable purpose and private inurement standards. Notably, these new provisions of the Affordable Care Act contain a built-in irony: If more people gain insurance coverage as health reform takes hold, fewer people will qualify for charity and hospitals will have more difficulty meeting their charity care obligations. Furthermore, if the United States were to achieve universal health insurance, would hospitals no longer qualify as "charitable" institutions? Whether federal tax exemption will continue to be a viable concept for healthcare organizations remains to be seen.

Taxation of Unrelated Business Income

Even if an organization meets the requirements for tax exemption, not all its income is tax exempt (see Legal Brief). When a 501(c)(3) charity earns revenue from a line of business that does not further its charitable purpose, that income is subject to unrelated business income taxation (UBIT) as though it were earned by a for-profit organization. Without UBIT, the charity would have an unfair competitive advantage over commercial entities that provide the same types of products or services.

So long as the unrelated activities do not constitute a substantial part of the charity's work, unrelated income does not threaten the organization's underlying tax-exempt status. What constitutes a "substantial part" has not been clearly defined, but a rule of thumb is that the IRS might challenge the tax-exempt status of a charity if its gross income from unrelated activities exceeds 50 percent of its total revenue. In addition, sales of goods or services to private parties below cost may also constitute private inurement and may jeopardize the tax-exempt status of the seller.[18]

Investment income—for example, income from dividends, interest, annuities, and research—is not taxable, but such operations as hospital gift shops; restaurants; parking lots; pharmacies; physicians' offices; and residences for interns, nurses, and other staff may generate taxable

Legal Brief

The taxation of exempt organizations' unrelated business income is governed by IRC §§ 511 to 515 and regulations found at 26 C.F.R. §§ 1.511-1 to 1.514(g)-1.

income. The fact that the income is used for hospital or charitable purposes does not exempt it from taxation. The test is whether the activity itself is substantially related to the charitable purpose of the tax-exempt institution. In other words, does it further the mission of the exempt organization, or is it simply an extra source of revenue? All the nuances of that question cannot be addressed here, but a hospital generally can avoid UBIT if it can show that it is conducting the business activity primarily for the convenience of patients. Whether sales to persons other than patients generate taxable income is a complex question that should be addressed with qualified tax counsel.

State and Local Property Taxes

ad valorem tax tax imposed in proportion to the value of the property being assessed

Some of the most interesting and financially consequential tax cases concern whether healthcare organizations' property should be assessed for **ad valorem tax**. A hospital, for example, typically sits on prime real estate, and given its structures and other improvements, the campus is often the most prominent and valuable property in the neighborhood. State and local authorities are understandably eager to generate tax revenue from those assets, but (as shown in this section) charities and governmental organizations—which are not taxed—do not offer a solution to communities' fiscal woes.

Governmental Property

Federal property is exempt from state and local taxes, and so is most property owned by state and local entities, depending on the relevant state constitution or statute. In some states, governmental ownership and control are sufficient to establish exemption, but other states require also that the property be used exclusively for a public purpose to justify exemption.[19]

In a 1986 Minnesota case, a medical clinic owned and operated by a municipal hospital was not exempt from taxation when it was staffed by physicians engaged in private practice on a fee-for-service basis. The board of the hospital and the physicians annually reviewed and agreed on the service fees charged to patients. Each doctor then received 60 percent of his gross accounts receivable. Noting that the issue hinged on whether the primary use of the facility was for public purposes or for private gain, the Minnesota Supreme Court denied the exemption; the facility was not being used exclusively for a public purpose.[20] (Today, this arrangement would raise fraud and abuse issues as well.)

Private Property

The exemption of private healthcare institutions' real estate and personal property from taxation depends on two main factors: (1) qualification as a charity and (2) use for a charitable purpose.

Qualification as a Charity

Like the property of any other business, the property of a for-profit health-care organization is fully taxable. If the owner claims to be a charity, state constitutional or statutory provisions determine exempt status.

In many states, a constitutional provision mandates tax exemption for property owned by charities. The legislature and courts cannot alter this requirement, although the courts have the power to interpret its meaning. Other state constitutions contain permissive exemptions, and a few state constitutions are silent on the matter. In either of these latter situations, the standards for tax-exempt status are for the legislature to determine.

The distinction between a mandatory constitutional provision and a permissive one (or none at all) is significant when, in the search for additional revenue, there is political pressure to restrict or reduce the number of ad valorem tax exemptions. This distinction was a factor in the iconoclastic decision of *Utah County v. Intermountain Health Care, Inc.*[21]

The Utah constitution had exempted from taxation all property owned by nonprofit entities and used exclusively for either religious worship or charitable purposes. In an attempt to "clarify" the constitutional language, the Utah legislature defined *charitable purposes* to mean "religious, hospital, educational, employee representation, or welfare purposes."[22] At issue in the case was whether the statutory definition impermissibly expanded the constitutional provision. The Supreme Court of Utah held that it did, saying that

> in ruling upon the validity of a statute which purports to define the meaning of a constitutional provision, we are obligated to scrutinize the language of the Constitution with considerable care. It is true . . . that a significant degree of deference is due to a legislative construction of the meaning of a constitutional term. But . . . [the Constitution] grants a charitable exemption and our statutes cannot expand or limit the scope of the exemption or defeat it. To the extent the statutes have that effect, they are not valid.[23]

After an exhaustive review of the meaning of *charity* and reaffirming a strict constructionist view that "taxation has been the rule and exemption has been the exception," the Supreme Court of Utah held that the 21-hospital Intermountain Health Care system had not proven its entitlement to relief from property taxes. The court found significant the fact that even though "no person in need of medical attention is denied care solely on the basis of a lack of funds," Intermountain Health Care's policy was to collect hospital charges from patients whenever possible. This ruling shook up comfortable assumptions and was a wake-up call for the healthcare sector. The shock waves that *Intermountain* created can still be felt today, as evidenced by *Provena* (presented later in The Court Decides).

Prior to *Intermountain*, provision of free care was not deemed a prerequisite for tax exemption, and few (if any) courts bothered to question that premise—at least not with any intellectual rigor. It was simply a given that caring for people is a charitable act, whether they have to pay for the care or not. As Justice Oliver Wendell Holmes Jr. wrote more than a hundred years ago, "It is one of the misfortunes of the law that ideas become encysted in phrases and thereafter for a long time cease to provoke further analysis."[24] Such was the case with the concepts of charity and charitable purpose.

For example, in the 1967 Nebraska case *Evangelical Lutheran Good Samaritan Society v. County of Gage,*[25] a home for the aged was organized as a not-for-profit corporation and required all residents to pay if they were able. Its rates were nearly the same as those charged by proprietary homes, and it operated at a profit in some years and at a deficit in others. The court held the real estate to be exempt, ruling in effect that charity should be defined in broader terms than merely almsgiving and relief of poverty.

Likewise, in *Central Board on Care of Jewish Aged, Inc. v. Henson,* the court of appeals of Georgia ruled in 1969 that a home for the elderly was exempt.[26] The home provided medical and nursing services to elderly persons of the Jewish faith. The residents' average age was nearly 83, and each resident paid a monthly charge based on financial ability—the maximum being $450. No applicant was refused admission because of inability to pay, and at all times a few residents were permitted to remain without paying. Deficits in annual operating expenses were covered by contributions from the Jewish Welfare Fund or individuals. The court wrote as follows: "The concept of charity is not confined to the relief of the needy and destitute, for aged people require care and attention apart from financial assistance, and the supply of this care and attention is as much a charitable and benevolent purpose as the relief of their financial wants."[27]

In 1981, the Massachusetts Supreme Judicial Court wrote,

> We recognize . . . that major changes in the area of health care, especially in modes of operation and financing, have necessitated changes as well in definitional predicates. The term "charitable," as applied to health care facilities, has been broadened since earlier times when it was limited mainly to almshouses for the poor. As a result, the promotion of health, whether through the provision of health care or through medical education and research, is today generally seen as a charitable purpose. Such a purpose is separate and distinct from the relief of poverty and no health organization need engage in "almsgiving" in order to qualify for exemption.[28]

Although these types of opinions give obeisance to the underlying principles, they merely rehash old definitions and apply those definitions to new facts. As shown again in a few pages, the situation has not changed much since Justice Holmes's day: Charity remains an encysted idea, and neither courts nor legislatures seem willing to question its continued pertinence to healthcare institutions in the twenty-first century.

Use for a Charitable Purpose

In general, an entity must own each parcel of land it wants exempted from taxation, and each parcel must qualify for exemption separately. The test of "ownership" is not as simple as it might appear because real estate law recognizes various types of land ownership and leasehold interests. All states grant exemption if the charity holds *fee simple* (complete) *legal title* to the land, and nearly all states likewise grant exemption if the charity holds *equitable title*. (Equitable title is held, for example, when one purchases land under a mortgage or an installment contract.) However, many states deny exemption to landowners who lease their land to a charitable corporation. In such cases, the charity has neither fee simple nor equitable title; it has merely obtained the right to possess and use the land by virtue of the lease. On the other hand, some states exempt such property from taxation because they believe that reducing the operating costs of charitable organizations is sound public policy.

Like Utah, most states require that tax-exempt property be *used exclusively* for charitable purposes. The meaning of this phrase has been the subject of thousands of disputes in venues from local taxing commissions to state supreme courts. For one thing, it usually means that vacant property and property owned for investment purposes do not qualify because they are not being *used* for charitable purposes. In other words, the use of the property determines the tax-exempt status; even charitable use of income derived from investment property does not qualify.

More contentious than *use* is the word *exclusive*. It raises issues about property owned by a charity but rented to or occupied by others, such as facilities used by medical staff members in their private practices. These situations, which are decided case by case and state by state, are usually analyzed by examining (1) how closely the use of the property relates to the primary purpose of the hospital and (2) the relative benefits to the respective parties.

In general, property is subject to taxation if a hospital rents it to private physicians or others and if the rent generates a profit in excess of the hospital's overhead (see The Court Decides: *Greater Anchorage Area Borough v. Sisters of Charity* at the end of this chapter).[29] A few states grant exemption for property rented to medical staff physicians for their private offices if the rent covers only the hospital's overhead costs, and in rare cases exemption may be permitted if the property is provided free of charge, such as when it serves as living quarters for a hospital chaplain.[30] However, other courts deny exemption in these situations even if the rent does not exceed the hospital's costs; they do so either (1) on the ground that it results in a private benefit and that therefore the exclusive-use test is not met or (2) on the ground that local statutes allow tax exemption only on land occupied by the hospital itself.[31] (Note that private inurement and fraud issues may also be implicated by less-than-market-value transactions. These subjects are covered later in this chapter and in chapter 15, respectively.)

Genesee Hospital v. Wagner is a frequently cited New York case that illustrates the issues of public policy raised by the lease of hospital-owned real estate.[32] The hospital built an office building next door for lease to private physicians. Rent paid by the doctors was set at market prices, but at first it did not cover operating costs. The New York statute requires that "real property owned by a corporation or association organized or conducted exclusively for . . . hospital . . . purposes . . . and used exclusively for carrying out . . . such purposes . . . shall be exempt from taxation."[33] However, the statute provides that "if any portion of such real property is not so used exclusively to carry out . . . such purposes but is leased or otherwise used for other purposes, such portion shall be subject to taxation and the remaining portion only shall be exempt."[34] At issue, then, was whether the office building was used exclusively for hospital purposes.

The trial court held that the building was exempt from taxation. Rather than give *exclusively* its literal meaning, the court considered whether the office building was "reasonably incident to the major purpose" of the hospital. Because the evidence clearly established that the hospital's concern was to maintain a "first-rate" medical center for both patient care and medical education rather than to benefit the private physicians personally, the trial court judge concluded that the hospital, its house staff, and patients benefited more from the use of the building than the private physicians did.[35] The public policy involved was made evident when the trial court concluded that the community views a modern hospital building to be an important investment if it enables a highly trained staff of attending physicians to work together.

On appeal, the decision was reversed and the office building was held to be taxable. The appellate court recognized that a professional building was an admirable addition to the community and that it enhanced the patient care and teaching functions of the hospital, but the facility was in direct competition with privately developed professional office buildings serving an identical function. Accordingly, the leased space did not qualify for exemption under the language of the New York statute (see also The Court Decides: *Barnes Hospital v. Collector of Revenue* at the end of this chapter).[36]

As in the area of unrelated business income, property tax issues are sometimes raised regarding cafeterias, gift shops, pharmacies, parking lots, and the like that a hospital owns and operates. Again, the legal issue is whether these activities are consistent with the requirement that they be used exclusively for charitable purposes. If such an activity is not conducted for commercial profit, and if it takes place in an area of the hospital building or the immediate premises not open to the general public, tax-exempt status is likely to be granted. If a cafeteria, gift shop, parking lot, or similar facility is not tax exempt, the hospital must determine whether local and state statutes permit *split-listing* of property for tax purposes if the related activity frequently takes place in some part of an institutional building. Split-listing essentially means that local tax authorities will list as taxable only the space that is not exempt and then grant the remainder of the hospital building tax-exempt status. Split-listing is permitted in most jurisdictions.[37] In states that do not allow it, hospitals should seek competent legal advice regarding nonexempt uses of the property.

With respect to vacant or unoccupied land, a court's decision turns on the exact language of the related state statute and judicial interpretation of that language. To confer tax exemption, some states require that the land be not only "used" for charitable purposes but also "occupied." Even if occupancy for a charitable purpose is not a statutory requirement, the meaning of *used* has to be determined. Vacant land held for possible use in the indefinite future but for which no plans for development exist would normally be taxable.[38] On the other hand, if plans for construction and development are well along, fund-raising is under way, and bids for construction have been received, the land—although still vacant, perhaps—is exempt in some jurisdictions.[39] Other states, however, may require actual use and occupancy before granting exemption.

Finally, note that to an increasing extent healthcare institutions are choosing to lease rather than purchase equipment and other types of personal property. Just as in states that require landowners to pay real estate taxes on property they lease to charities, leased personal property may also be subject to ad valorem taxation. In an Alaska case, a hospital's rental of beds, television sets, and X-ray equipment did not entitle the property's owner (the lessor) to an exemption. The exemption provisions did not apply because the lessor was presumably earning a profit, and thus the property was not being used "exclusively for non-profit, religious, [and] charitable purposes" as required by the state constitution and the relevant statute.[40]

Coming Full Circle

As noted at the beginning of this chapter, US courts and legislatures have struggled with tax exemption issues since the earliest days of the republic. The chapter now closes with one of the oldest and one of the newest cases to have entered the fray.

In 1860, the US Supreme Court was called on to interpret an 1851 Pennsylvania statute that revoked the tax exemption of Christ Church Hospital in Philadelphia. The hospital claimed that its exemption—granted by the legislature in 1833—was meant to be perpetual. But according to Justice John Archibald Campbell, "Perpetual is not synonymous to irrevocable,"[41] and using concepts almost identical to those in the twenty-first century decision discussed in the following paragraphs, he held that the Philadelphia hospital was not entitled to the exemption. Exemptions are special privileges, Justice Campbell said; they belong "to a class of statutes in which the narrowest meaning is to be taken," and they can be revoked at the pleasure of the state.[42]

In 2010—more than 150 years after *Christ Church Hospital* was decided—came *Provena Covenant Medical Center v. Department of Revenue*, which was mentioned briefly at the start of this chapter. Provena Covenant Medical Center (PCMC) is a modern, full-service Catholic hospital adjacent to the campus of the University of Illinois in Urbana. The details of the case are given in The Court Decides at the end of the chapter, but assume for now that PCMC is virtually indistinguishable in its operations from any hospital of its size in the country, whether for-profit or not-for-profit. It participates in Medicare and Medicaid, accepts most private health plans, and has a charity care policy for indigent patients. Consistent with its charitable mission, PCMC provides free care to persons in need, but it attempts to maintain a positive bottom line through appropriate billing and collection activities. The modest amount of charity care it provides is less than the value of its tax exemption ($1.1 million for the 2002 tax year).

After reviewing the definition of charity by tracing the term back to 1867, the Supreme Court of Illinois determined that PCMC was not entitled to an exemption. The court used some familiar concepts in reaching its conclusion:

- Taxation is the rule; exemption is the exception.
- The burden of proof is on the one seeking the exemption.
- Any doubt about the propriety of the exemption must be resolved in favor of the tax being paid.
- The way PCMC dispensed its "charity" did not differ substantially from the way a for-profit writes off bad debt.
- With few exceptions, PCMC provided services in exchange for compensation through insurance, Medicare, Medicaid, or self-payment by the patient.

The court summarized this last point as follows:

There was ample support for the Department of Revenue's conclusion that Provena failed to meet its burden of showing that it used the parcels [of land] in the PCMC complex actually and exclusively for charitable purposes. As our review of the undisputed evidence demonstrated, both the number of uninsured patients receiving free or discounted care and the dollar value of the care they received were **de minimus** [*sic*]. With very limited exception, the property was devoted to the care and treatment of patients in exchange for compensation through private insurance, Medicare and Medicaid, or direct payment from the patient or the patient's family.[43]

> **de minimis**
> inconsequential or of minor importance; a reference to the legal maxim *de minimis non curat lex* (Latin meaning "the law does not concern itself with trifles")

Provena applies criteria that have been established Illinois law for decades. It does not plow new legal ground, but it does churn up a lot of dust. Taxing authorities in other states are certain to use the lessons learned from the PCMC decision to plan or continue their own assaults on healthcare organizations' tax exemptions.

Summary

This chapter addresses the taxation of healthcare organizations, primarily not-for-profit corporations. All tax-exempt organizations are not-for-profit, but not all not-for-profits are tax exempt. The standards for income and property tax exemption are also discussed, as are the occasions in which some income of a tax-exempt organization may be taxable. The chapter raises the question of what it means to be a charity and what implications that designation may have under federal and state law. It closes with a review of a 2010 decision that, if followed by other states, augurs rough sailing ahead for nonprofit hospitals' property tax exemptions, especially if the Affordable Care Act significantly decreases the number of uninsured Americans.

Discussion Questions

1. How should the term *charity* be defined? What are the arguments against and in favor of counting the provision of healthcare in and of itself as charity?

2. Compare the structure and financing of today's "medical–industrial complex" to your mental image of the nineteenth- and early twentieth-century hospital. Outline your arguments—both pro and con—for this debate topic: *Resolved*, that government shall eliminate all favorable tax treatment for not-for-profit healthcare organizations.

3. Consider *Genesee Hospital*. Do you see any parallels between that case and *Charlotte Hungerford Hospital* (discussed in The Court Decides in chapter 6)? Both cases concern the use of hospital property for

a medical office building. In *Charlotte Hungerford Hospital*, the arrangement was upheld; in *Genesee Hospital*, it was not (in effect). Why were the cases decided differently?

4. Suppose the law requires that, for a property to be tax exempt, it must be used for exempt purposes. Suppose also that January 1 is the assessment date, and the use of the property on that date determines its exempt status for the coming year. In July 2016, a hospital buys a parcel of land near its main campus to build a facility for housing and maintaining its fleet of ambulances. Construction begins on December 1, 2016, and is completed in June 2017. The hospital starts using the building as an ambulance station on June 30, 2017. Should the land be considered exempt for 2016? What if construction had begun on January 2, 2017?

5. Discuss the future of property tax exemption in your state in the wake of decisions such as *Provena*.

The Court Decides

Greater Anchorage Area Borough v. Sisters of Charity
553 P.2d 467 (Alaska 1976)

Burke, J.

The central issue in this appeal is the tax-exempt status of a building owned by the Sisters of Charity of the House of Providence, under the provisions of Art. IX, Sec. 4, of the Constitution of Alaska and AS 29.53.020. *[Footnotes omitted.]*

The Sisters of Charity, a long-time healthcare provider in Alaska, erected the building in question, the Providence Professional Building, adjacent to their hospital on land deeded to them in 1959 by the United States for "hospital site, school and recreational purposes only." The construction of the Professional Building began in 1970; its first full year of operation was 1972.

The Professional Building has four floors, including a basement, and is connected by an underground tunnel to nearby Providence Hospital. Three floors are the subject of this appeal, since the parties agree that the basement and tunnel are used exclusively for hospital purposes and are, therefore, exempt from taxation.

The first, second and third floors are rented to doctors having hospital staff privileges at Providence Hospital, for use as their private office space. Approximately thirty-five doctors rent such space. These doctors, although enjoying staff privileges, are not employed by Providence Hospital, and their patients are not necessarily patients of the hospital. Thus, the actual use made of the

first, second and third floors is for office space by doctors engaged in the private practice of medicine.

. . .

A taxpayer claiming a tax exemption has the burden of showing that the property is eligible for the exemption. . . . [T]herefore, the burden is on the Sisters to show that the office space is exempt. . . . They must first show . . . that the property is "used exclusively for nonprofit . . . hospital . . . purposes." *[Quoting from the Alaska statute.]* . . . [W]e find as a matter of law, that the office space is not used exclusively for hospital purposes. . . . [W]hen the property in question is used even in part by non-exempt parties for their private business purposes, there can be no exemption.

. . .

The record indicates that the Sisters have performed a service to doctors and patients alike in constructing the Professional Building, and that healthcare at Providence has been benefited. In order to qualify for an exemption, however, the taxpayer must show, not benefits, but exclusive use. The use of the Professional Building for nonprofit hospital purposes is not exclusive. Therefore, we reverse and remand to the superior court for the entry of an order affirming the Board of Equalization's decision denying the Sisters' appeal. ■

The Court Decides

Barnes Hospital v. Collector of Revenue
646 S.W.2d 889 (Mo. Ct. App. 1983)

Pudlowski, J.

This appeal by Barnes Hospital involves taxation of Queeny Tower, a 17-story building connected to, used and owned by Barnes Hospital for the tax-exempt purposes of treating patients and providing them with care and services. Washington University Medical School, whose teaching facilities are located within the Barnes Hospital complex and whose faculty members comprise the medical staff of the hospital, leases Queeny Tower from Barnes. The part-time faculty subleases offices in Queeny Tower from Washington University for use in their private practice as well as for use in their teaching, research and Barnes Hospital functions.

. . .

The sole question raised is whether property owned by a tax exempt hospital and leased to the medical school for use by its faculty may be taxed where its part-time faculty members, also engaged in limited private practice, maintain their offices therein.

. . .

The first prerequisite for exemption is that the property be "used exclusively" for charitable purposes. Nowhere in its decision did the Missouri Supreme Court define the meaning of the statutory words "used exclusively" or "purposes." Thus, the initial proviso of the qualification articulated first in Franciscan, the statutory phrase "used exclusively," must be examined. The phrase could mean "solely" or "entirely" in its narrowest sense. We do not construe it in that sense.

. . .

. . . The statutory phrase "used exclusively" has reference to the primary and inherent use as against a mere secondary and incidental use. Our courts since Barnes have continued their reliance and acceptance of this definition.

. . .

The policy underlying the statute is to encourage charitable organizations. The meaning we attach to the language of the statute accords with the mandate in Barnes. Although it is the general rule that constitutional provisions exempting property are to be strictly construed, such provisions, though not subject to extension by construction or implication, are to be given a reasonable, natural and practical interpretation in light of modern conditions in order to effectuate the purpose for which the exemption is granted.

. . .

For the foregoing reasons, the judgment of the trial court is reversed and the cause remanded with directions that the decree of August 24, 1978, remain in full force and effect and that appellant's questioned property be removed from the tax rolls of St. Louis City and the City Collector be prohibited from levying tax or compelling payment thereon.

All concur. ∎

Discussion Questions

1. How can the *Greater Anchorage* (Alaska) and *Barnes Hospital* (Missouri) courts take two nearly identical tax laws, apply them to situations with virtually identical facts, and arrive at opposite conclusions? Are their decisions fair?

2. Which of the two interpretations do you find more persuasive?

3. Would *Barnes Hospital* have been decided differently if the property in question had been owned by a for-profit company but leased to the hospital for the same purposes?

4. What if a parking garage with daily or hourly fees and used by employees, patients, families, and visitors were located on a parcel of land owned by and adjacent to the hospital property? Would that use be exempt in Alaska or Missouri? Would it matter who accrued the revenue from the parking garage or what fees were charged? Does your answer change if the garage could also be used by patrons of local businesses that are not related to the hospital?

The Court Decides

Provena Covenant Medical Center v. Department of Revenue
236 Ill.2d 368, 925 N.E.2d 1131 (2010)

[As described in this chapter, the issue in this case is whether a certain Catholic hospital system, Provena Hospitals, had proven that it qualifies for property tax exemption for its Urbana, Illinois, hospital. The director of revenue had determined that the system had not sufficiently made its case and denied the exemption. On review, the circuit court reversed the director's decision, but an appellate court reinstated the denial. The hospital system now appeals to the state's highest court.

The system, which is the property owner, is itself exempt from federal income tax under IRC § 501(c)(3) and from various Illinois occupation and use taxes. None of these exemptions is determinative of the property tax issue. The opinion begins with some further background.]

Provena Hospitals owns and operates six hospitals, including Provena Covenant Medical Center (PCMC), a full-service hospital located in the City of Urbana. PCMC was created through the merger of Burnham City Hospital and Mercy Hospital. It is one of two

general acute care hospitals in Champaign/ Urbana and serves a 13-county area in east central Illinois. The services it provides include a 24-hour emergency department; a birthing center; intensive care, neonatal intensive care, and pediatrics units; surgical, cardiac care, cancer treatment, rehabilitation and behavioral health services; and home health care, including hospice. It offers case management services to assist older persons to remain in their homes and runs various support groups and health-related classes. It also provides smoking cessation clinics and screening programs for high cholesterol and blood pressure as well as pastoral care.

PCMC maintains between 260 and 268 licensed beds. Each year it admits approximately "10,000 inpatients and 100,000 outpatients." Some 60% of its inpatient admissions originate through the hospital's emergency room, which treats some 27,000 visitors annually.

PCMC provides an emergency department because it is required to do so by the [Illinois]

(continued)

(continued from previous page)

Hospital Emergency Service Act. Where emergency room services are offered, a certain level of health care is required to be provided to every person who seeks treatment there. That is so as a matter of both state and federal law. *[Citations omitted here and throughout.]*

Staffing PCMC are approximately 1,000 employees, 400 volunteers and 200 physicians. The physicians are not employed or paid by the hospital. . . . Provena Hospitals' employees do not work gratuitously. Everyone employed by the corporation, including those with religious affiliations, are paid for their services.* Compensation rates for senior executives are reviewed annually and compared against national surveys. Provena Health "has targeted the 75th percentile of the market for senior executive total cash compensation."

According to the record, PCMC's inpatient admissions encompass three broad categories of patients: those who have private health insurance, those who are on Medicare or Medicaid, and those who are "self-pay (uninsured)." PCMC has agreements with some private third-party payers which provide for payment at rates different from "its established rates." The payment amounts under these agreements cover the actual costs of care. The amounts PCMC receives from Medicare and Medicaid are not sufficient to cover the costs of care. Although PCMC has the right to collect a certain portion of the charges directly from Medicare and Medicaid patients and has exercised that right, there is still a gap between the amount of payments received and the costs of care for such patients. For 2002, PCMC calculated

---

This assertion is not literally true. Members of Catholic religious orders who have taken a vow of poverty are not themselves compensated for their services. Rather, their religious orders (the Sisters of Mercy, Alexian Brothers, etc.) are paid directly. The earnings are considered to be the income of the religious order and are not taxable to the individual.[44]

the difference to be $7,418,150 in the case of Medicare patients and $3,105,217 for Medicaid patients.

PCMC was not required to participate in the Medicare and Medicaid programs, but did so because it believed participation was "consistent with its mission." Participation was also necessary in order for Provena Hospitals to qualify for tax exemption under federal law. In addition, it provided the institution with a steady revenue stream.

[The court next reviews various facts relating to the system's and the hospital's financial performance, including budget items; expenses; net revenues; and policies relating to billing, collections, and charity care. The opinion contains the following findings, among others.]

In 2002 [the tax year in question], PCMC budgeted $813,694 for advertising. . . . The ads taken out by PCMC in 2002 covered a variety of matters, including employee want ads. None of its ads that year mentioned free or discounted medical care.

While not mentioned in PCMC's advertisements, a charity care policy was in place at the hospital, and the parties stipulated that PCMC's staff made "outreach efforts to communicate the availability of charity care and other assistance to patients." The charity care policy, which was shared with at least one other hospital under Provena Hospitals' auspices, provided that the institution would "offer, to the extent that it is financially able, admission for care or treatment, and the use of the hospital facilities and services regardless of race, color, creed, sex, national origin, ancestry or ability to pay for these services."

The charity policy was not self-executing. An application was required. Whether an application would be granted was determined by PCMC on a case-by-case basis using eligibility criteria based on federal poverty guidelines. . . .

PCMC's policy specified that the hospital would give a charity care application to anyone who requested one, but it was the patient's responsibility to provide all the information necessary to verify income level and other requested information. To verify income, a patient was required to present documentation "such as check stubs, income tax returns, and bank statements."

PCMC believed that its charity care program should be the payer of last resort. It encouraged patients to apply for charity care before receiving services, and if a patient failed to obtain an advance determination of eligibility under the program, normal collection practices were followed. PCMC would look first to private insurance, if there was any; then pursue any possible sources of reimbursement from the government. Failing that, the hospital would seek payment from the patient directly. . . .

The fact that a patient's account had been referred to collection did not disqualify the patient from applying to the charity care program. Applications would be considered "[a]t any time during the collection process." . . .

During 2002, the amount of aid provided by Provena Hospitals to PCMC patients under the facility's charity care program was modest. The hospital waived $1,758,940 in charges, representing an actual cost to it of only $831,724. This was equivalent to only 0.723% of PCMC's revenues for that year and was $268,276 less than the $1.1 million in tax benefits which Provena stood to receive if its claim for a property tax exemption were granted. The number of patients benefitting from the charitable care program was similarly small.

[The court next establishes the standard for review in cases such as this.] This standard is "significantly deferential." An administrative decision will be set aside as clearly erroneous only when the reviewing court is left with the definite and firm conviction that a mistake has been committed. . . . [T]his is not such a case.

Under Illinois law, taxation is the rule. Tax exemption is the exception. All property is subject to taxation, unless exempt by statute, in conformity with the constitutional provisions relating thereto. Statutes granting tax exemptions must be strictly construed in favor of taxation and courts have no power to create exemption from taxation by judicial construction.

The burden of establishing entitlement to a tax exemption rests upon the person seeking it. . . . If there is any doubt as to applicability of an exemption, it must be resolved in favor of requiring that tax be paid.

[Citing a 1968 decision, the court lists five "distinctive characteristics of a charitable organization." They are as follows:] (1) it has no capital, capital stock, or shareholders; (2) it earns no profits or dividends but rather derives its funds mainly from private and public charity and holds them in trust for the purposes expressed in the charter; (3) it dispenses charity to all who need it and apply for it; (4) it does not provide gain or profit in a private sense to any person connected with it; and (5) it does not appear to place any obstacles in the way of those who need and would avail themselves of the charitable benefits it dispenses. For purposes of applying these criteria, we defined charity as "a gift to be applied *** for the benefit of an indefinite number of persons, persuading them to an educational or religious conviction, for their general welfare—or in some way reducing the burdens of government."

. . .

Provena Hospitals plainly fails to meet the second criterion: its funds are not derived mainly from private and public charity and held in trust for the purposes expressed in the charter. They are generated, overwhelmingly, by providing medical services for a fee. While the corporation's consolidated statement of operations for 2002 ascribes $25,282,000 of Provena Hospitals'

(continued)

(continued from previous page)

$739,293,000 in total revenue to "other revenue," that sum represents a mere 3.4% of Provena's income, and no showing was made as to how much, if any, of it was derived from charitable contributions. The only charitable donations documented in this case were those made to PCMC, one of Provena Hospitals' subsidiary institutions, and they were so small, a mere $6,938, that they barely warrant mention.

Provena Hospitals likewise failed to show by clear and convincing evidence that it satisfied factors three or five. . . . While the record is filled with details regarding PCMC's operations, PCMC is but one of numerous institutions owned and operated by Provena Hospitals. It [PCMC] does not hold title to any of the property for which an exemption is sought. The actual owner is Provena Hospitals. As the Director of Revenue expressly concluded, however, "the record contains no information as to Provena Hospitals' charitable expenditures in 2002." The Director reasoned that without such information, it is simply "not possible to conclude that the true owner of the property is a charitable institution as required by Illinois law." We fully agree. The appellate court was therefore correct when it concluded that this aspect of the Department's decision was not clearly erroneous.

As detailed earlier in this opinion, eligibility for a charitable exemption under [Illinois law] requires not only charitable ownership, but charitable use. Specifically, an organization seeking an exemption . . . must establish that the subject property is "actually and exclusively used for charitable or beneficent purposes, and not leased or otherwise used with a view to profit." . . .

In rejecting Provena Hospitals' claim for exemption, the Department determined that the corporation also failed to satisfy this charitable use requirement. As with the issue of charitable ownership, the appellate court concluded that this aspect of the

Department's decision was not clearly erroneous. Again we agree.

[The court here returns to the 1968 Illinois decision, which had adopted the definition of charity from an 1893 case, which in turn had quoted an 1867 case from Massachusetts. See p. 442.]

Following Crerar, we explained *[in 1936]* that "[t]he reason for exemptions in favor of charitable institutions is the benefit conferred upon the public by them, and a consequent relief, to some extent, of the burden upon the State to care for and advance the interests of its citizens." *[Citing a 1927 case:]* "The reason for exempting certain property from public taxes arises from the fact that such property, in its use for charitable purposes, tends to lessen the burdens of government and to affect the general welfare of the public."

Conditioning charitable status on whether an activity helps relieve the burdens on government is appropriate. After all, each tax dollar lost to a charitable exemption is one less dollar affected governmental bodies will have to meet their obligations directly. If a charitable institution wishes to avail itself of funds which would otherwise flow into a public treasury, it is only fitting that the institution provide some compensatory benefit in exchange. While Illinois law has never required that there be a direct, dollar-for-dollar correlation between the value of the tax exemption and the value of the goods or services provided by the charity, it is a sine qua non of charitable status that those seeking a charitable exemption be able to demonstrate that their activities will help alleviate some financial burden incurred by the affected taxing bodies in performing their governmental functions. . . .

Even if Provena Hospitals were able to [show that it somehow reduced a burden on local government] there was ample support for the Department of Revenue's conclusion that Provena failed to [show] that it used the parcels in the PCMC complex actually and exclusively for charitable purposes. As our review of the undisputed evidence demonstrated, both the number of uninsured patients receiving free or discounted care and the dollar value of the care they received were de minimus. With very limited exception, the property was devoted to the care and treatment of patients in exchange for compensation through private insurance, Medicare and Medicaid, or direct payment from the patient or the patient's family.

To be sure, Provena Hospitals did not condition the receipt of care on a patient's financial circumstances. Treatment was offered to all who requested it, and no one was turned away by PCMC based on their inability to demonstrate how the costs of their care would be covered. The record showed, however, that during the period in question here, Provena Hospitals did not advertise the availability of charitable care at PCMC. Patients were billed as a matter of course, and unpaid bills were automatically referred to collection agencies. Hospital charges were discounted or waived only after it was determined that a patient had no insurance coverage, was not eligible for Medicare or Medicaid, lacked the resources to pay the bill directly, and could document that he or she qualified for participation in the institution's charitable care program. As a practical matter, there was little to distinguish the way in which Provena Hospitals dispensed its "charity" from the way in which a for-profit institution would write off bad debt.

[The opinion continues for another ten pages in which it dismisses the hospital's arguments that not a lot of charity is needed in this university town, that it provides other community benefits, and that it is entitled to a religious exemption because "it is, itself, a ministry of the Catholic Church." The penultimate substantive paragraph of the opinion reads:]

[T]he record clearly established that the primary purpose for which the PCMC property was used was providing medical care to patients for a fee. Although the provision of such medical services may have provided an opportunity for various individuals affiliated with the hospital to express and to share their Catholic principles and beliefs, medical care, while potentially miraculous, is not intrinsically, necessarily, or even normally religious in nature. We note, moreover, that no claim has been made that operation of a fee-based medical center is in any way essential to the practice or observance of the Catholic faith.

[The majority opinion then concludes:]
For the foregoing reasons, the Department of Revenue properly denied the charitable and religious property tax exemptions requested by Provena Hospitals in this case. The judgment of the appellate court reversing the circuit court and upholding the Department's decision is therefore affirmed.
. . .

[The majority opinion was written by an associate justice and joined by the chief justice and another member. Two justices did not participate. Two others joined in affirming the Director's decision that Provena failed to carry its burden of proof and that it is not entitled to a religious exemption, but they dissented from the majority's discussion of charitable use. The dissenting portion of the second opinion reads, in part, as follows:]

[T]he plurality holds that Provena Hospital's use of the property in 2002 was not a "charitable use" because the charity care provided was de minimus. . . . I disagree with this rationale. By imposing a quantum of care requirement and monetary threshold, the plurality is injecting itself into matters best left to the legislature.

The legislature did not set forth a monetary threshold for evaluating charitable use. We may not annex new provisions or add conditions to the language of a statute. . . .

(continued)

(continued from previous page)

I do not believe this court can, under the plain language of section 15-65, impose a quantum of care or monetary requirement, nor should it invent legislative intent in this regard. Setting a monetary or quantum standard is a complex decision which should be left to our legislature, should it so choose. The plurality has set a quantum of care requirement and monetary requirement without any guidelines. This can only cause confusion, speculation, and uncertainty for everyone: institutions, taxing bodies, and the courts. Because the plurality imposes such a standard, without any authority to do so, I cannot agree with it.

I also disagree with the plurality's conclusion that Provena Hospitals was "required to demonstrate that its use of the property helped alleviate the financial burdens faced by the county or at least one of the other entities supported by the county's taxpayers." Alleviating some burden on government is the reason underlying the tax exemption on properties, not the test for determining eligibility. Despite acknowledging this, the plurality converts this rationale into a condition of charitable status. I neither agree with this, nor do I believe that Provena Hospitals failed to show it alleviated some burden on government. . . .

While "lessening the burden of government" is a component of the definition of charity, it is inextricably tied to the public policy justifying the exemption itself and is not a requirement for demonstrating entitlement to the exemption. The plurality here errs in requiring Provena Hospitals to specifically demonstrate some burden of government it relieved. There is no such requirement. ■

Discussion Questions

1. As this *Provena* excerpt (about one-fourth of the total) shows, the case decision is long and complicated. It reflects the public policy struggles inherent in these issues. From what you have read, which of the two opinions (majority or partial dissent) do you feel is better reasoned, and why?
2. The court relies on—and quotes with approval—cases that are many decades (even more than a century) old. Why might those old cases not be relevant today?
3. Should the idea of charity be redefined to meet today's realities? Is it still a valid concept in the context of healthcare? If not, what would you recommend be changed?
4. Given what you know about other hospitals, to what extent do you think the Illinois court's rationale will serve as a blueprint for other states to revoke hospitals' tax exemptions?
5. How, if at all, can hospitals position themselves better to deal with property tax issues?

Notes

1. 26 U.S.C. § 501(c)(3).
2. Trustees of Dartmouth College v. Woodward, 17 U.S. 518, 562 (1819).
3. Trustees of Dartmouth College v. Woodward, 17 U.S. (4 Wheat.) 518 (1819). The same day this decision was announced (February 2,

1819), the US Supreme Court also decided a case involving a charity in *Trustees of the Philadelphia Baptist Ass'n v. Hart's Executors*, 17 U.S. (4 Wheat.) 1 (1819). The definition of *charity* was not at issue in that case, but its juxtaposition with *Dartmouth College* is interesting.

4. RUTH K. MCCLURE, CORAM'S CHILDREN: THE LONDON FOUNDLING HOSPITAL IN THE EIGHTEENTH CENTURY 205 (Yale University Press, 1981).

5. Duhaime's Law Dictionary, *Charity Definition* (accessed August 30, 2016), at http://www.duhaime.org/LegalDictionary/C/Charity.aspx.

6. 236 Ill.2d 368, 925 N.E.2d 1131 (2010).

7. 925 N.E.2d at 1147.

8. City of Philadelphia v. Masonic Home of Pennsylvania, 160 Pa. 572, 28 A. 954 (1894).

9. West Allegheny Hospital v. Board of Property Assessment, Appeals and Review, 500 Pa. 236, 455 A.2d 1170 (1982).

10. *See* Kansas Masonic Home v. Board of Commissioners, 81 Kan. 859, 106 P. 1082 (1910); *accord* Fitterer v. Crawford, 157 Mo. 51, 57 S.W. 532 (1900). In *Fitterer*, a home was denied tax exemption for other reasons.

11. Doctors Hospital v. Sexton, 267 A.D. 736, 48 N.Y.S.2d 201, 205 (1944), *aff'd*, 295 N.Y. 553, 64 N.E.2d 273 (1945). *See also* Bishop and Chapter of the Cathedral of St. John the Evangelist v. Treasurer of the City and County of Denver, 37 Colo. 378, 86 P. 1021 (1906) (a hospital may charge fees to all patients, and the amount received may exceed expenses).

12. 26 C.F.R. § 1.501(c)(3)-1(d)(2).

13. *See, e.g.*, Sonora Community Hosp. v. Commissioner, 397 F.2d 814 (9th Cir. 1968).

14. Rev. Rul. 383, 1969 C.B. 113.

15. 26 U.S.C. § 4958.

16. 26 U.S.C. § 501(r).

17. 26 U.S.C. § 501(r)(3)(B).

18. 26 C.F.R. § 1.512(a)-1(f). *See* United States v. Am. College of Physicians, 106 S. Ct. 1591 (1986) (income received by a medical organization from commercial advertisements in a professional journal is taxable as unrelated business income).

19. For example, Ohio Rev. Code Ann. § 5709.08 (page 1985) provides that "real or personal property belonging to the state or United States used exclusively for a public purpose, and public property used exclusively for a public purpose, shall be exempt from taxation." *See* Carney v. Cleveland, 173 Ohio St. 56, 108 N.E.2d 14 (1962).

20. City of Springfield v. Commissioner of Revenue, 380 N.W.2d 802 (Minn. 1986).

21. 709 P.2d 265 (Utah 1985).

22. 709 P.2d at 302, quoting from UTAH CODE ANN. § 59-2031.

23. 709 P.2d at 268.

24. Hyde v. United States, 225 U.S. 347, 391 (1911) (Holmes, J., dissenting).

25. 181 Neb. 831, 151 N.W.2d 446 (1967).

26. 120 Ga. App. 627, 629, 171 S.E.2d 747, 749 (1969).

27. *Id*. at 750.

28. Harvard Community Health Plan, Inc. v. Board of Assessors, 384 Mass. 536, 427 N.E.2d 1159 (1981).

29. 553 P.2d 467 (Alaska 1976).

30. Aultman Hosp. Ass'n v. Evatt, 140 Ohio St. 114, 42 N.E.2d 646 (1942) (residence for nurses was exempt); Sisters of Saint Mary v. City of Madison, 89 Wis. 2d 372, 278 N.W.2d 814 (1979) (rent-free residence provided for full-time hospital chaplain was exempt); Oakwood Hosp. Corp. v. Michigan State Tax Comm'n, 374 Mich. 524, 132 N.W.2d 634 (1965) (housing for interns and residents was exempt).

31. *See, e.g.*, Milton Hosp. v. Board of Tax Assessors, 360 Mass. 63, 271 N.E.2d 745 (1971); Medical Center of Vt., Inc. v. City of Burlington, 131 Vt. 196, 303 A.2d 468 (1973) (case was remanded to determine facts of whether physician's use of offices at noncommercial rental was primarily for hospital or private purposes); White Cross Hosp. Ass'n v. Warren, 6 Ohio St. 2d 29, 215 N.E.2d 374 (1966) (offices leased to physicians were not exempt); Doctors Hosp. v. Board of Tax Appeals, 173 Ohio St. 283, 181 N.E.2d 702 (1962) (housing for married staff paid a stipend by the hospital was not exempt); City of Long Branch v. Monmouth Medical Center, 138 N.J. Super. 524, 351 A.2d 756 (1976), *aff'd*, 73 N.J. 179, 373 A.2d 651 (1977) (housing for resident interns and nurses was exempt; space rented to private physicians at less than commercial rates is taxable).

32. Genesee Hosp. v. Wagner, 76 Misc. 2d 281, 350 N.Y.S.2d 582 (N.Y. Sup. Ct. 1973), *rev'd*, 47 A.D.2d 37, 364 N.Y.S.2d 934 (1975), *aff'd mem.*, 39 N.Y.2d 863, 352 N.E.2d 133, 386 N.Y.S.2d 216 (1976).

33. N.Y. Real Property Tax Law § 420-a(1)(a) (McKinney 1984).

34. N.Y. Real Property Tax Law § 420-a(2).

35. 76 Misc. 2d at 285–89, 350 N.Y.S.2d at 586–90.

36. Genesee Hosp. v. Wagner, 47 A.D.2d 37, 364 N.Y.S.2d 934 (1975). *Compare* Barnes Hosp. v. Leggett, 646 S.W.2d 889 (Mo. Ct. App.

1983) (teaching hospital's lease of space to part-time medical school faculty who also practiced privately does not destroy tax exemption because faculty provided free care to indigent hospital patients).

37. Sisters of Charity v. Bernalillo County, 93 N.M. 42, 596 P.2d 255 (1979) (pro rata taxation is allowed when office building and parking structure are used for both charitable and noncharitable purposes); Barnes Hosp. v. Leggett, 646 S.W.2d 899 (Mo. Ct. App. 1983) (constitutional provisions authorize exemption for portions of property used exclusively for charitable purposes).

38. *See, e.g.*, Oak Ridge Hosp. v. City of Oak Ridge, 57 Tenn. Ap. 487, 420 S.W.2d 583 (1967); Cleveland Memorial Medical Found. v. Perk, 10 Ohio St. 2d 72, 225 N.E.2d 233 (1967); Hillman v. Flagstaff Community Hosp., 123 Ariz. 124, 598 P.2d 102 (Ariz. 1979).

39. *See, e.g.*, Good Samaritan Hosp. Ass'n v. Glander, 155 Ohio St. 507, 99 N.E.2d 473 (1951); Cleveland Memorial Medical Found. v. Perk, 10 Ohio St. 2d 72, 255 N.E.2d 233 (1967).

40. Sisters of Providence in Washington, Inc. v. Municipality of Anchorage, 672 P.2d 446 (Alaska 1983); *accord* Kunes v. Samaritan Health Service, 121 Ariz. 413, 590 P.2d 1359 (Ariz. 1979) (to be exempt from ad valorem taxation, equipment must be owned).

41. Christ Church Hospital v. County of Philadephia, 65 U.S. (24 How.) 300, 302 (1860).

42. *Id.*

43. 925 N.E.2d 1149.

44. *See* IRS Pub. 517, which states, "If you are a member of a religious order and have taken a vow of poverty, you are already exempt from paying . . . tax on your earnings for ministerial services you perform as an agent of your church or its agencies. . . . Your earnings are considered the income of the religious order."

COMPETITION AND ANTITRUST LAW

13

More than three hundred years ago, the House of Lords (serving as the United Kingdom's highest court) addressed competition issues in a case involving contract-based restrictions on business:

> It is the privilege of a trader in a free country, in all matters not contrary to law, to regulate his own mode of carrying it on according to his own discretion and choice. If the law has regulated or restrained his mode of doing this, the law must be obeyed. But no power short of the general law ought to restrain his free discretion.[1]

In the centuries since, this and various other legal principles have evolved to promote competition and deter restrictive practices such as monopolies, combinations, cartels, conspiracies, price fixing, and group boycotts. These principles, both common law and statutory, are known as *competition law* in most of the developed world and as *antitrust law* in the United States (see Legal Brief on p. 470).

The first competition law statutes in the United States were the Sherman Antitrust Act (passed in 1890) and the Clayton and Federal Trade Commission Acts (both passed in 1914). These statutes and related provisions are summarized in exhibit 13.1. Together they constitute the basic competition

Legal Brief

The term *antitrust* evolved from the nineteenth-century practice of using trusts to destroy competitors and create monopolies. Barons of industry convinced or coerced the shareholders of competing companies to convey their shares to a board of trustees in exchange for dividend-paying certificates. The board would then manage all the companies in "trust" for the shareholders, in the process minimizing competition.

Eventually, *trust* was used to refer to monopolies in general. Standard Oil, US Steel, and Southern Pacific Railroad were prominent trusts. "Trust-busting" became a major policy and political issue in the late nineteenth and early twentieth centuries under presidents William McKinley and Theodore Roosevelt.

laws affecting US business today. Their application to healthcare organizations is the subject of this chapter.

The Sherman Act

Most healthcare antitrust litigation involves charges that the defendants have violated either Section 1 or Section 2 (or both) of the Sherman Act, originally known as the Sherman Antitrust Act. The substantive provision of Section 1 reads as follows: "Every contract, combination in the form of trust or otherwise, or conspiracy, in restraint of trade or commerce among the several states, or with foreign nations, is hereby declared to be illegal."[2] Thus, in 32 words Congress set the stage for more than 12 decades of litigation, and many millions of words have been written over the years to interpret this one sentence.

The illegality of a "contract, combination . . . or conspiracy" that restrains trade should be easy to grasp. Free markets are good; activities that inhibit free markets are bad. (Some people would contest this assumption, but we will take it as a given because Congress says so.) Harder to grasp is how to apply that proposition to an infinite number of situations involving possible restraints of trade (see Law in Action).

Law in Action

Because the Sherman Act applies only to restraints of trade or commerce, the standing assumption was that it did not apply to the practice of a profession. However, in the landmark case *Goldfarb v. Virginia State Bar Association,* the US Supreme Court ruled that a state bar association's minimum fee schedule for attorneys amounted to an illegal price-fixing arrangement.[74] The Supreme Court rejected the defendant's position that the antitrust laws do not apply to the "learned professions." Therefore, healthcare—whether provided by institutions such as hospitals or by physicians and other clinicians—is as subject to antitrust laws as are automobile manufacturers, the steel industry, software companies, and other businesses.

Section 2 of the Sherman Act is similarly terse. It reads as follows: "Every person who shall monopolize, or attempt to monopolize, or combine or conspire with any other person or persons, to monopolize any part of the trade or commerce among the several States, or with foreign nations, shall be deemed guilty of a felony."[3] Thus, both Sections 1 and 2 address *joint action*—an agreement or a conspiracy by two or more parties that restrains trade—and Section 2 adds the concept of *monopoly.*

Obviously, one cannot conspire with oneself, so an action by a single person

EXHIBIT 13.1

Federal Antitrust Law: Summary of Major Statutes and Principles

Statute/Principle	Main Topics	Comment
Sherman Antitrust Act		
In general	Federal power to regulate commerce and promote competition	Per se violations or rule-of-reason analysis
Section 1	Contracts, combinations, and conspiracies in restraint of trade	Needs two or more parties to conspire
Section 2	Monopolies, attempts to monopolize	Can be violated by one party
Clayton Act	Mergers and acquisitions; price discrimination; tying arrangements; overlapping directorships	Also protects labor union activities (e.g., strikes, agricultural boycotts); requires premerger notification to Federal Trade Commission and Department of Justice
Federal Trade Commission Act	Unfair competition and trade practices; false advertising; product labeling	Gives the Federal Trade Commission power to enforce the other statutes administratively and in civil suits
Jurisdictional issues	Interstate commerce	The activity must involve or affect interstate commerce for the federal government to have jurisdiction
	Labor organizations	Human labor is not a commodity or an article of commerce, thus the lawful activities of labor unions are not subject to the antitrust laws
Exemptions and immunities		
Statutory — McCarran-Ferguson Act	Exempts the business of insurance from antitrust laws	The business of insurance does not equal all activities of insurance companies; many people want the act repealed
Statutory — Healthcare Quality Improvement Act	Peer review of medical practice	Provides some antitrust immunity for professional review actions
Common law — Implied repeal		Not often a successful argument
Common law — State action		Narrowly construed
Common law — Noerr-Pennington doctrine	First Amendment right to petition government	Protects lobbying activities, efforts to influence government regulators

does not violate Section 1 of the Sherman Act. Likewise, a corporation, being a legal "person," cannot combine or conspire with itself even though it may act through numerous employees. In 1984, the Supreme Court took this line of reasoning one step further and held that a parent corporation could not agree or conspire with a wholly owned subsidiary corporation even if the two were considered separate legal entities for many other purposes. This decision "leaves untouched [by Section 1] a single firm's anticompetitive conduct (short of threatened monopolization) that may be indistinguishable in economic effect from the conduct of two firms."[4]

The analysis gets more interesting when two or more competitors in a given market unknowingly engage in parallel conduct, such as product pricing. The fact that competitors charge the same price for similar products does not prove a conspiracy. It may be circumstantial evidence for the jury to consider, but without actual proof that the parties conspired, identical pricing in itself does not violate Section 1 of the Sherman Act.[5] On the other hand, evidence showing that the competitors exchanged information and thereby stabilized prices is sufficient proof of a violation.[6] Whether competitors illegally colluded to restrain trade is determined on a case-by-case basis.

In contrast to Section 1, Section 2 of the Sherman Act can apply to a single business enterprise. In addition to prohibiting *combinations* (the term used in this chapter to describe merger, acquisition, and consolidation) that create a monopoly, the section prohibits actual monopolies and attempts to monopolize, even when they result from unilateral action.[7] Section 2 is violated when monopoly power—the power to control prices or exclude competition—exists as a result of "willful acquisition or maintenance of that power as distinguished from growth or development as a consequence of a superior product, business acumen, or historic accident."[8] In simple English, if the world beats a path to your door because you built a better mousetrap, you are not acting illegally, but if you take steps to keep other mousetrap manufacturers off the path, you are violating the law. As is so often the case, the principle is easy to state, but its application is not always free from ambiguity.

In a case alleging violation of the Section 2 monopolization provisions, a court must

1. determine the relevant market, both geographically and for the product;
2. decide whether the evidence shows control of prices or the exclusion of competitors; and
3. determine whether this monopoly power was acquired or maintained willfully.

The Clayton Act

Within a few years of the passage of the Sherman Act, the unintended consequences of its broad, vague language became apparent. For example, corporations used antitrust law to combat organized labor and criminalize union activities (see Law in Action). In 1914, Congress passed the Clayton Act to improve the regulatory scheme and correct some of the Sherman Act's deficiencies.

Among other provisions, the Clayton Act states flatly, "The labor of a human being is not a commodity or article of commerce," and it exempted "labor, agricultural, [and] horticultural organizations" from the antitrust laws.[9]

In addition, the Clayton Act requires companies to notify the Department of Justice (DOJ) and Federal Trade Commission (FTC) of any contemplated mergers or acquisitions above certain size criteria, and it prohibits

- price discrimination,
- tying arrangements (exclusive-dealing contracts),
- mergers and acquisitions that lessen competition, and
- interlocking director or officer positions in competing organizations.

The last point has seldom, if ever, been an issue for healthcare providers—presumably because it makes no sense to have a competitor's officer or board member occupying a similar position in one's own organization—but it was a technique companies once used to create a monopoly without the hassle of merging the corporations.

Price Discrimination

Part of the Clayton Act concerns discriminatory pricing practices, the purpose of which is to lessen competition or gain monopoly power. As amended over the years, it now reads, in part, as follows:

> [It is unlawful] to discriminate in price between different purchasers of commodities of like grade and quality . . . where the effect of such discrimination may be substantially to lessen competition or tend to create a monopoly in any line of

---

Law in Action

More than a century ago, the US Supreme Court decided *Loewe v. Lawlor*, better known as the Danbury Hatters' Case, 208 U.S. 274 (1908). A labor union boycotted the products of a nonunion hat manufacturer in Danbury, Connecticut. The manufacturer sued, arguing that the union's activities were an illegal combination in restraint of trade. The Supreme Court agreed; it let stand an injunction against the union and affirmed the trial court's award of triple damages.

The Clayton Act's protections for unions were a direct result of the outcry from labor in the wake of the Danbury Hatters' Case.

commerce, or to injure, destroy, or prevent competition with any person who either grants or knowingly receives the benefit of such discrimination.[10]

The statute specifically allows price differentials based on "the cost of manufacture, sale, or delivery resulting from the differing methods or quantities in which such commodities are . . . sold or delivered."[11] (The volume discount, therefore, remains legal.) Thus, prices are generally held to be lawful if set in good faith to meet competition and not to drive it out.

The section applies only to sales of commodities (i.e., merchandise, wares), so it does not cover intangible items such as patents, stocks, bonds, and healthcare services. It also does not bar price differentials when commodities sold are different in grade and quality or when they are sold to certain not-for-profit institutions (including hospitals) for their own use.

For example, in *Abbott Laboratories v. Portland Retail Druggists Association, Inc.*, several pharmaceutical manufacturers sold drugs to not-for-profit hospitals at lower prices than they charged commercial pharmacies. The pharmacies' trade association filed suit, believing that this pricing gave the hospitals an unfair commercial advantage. The key issue in the case was what the not-for-profit hospitals were doing with the drugs to qualify for the price differential. In other words, which purchases were for the hospitals' own use and which were for other purposes? The Supreme Court found that the following purchases qualified for the discount:

- Products used in treatment of inpatients, emergency patients, and outpatients seen on the premises
- Take-home prescriptions for those three categories of patients—to the extent that the prescriptions supplemented the treatment rendered at the hospital and were to be used for a limited time (e.g., small supplies of continuation medications given to patients at discharge)
- Drugs furnished to hospital employees, students, and members of the medical staff for their dependents' personal use[12]

On the other hand, except in emergencies when no other source of supply was available, the hospital was not permitted to use the drugs to refill prescriptions for its former patients or to sell them to walk-in customers.[13] The Supreme Court decided that use of the drugs for these purposes would give a hospital-based pharmacy an unfair advantage over commercial pharmacies.

Tying Arrangements and Exclusive-Dealing Contracts

Section 3 of the Clayton Act prohibits tying arrangements and contracts for exclusive dealing:

> It shall be unlawful for any person engaged in commerce . . . to lease or make a sale . . . of goods, wares, merchandise, machinery, supplies or other commodities . . . on the condition, agreement, or understanding that the lessee or purchaser thereof shall not use or deal in the goods [etc.] of a competitor . . . where the effect . . . may be to substantially lessen competition or tend to create a monopoly in any line of commerce.[14]

These prohibited restraints of trade—tying arrangements in particular—are discussed later in the chapter, but suffice it to say at this point that they do not apply to contracts of service and seldom apply to healthcare providers.

Mergers and Acquisitions

Corporate mergers, consolidations, and acquisitions are the subjects of Section 7 of the Clayton Act:

> No person engaged in commerce . . . shall acquire, directly or indirectly, the whole or any part of the stock . . . and no person subject to the jurisdiction of the Federal Trade Commission shall acquire the whole or any part of the assets of another person engaged also in commerce . . . where . . . the effect of such acquisition may be substantially to lessen competition, or to tend to create a monopoly.[15]

Section 7 essentially duplicates the Sherman Act's ban on monopolization and attempted monopolization, but this section is significant because (1) it is enforced by the FTC, which has no enforcement power under the Sherman Act, and (2) the Federal Trade Commission Act applies only to for-profit companies. For many years, therefore, the assumption was that Clayton Act Section 7 did not apply to mergers between nonprofit companies and that only the DOJ could prosecute such cases.

This assumption was challenged in the late 1980s when the FTC brought a monopoly case against the two largest hospitals in Rockford, Illinois, a city of 140,000 people about 90 miles northwest of downtown Chicago. Referring to Section 7, the defendants argued that the case had to be dismissed because they were not-for-profit corporations and thus not "subject to the jurisdiction of the [FTC]," as seemingly required by the statute. The US Court of Appeals disagreed.[16] Writing for a three-judge panel, the highly respected jurist Richard Posner reasoned that Section 7 refers not to the agency's powers under the Federal Trade Commission Act but to its jurisdiction to enforce the Clayton Act itself. Other courts agree with Judge Posner's reasoning (see Law in Action on the next page).[17] (The final outcome of the Rockford case is discussed later in the chapter, where rule-of-reason analysis is considered.)

The standards of the Sherman and Clayton acts are slightly different. Section 1 of the Sherman Act prohibits contracts, combinations, and

**Law in Action
(Judge Posner's Syllogism)**

Major premise: The Clayton Act gives the following government agencies authority to enforce its merger and acquisition provisions:

- The Surface Transportation Board, where applicable to common carriers
- The Federal Communications Commission, where applicable to radio and television
- The Secretary of Transportation, where applicable to air carriers
- The Federal Reserve System, where applicable to banks, banking associations, and trust companies
- The FTC, where applicable to "all other character of commerce"[75]

Minor premise: Not-for-profits are engaged in commerce.

Conclusion: The Clayton Act gives the FTC authority to enforce the Clayton Act's merger and acquisition provisions against not-for-profits even though the FTC could not enforce the Federal Trade Commission Act against the not-for-profits.

conspiracies in restraint of trade, and Section 2 prohibits monopolies or attempts to monopolize. While a corporate acquisition might not violate either of those provisions, its unintended effect might be to "substantially . . . lessen competition" or "tend to create a monopoly," which is the language of the Clayton Act. This fine distinction may be of academic interest only. As a practical matter, "the standard by which an acquisition is judged under the Sherman Act is similar, if not identical, to that under the Clayton Act."[18]

Two US Court of Appeals decisions in 2014 exemplify the effect that the Clayton Act can have on healthcare consolidation. The first involved a merger between two of the four hospital systems in the northwestern Ohio county that includes Toledo. The parties to the merger were ProMedica, by far that area's dominant hospital provider, and St. Luke's, an independent community hospital. The merger—which had been placed on hold pending the outcome of the FTC case—would have left ProMedica with a market share above 50 percent in one relevant product market (for primary and secondary care services) and above 80 percent in another (for obstetrical services). After the FTC found that this merger would adversely affect competition, the parties appealed to the Sixth Circuit.

The appeals court began by noting that Section 7 of the Clayton Act prohibits mergers "where in any line of commerce . . . the effect of such acquisition may be substantially to lessen competition, or to tend to create a monopoly."[19] After reviewing the facts in detail, the court upheld the FTC's order banning the merger.

The court felt the commission was correct in ruling that the consolidation was anticompetitive and likely to increase prices for acute care inpatient services and outpatient obstetric services. In addition, the court felt ProMedica had failed to rebut the presumption of illegality in that it did not show either that the merger would create efficiencies or enhance consumer welfare.

Two aspects of this case—the strong correlation between market share and price, and the degree to which this merger would further concentrate markets that are already highly concentrated—converge in a manner that fully supports the Commission's application of a presumption of illegality.

. . .

Once a merger is found illegal, "an undoing of the acquisition is a natural remedy." Here, the Commission found that divestiture would be the best means to preserve competition in the relevant markets. . . . We have no basis to dispute any of those findings. The Commission did not abuse its discretion in choosing divestiture as a remedy.

* * *

The Commission's analysis of this merger was comprehensive, carefully reasoned, and supported by substantial evidence in the record. The petition is denied.[20]

A similar case arose in Idaho when St. Luke's Health Systems of Nampa tried to acquire Saltzer Medical Group, the largest independent multispecialty physician group in the state. The FTC, the State of Idaho, and two local hospitals filed suit to block the acquisition, and the trial court found that the merger violated Section 7. The Ninth Circuit affirmed that decision.[21]

As the district court recognized, the job before us is not to determine the optimal future shape of the country's health care system, but instead to determine whether this particular merger violates the Clayton Act.

. . .

The district court expressly noted the troubled state of the U.S. health care system, found that St. Luke's and Saltzer genuinely intended to move toward a better health care system, and expressed its belief that the merger would "improve patient outcomes" if left intact. Nonetheless, the court found that the "huge market share" of the post-merger entity "creates a substantial risk of anticompetitive price increases" in the . . . market.[22]

St. Luke's and Saltzer had argued that the merger would result in greater efficiencies and that this should excuse the possible anticompetitive effects. The court did not agree: "We remain skeptical about the efficiencies defense in general and about its scope in particular. It is difficult enough in § 7 cases to predict whether a merger will have future anticompetitive effects without also adding to the judicial balance a prediction of future efficiencies." Accordingly, the judgment of the district court was affirmed and the merger was blocked.[23]

The Ohio and Idaho cases demonstrate a perceived tension between antitrust policy and the need to consolidate for greater efficiency and higher quality care. The Affordable Care Act (ACA) encourages consolidation, but it is clear that the FTC will continue to look critically at merger activity that arguably lessens competition or tends to create a monopoly.

The Federal Trade Commission Act

Congress passed the Federal Trade Commission Act in 1914, the same year the Clayton Act was passed. As noted earlier, this law is enforced by the FTC, an agency that has broad powers and that "deals with issues that touch the economic life of every American."[24]

Section 5 of the Federal Trade Commission Act empowers the FTC to regulate trade practices that are unfair or deceptive to consumers.[25] The FTC has brought numerous cases charging commercial advertisers with the following practices, some of which could apply to healthcare:

- Failing to reveal material facts about a product
- Making false claims and misrepresentations
- Offering misleading prices
- Disparaging a competitor's product by misleading or making untrue assertions
- Announcing unsupported endorsements by well-known persons
- Advertising a bargain to attract customers and then having only a higher-priced product available ("bait and switch")
- Conducting contests that award few of the prizes advertised
- Using overbearing methods in door-to-door sales

Jurisdiction, Exemptions, and Immunity
Congressional Authority: Regulating Interstate Commerce

The US Constitution gives Congress only certain powers, and all legislation must be in furtherance of one of those specified powers (see Legal Brief). In the case of competition laws, constitutional authority comes from the Commerce Clause—the power "to regulate Commerce with foreign Nations and among the several States." That power, however, does not

Legal Brief

In addition to regulation of interstate and foreign commerce, the US Constitution gives Congress the power to impose taxes, pay the government's debts, and provide for the common defense and general welfare. It has jurisdiction over naturalization, bankruptcy, admiralty, the federal judiciary, the District of Columbia, counterfeiting, copyright, and post offices. It has the power to declare and wage war, govern land and naval forces, and call forth militias. In furtherance of these and a few other enumerated responsibilities, Congress is authorized "to make all Laws which shall be necessary and proper for carrying into Execution the foregoing Powers, and all other Powers vested by this Constitution in the Government of the United States, or in any Department or Officer thereof."[76]

extend to *intra*state commerce. Where, then, do we draw the line between interstate and intrastate commerce?

The Constitution was written in the heyday of farmers, farriers, and other tradespeople, when commerce was truly local. Today, the "village blacksmith" can order his supplies by mail, telephone, or Internet; can have them shipped from anywhere in the world by land, sea, or air; and can pay for them through PayPal or an electronic funds transfer from a bank in Chicago, New York, or almost anyplace else. Thus, distinguishing between interstate and intrastate commerce today is not as simple as it might have been in President James Madison's time. Virtually every activity now affects or is affected by interstate commerce, and as a result Congress may regulate even local activities if they have a substantial harmful effect on interstate commerce.[26]

For many years, healthcare services were considered *intra*state commerce and thus were widely assumed to be exempt from federal antitrust statutes. A significant 1976 case proved that assumption wrong. In *Hospital Building Co. v. Trustees of Rex Hospital*,[27] the US Supreme Court held that an alleged conspiracy among a not-for-profit hospital, some hospital officials, and the head of the local health planning agency to prevent the relocation and expansion of a competing hospital had a substantial effect on interstate commerce.[28] A significant portion of the hospital's medicines and supplies, some of its patients, much of its revenue, and the contemplated financing for its planned expansion came from out-of-state sources. The Supreme Court concluded that these factors affected interstate commerce enough for the antitrust laws to apply.[29]

The lesson from *Hospital Building Co.* is that healthcare organizations today cannot avoid scrutiny by claiming that their conduct does not have a substantial effect on interstate commerce. Indeed, as the phenomenon of **medical tourism** becomes more common, healthcare has an international impact as well.

> **medical tourism**
> travel of people to another country to obtain medical treatment, usually because of cost considerations or the treatment's unavailability in their home country

Antitrust Exemptions

For 85 years after passage of the Sherman Act, the so-called learned professions (medicine and law, especially) were assumed to be exempt from the competition laws because they were not businesses in the traditional sense. This belief was shattered in 1975, when the Supreme Court explicitly held that the antitrust laws apply to attorneys and hospitals.[30] It noted that neither the nature nor the public service aspect of an occupation determines antitrust status. In 1982 came the coup de grâce—*Arizona v. Maricopa County Medical Society,* a case that involved an agreement among physicians to set maximum prices charged to beneficiaries of certain health plans.[31] Holding this practice to be price fixing—a per se violation of the Sherman Act—the Supreme Court demonstrated that the antitrust laws apply to the entire healthcare marketplace. The learned professions were exempt no more.

Nevertheless, a few antitrust exemptions (defenses, if you prefer) are available to healthcare organizations. Two are statutory: the McCarran-Ferguson Act and peer review immunity under the Health Care Quality Improvement Act. The other three—state action, Noerr-Pennington, and implied repeal—were created judicially. These exemptions are summarized in exhibit 13.2.

State Action

Of these exemptions, a special word is necessary about the principle of state action. We have seen the term in cases involving the Fifth and Fourteenth Amendments to the US Constitution, where the actions of a state (i.e., a governmental entity) take on special significance. The same is true in the arena of competition.

State and local governments regulate many business and economic activities in the interest of promoting health, safety, and public welfare. (Extensive state regulation of insurance was a major factor in the passage of the McCarran-Ferguson Act, for example.) Sometimes the state's regulatory requirements result in actions by private parties that restrain competition. In such a case, the state action doctrine may provide immunity from antitrust sanctions. In other words, "the state made me do it" is sometimes a defense to an antitrust claim.

The first case establishing this exemption was *Parker v. Brown*,[32] which involved California laws that restrained competition among raisin producers and increased market prices. The Supreme Court held that the state officials administering the law were exempt from antitrust claims because the program "derived its authority and efficacy from the legislative command of the state." Thirty-two years later, in *Goldfarb v. Virginia State Bar Association*,[33] the Supreme Court clarified this holding by saying that the restraint of trade must be *required* (not merely authorized) by the state acting in its sovereign capacity or must be conducted pursuant to a "clearly articulated and affirmatively expressed" state regulatory policy. Thus, the state action exemption has been narrowly construed: The state must either carry out the regulatory process itself or actively supervise the governmental body or private party doing so.

That few regulatory schemes in healthcare can meet these criteria is demonstrated by *FTC v. Phoebe Putney Health System* and *North Carolina State Bd. of Dental Exam'rs v. Federal Trade Comm'n*, both of which are excerpted in The Court Decides at the end of the chapter. In brief, *Phoebe Putney* involved the planned merger of two hospitals in rural southwest Georgia. One of the hospitals was owned by a state "hospital authority" (a state agency), which had formed two private not-for-profit corporations to manage the facility. When the FTC challenged the merger, the hospitals argued that they were covered by state-action immunity. The

Name	Provisions	Comment
McCarran-Ferguson Act, 15 U.S.C. §§ 1011–1015	The act exempts "the business of insurance" except for acts of boycott, coercion, or intimidation. The term *business of insurance* refers not to all aspects of an insurance company's operations but only those that involve spreading risk. See *Group Life and Health Insurance Co. v. Royal Drug Co.*, 440 U.S. 205 (1979).	The business of insurance involves underwriting risk. Unregulated prices for insurance might cause some companies to compete by charging rates that would not cover the actual risk. Those companies would be at risk of failure. State governments are, therefore, allowed to regulate the insurance business for the public good.
Health Care Quality Improvement Act of 1986, 42 U.S.C. §§ 11101 et seq.	The act provides qualified immunity for persons conducting professional review (peer review) activities that affect a physician's clinical privileges.	Refer to *Patrick v. Burget* in chapter 8, in which the US Supreme Court ruled that peer review activities are not immune from antitrust scrutiny. The Health Care Quality Improvement Act (HCQIA) was a direct response to that ruling.
State action doctrine	State regulation sometimes restricts or restrains competition and thus appears to run afoul of antitrust principles. When a defendant's anticompetitive conduct is required by a direct governmental mandate, the state action doctrine may exempt the conduct from antitrust scrutiny.	The restraint of trade must be the result of a clear and affirmatively expressed state regulatory policy, and the state must carry out the activity itself or actively supervise a private party doing so on the state's behalf. See the *Phoebe Putney* case at the end of this chapter.
Noerr-Pennington doctrine (See *Eastern Railroad Presidents Conference v. Noerr Motor Freight, Inc.*, 365 U.S. 127 [1961], and *United Mine Workers v. Pennington*, 381 U.S. 657 [1965])	The doctrine provides that lobbying to influence legislation or governmental regulation is exempt from the antitrust laws even if the result would be anticompetitive.	The doctrine is based on the First Amendment's provisions protecting free speech, especially political speech. The name refers to the names of the parties in two Supreme Court cases.
Implied repeal doctrine	This common-law principle that a new law prevails when it conflicts with an earlier statute, especially when the older law is more general, applies only if there is "clear repugnancy" between the two conflicting statutes and only if necessary to make the subsequent law work.	Implied repeal is disfavored and rarely applied. In the late 1970s, as an attempt to justify a trade-restraining conspiracy between a Blue Cross plan and a state health planning agency, it was argued that the 1974 health planning law was an implied repeal of portions of the antitrust laws. The Supreme Court was not amused.

EXHIBIT 13.2
Antitrust Exemptions of Relevance to Healthcare

Note: In addition to the exemptions listed, the Clayton Act created a safe harbor for labor and agricultural organizations; therefore, strikes and collective bargaining are not covered by the competition laws. Other exemptions not relevant to healthcare include those for professional sports and for newspaper publishers' joint operating agreements. 15 U.S.C. §§ 1291–1295 and 1801–1804.

Legal Brief

Free competition is a bedrock national economic policy. To prohibit individuals and corporations from restraining competition, while at the same time allowing states to do so, appears incongruous. It is understandable, however, given the federal nature of our governmental system and the long-standing battle over and respect for states' rights. (See, for example, the Tenth Amendment to the US Constitution.) The controversial nature of states' rights is perhaps one reason the state action exemption has been so narrowly construed.

Supreme Court disagreed, holding that state-action immunity is "disfavored" and must be clearly articulated and affirmatively expressed in order to apply. The North Carolina case was decided along similar lines, although more emphasis was placed on the anticompetitive aspects of the parties' conduct.

Thus, for state action to provide private parties with antitrust immunity, their actions must be "clearly articulated and affirmatively expressed as state policy" and must be "actively supervised by the State itself" (see Legal Brief).[34]

Sanctions and Enforcement of Antitrust Statutes

Federal law provides for severe civil and criminal penalties for antitrust violations:

> Every person who shall make any contract or engage in any combination or conspiracy hereby declared to be illegal shall be deemed guilty of a felony, and, on conviction thereof, shall be punished by fine not exceeding $100,000,000 if a corporation, or, if any other person, $1,000,000, or by imprisonment not exceeding 10 years, or by both said punishments, in the discretion of the court.[35]

Criminal prosecutions are initiated by the DOJ and are filed in the district that has jurisdiction over the defendants,[36] and either the DOJ or a state attorney general may bring civil actions seeking an injunction to stop illegal activity or break up monopolies. Civil litigation may be terminated by a *consent decree*—an agreement among the parties in which the defendants agree to eliminate the alleged illegal behavior without admitting guilt.[37] Consent decrees are often beneficial to all interested parties because modifying business practices is less costly than continuing to defend a case in court. Those who fail to abide by a consent decree or an injunction are subject to a fine of $10,000 per day.[38]

In addition, private parties—aggrieved competitors, usually—may file civil suits to enforce the Sherman Act. If successful, they may receive up to triple the amount of their actual damages.[39] They may also obtain an injunction and reimbursement for their attorneys' fees and court costs. This last provision encourages settlement because attorneys' fees in a major antitrust suit can amount to several million dollars. Needless to say, triple damages and reimbursement of attorneys' fees are strong deterrents.

Unlike the Sherman Act, the Clayton Act[40] is not a criminal statute. The civil remedies, however, are identical to those of the Sherman Act—the DOJ may seek an injunction or a consent decree; a state attorney general may seek an injunction or damages; and private parties may sue for triple damages, an injunction, or both.

The Federal Trade Commission Act[41] is enforced only by the FTC (see Legal Brief). It does not provide for private right of action, nor is the DOJ involved. Moreover, the act provides only for civil remedies. Because the FTC has investigatory authority over competition matters generally,[42] it is the primary enforcement agency of US competition law.

> **Legal Brief**
>
> As explained in the discussion of the Clayton Act, for many years the assumption was that the FTC had no jurisdiction over not-for-profit companies. Today, the consensus seems to be that it does have jurisdiction, but the issue is essentially moot because there is little substantive difference between the Clayton Act and the Sherman Act. The only practical difference is which agency will take the lead in prosecuting a particular enforcement action.

Rule-of-Reason Analysis and Per Se Violations

Shortly after the Sherman Act was passed, courts realized that not all contracts, combinations, or conspiracies in restraint of trade could be illegal—only unreasonable ones. Justice Louis D. Brandeis declaimed on this point back in 1918:

> Every agreement concerning trade, every regulation of trade, restrains. To bind, to restrain, is of their very essence. The true test of legality is whether the restraint imposed is such as merely regulates and perhaps thereby promotes competition or whether it is such as may suppress or even destroy competition. To determine that question the court must ordinarily consider the facts peculiar to the business to which the restraint is applied; its condition before and after the restraint was imposed; the nature of the restraint and its effect, actual or probable. The history of the restraint, the evil believed to exist, the reason for adopting the particular remedy, the purpose or end sought to be attained, are all relevant facts. This is not because a good intention will save an otherwise objectionable regulation or the reverse; but because knowledge of intent may help the court to interpret facts and to predict consequences.[43]

Whether as an advocate or a judge, Justice Brandeis was punctilious about mastering the complex facts of any case he undertook. His statement summarizes the approach he took to antitrust cases and is the foundation of what has come to be known as *rule-of-reason analysis*—a detailed, time-consuming examination of the issues, including the geographic and product markets involved. Ultimately, it is a case-by-case determination of the positive and negative effects the parties' actions have had or will have on competition.

The rule of reason is applied in most Section 1 cases, but some behavior is so clearly anticompetitive that a full-scale analysis is considered unnecessary. Therefore, over time the courts developed the *per se standard*. This abbreviated approach to restraint of trade is well summarized in this classic statement by Justice Hugo Black:

> There are certain agreements or practices which because of their pernicious effect on competition and lack of any redeeming virtue are conclusively presumed to be unreasonable and therefore illegal without elaborate inquiry as to the precise harm they have caused or the business excuse for their use. This principle of per se unreasonableness not only makes the type of restraints which are proscribed by the Sherman Act more certain to the benefit of everyone concerned, but it also avoids the necessity for an incredibly complicated and prolonged economic investigation. . . . Among the practices which the courts have heretofore deemed to be unlawful in and of themselves are *price fixing, division of markets, group boycotts, and tying arrangements.*[44] [Emphasis added.]

Competitor behaviors amount to automatic (per se) violations if they reflect any of the four practices specified in the last sentence of Justice Black's quote. In such cases, rule-of-reason analysis need not be applied and the plaintiff need not prove the restraint's actual effect on competition. The rule of reason, by contrast, places on the government or private plaintiff the burden of showing the actual anticompetitive effects of the challenged activity.

Applications to Healthcare

As discussed in the previous chapter (see p. 450), "ideas become encysted in phrases and thereafter for a long time cease to provoke further analysis."[45] This Holmesian aphorism may apply to certain assumptions that underlie antitrust policy.

As mentioned in a Legal Brief on page 470, the US competition laws date to the Industrial Revolution. A fair question, therefore, is whether the antediluvian principles of the Sherman Act (and other laws) are appropriate for the twenty-first century, especially in the healthcare arena. Senator John Sherman, brother of the famous Civil War General William Tecumseh Sherman and author of the antitrust law that bears his name, would no doubt be surprised that governmental regulators continue to pin the antitrust tail on today's healthcare donkey. But pin it they do, as shown by the 2013 case

Federal Trade Comm'n v. Actavis, Inc., among many other examples that could be cited.

This case—known casually as the "pay-for-delay case"—involved Solvay Pharmaceuticals, the maker of AndroGel. (AndroGel is a patented, brand-name prescription drug used to treat adult males with low testosterone levels.) When Actavis and another pharmaceutical company obtained patents for a generic drug modeled on AndroGel, Solvay sued them, claiming patent infringement. Rather than go to trial, however, the defendants entered into a "reverse payment" settlement with Solvay. In the settlement, the manufacturers of the generics agreed (1) not to bring their generic drugs to market for a specified number of years and (2) to promote AndroGel to physicians. In return, Actavis and the other manufacturer would receive millions of dollars from Solvay. In other words, they were being paid by Solvay to delay bringing their generic drugs to market.

The FTC filed suit, alleging that the agreement was an unlawful restraint of trade. The US Supreme Court held that this usual form of settlement, while not presumptively illegal, has the potential for genuine adverse effects on competition:

> We concede that settlement on terms permitting the patent challenger to enter the market before the patent expires would . . . bring about competition . . . , but settlement on the terms . . . at issue here—payment in return for staying out of the market—simply keeps prices at patentee-set levels, potentially producing the full patent-related $500 million monopoly return while dividing that return between the challenged patentee and the patent challenger. The patentee and the challenger gain; the consumer loses.[46]

The details of the complicated decision are not important here. Suffice it to say that the Supreme Court concluded that there was a risk of "significant anticompetitive effects" and remanded the case for further proceedings. The AndroGel case shows that antitrust law is alive and well in the healthcare arena—and not only with regard to combinations.

Some observers assert that healthcare markets are profoundly different from other markets and that normal antitrust analyses of market power and concentration are unsuitable. They argue that prices for hospital services are not simply a matter of supply and demand but are greatly influenced by factors outside hospitals' control, including

- Medicare and Medicaid programs' fee schedules,
- negotiated discounts for managed care plans,
- the aging of the patient population, and
- the cost of new drugs and medical technology.

Others—governmental regulators especially—contend that competition is as worthy a goal in healthcare as it is in any other field. They seek application of traditional antitrust principles to encourage competition, prevent monopolies or concentration of markets, and help control healthcare costs. This attitude prevailed throughout the 1980s and early 1990s when antitrust enforcement was a high priority, and it is seeing a revival today as regulators begin to reassert authority over the healthcare sector. (Exhibit 13.3 lists areas of antitrust concern for hospitals. See also Legal Decision Point.)

During the second half of the Bill Clinton administration and throughout the George W. Bush administration, regulators were less attentive to antitrust issues in healthcare and more concerned with mergers in other sectors and with international restraints of trade. The government had lost a string of hospital merger cases,[47] culminating in *FTC v. Butterworth Health Corp.*,[48] in which a court approved the combination of two of the four hospitals in Grand Rapids, Michigan, on the grounds of procompetitive effects, saying that

> [To permit] defendant hospitals to achieve the efficiencies of scale that would clearly result from the proposed merger would enable the board of directors of the combined entity to continue the quest for establishment of world-class health facilities in West Michigan, a course [that] the Court finds clearly and unequivocally would ultimately be in the best interests of the consuming public as a whole.[49]

After this 1996 decision was announced, hospital antitrust enforcement seemed to fall off the government's radar for a while, but it has picked up in recent years. Both the FTC and the DOJ have renewed aggressive enforcement against provider mergers they believed to be anticompetitive, challenging not just hospital transactions but also mergers and acquisitions of physician practices, drug companies, and even state licensing boards (see The Court Decides: *North Carolina State Bd. of Dental Exam'rs v. Federal Trade Comm'n* at the end of this chapter).

Legal Decision Point

Analyze how effective the activities listed in exhibit 13.3 (and the antitrust principles applied to them) have been in reducing the rising cost of US healthcare. Consider the root causes of cost increases and available alternatives to the way the healthcare system is financed.

Combinations Under the Sherman and Clayton Acts

Corporations grow and diversify through mergers and consolidations. In a merger, one corporation acquires the stock or assets of another company, which may then close or continue to operate in some other capacity. In a consolidation, two or more corporations join to form a new company and the predecessor corporations are dissolved. In casual conversation, *merger,*

Type of Activity	Possible Antitrust Concern
Health planning	Restraint of trade
Shared services	Price fixing, group boycott
Utilization review	Group boycott
Medical staff privileges	Group boycott
Third-party-payer contracts	Price fixing, group boycott, monopolization, tying arrangement
Managed care organizations	Price fixing, group boycott, monopolization, tying arrangement
Mergers and consolidations	Monopolization
State licensing boards	Group boycott
Pharmaceutical manufacturers	Price fixing, restraint of trade, monopolization

EXHIBIT 13.3
Antitrust Concerns for Healthcare

acquisition, and *consolidation* are often used interchangeably. As mentioned earlier, the word *combination* is used in this chapter to describe all three.

Four different competition law provisions bear on corporate combinations. Section 7 of the Clayton Act is the most significant,[50] but business combinations can also be challenged under Sections 1 and 2 of the Sherman Act[51] and Section 5 of the Federal Trade Commission Act.[52]

Business combinations are not per se violations, and some in fact promote competition, so actual or probable lessening of competition must be proven in cases brought under Sherman Act Section 1 (restraint of trade). Furthermore, Section 1 applies only to concerted action of two or more parties, not unilateral action. In contrast, Section 2—which prohibits monopolies, attempts to monopolize, and conspiracy to monopolize—can apply to unilateral action.[53] A Section 2 allegation must present three elements:

1. Proof of market power—the ability to exclude competitors or to fix or control prices, whether that ability is exercised or not
2. Definition of the relevant geographic and service markets
3. Proof that the defendant has achieved or is maintaining monopoly power willfully or unfairly

Size and the absence of competition alone do not prove the existence of an illegal monopoly. As the Supreme Court has stated, "Growth or development as a consequence of a superior product, business acumen, or historic accident" does not violate Section 2 of the Sherman Act.[54] (Recall the

Legal Brief

The prominence of Apple's iPhone and the struggles of Blackberry's products in the world of smartphones are examples of the "better mousetrap syndrome."

mousetrap analogy earlier in this chapter, and see Legal Brief.) Invention and innovation in a rapidly changing technological world encourage competition, and success in itself does not violate the principles of competition law.[55] For this reason, the Sherman Act is often difficult to enforce and the Clayton Act is used more often to challenge business combinations.

Section 7 of the Clayton Act prohibits combinations that "tend to create a monopoly." It applies only to combinations "in commerce." This standard may be more stringent than that of the Sherman Act, which applies to activity that "substantially affects commerce." The Clayton Act did not apply, for example, to the case of an out-of-state corporation doing business nationally that acquired two firms supplying local janitorial services in Southern California because the acquired companies were said not to be engaged in interstate commerce.[56] As a practical matter, the distinction between "in commerce" and "affecting commerce" is only an academic one.

If the behavior in question is not a per se violation, a rule-of-reason analysis requires (1) defining the product or service and (2) determining the geographic market for that product or service. This market analysis is followed by appraisal of the proposed combination's probable effect on competition.

In defining the product market, one must identify items that compete with each other and any interchangeable substitutes. If buyers are prone to substitute another product when the price of a certain item increases, the substitute must be included in the market. On the other hand, if the evidence shows that purchasers do not substitute comparable items when a given product's price increases, the targeted product stands alone as a market. (The phrase used in appraising this factor is *cross elasticity of demand*.)

The market must be defined in relation to the facts of each case. For example, in one case, the Supreme Court held that cellophane (cellulose film used in food packaging and other industrial applications) competes with other types of flexible packaging materials. Because the defendant possessed only 18 percent of the market for packaging materials, it had not committed an antitrust violation even though it had nearly 75 percent of the market for cellophane.[57] In other words, demand was elastic—if the price for cellophane went up, other packaging products would substitute.

Obviously, definition of the market has a profound effect on the outcome of a case. An expansive definition includes more competitors and makes the market area appear less concentrated and the combination less monopolistic.

In a merger case from Roanoke, Virginia, for example, the court noted that one hospital in question drew 27 percent of its patients from 14 counties, including three counties in West Virginia. It also appeared to draw at least 100 patients per year from each of six other counties. The second hospital drew about 18 percent of its patients from eight counties outside Roanoke. In the geographic area thus described, about 20 other hospitals provided primary—and, in some cases, secondary—care. On the basis of this analysis, the court concluded that the two merging hospitals were competing with the hospitals in those surrounding counties, and it approved the merger. The court also found that the merger "would probably improve the quality of healthcare in western Virginia and reduce its cost and will strengthen competition between the two large hospitals that would remain in the Roanoke area."[58]

In contrast to the Roanoke decision stands *United States v. Rockford Memorial Corporation*,[59] a decision by the esteemed appellate court Judge Richard Posner that involved the two largest hospitals in Rockford, Illinois. If allowed to merge, the two would have controlled as much as 72 percent of the market for inpatient services, and they and the area's other large hospital (which was not party to the proposed combination) would have controlled about 90 percent. Unlike the judge in the Roanoke case, Judge Posner refused to generalize about the shift of traditional hospital services to outpatient settings:

> If a firm has a monopoly of product X, the fact that it produces another product, Y, for which the firm faces competition is irrelevant to its monopoly unless the prices of X and Y are linked. For many services provided by acute-care hospitals, there is no competition from other sorts of provider. If you need a kidney transplant, or a mastectomy, or if you have a stroke or a heart attack or a gunshot wound, you will go (or be taken) to an acute-care hospital for inpatient treatment. The fact that *for other services* you have a choice between inpatient care at such a hospital and outpatient care elsewhere places no check on the prices of the services we have listed, for their prices are not linked to the prices of services that are not substitutes or complements. If you need your hip replaced, you can't decide to have chemotherapy instead [just] because it's available on an outpatient basis at a lower price.[60] [Emphasis added.]

Having concluded that the relevant product market was inpatient, acute care services only, Judge Posner turned to the geographic market analysis. Although he accepted the trial court's finding that the service area was a large portion of northern Illinois and southern Wisconsin, 87 percent of the hospitals' admissions were from Rockford, the rest of the county in which it is located, and "pieces of several other counties." This larger service area contained six

Law in Action

It is always possible to take pot shots at a market definition (we have just taken one), and the defendants do so with vigor and panache. Their own proposal, however, is ridiculous—a ten-county area in which it is assumed (without any evidence and contrary to common sense) that Rockford residents, or third party payers, will be searching out small, obscure hospitals in remote rural areas if the prices charged by the hospitals in Rockford rise above competitive levels. Forced to choose between two imperfect market definitions, the defendants' and the district judge's (the latter a considerable expansion of the government's tiny proposed market) . . . we choose the less imperfect, the district judge's.[77]

—Judge Richard Posner

hospitals in all, but "90 percent of Rockford residents who are hospitalized are hospitalized in Rockford itself." Thus, on behalf of the three-judge appellate panel, Judge Posner declared that "for the most part hospital services are local," and he affirmed the trial court's injunction prohibiting the combination (see Law in Action).[61]

The *Rockford* court's analysis has since become the majority view: The relevant product market in hospital combination cases is usually general, acute care hospital services. Nevertheless, the Roanoke and Rockford cases illustrate the difference that geography, demographics, and product definition can make in a rule-of-reason analysis. They also illustrate why the outcome of hospital antitrust cases is often difficult to predict: "These decisions require factual judgments regarding what the future may hold in an industry undergoing revolutionary change. Like pilots landing at night aboard an aircraft carrier, courts are aiming for a target that is small, shifting and poorly illuminated."[62] That comment was made more than three decades ago. How prescient it was given this era of healthcare reform!

After the relevant product and geographic markets have been determined, the competitive effect of a combination must be predicted. The goal is to determine whether the effect of the combination, in the words of the Clayton Act, "may be substantially to lessen competition or tend to create a monopoly." Among the important factors to consider in evaluating the potential competitive effect of a combination are the following:

- Whether competing firms or potential competitors have been eliminated from the market
- Whether the acquisition of a relatively small but locally dominant firm by a larger organization makes the acquired company even more dominant
- Whether the combination may lead the firms to buy each other's products and thereby harm competitors
- What has happened to the competitive environment in situations in which combinations have already occurred

The focus is on the future and potential adverse effects on competition. A combination can be challenged long after the transaction occurs because the statute of limitations does not begin to run until anticompetitive effects are felt.[63] The statute itself provides neither a quantitative nor qualitative means of determining whether competition has changed. Each combination has to be viewed functionally in the context of the particular industry.

Horizontal Combinations

Horizontal combinations are likely to have the most significant effects on competition. To judge a combination's effect, the federal regulatory agencies (DOJ, FTC) and the courts generally use a mathematical formula—the Herfindahl-Hirschman Index (HHI)—to measure market concentration.[64] The HHI is calculated by squaring each firm's (hospital's or other entity's) market share and summing the squares. For example, a market consisting of four firms with market percentages of 30, 30, 20, and 20, respectively, has an HHI of 2,600 ($30^2 + 30^2 + 20^2 + 20^2 = 2,600$). The HHI can range from 10,000 (in the case of a pure monopoly) to a number approaching zero (in the case of an atomistic market).

On the basis of the post-combination HHI value, markets are classified into three types:

1. Unconcentrated: HHI below 1,500
2. Moderately concentrated: HHI between 1,500 and 2,500
3. Highly concentrated: HHI above 2,500

The agencies then compare the precombination and postcombination HHI scores. The higher the postcombination market type and the greater the increase in the HHI, the greater the likelihood that the agencies will request additional information and further investigate the combination.

Vertical Combinations

Unlike horizontal combinations, vertical combinations—the union of a vendor and a customer—do not directly eliminate a competitor; instead, they ensure the availability of supplies to the customer and perhaps solidify sales of the vendor's product. The problem from the standpoint of competition law is that the vertical combination may

- foreclose the customer's competitors from their source of supply;
- foreclose the vendor's competitors from access to the market (or a substantial portion of it); or
- force actual or potential competitors into vertical arrangements of their own, which may in turn have anticompetitive effects.[65]

Although not a healthcare case, Ford Motor Company's acquisition of Autolite in the early 1960s is a simple illustration of a vertical combination.

Autolite manufactured spark plugs, an essential component of automobiles. The Supreme Court held that the combination violated the Clayton Act because it eliminated Ford as a potential spark plug manufacturer and removed it from the market as a significant buyer of other manufacturers' products. The argument that the combination made Autolite more competitive was irrelevant.[66]

An example of a vertical combination in healthcare involved the two-hospital town of Vicksburg, Mississippi. One of the hospitals agreed to acquire the two largest physician clinics in the area. The other hospital filed suit, alleging that this vertical combination would cause the physician clinics to shift their patient admissions to the defendant hospital and would give that hospital monopoly power for managed care contracts. After giving the case serious analysis (the opinion runs about 20,000 words, plus footnotes), the trial court judge ruled, "The challenged merger is neither the product of a concerted effort to monopolize nor likely to stifle competition to any substantial degree in the relevant markets."[67]

Another form of business combination prevalent in the healthcare arena is the *joint venture*—an association of two or more firms meant to accomplish a defined economic goal. A joint venture has many attributes of a partnership, but it may be set to end when it completes its project or accomplishes its economic goal. Joint ventures are subject to the same scrutiny under the competition laws as other types of combined activity (see Law in Action). The courts evaluate all relevant factors in deciding whether the venture is likely to lessen competition.[68] A joint venture is usually approved if the defined goal of the agreement is legitimate and if the market share involved is relatively small.

Law in Action

In some circumstances, both parties to a proposed combination (or merger) must report the pending transaction to the government.[78] The details of the requirement are not important here; suffice it to say that precombination notification is often required because it enables the government to review the implications of an agreement or an offer to combine before the transaction is completed. If the government concludes that the transaction is likely an antitrust violation, it can seek a preliminary injunction to halt the deal pending further investigation.

Summary of Rule-of-Reason Analysis

In a Clayton Act case, the plaintiff—whether the government or a private party—bears the burden of proving the defendant's share of the market and the market's concentration values. The plaintiff must also show that the combination is likely to have an anticompetitive effect.[69] This standard of proof in turn necessitates a broad and expansive factual inquiry beyond statistical calculation of market share, HHI, and so forth.

The rule-of-reason analysis, then, permits the use of subjective judgment in evaluating the facts presented in court and the likely effect of the proposed combination. The courts require that all relevant economic factors and probabilities be considered when the Clayton Act is used as the basis for challenging a combination. Among these factors are the following:

- Ease of entry into a market
- Economic health of the particular industry
- Characteristics of the products involved
- Availability of substitute products
- Nature of consumer demand
- Possible procompetitive effects

For example, in *FTC v. Butterworth* (mentioned earlier), the government sought to enjoin the combination of two of the four hospitals in Grand Rapids, Michigan. When the case began, the two facilities had approximately 75 percent of the general, acute care hospital beds in the region; after the merger, the facilities would control about two-thirds of the total market for general inpatient services and make Grand Rapids a highly concentrated market. Despite this prediction, the federal district court refused to stop the transaction. It found a number of salient points persuasive:

1. Evidence from economists showed that higher market concentration does not correlate to higher healthcare costs but in fact could lower prices.
2. Both organizations were community-based, not-for-profit corporations whose boards comprised local business leaders who had an interest in providing high quality at low cost.
3. The boards of the two hospitals issued formal assurances to the community that the purpose of the combination was to reduce costs and pass the savings along to consumers.
4. The merger would most likely temper the growing influence of managed care organizations, stabilize managed care rates, and reduce cost shifting.
5. The combination would help prevent a "medical arms race" through significant efficiencies and lower capital expenditures.

Although it would be inappropriate to generalize, given that the rule-of-reason approach by its very nature requires a determination based on the facts and circumstances of each individual case, these are the kinds of factors that will be taken into account.

Antitrust Safety Zones

Periodically, the DOJ and the FTC issue joint statements explaining their antitrust enforcement policies. These policy papers can be found on the FTC website (http://www.ftc.gov). The latest policy statement created a *safety zone* for accountable care organizations (ACOs) that participate in the Shared Savings Program under the ACA.[70] Safety zones "describe conduct that the agencies will not challenge under the antitrust laws, absent extraordinary circumstances."[71] The safety zones for general healthcare transactions are as follows:

- Combinations involving a small hospital
- Joint ventures to purchase expensive or high-tech equipment or to provide certain expensive services
- Collective efforts to share non-fee-related information (e.g., medical data)
- Arrangements to provide fee-related information to purchasers of health services
- Participation in surveys regarding prices, wages, salaries, and benefits under certain circumstances
- Group purchasing arrangements that meet certain conditions
- Physician network joint ventures that involve certain types of risk sharing
- Certain multiprovider network arrangements, if efficiencies that benefit consumers might result

All of the safety zones, whether for ACOs or general healthcare transactions, have preconditions and are described narrowly so as not to foreclose agency action unnecessarily. The authors of the statements are also careful to note that actions that fall outside the antitrust safety zones are not necessarily anticompetitive and may actually be procompetitive.

Underscoring this viewpoint, an assistant US attorney general made the following remarks to a joint meeting of the American Bar Association and American Health Lawyers Association:

> There can be no doubt that vigorous yet responsible antitrust enforcement is crucial if we are to benefit from innovation and efficiency in our health care delivery system and reduce rising health care costs in both the public and private sectors.
>
> The US population is aging, with the baby boomers once again transforming the demographic landscape as they reach 65. These changing demographics demand that we devise ways to treat even greater numbers of increasingly sick patients more efficiently and affordably. Unquestionably, that will lead to additional interest in integrating what most observers say is now a fragmented health care delivery system.
>
> There does not seem to be serious dispute that clinical integration and coordinated care have the potential to decrease costs and improve quality. The key is whether we can gain those benefits without sacrificing meaningful competition.

The answer to that question is undoubtedly "yes." The Health Care Policy Statements and business reviews of the federal antitrust enforcement agencies make clear that the antitrust is not an impediment to the formation of innovative, integrated health care delivery systems and genuine increases in provider efficiency.[72]

Expectations for Future Enforcement Activities

Consolidation of providers will continue as the ACA is implemented, as will antitrust enforcement activity in connection with hospital, health plan, and physician transactions (see Law in Action). Exclusive contracting by large providers will be just one of many contracting issues, and the balance of power between dominant providers and large health plans will present novel antitrust concerns. Collective negotiations by competing providers have always raised antitrust issues, but many providers are either ignorant of the antitrust consequences or will choose to ignore them.

Although few ACOs have thus far sought the voluntary antitrust review that is available to them, they must understand the antitrust implications of their activities when contracting with commercial payers. The FTC–DOJ joint statement on the antitrust aspects of ACOs sets forth the enforcement agencies' views on market power and appropriate and inappropriate contracting practices.[73]

The *N.C. State Board of Dental Examiners* case showed that state licensing boards that consist of competing providers must be aware they can violate the antitrust laws when their activities restrain competition. And finally, the Supreme Court decision in the AndroGel pay-for-delay case will have significant implications for pharmaceutical manufacturers.

In sum, the enforcement agencies continue to believe in their mission to protect competition. As health reform takes hold, antitrust issues will be an important part of the healthcare scene.

Summary

This chapter reviews the basic concepts of competition (antitrust) law, including laws against restraints of trade, monopolization, and price discrimination. It distinguishes among per se violations—division of markets, price fixing, group boycotts, and tying arrangements—and shows how cases that do not fit one of those categories are decided on the basis of a rule-of-reason analysis specific to the anticompetitive effects of each set of facts. Exemptions from the antitrust laws include implied repeal, state action,

Law in Action

As the ACA is implemented in the next few years, students may wish to consider to what extent it remains true that "antitrust is not an impediment" to greater efficiency and clinical integration.

Noerr-Pennington, and the business of insurance doctrines. This chapter reviews the factors used in defining the appropriate market for individual cases, and it concludes with a discussion of what to expect in the coming years, especially now that the ACA has begun to be implemented.

Discussion Questions

1. Name and describe the per se violations of antitrust law.
2. Define the rule of reason and describe when it is used.
3. In today's economy, what are some examples of intrastate commerce? In other words, what business does not affect interstate commerce?
4. How would you define the geographic and product markets of large healthcare organizations such as the Mayo Clinic, Cleveland Clinic, Kaiser Permanente, and Johns Hopkins? What are the barriers that keep new competitors from entering those markets?
5. How, if at all, does the phenomenon of medical tourism affect your perception of the market for healthcare services (see chapter 15)?

The Court Decides

Federal Trade Comm'n v. Phoebe Putney Health System
133 S.Ct. at 1003, __ U.S. __ (2013)

SOTOMAYOR, J., delivered the opinion for a unanimous Court.

Under this Court's state-action immunity doctrine, when a local governmental entity acts pursuant to a clearly articulated and affirmatively expressed state policy to displace competition, it is exempt from scrutiny under the federal antitrust laws. In this case, we must decide whether a Georgia law that creates special-purpose public entities called hospital authorities and gives those entities general corporate powers, including the power to acquire hospitals, clearly articulates and affirmatively expresses a state policy to permit acquisitions that substantially lessen competition. . . .

In 1941, the State of Georgia amended its Constitution to allow political subdivisions to provide health care services. . . . Under the Law, a hospital authority "exercise[s] public and essential governmental functions" and is delegated "all the powers necessary or convenient to carry out and effectuate" the Law's purposes.

In the same year that the Law was adopted, the city of Albany and Dougherty County established the Hospital Authority of Albany-Dougherty County (Authority) and the Authority promptly acquired Phoebe Putney Memorial Hospital (Memorial), which has been in operation in Albany since 1911. In 1990, the Authority restructured its operations by forming two private nonprofit corporations to manage Memorial: Phoebe Putney Health System, Inc. (PPHS), and its subsidiary, Phoebe Putney Memorial Hospital, Inc. (PPMH). The Authority leased Memorial to PPMH for $1 per year for 40 years. Under the lease, PPMH has exclusive authority over the operation of Memorial. . . .

Memorial is one of two hospitals in Dougherty County. The second, Palmyra Medical Center (Palmyra), was established in Albany in 1971 and is located just two miles from Memorial. . . . Together, Memorial and Palmyra account for 86 percent of the market for acute-care hospital services provided to commercial health care plans and their customers in the six counties surrounding Albany. Memorial accounts for 75 percent of that market on its own.

In 2010, PPHS began discussions with HCA [Palmyra's owner] about acquiring Palmyra. Following negotiations, PPHS presented the Authority with a plan under which the Authority would purchase Palmyra with PPHS controlled funds and then lease Palmyra to a PPHS subsidiary for $1 per year under the Memorial lease agreement. The Authority unanimously approved the transaction.

[After the FTC challenged the merger, both a federal district court and the Eleventh Circuit held that the transaction was immune from antitrust liability under the "state action" exemption. The Supreme Court granted certiorari.]

In *Parker* v. *Brown,* this Court held that because "nothing in the language of the Sherman Act or in its history" suggested that Congress intended to restrict the sovereign capacity of the States to regulate their economies, the Act should not be read to bar States from imposing market restraints "as an act of government." Following *Parker,* we have held that under certain circumstances, immunity from the federal antitrust laws may extend to nonstate actors carrying out the State's regulatory program.

(continued)

(continued from previous page)

But given the fundamental national values of free enterprise and economic competition that are embodied in the federal antitrust laws, "state-action immunity is disfavored, much as are repeals by implication." Consistent with this preference, we recognize state-action immunity only when it is clear that the challenged anticompetitive conduct is undertaken pursuant to a regulatory scheme that "is the State's own."

. . .

Our case law makes clear that state-law authority to act is insufficient to establish state-action immunity; the substate governmental entity must also show that it has been delegated authority to act or regulate anticompetitively. . . .

We have no doubt that Georgia's hospital authorities differ materially from private corporations that offer hospital services. But nothing in the Law or any other provision of Georgia law clearly articulates a state policy to allow authorities to exercise their general corporate powers, including their acquisition power, without regard to [the] negative effects on competition. . . .

We hold that Georgia has not clearly articulated and affirmatively expressed a policy to allow hospital authorities to make acquisitions that substantially lessen competition. The judgment of the Court of Appeals is reversed, and the case is remanded for further proceedings consistent with this opinion. ∎

Discussion Questions

1. Research and explain the community of Albany-Dougherty County and the corporate structure involved in this case. Who do you suppose were the officials in the various corporate entities?
2. Explain how the transaction was structured, and why.
3. The federal trial court was the US District Court for the Middle District of Georgia; the Court of Appeals was the Eleventh Circuit, which sits in Atlanta. Considering the locations of and incumbent judges on these courts, why might the Supreme Court have a different worldview and a different perspective on the policy aspects of this issue?

The Court Decides

North Carolina State Bd. of Dental Exam'rs v. Federal Trade Comm'n
___ U.S. ___ (2015)

JUSTICE KENNEDY delivered the opinion of the Court, in which ROBERTS, C. J., and GINSBURG, BREYER, SOTOMAYOR, and KAGAN, JJ., joined. ALITO, J., filed a dissenting opinion, in which SCALIA and THOMAS, JJ., joined.

This case arises from an antitrust challenge to the actions of a state regulatory board. A majority of the board's members are engaged in the active practice of the profession it regulates. The question is whether the board's actions are protected from Sherman Act regulation under the doctrine of state-action antitrust immunity, as defined and applied in this Court's decisions beginning with *Parker v. Brown*, 317 U. S. 341 (1943).

[North Carolina law provides that the State Board of Dental Examiners is "the agency of the State for the regulation of the practice of dentistry." The Board's principal duty is to create, administer, and enforce a licensing system for dentists; and six of its eight members must be licensed, practicing dentists.

The act does not specify that teeth whitening is "the practice of dentistry," but dentists started providing the service in the 1990s. By 2003, cosmetologists and other nondentists started charging lower prices for the same services, and the dental board began to issue cease-and-desist letters warning that the unlicensed practice of dentistry is a crime. This and other threatening actions led nondentists to stop offering teeth whitening services, but some of them complained to the Federal Trade Commission (FTC), which began an investigation.

In 2010 the FTC filed administrative charges alleging that the dental board's concerted action to exclude nondentists from the market for teeth whitening amounted to an anticompetitive and unfair method of competition under the Federal Trade Commission Act. The dental board moved to dismiss the complaint on the ground of "state-action immunity," but the FTC denied that motion, ruling that even if the board had acted pursuant to a clearly articulated state policy, it must be actively supervised by the state to claim immunity, which it was not. This ruling was ultimately affirmed by the US Court of Appeals for the Fourth Circuit, and a petition for certiorari to the Supreme Court followed.]

Federal antitrust law is a central safeguard for the Nation's free market structures. In this regard it is "as important to the preservation of economic freedom and our free-enterprise system as the Bill of Rights is to the protection of our fundamental personal freedoms." The antitrust laws declare a considered and decisive prohibition by the Federal Government of cartels, price fixing, and other combinations or practices that undermine the free market.

The Sherman Act serves to promote robust competition, which in turn empowers the States and provides their citizens with opportunities to pursue their own and the public's welfare. The States, however, [sometimes may] impose restrictions on occupations, confer exclusive or shared rights to dominate a market, or otherwise limit competition to achieve public objectives. If every duly enacted state law or policy were required to conform to the mandates of the Sherman Act, thus promoting competition at the expense of other values a State may deem fundamental, federal antitrust law would impose an impermissible burden on the States' power to regulate.

For these reasons, the Court in *Parker v. Brown* interpreted the antitrust laws to confer immunity on anticompetitive conduct by the States when acting in their sovereign capacity. That ruling recognized Congress's purpose to respect the federal balance and to "embody in the Sherman Act the federalism principle that the States possess a significant measure of sovereignty under our Constitution."

In this case the Board argues [that] its members were invested by North Carolina with the power of the State and that, as a result, the Board's actions are cloaked with *Parker* immunity. This argument fails, however. A nonsovereign actor controlled by active market participants—such as the Board—enjoys *Parker* immunity only if it satisfies two requirements: "first that 'the challenged restraint . . . be one clearly articulated and affirmatively expressed as state policy,' and second that 'the policy . . . be actively supervised by the State.'" *[Citing the Phoebe Putney case, excerpted beginning on*

(continued)

(continued from previous page)

p. 497] . . . Here, the Board did not receive active supervision by the State when it interpreted the Act as addressing teeth whitening and when it enforced that policy by issuing cease-and-desist letters to nondentist teeth whiteners.

. . .

Limits on state-action immunity are most essential when the State seeks to delegate its regulatory power to active market participants, [because] established ethical standards may blend with private anticompetitive motives in a way difficult even for market participants to discern. Dual allegiances are not always apparent to an actor. In consequence, active market participants cannot be allowed to regulate their own markets free from antitrust accountability. Indeed, prohibitions against anticompetitive self-regulation by active market participants are an axiom of federal antitrust policy.

. . .

[Citing Phoebe Putney *and other cases, Justice Kennedy discusses the reasons to limit a state's ability to delegate regulatory power to "active market participants."]*

[L]imits on delegation must ensure that "[a]ctual state involvement, not deference to private price-fixing arrangements under the general auspices of state law, is the precondition for immunity from federal law." And [the] active supervision requirement, in particular, is an essential condition of state-action immunity when a nonsovereign actor has "an incentive to pursue [its] own self-interest under the guise of implementing state policies." . . . [T]he need for supervision [by the state] turns not on the formal designation given by States to regulators but on the risk that active market participants will pursue private interests in restraining trade.

State agencies controlled by active market participants, who possess singularly strong private interests, pose the very risk of self-dealing [that the] supervision requirement was created to address.

. . .

By statute, North Carolina delegates control over the practice of dentistry to the Board. The Act, however, says nothing about teeth whitening, a practice that did not exist when [the law] was passed. After receiving complaints from other dentists about the nondentists' cheaper services, the Board's dentist members—some of whom offered whitening services—acted to expel the dentists' competitors from the market. In so doing the Board relied upon cease-and-desist letters threatening criminal liability, rather than any of the powers at its disposal that would invoke oversight by a politically accountable official. With no active supervision by the State, North Carolina officials may well have been unaware that the Board had decided teeth whitening constitutes "the practice of dentistry" and sought to prohibit those who competed against dentists from participating in the teeth whitening market. Whether or not the Board exceeded its powers under North Carolina law, there is no evidence here of any decision by the State to initiate or concur with the Board's actions against the nondentists.

. . .

The Sherman Act protects competition while also respecting federalism. It does not authorize the States to abandon markets to the unsupervised control of active market participants, whether trade associations or hybrid agencies. If a State wants to rely on active market participants as regulators, it must provide active supervision if state-action immunity under *Parker* is to be invoked.

The judgment of the Court of Appeals for the Fourth Circuit is affirmed. ■

Discussion Questions

1. What does Justice Kennedy mean by the term "active market participants"?
2. What kind of "active supervision" might the state have engaged in to yield a different outcome to this litigation?
3. In every state there are professional licensing boards similar to the North Carolina dental board. How, if at all, does this decision hamper state boards that license physicians, nurses, and other healthcare professionals?
4. Compare this decision with that of the court in *Phoebe Putney* to the case of *Patrick v. Burget* in chapter 8 (beginning on p. 266). How are they similar, and where do they differ?
5. By virtue of the HCQIA, which was passed in response to *Patrick*, "active market participants" involved in peer review are immune from liability. How are the actions of the members of the North Carolina dental board different?

Notes

1. Mitchel v. Reynolds, 1 P. Wms. 181, 24 Eng. Rep. 347 (1711), quoted in National Soc. of Prof. Engineers v. United States, 435 U.S. 679 (1978).
2. 15 U.S.C. § 1.
3. 15 U.S.C. § 2.
4. Copperweld Corp. v. Independence Tube Co., 467 U.S. 752, 775 (1984).
5. Theatre Enterprises v. Paramount Film Distributing Corp., 346 U.S. 537 (1954).
6. United States v. Container Corp., 393 U.S. 333 (1969).
7. 15 U.S.C. § 2.
8. United States v. Grinnell Corp., 384 U.S. 563, 570–71 (1966).
9. 15 U.S.C. § 17.
10. 15 U.S.C. § 13(a).
11. *Id.*
12. 425 U.S. 1 (1976).
13. *Id.* at 15, 17–18.
14. 15 U.S.C. § 14.
15. 15 U.S.C. § 18.
16. United States v. Rockford Memorial Corp., 898 F.2d 1278 (7th Cir., 1990), *cert. denied*, 498 U.S. 920 (1990).

17. *See, e.g.*, FTC v. University Health, Inc., 938 F.2d 1206 (11th Cir. 1991), FTC v. Freeman Hosp., 69 F.3d 260, 266–67 (8th Cir. 1995), *and* FTC v. Butterworth Health Corp., 946 F. Supp. 1285 (W.D. Mich. 1996). In *FTC v. Butterworth,* the opinion states, "Defendant hospitals do not seriously question the FTC's authority to challenge the proposed merger at this stage of the proceedings, which authority is presumed."

18. McCaw Personal Communications v. Pacific Telesis Group, 645 F. Supp. 1166, 1173 (N.D. Cal., 1986).

19. 15 U.S.C. § 18.

20. ProMedica Health Syst., Inc. v. Federal Trade Comm'n, ___ F. 3d ___ (6th Cir., 2014), *cert denied* ___ U.S. ___, May 4, 2015.

21. Saint Alphonsus Med. Center-Nampa Inc. v. St. Luke's Health Sys., Ltd., 778 F.3d 775 (9th Cir., 2015).

22. *Id.* at 782.

23. *Id.* at 790.

24. Fed. Trade Comm'n, *About the FTC* (accessed September 1, 2016), at http://www.ftc.gov/ftc/about.shtm.

25. 15 U.S.C. § 45(a).

26. *See, e.g.*, Heart of Atlanta Motel, Inc. v. United States, 379 U.S. 241 (1964), in which the Court wrote, "If it is interstate commerce that feels the pinch, it does not matter how [local is] the operation which applies the squeeze." *Id.* at 258, quoting United States v. Women's Sportswear Mfrs. Ass'n, 336 U.S. 460, 464 (1949).

27. 425 U.S. 738 (1976), reversing and remanding, 511 F.2d 678 (4th Cir. 1975). As noted in the chapter, the Sherman Act prohibits "[e]very contract, combination . . . or conspiracy, in restraint of trade or commerce among the several States." 15 U.S.C. § 1. The act also forbids the monopolizing of "any part of the trade or commerce among the several States." 15 U.S.C. § 2.

28. 425 U.S. at 744.

29. *Id.* at 746–47.

30. *See* Goldfarb v. Va. State Bar Ass'n, 421 U.S. 773 (1975) ("the nature of an occupation, standing alone, does not provide sanctuary from the Sherman Act . . . nor is the public service aspect of professional practice controlling in determining whether § 1 includes professions"), *and* Hosp. Bldg. Co. v. Trustees of Rex Hosp., 425 U.S. 738 (1976).

31. 457 U.S. 332 (1982).

32. 317 U.S. 341 (1943).

33. 421 U.S. 773 (1975).

34. N.C. Bd. of Dental Exam'rs v. Fed. Trade Comm'n., __ F.3d __ (4th Cir., 2013).

35. 15 U.S.C. § 1.

36. 15 U.S.C. § 15a.

37. 15 U.S.C. § 16(b).

38. 15 U.S.C. § 18a(g).

39. 15 U.S.C. § 15.

40. 15 U.S.C. §§ 12–27.

41. 15 U.S.C. §§ 41–58.

42. 15 U.S.C. § 46.

43. Board of Trade of the City of Chicago v. United States, 246 U.S. 231 (1918).

44. Northern Pac. Ry. Co. v. United States, 356 U.S. 1, 5 (1958) (opinion of the Court by Justice Hugo Black).

45. Hyde v. United States, 225 U.S. 347 (1912).

46. Fed. Trade Comm'n v. Actavis, Inc., 133 S.Ct. 2223, 2235-36 (2013).

47. *See, e.g.*, FTC v. Freeman Hosp., 911 F. Supp. 1213 (W.D. Mo.), *aff'd* 69 F.3d 260 (8th Cir. 1995); United States v. Mercy Health Services, 902 F. Supp. 968 (N.D. Iowa 1995); United States v. Carilion Health System, 707 F. Supp. 840 (W.D. Va. 1989), *aff'd* 892 F.2d 1042 (1989).

48. 946 F. Supp. 1285 (1996).

49. *Id.* at 1302.

50. 15 U.S.C. § 18.

51. 15 U.S.C. § 1, 2.

52. 15 U.S.C. § 45.

53. 15 U.S.C. § 2.

54. United States v. Grinnell Corp., 384 U.S. 563, 571 (1966).

55. Berkey Photo, Inc. v. Eastman Kodak Co., 603 F.2d 263 (2d Cir. 1979) (there is no duty to disclose the introduction of new products in advance); ILC Peripherals Leasing Corp. v. International Business Mach. Corp., 458 F. Supp. 423 (N.D. Cal. 1978) (defendant's introduction of new technology at lower prices does not constitute monopolization).

56. United States v. Am. Bldg. Maint. Indus., 422 U.S. 271 (1975).

57. United States v. E.I. du Pont de Nemours Co., 351 U.S. 377 (1956).

58. U.S. v. Carilion Health System, 707 F. Supp. 840, 846 (1989).

59. 898 F.2d 1278 (7th Cir. 1990).

60. *Id.* at 1284.

61. Quotes in this section drawn from 898 F.2d 1284–1285.

62. Thomas Greany, *Night Landings on an Aircraft Carrier: Hospital Mergers and Antitrust Law*, 23 AM. J. L. & MED. 191 (1977). The author's thesis is that "courts deciding hospital merger cases are asked to make exceedingly fine-tuned appraisals of complex economic relationships."

63. United States v. E.I. du Pont de Nemours Co., 353 U.S. 586 (1957) (defendant's ownership of 23 percent of stock in General Motors Corp. could be challenged 35 years after the acquisition).

64. This entire HHI discussion is adapted from Dept. of Justice & Fed. Trade Comm'n, *Horizontal Merger Guidelines* (published August 19, 2010), at http://www.justice.gov/atr/public/guidelines/hmg-2010. html. As its title suggests, the *Guidelines* document does not cover vertical integration or other types of nonhorizontal combinations.

65. Fruehauf Corp. v. FTC, 603 F.2d 345, 352–54 (1979).

66. Ford Motor Co. v. United States, 405 U.S. 562 (1972).

67. HTI Health Services v. Quorum Health Group, 960 F. Supp. 1104 (S.D. Miss., 1997).

68. United States v. Penn-Olin Chem. Co., 378 U.S. 158 (1964).

69. United States v. General Dynamics Corp., 415 U.S. 486 (1974).

70. 76 Fed. Reg. 67026, October 28, 2011.

71. Dept. of Justice & Fed. Trade Comm'n, *Statements of Antitrust Enforcement Policy in Health Care* (published August 1996), at https://www.justice.gov/atr/statements-antitrust-enforcement-policyin-health-care.

72. Christine A. Varney, Asst. Atty. Gen., Antitrust Div., US Dept. of Justice, *Antitrust and Healthcare* (published May 24, 2010), at http://www.justice.gov/atr/public/speeches/258898.htm#_ftn12, *citing* Dept. of Justice & Fed. Trade Comm'n, *Statements of Antitrust Enforcement Policy in Health Care, Statement 8* (published August 1996), at https://www.justice.gov/atr/statements-antitrust-enforcement-policy-health-care#CONTNUM_61.

73. 76 Fed. Reg. 67026 (Oct. 28, 2011).

74. 421 U.S. 773 (1975). *See also* Boddicker v. Arizona State Dental Ass'n, 549 F.2d 626 (9th Cir. 1977), *cert. denied*, 434 U.S. 825 (1978); Am. Medical Ass'n v. FTC, 638 F.2d 443 (2d Cir. 1980).

75. 15 U.S.C. § 21(a).

76. U.S. CONST. art. 1, § 8.

77. U.S. v. Rockford Memorial Corp., 898 F.2d 1278 (7th Cir. 1990).

78. 15 U.S.C. § 18a.

ISSUES OF REPRODUCTION AND BIRTH

After reading this chapter, you will

- understand that voluntary sterilization is seldom a significant legal issue except, perhaps, for those with religious objections;
- appreciate the difference between wrongful life cases and wrongful birth cases;
- be aware of the issues involved in "artificial parenting," in vitro fertilization, and stem cell technology;
- have a better appreciation for abortion as a legal and public policy issue; and
- understand the hospital's proper role in reproductive matters.

C ourts of law are often asked to apply legal principles to social, moral, and ethical controversies. Although the issues are virtually intractable and the courts seem imperfectly constructed to resolve them, every **justiciable** case must be decided. This chapter reviews some of the most vexing issues ever brought to court: sterilization, wrongful birth and wrongful life, other reproduction issues, and abortion.

justiciable
capable of being settled by a court of law

Sterilization

Sterilization is a surgical procedure intended to prevent procreation. For men the most common procedure is a *vasectomy*, while for women it is a *salpingectomy* (tubal ligation). Voluntary sterilizations are performed on patients who are competent to understand the procedure and its consequences and have given fully informed consent. Patients who receive involuntary sterilizations have not given informed consent because they are incompetent or because the state has declared the sterilization compulsory. Involuntary sterilizations were once performed as eugenic measures to protect society from allegedly inheritable disability, but eugenic sterilizations are now almost universally condemned (see discussion of *Buck v. Bell* later in the chapter).

Voluntary Sterilization

The term *sterilization* is reserved for surgery intended to eliminate the ability to reproduce. A therapeutic procedure that incidentally results in sterility is not considered a sterilization and presents few legal issues, assuming proper informed consent was given. For example, a hysterectomy (removal of the uterus), an oophorectomy (removal of the ovaries), or an orchiectomy (removal of the testes) to treat cancer is simply an operation that unavoidably makes one unable to procreate.

Contraceptive sterilization, however, has not always been lawful in all jurisdictions. For many years, at least two states—Connecticut and Utah—expressly prohibited intentional sterilization. In Utah, the statutory language seemed to prohibit all sterilizations, but when the law was challenged, the Utah Supreme Court ruled that it applied only to institutionalized patients because it was part of the Utah Code that deals with state institutions.[1] Voluntary sterilization of other patients was decriminalized.

Connecticut's law prohibited the use of contraceptives (e.g., prophylactics) and banned counseling about their use. Voluntary contraceptive sterilization was thus prohibited by implication. This statute was declared unconstitutional in the landmark case *Griswold v. Connecticut,* in which the US Supreme Court ruled that the statute invaded a "zone of privacy created by several fundamental constitutional guarantees" protected by the due process clause of the Fourteenth Amendment.[2] (This viewpoint was not unanimous; see Law in Action.) Another Connecticut statute authorizing sterilizations for eugenic purposes was repealed in 1971.

Contraceptives aside, most states' laws have always been silent on the matter of sterilization. Modern mores and ideas about family planning have firmly established voluntary sterilization as a matter of personal choice. Thus, no significant legal barriers obstruct sterilization for convenience, although in some quarters—particularly the Roman Catholic Church and certain other religious organizations—there is significant moral objection to contraception generally and to being required to pay for its coverage under health plans.

The procedure's legality notwithstanding, sterilization raises legal issues concerning informed consent. Sterilization is usually irreversible; it permanently deprives the patient of the ability to procreate. Some individuals, especially young people, may not fully understand the consequences of the procedure, and others may misunderstand the operation (e.g., its irrevocability) or whether insurance will pay for it. For these reasons, full informed consent is particularly necessary to ensure not only that the patient fully comprehends the operation but also that no duress, coercion, or deception has been used to elicit that consent.

Federal regulations govern sterilizations performed under programs administered by the Public Health Service.[3] They establish specific consent requirements and permit sterilizations only of competent, voluntarily consenting individuals who are at least 21 years old and not institutionalized. They also specify the information patients must be given before they consent: the nature, the risks, the alternatives, and the irreversibility of the procedure. Although these regulations do not apply directly to private hospitals, they could be considered the standard of care should litigation arise, and they can serve as the benchmark for developing hospital policy.

In addition, some states have laws governing voluntary sterilizations. Healthcare providers must be fully aware of both the state and any applicable federal laws governing sterilizations, and they should set up procedures to ensure compliance. Even in the absence of legislation, the provider's policies and actions should make certain that the patient's consent is fully informed.

Eugenic Sterilization and Sterilization of Incompetent Persons

Eugenics is the study of hereditary improvement by selective breeding. Thus, eugenic sterilization refers to surgery on persons thought to be of unsound mind or otherwise unfit to be parents because of presumably inheritable disabilities. Approximately half of the states have never enacted statutes authorizing eugenic sterilization, and in another dozen or so states, the laws that once permitted the procedure have been repealed altogether or in part. In the few states whose statutes remain on the books, the procedure is strongly disfavored and rarely used.

Compulsory sterilization statutes typically applied only to persons confined to state institutions (e.g., hospitals for the mentally ill, "training schools," prisons). They usually identified the persons subject to the law as "insane," "feeble minded," "a habitual criminal," "mentally defective," "a sexual psychopath," and similar pejoratives presumably meaningful to medical science at one time but offensive to most observers today.

The famous Supreme Court case *Buck v. Bell*,[4] decided in 1927 and roundly criticized today, established the constitutionality of these statutes. Carrie Buck had been committed to the Virginia "colony" for epileptics and

Law in Action

Since 1879 Connecticut has had on its books a law which forbids the use of contraceptives by anyone. I think this is an uncommonly silly law. As a practical matter, [it] is obviously unenforceable. . . . But we are not asked in this case to say whether we think this law is unwise, or even asinine. We are asked to hold that it violates the United States Constitution. And that I cannot do.

. . . What provision of the Constitution [makes] this state law invalid? The Court says it is the right of privacy "created by several fundamental constitutional guarantees." With all deference, I can find no such right of privacy in the Bill of Rights, in any other part of the Constitution, or in any case ever before decided by this Court.

—Justice Potter Stewart, dissenting (with Justice Hugo Black) in *Griswold* 381 U.S. 479 at 527, 530

the "feeble minded." She was the daughter of a "feeble-minded" mother who had also been confined to the institution. At age 17, Carrie had given birth to an illegitimate child, the product of rape by a relative of her foster parents. In concert with the author of a new eugenics law, and with the collusion of Carrie's court-appointed attorney (who apparently conducted a purposefully inadequate defense), the institution's superintendent filed a test case to have Carrie sterilized.

After the trial court ordered a salpingectomy and Virginia's highest court upheld the law, the case went to the US Supreme Court, where it was again upheld—by an 8–1 vote—in an opinion by Justice Oliver Wendell Holmes Jr., one of the titans of American jurisprudence (see Law in Action). By analogy to mandatory vaccination programs, the statute was held to be constitutional under the state's power to regulate the health and welfare of its residents.

In fact, Carrie was not mentally disabled, and her mother was only mildly so. Carrie's daughter was only one month old when she was labeled "mentally defective" by a Red Cross nurse. She died of the measles in 1932 and had by that time completed the second grade. Carrie lived into old age and married twice, but of course she bore no other children.

In contrast to *Buck*, in 1942 the Supreme Court held unconstitutional an Oklahoma statute that authorized sterilization of "habitual criminals" but exempted individuals described as "embezzlers." The Supreme Court's rationale was that the exemption was an unreasonable classification in violation of the equal protection clause of the Fourteenth Amendment— there being no logical difference between embezzlers and other kinds of criminals (see The Court Decides at the end of this chapter).[5] The Supreme Court also recognized procreation as a fundamental constitutional right, thus subjecting the statute to strict scrutiny regarding equal protection. *Buck*, therefore, is no longer a valid precedent, although it has never been explicitly overruled.

Eugenic sterilization statutes have been much criticized. One underlying

---

Law in Action

To support his controversial ruling that the state's interest in a "pure" gene pool outweighed the individual's interest in bodily integrity, Justice Holmes wrote:

> We have seen more than once that the public welfare may call upon the best citizens for their lives. It would be strange if it could not call upon those who already sap the strength of the State for these lesser sacrifices, often not felt to be such by those concerned, in order to prevent our being swamped with incompetence. It is better for all the world, if instead of waiting to execute degenerate offspring for crime, or to let them starve for their imbecility, society can prevent those who are manifestly unfit from continuing their kind. The principle that sustains compulsory vaccination is broad enough to cover cutting the Fallopian tubes. *Three generations of imbeciles are enough.*[100] (Italics added.)

One might say about Justice Holmes that he was not always right, but he was never in doubt.

premise for the procedure—that traits such as mental illness and criminality are hereditary—has been largely discredited by the scientific community.[6] With support for the statutes undermined, they are unlikely to withstand constitutional scrutiny today. The New Jersey Supreme Court summarized well the attitude of many:

> It cannot be forgotten . . . that public attitudes toward mental impairment and the handicapped in general have sometimes been very different. We must always remain mindful of the atrocities that people of our own [twentieth] century and culture have committed upon their fellow humans. We cannot adequately express our abhorrence for the kind of ideology that assigns vastly differing value to the lives of human beings because of their innate group characteristics or personal handicaps.[7]

As shown later in this chapter, the concepts of personal privacy and autonomy in matters of reproduction underlying the *Griswold* (contraceptives) and *Skinner* (involuntary sterilization) decisions formed a stepping stone for the short jump to abortion rights in 1973.

Wrongful Birth and Wrongful Life

Sterilization and abortion procedures sometimes fail. (Abortion is discussed later in this chapter.) *Speck v. Finegold*[8] was a rare case in that both procedures failed in one dazzling sequence of events involving the same couple.

Mr. Speck suffered from a genetic disease known as neurofibromatosis (see "Neurofibromatosis"). After passing the disease on to two of his children, and fearing that future offspring would be similarly afflicted, he decided to have a vasectomy. Dr. Finegold performed the procedure in early 1974 and assured Mr. Speck that he could engage in sexual relations with his wife without "contraceptive devices." Mrs. Speck became pregnant anyway. Under her new "right to choose" (*Roe v. Wade* had been decided the previous year), she consulted Dr. Schwartz and underwent an abortion procedure that Dr. Schwartz told her was successful. It was not, and Mrs. Speck was still pregnant. (The opinion does not explain how a physician could

Neurofibromatosis

Neurofibromatosis is a genetic disease characterized by usually benign tumors of the nerve fibers (neurofibromas) on and under the skin. The disease is sometimes accompanied by bone deformity and a predisposition to cancers, especially of the brain, and is also called multiple neurofibroma, neuromatosis, Recklinghausen's Disease, and von Recklinghausen's Disease.

Joseph Merrick (the famous "elephant man") was once thought to have been afflicted with neurofibromatosis, but the consensus today is that he suffered from the rare Proteus Syndrome.

Proteus Syndrome is discussed at http://ghr.nlm.nih.gov/condition/proteus-syndrome. For more information on specific neurological diseases, search http://www.ninds.nih.gov.

think he had aborted a pregnancy when in fact he had not.) In April 1975, Mrs. Speck gave birth to a third child, Francine, who also was afflicted with neurofibromatosis.

This bizarre case turned on five central questions: Did the Specks have valid causes of action against the physicians who performed the operations? If so, what were their damages? Could they recover for mental distress and the costs of raising Francine? Would the amount of damages be different if she had been born healthy? (The Specks strove to ensure they would not have a third child, healthy or not.) Did Francine have a right to recover damages?

In the decision by a Pennsylvania appellate court, as modified by the state's supreme court, the ultimate answers were (1) regular principles of tort law apply and (2) if negligence were proven, the Specks would be entitled to recover for the costs of care and treatment of Francine and for their own mental distress. The high court split evenly on the issue of whether Francine had a legally cognizable injury for what has become known as "wrongful life." The opinion states, somewhat turgidly, "The Court being evenly divided on the question of whether an infant plaintiff can bring an action in the circumstances of this case, the Order of the Superior Court that the infant plaintiff's cause of action is not legally cognizable is affirmed."[9]

Many courts before and since *Speck* have addressed wrongful birth and wrongful life cases. The term *wrongful birth* is typically used in suits by parents for the birth of a child born with a disability. *Wrongful life* cases are brought on behalf of the child, claiming that but for negligence the child would not have been born. Some cases in which the defendant's alleged negligence led to an unwanted pregnancy have been labeled *wrongful conception*. The first such case might be one that occurred in 1934 when a physician in Minnesota performed a negligent sterilization procedure on a patient who later became pregnant.[10] After she delivered a healthy child, her husband sued for medical expenses and anxiety. His case was dismissed because he alleged deceit, not negligence, so proof of fraudulent intent was required; in addition, the court ruled he had suffered no damage.

Not all courts use the same terminology, and "wrongful birth" or even "wrongful parentage" is sometimes an umbrella term for all such actions. Terminology aside, these cases are the result of two simultaneous developments: (1) the legal recognition of parents' right to decide whether to conceive or abort, and (2) the great advances in medical science that make genetic testing and counseling a commonplace medical practice. The following are examples of circumstances in which legal actions have been taken:

- Unsuccessful implementation of contraceptive measures, including negligently performed sterilizations (as in *Speck*)
- Failure to provide genetic counseling or testing when warranted
- Failure to diagnose and inform the patient of pregnancy

- Failure to detect and warn the patient of diseases, such as rubella or genetic defects, early enough to permit abortion
- Negligence in performing an abortion

These failures led to the birth of a disabled child or one who was healthy but unplanned. The circumstances are all types of medical negligence, but they share a distinguishing feature: If the physician had not been negligent, the child would not have been born or would have been born without a disability. Wrongful life cases, in particular, cause considerable legal, ethical, and philosophical angst because the plaintiffs claim that the child's very existence is the injury.

Duty, Breach, and Causation

To succeed in any malpractice case, the plaintiff must prove a duty of care, a breach of that duty, an injury proximately caused by the breach, and legally recognized damages. In the wrongful birth and wrongful life arena, the courts have had little difficulty discerning duty and breach and only slightly more trouble with causation, but they have struggled mightily with the measure of damages, especially in wrongful life cases.

Courts in virtually all jurisdictions have held that physicians owe a duty of care to the parents and even to the unborn child in wrongful life and wrongful birth cases. For example, in *Turpin v. Sortini,* the parents of a little girl were told she had normal hearing when in fact she was deaf from a hereditary condition.[11] The couple's next child was also deaf. The court held that the professional who tested the first child's hearing had a duty not only to the parents but also to the second child because he should have discovered and thus foreseen that the ailment would be inherited by other children.

The physician's duty in these and other medical malpractice cases was to conform to the generally accepted standards of care exercised by other physicians in similar circumstances at the time of the alleged malpractice. For example, in 1969, a physician allegedly failed to tell his patients of the risk that their baby would be afflicted with cri du chat syndrome, a chromosomal disorder that causes severe intellectual disability, among other conditions (see "Cri du Chat Syndrome" on p. 512). The doctor did not perform amniocentesis. The parents sued for damages after their child was born with the condition, but their suit was rejected because "on the bases of the patient's medical history and the state of medical knowledge regarding the use of the amniocentesis test in 1969, the defendants' failure to perform the test was no more than a permissible exercise of medical judgment and not a departure from then accepted medical practice."[12]

In contrast, in 1974, a physician was held liable after he failed to advise his 37-year-old pregnant patient that the risk of bearing a child with Down syndrome is greater for women older than 35 and did not inform her of the

Cri du Chat Syndrome

Cri du chat syndrome gets its name from the French phrase meaning "cry of the cat" because of the distinctive mewing sound made by infants with the disorder, which is ascribed to abnormal development of the larynx. The cry becomes less distinctive with age. Babies with cri du chat syndrome are often underweight at birth. The disorder is also characterized by distinctive facial features, small head size (microcephaly), low birth weight, weak muscle tone, a round face, low-set ears, strabismus (a condition in which the eyes do not point in the same direction), and facial asymmetry. Cardiac malformations may occur and affect the vital prognosis. The severity of the condition varies depending on the amount of missing DNA material.

In terms of development and behavior, severe intellectual disability is typical of people with this syndrome. They have difficulty expressing themselves verbally and often use signing to communicate, and they are commonly hypersensitive to noise. In addition, some have autistic traits, such as repetitive behaviors and obsessions with certain objects, and many seem to enjoy pulling hair. They tend to be happy children and sometimes are described as loving and sociable. For more information, see http://www.nlm.nih.gov/medlineplus/ency/article/001593.htm.

availability of amniocentesis to detect the defect. The court reasoned that amniocentesis was then an accepted medical practice, abortion was recognized as a patient's right, and genetic counseling had become customary.[13] In fact, because genetic testing can now reveal many types of birth defects, the standard of care today requires that prospective at-risk parents be counseled about available tests and medical alternatives, such as abortion.[14] Courts have held that physicians are not required to recommend abortion, but they must at least inform patients of the facts and available alternatives or refer patients to another practitioner early enough to ensure that the patient has recourse to a number of solutions.

Liability has also been found for the following prenatal injuries in wrongful birth cases:

- Failure to diagnose rubella in a pregnant woman whose child was born with a disability[15]
- Failure to diagnose cystic fibrosis in the parents' first child, thus leaving the parents unaware of the risk that a second child would be similarly afflicted[16]
- A mistake resulting in the birth of a healthy but unwanted child[17]
- Failure to inform the patient that the drug she was taking to control her epilepsy could cause birth defects[18]

Even if a plaintiff has a cognizable claim, the suit must be brought within the applicable limitations period, which traditionally begins at the time of the alleged negligence. Because pregnancy and birth may occur years after an allegedly negligent sterilization procedure, however, the tendency of recent decisions is to hold that the period begins at the time the breach of duty is discovered or should have been discovered. In other words, the statute of limitations runs from the time pregnancy is confirmed.[19] (Application of the "discovery rule" to cases of wrongful birth follows the development of the rule in other malpractice situations. In a case involving congenital birth defects, the limitations period begins to run on the date the disabilities become known to the parents—whether it be the date of the child's birth or, because of prenatal testing, an earlier date.[20])

Damages

As one can see, the courts have little difficulty with questions of duty, breach, and causation in wrongful birth cases. Most have upheld the parents' cause of action, finding proximate cause in the fact that but for the physician's negligence, the child would not have been born or would not have suffered the prenatal injury.[21] However, the courts have struggled with the question of damages and have come to widely inconsistent conclusions, especially in wrongful life cases. The proper measure of damages is difficult to determine because public policy values life and generally views the birth of a child as a blessing.

Virtually all courts that recognize a cause of action for wrongful birth have allowed parents to recover expenses for the pregnancy and childbirth, even when the child was healthy.[22] Other damages, such as lost wages, have also been held recoverable.[23] Damages for the woman's pain and suffering as a result of the pregnancy and birth have been allowed,[24] as have damages for the husband's loss of consortium.[25]

The courts disagree, however, on the subject of damages for the parents' emotional distress. In cases concerning children born with a serious disease or disability, some have permitted compensation for mental distress. For example, in one Virginia case, a man's blood was mislabeled and the couple did not discover that he was a carrier of Tay-Sachs disease (a usually fatal genetic disorder) until their child was born with it. Damages were allowed for the emotional distress the parents experienced as a result of the child's suffering and death.[26] In another case involving Tay-Sachs, however, the court denied damages for emotional harm, arguing that the child suffered the injury, not the parents.[27] A New Hampshire case took a middle ground and permitted damages for the parents' "tangible pecuniary losses, such as medical expenses or counseling fees."[28]

Claims for the expense of raising a disabled child are more controversial. Almost all jurisdictions view the birth of a child, even one with disabilities, as an occasion of some benefit and joy to the parents. A traditional rule of tort law—the *benefit rule*—requires that any damages awarded to an injured plaintiff be reduced by the value of any benefit that the tortfeasor bestowed on the plaintiff. Most courts, even those allowing the costs of child rearing in wrongful birth cases, require the jury to offset the parents' damages with the benefits of having the child.[29] (Some juries find that these benefits outweigh the costs of rearing the child and therefore deny any child-rearing costs,[30] a somewhat surprising finding given the indeterminate, metaphysical nature of the calculus involved.)

In *Cockrum v. Baumgartner,* a negligent sterilization failed to prevent pregnancy, and an unwanted but healthy child was the result.[31] The court recognized the parents' cause of action for wrongful birth because the decision not to have a child is a legally protected right and its violation cannot be ignored. Noting that damage awards are an effective recognition of legal rights, the court allowed the costs of raising the child. It held that the benefit rule applies only if the benefit is to the same interest that was harmed. The court found that the emotional benefits of child rearing are separate from the injured financial interests of the parents. The extraordinary costs of raising a disabled child—payments for institutional or other specialized care, medical expenses, and special education and training—have generally been allowed. These amounts are determined by identifying the extra expenses beyond what would be spent on a healthy child.[32] Even in these cases, some courts have held that the advantages of parenthood and the value of the child's life outweigh the burdens of child rearing.[33]

Wrongful Life

In contrast to wrongful birth cases, only California, Washington, New Jersey, and Maine permit a cause of action for wrongful life. No such action has been allowed on behalf of a healthy child who was unwanted or illegitimate because the courts have found that the child suffered no injury.[34] Even when the child suffered from a grave disease or birth defect, most courts have repeatedly refused to recognize a cause of action on several grounds:

- The professional negligence was not the cause of the disease or injury.
- Life, even one that is impaired, is not considered a legal injury.
- Damages for an impaired life, as opposed to no life, cannot be determined.[35]

The purpose of compensatory damages is to restore the plaintiffs to the position they would have occupied had there been no negligence. In wrongful life cases, that position would be nonexistence: But for the defendant's negligence, the child would not have been born. Most courts have held that no one can determine the value of nonexistence, and therefore such actions fail, lacking the necessary requirements of proximate cause and legally compensable injury. Courts also have held that there is no fundamental right to be born healthy,[36] and some courts believe that allowing a cause of action for wrongful life would diminish the value of human life and would be contrary to society's goal of protecting, preserving, and improving the quality of human existence.[37]

A few states do recognize a cause of action for wrongful life; California was the first. In *Curlender v. Bio-Science Laboratories, Inc.,* the plaintiff was a child born with Tay-Sachs disease, allegedly as a result of negligent testing to determine whether the parents were carriers.[38] The child was mentally and physically disabled and had a life expectancy of only four years. Finding a "palpable injury," a California court of appeals held that the child could recover damages for pain and suffering and pecuniary loss because of her impaired condition. The costs of care were awarded as damages, but only once—not to both the parents and the child. Two years later, the California Supreme Court recognized another child's cause of action for wrongful life in *Turpin v. Sortini* and rejected the argument that such actions were against public policy.[39] According to the court, it was "hard to see how an award of damages to a severely disabled or suffering child would 'disavow' the value of life or in any way suggest that the child is not entitled to the full measure of legal and nonlegal rights and privileges accorded to all members of society."[40] According to the court's finding, one could not say as a matter of law that an impaired life is always preferable to no life.

A California statute recognizes the fundamental right of adults to control medical decisions, including the decision to withdraw or withhold life-sustaining procedures.[41] By analogy, the *Turpin* court found that these parents were prevented from making an informed and meaningful choice whether to conceive or bear a disabled child and that the choice was partly on behalf of the child. Although the court agreed with other opinions that general damages are impossible to assess, it found that the extraordinary expenses of caring for a disabled child were not speculative. It held that it was illogical to permit the parents but not the child to recover for the costs of medical care related to the disability. Otherwise, the court stated, the child's receipt of necessary medical expenses depended on whether the parents sued and recovered damages or whether the expenses were incurred when the parents were still legally responsible for the child's care (see Law in Action).

The Washington Supreme Court also found that a child should have a cause of action for wrongful life. In *Harbeson v. Parke-Davis, Inc.*, it held that imposing liability for wrongful life would promote social objectives—such as genetic counseling and prenatal testing—and would discourage malpractice.[42] The court had no difficulty finding the requisite proximate cause:

It is clear in the case before us that, were it not for negligence of the physicians [in not advising the mother of the danger of taking a certain drug during pregnancy], the minor plaintiffs would not have been born, and would consequently not have suffered fetal hydantoin syndrome. More particularly, the plaintiffs would not have incurred the extraordinary expenses resulting from that condition.[43]

Law in Action

In *Turpin*, the negligence was failure to adequately diagnose the deafness of the plaintiffs' first daughter as hereditary. As a result, the plaintiffs' second daughter was born with the same condition. The girls were named Hope and Joy.

The distinction between the parents' and the child's causes of action is important. Awards to the parents cover only their expenses during the time they are legally responsible for the child—for example, until the age of majority. The child's damages, however, may continue throughout life—perhaps many years beyond the age of majority.

Some states have passed laws concerning actions for wrongful life and wrongful birth. In *Curlender*, discussed earlier, the California court of appeals said in dictum that children born with birth defects should be allowed to sue their parents for their pain and suffering if the parents foresaw the defect and chose not to abort. The California legislature quickly responded with a statute outlawing such a case lest parents feel pressured to abort or prevent conception.[44] Minnesota went further with legislation prohibiting actions for wrongful birth and wrongful life that claim "but for the alleged negligence a child would have been aborted."[45] The statute does permit actions for failure of a contraceptive method or a sterilization procedure and for failure to diagnose a disease or defect that could have been prevented or cured if detected early enough. Abortion is not viewed as a prevention or cure, however, and neither the failure nor the refusal of anyone to perform or obtain an abortion constitutes a defense in any action or is a consideration in the award of damages.[46] Maine is the only state to approve of wrongful life actions by statute. (See Legal Brief for the section of Maine's Health Security Act that addresses both wrongful life and wrongful birth).

Wrongful birth and wrongful life cases show that as medical knowledge and technology expand, the duty of the physician also grows—not only to perform tests and procedures with necessary care but also to provide genetic counseling. In addition to performing all duties carefully, physicians should carefully document in the medical record any discussions with

Legal Brief
Me. Rev. Stat. Title 24, § 2931

1. **Intent.** It is the intent of the Legislature that the birth of a normal, healthy child does not constitute a legally recognizable injury and that it is contrary to public policy to award damages for the birth or rearing of a healthy child.

2. **Birth of healthy child; claim for damages prohibited.** No person may maintain a claim for relief or receive an award for damages based on the claim that the birth and rearing of a healthy child resulted in damages to him. A person may maintain a claim for relief based on a failed sterilization procedure resulting in the birth of a healthy child and receive an award of damages for the hospital and medical expenses incurred for the sterilization procedures and pregnancy, the pain and suffering connected with the pregnancy and the loss of earnings by the mother during pregnancy.

3. **Birth of unhealthy child; damages limited.** Damages for the birth of an unhealthy child born as the result of professional negligence shall be limited to damages associated with the disease, defect or handicap suffered by the child.

4. **Other causes of action.** This section shall not preclude causes of action based on claims that, but for a wrongful act or omission, maternal death or injury would not have occurred or handicap, disease, defect or deficiency of an individual prior to birth would have been prevented, cured or ameliorated in a manner that preserved the health and life of the affected individual.

patients about possible genetic and other risks to patients' unborn children or children who have not yet been conceived and about the availability of appropriate preconception or prenatal testing, therapies, and alternatives. The documentation also should cover the patient's decision concerning the risks, testing, and alternatives. Recording informed consent for medical treatment is essential in any circumstance but is especially so in the important and constitutionally protected matter of procreation.

Other Reproduction Issues

Other than abortion, two reproduction-related issues deserve note: (1) the use of stem cells in medical treatment and research and (2) assisted reproductive technology.

Use of Stem Cells in Medical Treatment and Research

Stem cells are basic units of living matter that, remarkably, have the potential to develop into many types of cells in the human body. They also serve as a kind of internal repair system, dividing virtually without limit to replenish other cells as long as the person is still alive. Stem cells renew themselves through mitosis and, under certain conditions, can be induced to become tissue- or organ-specific cells with special functions.

Until recently, scientists worked primarily with embryonic stem cells—those created for reproductive purposes through in vitro fertilization (IVF) and then donated for research with the informed consent of the donor. In the first decade of the twenty-first century, however, it was discovered that some specialized adult cells could be genetically reprogrammed to assume a stem cell–like state. Additional research is needed, but these "induced pluripotent stem cells" avoid many of the moral objections to embryonic stem cell research and could serve as useful tools in repairing human tissue and treating disease. They are already being used by pharmaceutical companies to develop new drugs.[47]

Research reveals few judicial decisions that involve stem cell technology. Of those that do, most are concerned with side issues, mention the topic only in obiter dicta, or concern questions of public policy and politics. For example, because the process may involve destruction of human embryos, the George W. Bush administration limited federal funding for embryonic stem cell research to lines of cells from embryos that had already been destroyed and were derived by private or foreign researchers. President Barack Obama lifted that limitation, and challenges to his action have been unsuccessful.[48]

In 2006, Missouri voters passed a constitutional amendment that prohibits the cloning of human beings but "ensures that Missouri patients have access to stem cell therapies and cures, that Missouri researchers can conduct stem cell research in the state, and that all such research is conducted safely and ethically." These provisions were the subject of two appellate court rulings concerning technical aspects of the ballot language.[49] They have not been the focus of any substantive judicial decision in the years since the amendment passed. In the future, we may see more legislation or litigation on issues related to stem cells, especially stem cell research.[50]

Assisted Reproductive Technology

Assisted reproductive technology (*ART*) is a generic term that refers to artificial methods of achieving pregnancy. ART is used often in cases of infertility, but fertile couples also may be treated if they have contraindications to a normal pregnancy (e.g., genetic or communicable disease factors). According to the Centers for Disease Control and Prevention (CDC),

> ART includes all fertility treatments in which both eggs and sperm are handled. In general, ART procedures involve surgically removing eggs from a woman's ovaries, combining them with sperm in the laboratory [i.e., IVF], and returning them to the woman's body or donating them to another woman. They do not include treatments in which only sperm are handled (i.e., intrauterine—or artificial—insemination) or procedures in which a woman takes medicine only to stimulate egg production without the intention of having eggs retrieved.[51]

The CDC reports that as many as 10 percent of women of reproductive age in the United States have some form of medical consultation or test regarding infertility at some time in their lives, and about 2 percent have an infertility-related medical appointment in a given year. Given the prevalence of infertility and the publicity ART has received since the first "test tube baby" was born in 1978, the number of ART procedures (called "cycles") has steadily increased. In 2013 (the latest data available), more than 190,000 ART cycles were performed at 467 reporting fertility clinics in the United States. These procedures engendered more than 54,000 live births resulting in nearly 68,000 infants.[52]

In addition, the US Supreme Court's landmark decision in *Obergefell v. Hodges*, 576 U.S. ___ (2015), which established the fundamental constitutional right of same-sex couples to marry, will undoubtedly lead to an increased number of children born through assisted reproductive technologies.

Artificial Insemination

Artificial insemination (*AI*) is the process by which sperm is placed into the female's reproductive tract by means other than sexual intercourse. AI involves sperm (fresh or frozen) from a woman's husband or another man (a known or anonymous donor). Couples in which the male is unable to fertilize normally or women who have no male partner may use AI to conceive. It also may be used to impregnate a woman who has agreed to carry a baby to term for another woman through gestational surrogacy.

Gestational Surrogacy

A "gestational surrogate" is a woman who—usually for a fee—agrees to carry a fetus to term for a couple or another woman. The embryo from which the fetus grows may be conceived through ART, may be conceived normally for later adoption (e.g., by the genetic father's spouse), or may be conceived normally and then transferred to the surrogate because the natural mother is at risk of miscarriage. If AI or IVF is used, the sperm may or may not be that of the husband of the egg-bearing woman, and the egg may or may not be that of the wife of the sperm donor. The genetic parents (whose identities may or may not be known) can be different than the adoptive parent(s) for whom the surrogate mother carries the child.

Many of the legal issues that arise in ART cases concern the numerous permutations of the relationships involved (see Legal Brief). For example, in the 1988 case *In re Baby M*,[53] the Supreme Court of New Jersey was asked to determine parental status after a surrogate mother reneged on her contract to surrender the child after birth. The contract was between Mary Beth Whitehead and William Stern, whose wife was infertile. It provided that, for a fee of $10,000, Ms. Whitehead would be inseminated with Mr. Stern's sperm, would conceive a child and carry it to term, and would give the child over for Mrs. Stern to adopt. (Mr. Stern, the sperm donor, would be recognized as the natural father.)

The Sterns filed suit when Ms. Whitehead failed to abide by the agreement. The trial court determined that the surrogacy contract was valid, but the New Jersey Supreme Court disagreed. It held that the contract conflicted with New Jersey laws prohibiting the use of money in connection with adoptions. According to the court, "The contract's basic premise, that the natural parents can decide in advance of birth which one is to have custody of the child, bears no relationship to the law that the child's best interests shall determine custody."[54] The court continued as follows:

Legal Brief

Artificial reproductive technologies are a blessing to couples who are otherwise unable to have children, and their success rate has increased dramatically in recent years. Technology aside, the ultimate success of the endeavor depends on complex interpersonal relationships that can fail in numerous ways because at least seven people may be directly involved:

1. Sperm donor (genetic father)
2. Egg donor (genetic mother)
3. Spouse or partner of sperm donor
4. Spouse or partner of egg donor
5. Birth mother (genetic mother or gestational surrogate)
6. Gestational surrogate's husband or partner, who may or may not be the sperm donor
7. Baby

Given this number of individuals and their various egos, expectations, fears, and levels of understanding, it is no wonder that disputes among the parties can lead to litigation.

> This is the sale of a child, or, at the very least, the sale of a mother's right to her child, the only mitigating factor being that one of the purchasers is the father. Almost every evil that prompted the prohibition on the payment of money in connection with adoptions exists here.[55]

The court next needed to settle the issue of who should have custody of Baby M. It held that the claims of the genetic father (Mr. Stern) and the natural mother (Ms. Whitehead) were entitled to equal weight and that the child's best interests would be the deciding factor. Weighing the personalities, financial situations, and family lives of the parties, the court gave custody to the Sterns but allowed Ms. Whitehead visitation rights.

A Kentucky case appears to contradict *Baby M* (see Legal Decision Point). In the 1986 decision *Surrogate Parenting Associates, Inc. v. Commonwealth ex rel. Armstrong*,[56] the state attorney general sued a company that arranged surrogate motherhood for infertile couples. The suit alleged that the defendant's activities violated a state statute prohibiting the sale or purchase of "any child for the purpose of adoption," but the court disagreed. It held that the activities of Surrogate Parenting Associates (SPA) did not constitute buying and selling babies because "there are fundamental differences between the surrogate parenting procedure in which SPA participates and the buying and selling of children as prohibited by [law]."[57] The court wrote approvingly of SPA's services:

> We have no reason to believe that the surrogate parenting procedure . . . will not, in most instances, proceed routinely to the conclusion desired by all of the parties at the outset — a woman who can bear children assisting a childless couple to fulfill their desire for a biologically-related child.[58]

Another example of the kinds of disputes that arise from what we might call "assisted parenting" is *Davis v. Davis*.[59] The case began as a divorce action in which the parties—appellee Junior Lewis Davis and his wife, the appellant Mary Sue Davis—agreed on all settlement terms except the disposition of seven frozen embryos that were the product of IVF. Mrs. Davis had asked for custody of the embryos so that she could become pregnant after the divorce. She later changed her mind and stated that she wanted to donate them to another couple for implantation. Mr. Davis did not agree with either approach. The trial court held that the embryos were "human beings" from the moment of conception, and it awarded custody to Mrs. Davis. The intermediate appellate court reversed the decision, holding that Mr. Davis had a constitutional right not to beget a child in

Legal Decision Point

How do you think the Kentucky court would have decided the *Baby M* case?

this manner and that the state had no compelling interest to overrule either party's wishes.

The Supreme Court of Tennessee then heard the case. It began by addressing the issue of whether the embryos were persons or property in the eyes of the law. It concluded that neither Tennessee law nor the US Constitution would consider them persons but that because of their potential to become human beings they deserved greater respect than that which is given to material property. Thus, the court set aside the persons versus property issue to focus on the essential question of whether the Davises would become parents. In balancing the parties' interests, the court found that to grant Mrs. Davis's wish could result in unwanted fatherhood for Mr. Davis. This outcome, the court held, would be a greater financial and psychological burden than Mrs. Davis's disappointment in knowing that the IVF procedures she underwent were to no avail and that the embryos would never become children.

The Uniform Parentage Act

Cases such as *Baby M, Davis v. Davis*, and others[60] raised significant questions that were inconceivable (pun intended) for most of human history: Who is the legal mother when ART is involved? Who is the legal father? What, if any, are the parental rights and obligations of the sperm and egg donors? Must someone pay child support? Is a gestational surrogacy contract valid and enforceable? Must the child be adopted by someone, and if so, who is eligible to adopt?

Such questions prompted the federal government to require states to establish procedures concerning parentage, paternity, genetic testing, child support, and related issues as a condition of their receipt of federal funds for "welfare" programs (Temporary Assistance for Needy Families).[61] In furtherance of this goal, the Uniform Law Commission approved in 2000 and revised in 2002 the Uniform Parentage Act (UPA), which as of early 2016 has been adopted in some form by at least eleven states. (The text of the UPA can be accessed by searching the Uniform Law Commission website: http://www.uniformlaws.org.)

In addition, while all states now have some type of parentage laws that addresses these issues, the UPA is only a *model* law and thus state laws vary widely. To say there is uniformity is a gross misconception. For example, some states permit surrogate contracts, others permit them only for heterosexual couples, and still others expressly forbid them. Where surrogacy is permitted, how to list parentage on the birth certificate may be an issue, and in some states even adoption by lesbians and gay males is not permitted. Thus, as is often the case in our federal system of government, assisted reproductive technologies present a patchwork quilt of conflicting provisions about which generalizing is impossible.

> *It perhaps is not generally appreciated that the restrictive criminal abortion laws in effect in a majority of States today are of relatively recent vintage.*
>
> —*Roe v. Wade*, 410 U.S. 113, 129 (1973)

Abortion

Our discussion now turns to what has been the most socially divisive and perhaps most judicially difficult reproduction issue of all: abortion.

Before the nineteenth century, English and US laws did not prohibit induced abortion—at least in the early stages of pregnancy. Some scholars maintain that English law never regarded abortion of a quickened fetus (one that has made movements the mother can feel) as a criminal act; others disagree. Accordingly, American courts that decide cases pursuant to the common law reached different conclusions. Some held that an abortion of a quickened fetus was criminal—at least a misdemeanor—but others ruled that an abortion, regardless of the stage of pregnancy, was not a crime.[62] In any event, the matter soon became a question solely of statutory law because a generally accepted principle in Anglo-American jurisprudence is that criminal law must be established by statute and not by common-law judicial decision.

The English Parliament enacted the first restrictive abortion statute in 1803.[63] It provided that a willful abortion of a quickened fetus was a capital crime and established lesser penalties for abortions performed during earlier stages of pregnancy. If the surgery was performed in good faith to preserve the life of the mother, however, no criminal act had been committed.[64]

American jurisdictions passed their first restrictive abortion statutes in the early 1800s. Connecticut was the first state to do so when, in 1821, it passed a statute that accepted the English distinction between a quickened and a nonquickened fetus. Similarly, an 1828 New York statute provided that an abortion after quickening was manslaughter but was a misdemeanor at an earlier stage. An exception to manslaughter was made for abortions performed to preserve the life of the mother.

By the late 1860s, nearly all states had enacted restrictive abortion statutes of some type, and most statutes in time abandoned the distinction between a quickened and nonquickened fetus. By the end of the 1950s, these statutes could be categorized as follows:

- Laws that banned all abortions regardless of the stage of pregnancy and regardless of the reason for the procedure
- Laws that permitted termination of pregnancy to preserve the mother's life while prohibiting termination under all other circumstances
- Laws that permitted abortion to preserve the mother's health, providing that only a physician could perform the procedure (in some states, only after consulting with other physicians) and providing proper medical safeguards

During the 1960s, however, a trend to relax these state laws developed, and by the time of the US Supreme Court's abortion decisions in 1973 about a third of the states had adopted a model abortion law that permitted a licensed physician to terminate a pregnancy when there was "substantial risk that continuance of pregnancy would gravely impair the physical or mental health of the mother or that the child would be born with grave physical or mental defects or that the pregnancy resulted from rape, incest, or other felonious intercourse."[65] Under this model law, termination of pregnancy under circumstances other than those described was a third-degree felony if performed before the twenty-sixth week (roughly the end of the second trimester) and was a first-degree felony if performed thereafter. The law further required that all abortions take place in a licensed hospital (unless an emergency existed and such facilities were not available) and that at least two physicians certify in writing the circumstances justifying the surgery. Some jurisdictions added the following requirements:

- The patient had to be a resident of the state for a specified time before the surgery.
- The attending physician was required to obtain the concurrence of the hospital's medical staff committee.
- The hospital where the surgery was to be performed had to be accredited by The Joint Commission.

By the end of 1970, liberalization of the law in New York, Washington, Hawaii, and Alaska had gone much further than the model abortion law. These states had adopted the principle of "abortion on demand," at least up to a statutorily designated stage of pregnancy. (New York, Hawaii, and Alaska accomplished this change by statute, and Washington did so by public referendum.) These states imposed certain restrictions; for example, the procedure had to be performed by a licensed physician in a licensed or accredited hospital, or the woman was required to establish a period of residency in the state before she would be eligible for an abortion.

In January 1973, landmark abortion cases addressed a fundamental constitutional issue: Does a woman have a right to decide for herself, without governmental regulation, whether to bear a child? Given the aspects of personal privacy and autonomy that the US Supreme Court recognized in cases involving contraception and sterilization, the answer is not surprising.

The Roe and Doe Cases

Roe v. Wade[66] concerned the constitutionality of a restrictive Texas statute that permitted abortions only to save the life of the mother. The companion case, *Doe v. Bolton*,[67] questioned Georgia's somewhat more permissive legislation.

When fundamental individual rights are involved, a state must typically convince the court that there is a compelling interest to justify the restraint on those rights. Because an individual's right of privacy is fundamental, the *Roe* and *Bolton* cases employed the compelling interest test when ruling on the constitutionality of the Texas and Georgia abortion statutes.

In *Roe*, the US Supreme Court held that the Texas statute violated the due process clause of the Fourteenth Amendment because the individual's right of privacy trumped the state's interest in promoting the general welfare. However, the court did recognize two state interests that would justify some regulation: protecting the life and health of pregnant women and protecting the "potentiality of human life." The longer a pregnancy lasts, the more heavily these interests weigh against the woman's right of privacy.

According to the *Roe* decision, during the first trimester of pregnancy the health risk posed by abortion is less than the risk of childbirth. Thus, in the first trimester, the state's interest in maternal and fetal health does not outweigh the right of privacy and states may restrict abortions only as they might regulate other surgical procedures—for example, by requiring that they be performed by licensed physicians.[68] Essentially, the decision to perform an abortion during the first trimester of pregnancy was left to the discretion of the patient and her physician.

The Supreme Court next found that during the second trimester the risk to the woman is greater and the state's interest in protecting health becomes more compelling. At this stage, restrictions to protect health are permissible as long as they do not unreasonably interfere with the woman's right to make her own decision. Finally, the court held that the state's interest in protecting potential life becomes compelling when the fetus is viable (capable of surviving outside the womb)—at about 28 weeks after conception. From that stage forward, a state may proscribe abortions altogether except to protect the life or health of the mother.[69]

Doe v. Bolton involved the constitutionality of Georgia's "liberalized" abortion statute patterned after the model abortion law mentioned earlier. The statute permitted termination of pregnancy when it endangered the woman's life or injured her health; when the baby was likely to be born with grave, permanent disabilities; or when conception resulted from rape. In the interest of protecting the patient's health and well-being, however, the law required physicians to exercise their "best clinical judgment" when recommending an abortion. It also required that the physician's judgment be confirmed in writing by two other physicians, that the procedure be carried out in a licensed hospital accredited by The Joint Commission, and that it be approved by a medical staff committee. Further, the patient had to establish Georgia residency to be eligible for the abortion.

The Supreme Court upheld the statutory requirement that the "best clinical judgment" of the patient's physician be exercised when considering abortion, but it struck down the other procedural requirements and the residency requirement, holding that they unduly restricted the rights of doctors and patients to decide. The requirement for confirmation of the physician's judgment was singled out for particular disapprobation. "No other voluntary medical or surgical procedure for which Georgia requires confirmation . . . has been cited to us," the opinion states. "If a physician is licensed . . . he is recognized by the State as capable of exercising acceptable clinical judgment. . . . Required acquiescence by co-practitioners has no rational connection with a patient's needs and unduly infringes on the physician's right to practice."[70]

The Supreme Court did recognize that the state might, if it wished, require that abortions after the first trimester be performed at licensed facilities and that the state might also promulgate reasonable standards consistent with its legitimate interest in protecting maternal health.[71] The residency requirement was ruled an invasion of the constitutionally protected right to travel included in the privileges and immunities clause of Article IV of the US Constitution.

State Regulation of Abortion After 1973

In the years since *Roe* and *Bolton*, the Supreme Court has issued further guidance on judicial review of state abortion regulation and has examined on a case-by-case basis the constitutionality of state and local abortion regulations that attempted to limit a woman's right to choose. Restrictions that have been held constitutional include the following:

- Requirement that any tissue removed following an abortion—whether in a hospital or clinic—be submitted to a pathologist (upheld because it placed a "relatively insignificant burden" on a woman's decision on abortion, was "reasonably related to generally accepted medical standards," and furthered "important health-related state concerns")[72]
- Record keeping and reporting requirements—provided that they are not unduly burdensome, that they protect confidentiality, and that the facts are legitimately related to the state's health interest[73]
- Statute requiring that second-trimester abortions be performed in licensed clinics (upheld as a reasonable means of furthering the state's compelling interest in maternal health)[74]
- Requirement for written informed consent[75]

Restrictions that have been struck down include the following:

- Pennsylvania Abortion Control Act's detailed reporting for each abortion performed at any stage of pregnancy[76]
- Ordinance that required, among other mandates, that all abortions after the first trimester take place in a hospital

- Requirement that a waiting period elapse between the woman's consent to an abortion and the abortion procedure (struck down because it served no legitimate state interest)
- Requirements that certain specific information be given to the woman before obtaining her written consent and that a physician inform a patient that "the unborn child is a human life from the moment of conception"
- Requirement that counseling be given only by the attending physician[77]
- State ban on "partial birth abortion," although a later federal ban was upheld[78]

In *Roe*, the Supreme Court held that a state could criminalize all abortions (except those necessary to preserve the mother's life or health) after the fetus becomes viable because at that point the state's interest in protecting the potentiality of human life becomes compelling. It found that the medical community considers a fetus to be "viable" if it is potentially able to live outside the mother's womb, even though with some artificial aid, and the court stressed that the "abortion decision in all its aspects is inherently, and primarily, a medical decision," and it left determination of the point of viability "flexible for anticipated advancements in medical skill."[79]

In 1973, medical science recognized a relatively clear division of pregnancy: the inherent risk of pregnancy increased after the first three months, and fetal viability occurred at about the end of the second three months. This trimester structure was therefore used to determine when the state's interests outweighed those of the woman and therefore the point at which the state could place restrictions on abortions.

Many critics dispute the soundness of this approach. As Justice Sandra Day O'Connor noted in the *City of Akron* case ten years later:

> The *Roe* framework ... is clearly on a collision course with itself. As the medical risks of various abortion procedures decrease, the point at which the State may regulate for reasons of maternal health is moved further forward to actual childbirth. As medical science becomes better able to provide for the separate existence of the fetus, the point of viability is moved further back toward conception. . . . The *Roe* framework is inherently tied to the state of medical technology that exists whenever particular litigation ensues.[80]

Indeed, these kinds of advances have occurred. In 1973, a fetus was considered viable at about 28 weeks after conception; since then, the lives of infants born at 20 weeks or even earlier can be saved as a result of new medical science. Some abortions, however, such as those requested when genetic diseases or defects are diagnosed, cannot be performed before 18 to 20 weeks because amniocentesis—the procedure that reveals the disease or defect—cannot always be performed before that time. Furthermore, some attempted abortions actually result in live births, although depending on gestational age, a fetus that survives an abortion may not be capable of living more than momentarily outside the womb.

The question of viability thus raises a number of issues, not all of which have been (or are capable of being) addressed by the legislatures or courts. If abortions are criminal after viability, who determines viability? Who decides whether the abortion was necessary to protect the mother's life or health? What does "health" encompass? Even if the abortion is medically necessary, must the physician use the method most likely to preserve the life of the fetus? What duty of care is owed to the fetus who survives an abortion?

These remain perplexing questions with no clear answers. In seeking to protect the life of the viable fetus, for example, some states have imposed a requirement that a second physician be present to attend to the child at all postviability abortions. The Supreme Court upheld this requirement in *Planned Parenthood Association of Kansas City, Missouri, Inc. v. Ashcroft* as reasonably furthering the state's compelling interest in protecting the lives of viable fetuses.[81] The Supreme Court also requires that there be an exception to the second physician requirement in case of a medical emergency that threatens the mother's health. Because there was no emergency exception in the Pennsylvania statute as amended in 1982, the Supreme Court found that law unconstitutional as well.[82]

Missouri was the focus of another landmark abortion case, *Webster v. Reproductive Health Services*,[83] decided in 1989. In *Webster*, the Supreme Court addressed four provisions of a Missouri statute:

1. Preamble declaring that life begins at conception and that "unborn children have protectable interests in life, health, and well-being"
2. Prohibition on the use of public facilities or employees to perform abortions
3. Prohibition on public funding of abortion counseling
4. Requirement that physicians conduct viability tests before performing abortions

The court declined to wade into the philosophical quagmire of when life begins but it upheld the other three provisions. The significance of *Webster*, however, is not so much its specific holdings but its language calling *Roe*'s trimester analysis into doubt:

We think that the doubt cast upon the Missouri statute . . . is not so much a flaw in the statute as it is a reflection of the fact that the rigid trimester analysis of the course of a pregnancy enunciated in *Roe* has resulted in subsequent cases making constitutional law in this area a virtual Procrustean bed. . . .

In the first place, the rigid *Roe* framework is hardly consistent with the notion of a Constitution cast in general terms as ours is, and usually speaking in general principles, as ours does. The key elements of the *Roe* framework—trimesters and viability—are not found in the text of the Constitution or in any place else one would expect to find a constitutional principle. Since the bounds of the inquiry are essentially indeterminate, the result has been a web of legal rules that have become increasingly intricate, resembling a code of regulations rather than a body of constitutional doctrine. As Justice White has put it, the trimester framework has left this Court to serve as the country's "ex officio medical board with powers to approve or disapprove practices and standards throughout the United States."

In the second place, we do not see why the State's interest in protecting potential human life should come into existence only at the point of viability, and that there should therefore be a rigid line allowing state regulation after viability but prohibiting it before viability.[84]

Because no clear majority of justices was prepared to overrule *Roe*, the quoted language is dictum. It is dictum, however, that has greatly encouraged the antiabortion forces who await the day *Roe* is overturned. That opportunity seemed to come in 1992 in *Planned Parenthood of S.E. Pennsylvania v. Casey*, which involved a Pennsylvania law containing numerous provisions the plaintiffs contended were obstacles to a woman's choice of abortion, including a requirement that informed consent be provided at least 24 hours prior to the procedure and be accompanied by certain clinical information. It also required parental or judicial consent for a minor's abortion and gave a narrow definition of "medical emergency," thus allowing these requirements to be avoided in certain situations.[85]

Supporters of the law, including the Commonwealth of Pennsylvania and the federal government, not only asked that the statute be upheld but also urged that *Roe* be reversed. A widely divided Supreme Court declined to do so. It upheld the first two provisions, stating that they did not constitute an "undue burden" on a woman's right to choose, but it struck down others as overly burdensome and too narrowly written. Note that by upholding the provision regarding minors, the court implicitly affirmed the general rule that a state may require parental consent for a minor's abortion if the minor also has an option to seek judicial approval if she does not wish to seek or cannot obtain a parent's consent.

In the course of announcing the decision, Justice O'Connor's lead opinion famously declared, "Liberty finds no refuge in a jurisprudence of doubt." From this strong affirmation of the principle of stare decisis, the Supreme Court upheld *Roe*'s essential holdings. *Roe* did not escape unscathed, however. In her opinion, Justice O'Connor wrote, "We reject the rigid trimester framework of *Roe v. Wade*." Instead of trimesters, the opinion focused on the concept of fetal viability:

> The concept of viability . . . is the time at which there is a realistic possibility of maintaining and nourishing a life outside the womb, so that the independent existence of the second life can in reason and all fairness be the object of state protection that now overrides the rights of the woman.

The opinion continued on this point: "The woman's right to terminate her pregnancy before viability is the most central principle of *Roe v. Wade*. It is a rule of law and a component of liberty we cannot renounce."

On the question of rejecting *Roe*'s trimester framework, Justice O'Connor did not speak for a majority of the justices. The judgment of the Supreme Court was announced in the opinion Justice O'Connor authored, which was joined by Justice Anthony Kennedy and Justice David Souter, but even Justice Kennedy did not concur in the dictum regarding trimesters. Justice Harold ("Harry") Blackmun and Justice John Paul Stevens joined in portions of the O'Connor opinion, thus providing the five votes necessary for the particular actions ultimately taken ("affirmed in part" and "reversed in part"), but they also joined Chief Justice William Rehnquist and Justices Byron White, Antonin Scalia, and Clarence Thomas in dissenting from at least a part of the lead opinion. Furthermore, the latter four members of the Supreme Court would have reexamined *Roe*'s principle that abortion is a fundamental right, concluded that the abortion choice is not a constitutional right at all, and urged that the statute be upheld in its entirety.

The Casey *Case and Its Aftermath*

Casey is a long and complicated decision that includes numerous written opinions, some of them reflecting what seem to be personal tensions among the justices, and it provides no clear majority position on some of the more significant abortion-related issues. *Casey* and this chapter's lengthy discussion demonstrate the complexity of these issues, which have been contentious and divisive for decades and show no sign of being resolved anytime soon.

In one of his final remarks on the subject, Justice Blackmun, author of the majority opinion in *Roe*, wrote the following:

> In one sense, the Court's approach [in *Casey*] is worlds apart from that of the Chief Justice and Justice Scalia [two of the dissenters]. And yet, in another sense, the distance between the two approaches is short—the distance is but a single vote.
>
> I am 83 years old. I cannot remain on this Court forever, and when I do step down, the confirmation process for my successor well may focus on the issue

before us today. That, I regret, may be exactly where the choice between the two worlds will be made.[86]

Contrary to Justice Blackmun's prediction, his successor's confirmation process did not overly focus on abortion, and the new justice, Stephen G. Breyer, summed up the status of abortion law in a decision issued in 2000:

Aware that constitutional law must govern a society whose different members sincerely hold directly opposing views, and considering the matter in light of the Constitution's guarantees of fundamental individual liberty, this Court, in the course of a generation, has determined and then redetermined that the Constitution offers basic protection to the woman's right to choose.[87]

Thus, stare decisis proved a formidable principle for constancy as the Supreme Court once again declined to overrule *Roe*. This stability is reflected in the fact that relatively few cases have reached the high court for more than two decades. *Ayotte v. Planned Parenthood of Northern New England* raised serious questions about a New Hampshire parental notice statute that failed to contain a medical emergency exception.[88] The case was remanded for further consideration, and before the lower courts could fashion a proper remedy, the state legislature repealed the law in its entirety.

In *Gonzales v. Carhart*, the Supreme Court upheld the federal partial-birth abortion law on procedural grounds.[89] In doing so, it reaffirmed the essential holdings of *Casey*—that a woman has a right to choose, the state has some power to restrict abortions after viability, and the state has legitimate interests in protecting the health of the woman and the life of the fetus. Because the specific procedure involved in *Carhart* is performed only rarely and the statute's scope is narrow, however, the opinion may have only limited precedential value.

After these cases were handed down, rather than continuing to launch frontal assaults on *Roe v. Wade*, abortion opponents turned to state legislatures to try restricting the procedure incrementally by statute. A new Texas law was a prime example, and the most recent Supreme Court decision—*Whole Woman's Health v. Hellerstedt*[90]—is the result.

In 2013 the Texas legislature passed a law that required physicians who perform abortions to have admitting privileges at a hospital within 30 miles of the abortion facility. It also required the facility to meet the standards of a licensed ambulatory surgical center (ASC). Once the admitting privileges provision began to be enforced, the number of facilities doing abortions in Texas dropped in half—to about 20—and would have fallen to seven or eight had the surgical center provision taken effect. Furthermore, given the state's size, fewer facilities meant that the number of women of reproductive age living a long distance from an abortion clinic increased exponentially. For example, it was estimated that the number living more than 200 miles from a provider increased from 10,000 to 290,000 after the privileges provision went into effect and would have increased to three-quarters of a million if the ASC requirement had been upheld.

The law was challenged immediately, and in 2016 the Supreme Court concluded that both the admitting privileges and surgical center requirements violate the Constitution because they place a substantial obstacle in the path of women seeking an abortion and constitute an undue burden on abortion access. The court also found that neither requirement yielded any significant health benefit when compared to the state's prior, less restrictive law.

Given that the "directly opposing views" Justice Breyer referred to persist, there is little chance that abortion will totally disappear from the judicial radar screen. However, in light of *Whole Woman's Health*, it may be some time before the issue again confronts the Supreme Court.

Hospitals' Role in Reproduction Issues

Are healthcare institutions legally required to make abortion and sterilization services available to their patients? As usual, the answer is not clear.

Some state and federal statutes contain a *conscience clause* that permits hospitals and physicians to refuse to perform abortions on moral or religious grounds. (This clause was discussed by way of dictum in *Doe v. Bolton*.) In the absence of such a clause, the legal issue is whether hospitals that refuse to provide abortions or sterilizations are either acting in the name of the state in denying the patient due process and equal protection of law—and thus violating the Fourteenth Amendment—or acting "under color of law" and denying civil rights. As emphasized repeatedly in various contexts throughout this book, the Fourteenth Amendment applies to state action; therefore, a state or an institution acting on its behalf may not prevent an individual from exercising constitutional or statutorily protected rights.

One point seems to be well settled: A hospital owned and operated by federal, state, or municipal government may not refuse to permit abortions and sterilizations that are lawful surgical procedures.[91] Whether the law may require a private hospital to furnish reproductive services is a more difficult question, but the weight of authority holds that the institution's moral and religious convictions should be respected. Thus, a private hospital need not provide abortion or sterilization services, even if it has been funded to a significant extent by federal money and receives such benefits as a tax exemption.[92] The leading case on this question is *Doe v. Bellin Memorial Hospital*,[93] decided by a federal court of appeals shortly before *Roe* and *Bolton*. As a private hospital, Bellin Memorial could prevent its staff physicians from performing legally permissible abortions because no state action was involved. Similarly, relying on *Doe v. Bellin, Allen v. Sisters of St. Joseph* held that a Catholic institution could ban a voluntary sterilization procedure.[94]

In *Watkins v. Mercy Medical Center*, a physician brought suit against a Catholic hospital that forbade abortions and sterilizations.[95] A federal district court upheld the hospital's policy, saying that state action was not indicated merely by receipt of governmental money, state licensure, or tax exemption. Significant in this decision was the Health Programs Extension Act of 1973, which specifically provides that receipt of Hill-Burton money does not require a hospital to provide abortions or sterilizations as long as refusal is founded on religious beliefs or moral conviction.[96] (Although Mercy Medical Center was not required to permit the plaintiff physician to perform the desired surgical procedure, it could not terminate a medical staff appointment solely on the basis of the physician's personal beliefs.) Most decisions pertaining to private hospitals have similarly held that no state action is involved under the Fourteenth Amendment and that voluntary institutions that prohibit abortion and sterilization are not denying patients' civil rights.[97]

As mentioned, many states have specific conscience clauses to protect institutions' and individuals' moral or religious convictions. Most of these state laws relate only to abortions. They purportedly apply to all hospitals—governmental and private—but some are made applicable only to hospitals owned and operated by churches or religious orders. (The provisions of the Georgia statute discussed earlier were implicitly upheld in the case of *Bolton*.) Provisions pertaining to an individual's right of refusal to participate seem clearly constitutional. Perhaps the same can be said of the statutes recognizing the moral and religious convictions of a private sectarian hospital, as they are valuable rights to be protected in a free society.

A related issue is whether a state may deny Medicaid payments for elective or medically necessary abortions rendered to indigent patients. The eponymous Hyde Amendment, the first version of which was passed in 1976 and since has been renewed annually, denies federal funding of abortions except to save the mother's life or in cases of rape or incest. The Supreme Court has ruled that the Medicaid law does not require a state participating in the Medicaid program to fund either elective nontherapeutic abortions[98] or medically necessary abortions[99] as a condition of participation. Because a private hospital need not provide abortion services, hospitalized patients who are refused abortion or sterilization should be fully informed of their condition and provided with sound medical advice indicating where proper and appropriate care can be obtained.

Additional legal issues concern hospitals that do perform abortions and sterilizations. Most state statutes criminalize third-trimester abortions that are not necessary to preserve the life or health of the mother. A hospital has a duty to prevent criminal acts from occurring on its premises; hence, counsel must carefully advise the hospital and its medical staff about the current legal status of pregnancy terminations. Administrative policies and procedures must be developed to make sure that the institution and its staff perform their duties in a lawful manner.

Summary

Issues of reproduction are sensitive and often contentious. This chapter reviews many of the legal questions regarding sterilization, wrongful life, wrongful birth, surrogate parenting, IVF, stem cell research, and abortion. It discusses hospitals' role in reproduction issues—whether hospitals can be required to provide such services and when they can expect government programs to pay for the procedures if they do provide them. It also points out that abortion-related issues will continue to be subjects of judicial review and that the number of cases considering stem cell research will increase.

Discussion Questions

1. In *Griswold*, Justice Stewart skewered the majority for asserting that the Ninth Amendment of the US Constitution supported its decision to overturn the Connecticut contraception statute. He wrote, "The idea that a federal court could ever use the Ninth Amendment to annul a law passed by the elected representatives of the people of the State of Connecticut would have caused James Madison no little wonder." What does the Ninth Amendment say, and why would Justice Stewart say that President Madison, in particular, would be perplexed by its use to justify the majority's opinion?

2. Can the *Buck* and *Skinner* decisions be reconciled?

3. In *Turpin v. Sortini*, the California Supreme Court said it was difficult to understand how awarding damages to a child who would not have been born if not for the defendants' negligence "would disavow the value of life." *Depreciate* is probably more apt than *disavow* in the context of that sentence. Can you construct the moral argument that as a public policy matter, such an award would depreciate the value of human life?

4. Summarize the state of the law following the Supreme Court's decision in *Casey*.

5. What is the difference between a wrongful life case and a wrongful birth case? How is the measurement of damages in wrongful life cases different from that in wrongful birth cases?

6. What kinds of legal issues do you think stem cell research and genetic therapies will present in the coming years?

The Court Decides

Skinner v. Oklahoma ex rel. Attorney General
316 U.S. 535 (1942)

Mr. Justice Douglas delivered the opinion of the Court.

This case touches a sensitive and important area of human rights. Oklahoma deprives certain individuals of a right which is basic to the perpetuation of a race—the right to have offspring. Oklahoma has decreed the enforcement of its law against petitioner, overruling his claim that it violated the Fourteenth Amendment. Because that decision raised grave and substantial constitutional questions, we granted the petition for certiorari.

The statute involved is Oklahoma's Habitual Criminal Sterilization Act. That Act defines an "habitual criminal" as a person who, having been convicted two or more times for crimes "amounting to felonies involving moral turpitude," either in an Oklahoma court or in a court of any other State, is thereafter convicted of such a felony in Oklahoma and is sentenced to a term of imprisonment in an Oklahoma penal institution. Machinery is provided for the institution by the Attorney General of a proceeding against such a person in the Oklahoma courts for a judgment that such person shall be rendered sexually sterile. Notice, an opportunity to be heard, and the right to a jury trial are provided. The issues triable in such a proceeding are narrow and confined.

If the court or jury finds that the defendant is an "habitual criminal" and that he "may be rendered sexually sterile without detriment to his or her general health," then the court "shall render judgment to the effect that said defendant be rendered sexually sterile" by the operation of vasectomy in case of a male, and of salpingectomy in case of a female. Only one other provision of the Act is

material here, and [it] provides that "offenses arising out of the violation of the prohibitory laws, revenue acts, embezzlement, or political offenses, shall not come or be considered within the terms of this Act."

Petitioner was convicted in 1926 of the crime of stealing chickens, and was sentenced to the Oklahoma State Reformatory. In 1929 he was convicted of the crime of robbery with firearms, and was sentenced to the reformatory. In 1934 he was convicted again of robbery with firearms, and was sentenced to the penitentiary. He was confined there in 1935 when the Act was passed. In 1936 the Attorney General instituted proceedings against him. Petitioner in his answer challenged the Act as unconstitutional by reason of the Fourteenth Amendment. A jury trial was had. The court instructed the jury that the crimes of which petitioner had been convicted were felonies involving moral turpitude, and that the only question for the jury was whether the operation of vasectomy could be performed on petitioner without detriment to his general health. The jury found that it could be. A judgment directing that the operation of vasectomy be performed on petitioner was affirmed by the Supreme Court of Oklahoma by a five to four decision.

Several objections to the constitutionality of the Act have been pressed upon us. It is urged that the Act cannot be sustained as an exercise of the police power, in view of the state of scientific authorities respecting inheritability of criminal traits. It is argued that due process is lacking because, under this Act, unlike the Act upheld in *Buck v.*

(continued)

(continued from previous page)

Bell, the defendant is given no opportunity to be heard on the issue as to whether he is the probable potential parent of socially undesirable offspring. It is also suggested that the Act is penal in character and that the sterilization provided for is cruel and unusual punishment and [violates] the Fourteenth Amendment. We pass those points without intimating an opinion on them, for there is a feature of the Act [that] clearly condemns it. That is, its failure to meet the requirements of the equal protection clause of the Fourteenth Amendment.

We do not stop to point out all of the inequalities in this Act. A few examples will suffice. In Oklahoma, grand larceny is a felony. Larceny is grand larceny when the property taken exceeds $20 in value. Embezzlement is punishable "in the manner prescribed for feloniously stealing property of the value of that embezzled." Hence, he who embezzles property worth more than $20 is guilty of a felony. A clerk who appropriates over $20 from his employer's till and a stranger who steals the same amount are thus both guilty of felonies. If the latter repeats his act and is convicted three times, he may be sterilized. But the clerk is not subject to the pains and penalties of the Act no matter how large his embezzlements nor how frequent his convictions. A person who enters a chicken coop and steals chickens commits a felony; and he may be sterilized if he is thrice convicted. If, however, he is a bailee of the property and fraudulently appropriates it, he is an embezzler. Hence, no matter how habitual his proclivities for embezzlement are and no matter how often his conviction, he may not be sterilized. Thus, the nature of the two crimes is intrinsically the same and they are punishable in the same manner. *[Paragraph break added.]*

Furthermore, the line between them follows close distinctions—distinctions comparable to those highly technical ones which shaped the common law as to "trespass" or "taking." There may be larceny by fraud rather than embezzlement even where the owner of the personal property delivers it to the defendant, if the latter has at that time "a fraudulent intention to make use of the possession as a means of converting such property to his own use, and does so convert it." If the fraudulent intent occurs later and the defendant converts the property, he is guilty of embezzlement. Whether a particular act is larceny by fraud or embezzlement thus turns not on the intrinsic quality of the act but on when the felonious intent arose—a question for the jury under appropriate instructions.

It was stated in *Buck v. Bell* that the claim that state legislation violates the equal protection clause of the Fourteenth Amendment is "the usual last resort of constitutional arguments." Under our constitutional system the States in determining the reach and scope of particular legislation need not provide "abstract symmetry." They may mark and set apart the classes and types of problems according to the needs and as dictated or suggested by experience. It was in that connection that Mr. Justice Holmes, speaking for the Court in [another case] stated, "We must remember that the machinery of government would not work if it were not allowed a little play in its joints."

. . .

But the instant legislation runs afoul of the equal protection clause. . . . We are dealing here with legislation which involves one of the basic civil rights of man. Marriage and procreation are fundamental to the very existence and survival of the race. The power to sterilize, if exercised, may have subtle, far-reaching and devastating effects. In evil or reckless hands it can cause races or types which are inimical to the dominant group to wither and disappear. There is no redemption for the individual whom the law touches. Any experiment which the State conducts is to his irreparable injury. He is forever deprived of a basic liberty. We mention these matters not to re-examine the scope of the police power of the States. We advert to them merely in emphasis of our view that strict scrutiny of the classification which a State makes in a sterilization law is essential, lest unwittingly, or otherwise, invidious discriminations are made against groups or types of individuals in violation of the constitutional guaranty of just and equal laws. The guaranty of "equal protection of the laws is a pledge of the protection of equal laws." When the law lays an unequal hand on those who have committed intrinsically the same quality of offense and sterilizes one and not the other, it has made as invidious a discrimination as if it had selected a particular race or nationality for oppressive treatment. Sterilization of those who have thrice committed grand larceny, with immunity for those who are embezzlers, is a clear, pointed, unmistakable discrimination. Oklahoma makes no attempt to say that he who commits larceny by trespass or trick or fraud has biologically inheritable traits which he who commits embezzlement lacks. *[Paragraph break added.]*

Oklahoma's line between larceny by fraud and embezzlement is determined, as we have noted, "with reference to the time when the fraudulent intent to convert the property to the taker's own use" arises. We have not the slightest basis for inferring that that line has any significance in eugenics, nor that the inheritability of criminal traits follows the neat legal distinctions which the law has marked between those two offenses. In terms of fines and imprisonment, the crimes of larceny and embezzlement rate the same under the Oklahoma code. Only when it comes to sterilization are the pains and penalties of the law different. The equal protection clause would indeed be a formula of empty words if such conspicuously artificial lines could be drawn. In *Buck v. Bell* the Virginia statute was upheld though it applied only to feeble-minded persons in institutions of the State. But it was pointed out that "so far as the operations enable those who otherwise must be kept confined to be returned to the world, and thus open the asylum to others, the equality aimed at will be more nearly reached." Here there is no such saving feature. Embezzlers are forever free. Those who steal or take in other ways are not. If such a classification were permitted, the technical common law concept of a "trespass" based on distinctions which are "very largely dependent upon history for explanation" could readily become a rule of human genetics.

It is true that the Act has a broad severability clause. But we will not endeavor to determine whether its application would solve the equal protection difficulty. The Supreme Court of Oklahoma sustained the Act without reference to the severability clause. We have therefore a situation where the Act as construed and applied to petitioner is allowed to perpetuate the discrimination which we have found to be fatal. Whether the severability clause would be so applied as to remove this particular constitutional objection is a question which may be more appropriately left for adjudication by the Oklahoma court. That is reemphasized here by our uncertainty as to what excision, if any, would be made as a matter of Oklahoma law. It is by no means clear whether, if an excision were made, this particular constitutional difficulty might be solved by enlarging on the one hand or contracting on the other the class of criminals who might be sterilized.

Reversed. ■

(continued)

(continued from previous page)

Discussion Questions

1. What does *ex rel.* mean in the caption of the case?
2. What does Justice Douglas mean when he talks about a "severability clause" in the statute?
3. The opinion takes pains to distinguish *Buck v. Bell* from the present case. Are you persuaded by Justice Douglas's discussion, or has he effectively overruled *Buck* without saying so?
4. In the 1930s, Hereditary Health Courts were established in Nazi Germany to enforce sterilization laws on individuals suspected of hereditary diseases and other "defects." See generally, Robert J. Lifton, The Nazi Doctors: Medical Killing and the Psychology of Genocide (Basic Books 1986), 22–44. Should forced sterilization—whether for eugenic reasons or otherwise—ever be allowed? If so, under what circumstances and controls?

Notes

1. Parker v. Rampton, 28 Utah 2d 36, 497 P.2d 848 (1972).
2. 381 U.S. 479 (1965). *See also* Eisenstadt v. Baird, 405 U.S. 438 (1972) (unmarried persons have the same constitutional right to privacy with respect to contraceptive measures as married persons have).
3. 42 C.F.R. §§ 50.201–50.210.
4. 274 U.S. 200 (1927).
5. Skinner v. Oklahoma, 316 U.S. 535 (1942).
6. *See, e.g.,* North Carolina Ass'n for Retarded Children v. State of N.C., 420 F. Supp. 451, 454 (1976), in which the court made a finding of fact that "[m]ost competent geneticists now reject social Darwinism and doubt the premise implicit in Mr. Justice Holmes' incantation that '. . . three generations of imbeciles is enough.' . . . [P]revalent medical opinion views with distaste even voluntary sterilizations for the mentally retarded and is inclined to sanction it only as a last resort and in relatively extreme cases. In short, the medical and genetical experts are no longer sold on sterilization to benefit either retarded patients or the future of the Republic."
7. In re Grady, 85 N.J. 235, 245, 426 A.2d 467, 472 (1981). *See also* Burgdorf and Burgdorf, *supra* note 100.
8. Speck v. Finegold, 268 Pa. Super. 342, 408 A.2d 496 (1979), *modified*, 497 Pa. 77, 439 A.2d 110 (1979).

9. 497 Pa. at 80, 439 A.2d at 112.

10. Christensen v. Thornby, 192 Minn. 123, 255 N.W. 620 (1934).

11. 31 Cal. 3d 220, 182 Cal. Rptr. 337, 643 P.2d 954 (1982).

12. Johnson v. Yeshiva Univ., 42 N.Y.2d 818, 820, 396 N.Y.S.2d 647, 648, 364 N.E.2d 1340, 1341 (1977).

13. Becker v. Schwartz, 46 N.Y.2d 401, 413 N.Y.S.2d 895, 386 N.E.2d 807 (1978).

14. Examples of wrongful birth actions for negligence in genetic counseling, testing, or diagnosis include (among others) cases involving Down syndrome. *See, e.g.*, Call v. Kezirian, 135 Cal. App. 3d 189, 185 Cal. Rptr. 103 (1982); Berman v. Allan, 80 N.J. 421, 404 A.2d 8 (1979); Azzolino v. Dingfelder, 71 N.C. App. 289, 322 S.E.2d 567 (1984), *review granted*, 327 S.E.2d 887 (1985); Phillips v. United States, 508 F. Supp. 537 (D.S.C. 1980), 508 F. Supp. 544 (D.S.C. 1981). Regarding Tay-Sachs disease, *see, e.g.*, Curlender v. Bio-Science Laboratories, 165 Cal. Rptr. 477, 106 Cal. App. 3d 811 (1980); Goldberg v. Ruskin, 128 Ill. App. 3d 1029, 471 N.E.2d 530 (1984); Gildiner v. Thomas Jefferson Univ. Hosp., 451 F. Supp. 692 (E.D. Pa. 1978).

15. Smith v. Cote, 128 N.H. 231, 513 A.2d 341 (1986); Dumer v. St. Michael's Hosp., 69 Wis. 2d 766, 233 N.W.2d 372 (1975).

16. Schroeder v. Perkel, 87 N.J. 53, 432 A.2d 834 (1981).

17. Troppi v. Scarf, 31 Mich. App. 240, 187 N.W.2d 511 (1971).

18. Harbeson v. Parke-Davis, Inc., 98 Wash. 2d 460, 656 P.2d 483 (1983).

19. Hackworth v. Hart, 474 S.W.2d 377 (Ky. 1971); Hays v. Hall, 488 S.W.2d 412 (Tex. 1972); Vilord v. Jenkins, 226 So. 2d 245 (Fla. Dist. Ct. App. 1969); Teeters v. Currey, 518 S.W.2d 512 (Tenn. 1974).

20. Blake v. Cruz, 108 Idaho 253, 698 P.2d 315 (1984).

21. Courts have uniformly rejected the claim that the parents have a duty to mitigate damages by obtaining an abortion or placing the child for adoption. *See, e.g.*, Jones v. Malinowski, 299 Md. 257, 473 A.2d 429 (1984), *and* Cockrum v. Baumgartner, 99 Ill. App. 3d 271, 425 N.E.2d 968 (1981), *cert. denied*, 464 U.S. 846 (1983), *rev'd on other grounds*, 447 N.E.2d 385 (1983). In one case of a negligent sterilization, the defendants claimed that the husband's sexual relations with his wife were an "intervening cause" of the pregnancy that should relieve the defendants of responsibility. The court was not amused. Custodio v. Bauer, 251 Cal. App. 2d 303, 59 Cal. Rptr. 463 (1967).

22. *See, e.g.*, Nolan v. Merecki, 88 A.D.2d 1021, 451 N.Y.S.2d 914 (1982).

23. *See, e.g.,* Troppi v. Scarf, 31 Mich. App. 240, 187 N.W.2d 511 (1971), *and* Ziemba v. Sternberg, 45 A.D.2d 230, 357 N.Y.S.2d 265 (1974).

24. *See, e.g.,* Bushman v. Burns Clinic Medical Center, 83 Mich. App. 453, 268 N.W.2d 683 (1978), *and* Sorkin v. Lee, 434 N.Y.S.2d 300, 78 A.D.2d 180 (1980).

25. *See, e.g.,* Bushman, *supra* note 24; James G. and Lurana G. v. Caserta, 332 S.E.2d 872 (Sup. Ct. App. W. Va. 1985); Sorkin v. Lee, 434 N.Y.S.2d 300, 78 A.D.2d 180 (1980).

26. Naccash v. Burger, 223 Va. 406, 290 S.E.2d 825 (1982). Other cases permitting recovery for emotional distress include Berman v. Allan, 80 N.J. 421, 404 A.2d 8 (1979); Blake v. Cruz, 108 Idaho 253, 698 P.2d 315 (1984).

27. Howard v. Lecher, 53 A.D.2d 420, 386 N.Y.S.2d 460 (1976), *aff'd,* 42 N.Y.2d 109 (1977). *See also* Becker v. Schwartz, 46 N.Y.2d 401, 413 N.Y.S.2d 895, 386 N.E.2d 807 (1978) (damages for emotional harm would be too speculative), *and* Goldberg v. Ruskin, 84 Ill. Dec. 1 (1984), *modified,* 128 Ill App. 3d 1029, 471 N.E.2d 530 (1984) (parents failed to allege that they suffered physical injury and therefore could not recover damages for emotional harm).

28. Smith v. Cote, *supra* note 15.

29. *See, e.g.,* Ochs v. Borelli, 187 Conn. 253, 445 A.2d 883 (1982).

30. *See, e.g.,* Rieck v. Medical Protective Co., 64 Wis. 2d 514, 219 N.W.2d 242 (1974) (failure to make a timely diagnosis of pregnancy). Other cases denying costs of raising a healthy child include Wilczynski v. Goodman, 73 Ill. App. 3d 51, 29 Ill. Dec. 216, 391 N.E.2d 479 (1979) (negligent performance of therapeutic abortion); Public Health Trust v. Brown, 388 So. 2d 1084 (Fla. App. 1980) (failed sterilization); Wilbur v. Kerr, 275 Ark. 239, 628 S.W.2d 568 (1982) (husband had not one but two unsuccessful vasectomies); Sorkin v. Lee, 434 N.Y.S.2d 300, 78 A.D.2d 180 (1980) (failed tubal ligation).

31. 99 Ill. App. 3d 271, 425 N.E.2d 968 (1981).

32. *See, e.g.,* Blake v. Cruz, 108 Idaho 253, 698 P.2d 315 (1984); Goldberg v. Ruskin, 84 Ill. Dec. 1 (1984), *modified,* 128 Ill. App. 3d 1029, 471 N.E.2d 530 (1984); Schroeder v. Perkel, 87 N.J. 53, 432 A.2d 834 (1981); Jacobs v. Theimer, 519 S.W.2d 846 (Tex. 1975).

33. *See, e.g.,* Berman v. Allan, 80 N.J. 421, 404 A.2d 8 (1979).

34. *See, e.g.,* Still v. Gratton, 55 Cal. App. 3d 698, 127 Cal. Rptr. 652 (1976); Zepeda v. Zepeda, 41 Ill. App. 2d 240, 190 N.E.2d 849 (1963), *cert. denied,* 379 U.S. 945 (1964); Williams v. State, 25 A.D.2d 906, 269 N.Y.S.2d 786 (1966).

35. *See, e.g.,* Elliot v. Brown, 361 So. 2d 546 (Ala. 1978); DiNatale v. Lieberman, 409 So. 2d 512 (Fla. App. 1982); Blake v. Cruz, 108 Idaho 253, 698 P.2d 315 (1984); Goldberg v. Ruskin, 84 Ill. Dec. 1 (1984), *modified*, 128 Ill. App. 3d 1029, 471 N.E.2d 530 (1984); Whit v. United States, 510 F. Supp. 146 (D. Kansas 1981); Eisbrenner v. Stanley, 106 Mich. App. 357, 308 N.W.2d 209 (1981); Berman v. Allan, 80 N.J. 421, 404 A.2d 8 (1979); Becker v. Schwartz, 46 N.Y.2d 401, 413 N.Y.S.2d 895, 386 N.E.2d 807 (1978); Gildiner v. Thomas Jefferson Univ. Hosp., 451 F. Supp. 692 (E.D. Pa. 1978); Phillips v. United States, 508 F. Supp. 537 (D.S.C. 1980), 508 F. Supp. 544 (D.S.C. 1981); Nelson v. Krusen, 678 S.W.2d 918 (Tex. 1984); Dumer v. St. Michael's Hosp., 69 Wis. 2d 766, 233 N.W.2d 372 (1975).

36. Becker v. Schwartz, 46 N.Y. 2d 401, 413 N.Y.S.2d 895, 386 N.E.2d 807 (1978).

37. Blake v. Cruz, 108 Idaho 253, 698 P.2d 315 (1984).

38. 106 Cal. App. 3d 811, 165 Cal. Rptr. 477 (1980).

39. 31 Cal. 3d 220, 182 Cal. Rptr. 337, 643 P.2d 954 (1982).

40. *Id.* at 233, 182 Cal. Rptr. at 344–45, 643 P.2d at 961–62.

41. Cal. Health & Safety Code § 7186 (Supp. 1986). The court also cited Matter of Quinlan, 70 N.J. 10, 355 A.2d 647 (1976), *cert. denied*, 429 U.S. 922 (1976), *and* Superintendent of Belchertown State School v. Saikewicz, 373 Mass. 728, 370 N.E.2d 417 (1977), recognizing that an individual has the right to decide whether life is preferable to death under certain circumstances.

42. 98 Wash. 2d 460, 656 P.2d 483 (1983).

43. *Id.* at 483, 656 P.2d at 497. Other cases permitting a wrongful life action include Call v. Kezirian, 135 Cal. App. 3d 189, 185 Cal. Rptr. 103 (1982); Azzolino v. Dingfelder, 71 N.C. App. 289, 322 S.E.2d 567 (1984), *review granted*, 313 N.C. 327, 327 S.E.2d 887 (1985); Procanik v. Cillo, 97 N.J. 339, 478 A.2d 755 (1984). These cases followed *Turpin* in permitting special damages for extraordinary expenses but denying general damages.

44. Cal. Civil Code § 43.6(a) (1982): "No cause of action arises against a parent of a child based upon the claim that the child should not have been conceived or, if conceived, should not have been allowed to have been born alive."

45. Minn. Stat. Ann. § 145.424, subds. 1 & 2 (West Supp. 1986). In light of the constitutional right of reproductive freedom, this statute may not be constitutional.

46. Minn. Stat. Ann. § 145.424, subd. 3. The California statute has a similar provision, Cal. Civil Code § 43.6(b) (1982).

47. For background information on stem cells, *see* National Institutes of Health, *Stem Cell Basics* (modified March 31, 2015), at http://stemcells.nih.gov/info/basics1.htm.

48. *See* Doe v. Obama, 670 F. Supp. 2d 435, 437 (2009), *and* Sherley v. Sebelius, No. 11-5241 (D.C. Cir. 2012).

49. Missourians Against Cloning v. Carnahan, 190 S.W.3d 451 (Mo. App., 2006) and Cures Without Cloning v. Pund, 259 S.W.3d 76 (Mo. App., 2008).

50. For further information, *see* National Institutes of Health, *Stem Cell Information* (modified August 8, 2016), at http://stemcells.nih.gov.

51. Centers for Disease Control and Prevention, *What Is Assisted Reproductive Technology?* (updated November 14, 2014), at http://www.cdc.gov/art/whatis.html.

52. These and related statistics, including ART success rates, are updated periodically at the Centers for Disease Control and Prevention website, http://www.cdc.gov/art.

53. 109 N.J. 396, 537 A.2d 1227 (1988).

54. *Id.* at 435.

55. *Id.* at 437–38.

56. 704 S.W.2d 209 (Ky. 1986).

57. *Id.* at 211.

58. *Id.* at 213–14.

59. 842 S.W.2d 588 (Tenn. 1992).

60. *See, e.g.,* In re C.K.G., 173 S.W.3d 714 (Tenn. 2005) (child support for three children born via IVF with donor eggs and the man's sperm; the birth mother and genetic father were unmarried), *and* In re K.M.H., 169 P.3d 1025 (Kans. 2007) (parental rights and paternity dispute involving twins who were the product of artificial insemination of an unmarried woman with sperm from a male friend).

61. 42 U.S.C. §§ 654, 666.

62. *See* Roe v. Wade, 410 U.S. 113, notes 27–28 (1973).

63. Lord Ellenborough's Act, 42 Geo. 3, c. 58. Parliament reversed this position by enacting a liberal abortion bill in 1967.

64. This brief summary was adapted from the US Supreme Court's decision in *Roe v. Wade.* For the Supreme Court's full historical background, *see* 410 U.S. at 129–47.

65. Model Penal Code § 230.3(2) (1962).

66. 410 U.S. 113 (1973).

67. 410 U.S. 179 (1973).

68. Such a requirement is clearly constitutional; most abortions are, after all, surgical procedures. May v. State of Ark., 254 Ark. 194,

492 S.W.2d 888 (1973), *cert. denied*, 414 U.S. 1024 (1973). This decision was rendered after the *Roe* and *Bolton* cases. *See also* State v. Norflett, 67 N.J. 268, 337 A.2d 609 (1975).

69. Note that the court in *Roe* did not decide when life begins or when the fetus becomes a "person." Physicians, theologians, and philosophers have long debated these questions. Rhode Island legislation, enacted after the landmark Supreme Court cases, declared that life begins at conception and that accordingly abortion at any stage of pregnancy is criminal. This law was declared unconstitutional, even though the *Roe* case had sidestepped this particular question. Doe v. Israel, 358 F. Supp. 1193 (D.R.I. 1973), *cert. denied*, 416 U.S. 993 (1974). Hence, the constitutional right to have an abortion, as articulated by *Roe*, may not be avoided by a state statute expressing another philosophy or other grounds that attempt to circumvent individual rights. Further, the *Roe* and *Bolton* decisions have been held to apply retroactively. A criminal conviction of a physician under an abortion statute now declared unconstitutional must be vacated even if it preceded the Supreme Court decision. State v. Ingel, 18 Md. App. 514, 308 A.2d 223 (1973).

70. 410 U.S. 179, 199 (1973), *reh'g denied*, 410 U.S. 959 (1973).

71. Many took this statement to mean that states could require that second-trimester abortions be performed only in hospitals. However, such a requirement was later found unconstitutional. City of Akron v. Akron Center for Reproductive Health, Inc., 462 U.S. 416 (1983).

72. Planned Parenthood Ass'n of Kansas City, Mo., Inc. v. Ashcroft, 462 U.S. 476 (1983).

73. *See* Planned Parenthood of Central Mo. v. Danforth, 428 U.S. 52 (1976).

74. Simopoulos v. Virginia, 462 U.S. 506 (1983).

75. Planned Parenthood of Central Mo. v. Danforth, 428 U.S. 52 (1976).

76. Pa. Cons. Stat. Ann. §§ 3211(a), 3214(h) (Purdon 1983). The statute was ruled unconstitutional in Am. College of Obstetricians v. Thornburgh, 106 S. Ct. 2169, 2182 (1986). Physicians had to sign and file a report the following month identifying themselves and naming the hospital or clinic; the referring physician, agency, or service; the woman's place of residence, age, race, and marital status; the number of her prior pregnancies; the date of her last menstrual period; the probable gestational age of the unborn child; the "length and weight of the aborted unborn child"; the method of payment for the procedure; and the basis for "any medical judgment that a medical emergency existed" and for the physician's determination "that a child is not viable."

77. Each of the previous four points was decided in City of Akron v. Akron Center for Reproductive Health, Inc., 462 U.S. 416 (1983) at 456, 458 (O'Connor, J., dissenting).

78. Stenberg v. Carhart, 530 U.S. 914 (2000). The federal partial-birth abortion ban was upheld in Gonzales v. Carhart, 550 U.S. 124 (2007).

79. Colautti v. Franklin, 439 U.S. 379, 387 (1979) (quoting Roe v. Wade, 410 U.S. at 160, 166).

80. City of Akron v. Akron Center for Reproductive Health, Inc., *supra* note 77.

81. 462 U.S. 476 (1983).

82. Thornburgh v. Am. College of Obstetricians and Gynecologists, 476 U.S. 747, 106 S. Ct. 2169 (1986).

83. 492 U.S. 490 (1989).

84. *Id.* at 517–19.

85. 505 U.S. 833 (1992).

86. *Id.* at 936.

87. Stenberg v. Carhart, *supra* note 78.

88. 546 U.S. 320 (2006).

89. 550 U.S. 124 (2007).

90. Whole Woman's Health v. Hellerstedt, __U.S. __ (June 27, 2016).

91. *See, e.g.*, Hathaway v. Worcester City Hospital, 475 F.2d 701 (1st Cir. 1973), *appeal for stay of mandate denied*, 411 U.S. 929 (1973), reversing the federal district court, which had held that the patient possessed no constitutional right to have a sterilization performed in a city hospital. 341 F. Supp. 1385 (D. Mass. 1972). The decision of the court of appeals was rendered after the *Roe* and *Bolton* cases.

92. Taylor v. St. Vincent's Hosp., 369 F. Supp. 948 (D. Mont. 1973), *aff'd*, 523 F.2d 75 (9th Cir. 1975), *cert. denied*, 424 U.S. 948 (1976).

93. 479 F.2d 756 (7th Cir. 1973).

94. 361 F. Supp. 1212 (N.D. Tex. 1973), *appeal dismissed*, 490 F.2d 81 (5th Cir. 1974). Moreover, the district court's decision was rendered moot because the patient in fact obtained sterilization at another hospital.

95. 364 F. Supp. 799 (D. Idaho 1973), *aff'd*, 520 F.2d 894 (9th Cir. 1975).

96. Health Programs Extension Act, 42 U.S.C.A. § 300a-7 (1973). Where nothing in the record proves that a private hospital's policy of prohibiting abortions is based on institutional religious beliefs

or moral convictions, the Health Programs Extension Act does not apply. Moreover, a private hospital is engaged in "state action" when it has received Hill-Burton and other governmental funds. Doe v. Charleston Area Medical Center, 529 F.2d 638 (4th Cir. 1975).

97. *See also* Chrisman v. Sisters of St. Joseph of Peace, 506 F.2d 308 (9th Cir. 1974) (Health Programs Extension Act, 42 U.S.C.A. § 300a-7 is constitutional); Greco v. Orange Memorial Hosp., 374 F. Supp. 227 (E.D. Tex. 1974), *aff'd*, 513 F.2d 873 (5th Cir. 1975), *cert. denied*, 423 U.S. 1000 (1975) (a private hospital is not engaged in "state action," even though it receives a significant amount of governmental funds; thus, it may bar abortions). The denial of certiorari by the Supreme Court in effect permits conflicting decisions on state action to remain, without resolving the issue on constitutional merits.

98. Beal v. Ann Doe, 432 U.S. 438 (1977); moreover, the equal protection clause of the Fourteenth Amendment does not require a state participating in the Medicaid program to pay expenses of nontherapeutic abortions for indigent women even though it does pay expenses of childbirth. Maher v. Roe, 432 U.S. 464 (1977).

99. Harris v. McRae, 448 U.S. 297 (1980), *reh'g denied*, 448 U.S. 917 (1980). The court also held that the Hyde Amendment does not violate due process, equal protection under the Fifth Amendment, or the Establishment Clause of the First Amendment.

100. Judge Posner says of this quote from Justice Holmes: "[It] would be a poorly reasoned, a brutal, and . . . a vicious opinion even if Carrie Buck really had been an imbecile. [Nevertheless,] it is a first-class piece of rhetoric." RICHARD POSNER, LAW AND LITERATURE 273 (Harvard University Press 1998). For more commentary on this case, *see* Robert Burgdorf and Marcia Burgdorf, *The Wicked Witch Is Almost Dead: Buck v. Bell and the Sterilization of Handicapped Persons*, 50 TEMPLE L. Q. 995 (1977).

FRAUD LAWS AND CORPORATE COMPLIANCE 15

After reading this chapter, you will

- understand the basic federal laws relating to healthcare fraud and abuse and how the Affordable Care Act has affected them,
- be able to identify the most significant statutes relating to fraud and abuse in federal healthcare payment programs,
- know how the concepts of kickback and self-referral affect hospital operations, and
- recognize the benefits of maintaining an active corporate integrity program.

Healthcare is a multitrillion-dollar field and thus a prime target for malefactors who want to defraud insurance companies and the government. This chapter discusses the laws aimed at curbing healthcare fraud, the enforcement and application of those laws, and how the Affordable Care Act of 2010 (ACA) changed the law enforcement climate.

In addition, the chapter explores the Foreign Corrupt Practices Act (FCPA), a statute first enacted in 1977 but which has become more prominent in healthcare compliance circles recently because of medical tourism and international commerce. The FCPA, according to the Department of Justice, "was enacted for the purpose of making it unlawful for certain classes of persons and entities to make payments to foreign government officials to assist in obtaining or retaining business."[1] Today, the act also applies to foreign companies and individuals doing business in the United States.

The role that corporate integrity programs play in promoting legal compliance and business ethics in a well-run healthcare organization is also discussed in this chapter. Upright organizations must be sensitive to the potential for their employees to be involved in fraud, abuse, and other illicit conduct. They must work to maintain high ethical principles not only because an image of moral respectability is good for business but also because such conduct is simply the right thing to do.

The Enforcement Climate

In general, the factors contributing to the rising costs of healthcare include the following:

- Research and development for new drugs and technology
- Administrative cost of myriad insurance plans
- Increased demand for treatment of chronic diseases
- Aging population

The Centers for Medicare & Medicaid Services (CMS) maintains official estimates of total healthcare spending in the United States back to 1960. These data reflect "annual US expenditures for health care goods and services, public health activities, program administration, the net cost of private insurance, and research and other investment related to health care."[2] In 2014 (the latest year for which data were available at time of writing), total US healthcare spending reached $3.0 trillion, which translates to more than $9,500 per person and 17.5 percent of the nation's gross domestic product (see exhibits 15.1 and 15.2).

EXHIBIT 15.1
The Nation's Health Dollar ($3.0 Trillion), Calendar Year 2014: Where It Came From

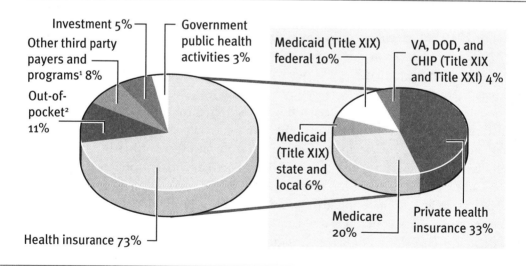

[1] Includes worksite health care, other private revenues, Indian Health Service, workers' compensation, general assistance, maternal and child health, vocational rehabilitation, Substance Abuse and Mental Health Services Administration, school health, and other federal and state local programs.

[2] Includes copayments, deductibles, and any amounts not covered by health insurance.

Note: Sum of pieces may not equal 100% due to rounding.

Source: Centers for Medicare & Medicaid Services, Office of the Actuary, National Health Statistics Group.

EXHIBIT 15.2

The Nation's Health Dollar ($3.0 Trillion), Calendar Year 2014: Where It Went

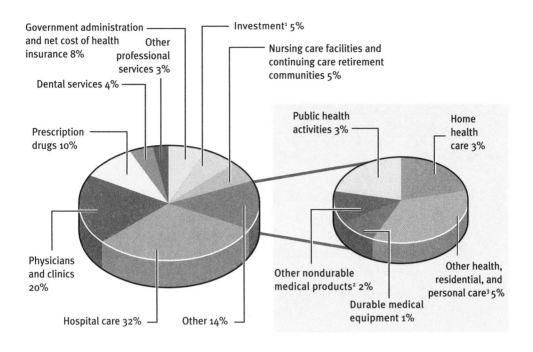

¹ Includes Research (2%) and Structure and Equipment (4%).

² Includes expenditures for residential care facilities, ambulance providers, medical care delivered in nontraditional settings (such as community centers, senior citizen centers, schools, and military field stations), and expenditures for Home and Community Waiver programs under Medicaid.

Note: Sum of pieces may not equal 100% due to rounding.

Source: Centers for Medicare & Medicaid Services, Office of the Actuary, National Health Statistics Group.

Total national health expenditures are expected to continue to rise slightly faster than GDP and to reach about 19.6 percent by 2024, at which time federal, state, and local governments are projected to finance 47 percent of national health spending. These increases will reflect the net result of population aging, a generally improving economy, and the results of the ACA's reduction in the number of uninsured individuals. Although this health spending growth is faster than in the recent past, it is still slower than the growth rate experienced over the three decades preceding the Great Recession.[3]

Because the government is such a large purchaser of healthcare services, it is an obvious target for fraud. Thus, elimination of fraud and waste in these programs is a high priority for law enforcement and policymakers.[4] Each year, more resources are allocated to the Department of Justice (DOJ), the Federal Bureau of Investigation, the Offices of the United States Attorneys, the Department of Health and Human Services (HHS) Office of

Inspector General, and other enforcement agencies. State attorneys general conduct their own investigations and prosecutions, often working closely with federal officials. Private individuals who have firsthand knowledge of fraud are permitted to sue on behalf of the government and to collect a percentage of any proceeds recovered.

The ACA places even more emphasis on fraud prevention. It contains numerous provisions aimed at enhancing the integrity of government programs, including a title of more than 100 legislative pages under the heading "Transparency and Program Integrity." The impact of this legislation is considered in the ensuing discussion. The most significant changes affect the False Claims Act, the antikickback statute, and the Stark physician self-referral law.

Verdicts and settlements in civil fraud cases can amount to tens or even hundreds of millions of dollars (see exhibit 15.3), and offenders convicted of criminal offenses can receive massive fines and lengthy jail terms.

In *United States v. Lorenzo*, for example, a dentist billed Medicare for "consultations" on nursing home residents. Medicare does not cover dental services, and Dr. Lorenzo's examinations, according to the court, "were nothing more than the oral cancer screening that previously had been done as part of a routine dental examination. None of these examinations had been conducted at the request of an attending physician or because of a specifically identified medical concern."[5] The government proved that Dr. Lorenzo had submitted 3,683 false claims and, as a result, had received overpayments totaling $130,719.20. The court assessed damages of approximately $19 million, nearly 150 times the amount of the fraud.

A second example involved Dr. Krizek, a psychiatrist trained at the Charles University in Prague (former Czechoslovakia) and Beth Israel

	Defendant's Name	Allegation	Settlement
EXHIBIT 15.3 Top Five Healthcare Fraud Settlements of 2014	DaVita Healthcare Partner	Kickbacks	$400 million
	Endo Health Solutions and Endo Pharmaceuticals	Marketed drug for off-label uses	$192.7 million
	Amedisys	False billing	$150 million
	Omnicare	Kickbacks; false claims	$124.2 million
	GlaxoSmithKline	Inaccurate advertising	$105.0 million

Source: Data from *Largest Healthcare Fraud Settlements from 2014*, MODERN HEALTHCARE, MAY 9, 2015, 34.

Hospital in New York City. Dr. Krizek had been practicing in Washington, DC, for 21 years when the government brought a false claims case against him. According to the court, Dr. Krizek was a "capable and competent physician," many of whose patients suffered from "horribly severe psychiatric disorders and often suffered simultaneously from other serious medical conditions."[6] The prosecution could not prove that Dr. Krizek rendered inappropriate care, but numerous false claims allegations were his downfall.

The evidence showed that the doctor charged the government for a full face-to-face session—45 to 50 minutes—regardless of whether he spent 20 minutes or two hours with a patient. He argued that even if he spent only half an hour with the patient in person, he considered related services—such as medication management and discussions with other staff—to be part of patient care and therefore thought he had not harmed the government. One piece of evidence showed that his practice submitted 23 claims for full sessions in a single day, so the court was impressed with neither Dr. Krizek's argument nor his management skills: "While Dr. Krizek was a dedicated and competent doctor . . . his billing practices, or at a minimum his oversight of [the] billing system, was seriously deficient. Dr. Krizek knew little or nothing of the details of how the bills were submitted [on his behalf]."[7] The court concluded that

> Dr. Krizek must be held accountable for his billing system along with those who carried it out. . . . The Court . . . will hold the defendants liable under the False Claims Act on those days where claims were submitted in excess of the equivalent of twelve . . . claims (nine patient-treatment hours) in a single day and where the defendants cannot establish that Dr. Krizek legitimately devoted the claimed amount of time to patient care on the day in question.[8]

Among the many interesting aspects of the various *Krizek* court opinions (four in all), perhaps the most noteworthy is the trial court's displeasure with how the government handled the case. After more than four years of litigation, the judge slammed the door in 1998 with this parting shot:

> The Government insists on pursuing a case that should long have been over. If the Court acceded to all of the Government's requests, this litigation would proceed well into the next century. The Government has won its case and gained a substantial recovery. Dr. Krizek is now retired and is no longer practicing psychiatry. Although apparently a fine physician, he is now a broken man. Not only is he out of the medical profession, but also he is suffering from the advanced stages of cancer. The Government refuses to let go of this case. When it began its case, the Government was seeking over $80 million worth of damages, a figure that the Court of Appeals declared was "astronomical." Despite the fact that Dr. Krizek is

incapable of paying such a sum, the Government continues to relentlessly pursue Dr. Krizek, who is at this point a broken and sick man. The Government's pursuit of Dr. Krizek is reminiscent of Inspector Javert's quest to capture Jean Valjean in Victor Hugo's *Les Miserables*. While the Government's vigor in pursuing violators of the law is to be commended, there comes a point when a civilized society must say enough is enough. That point has been reached in this case.[9]

Notwithstanding the overly zealous prosecution of Dr. Krizek, his and other cases demonstrate the seriousness with which the government views fraud and abuse. Under the joint direction of the attorney general and the secretary of HHS, the federal Health Care Fraud and Abuse Control Program recovers more than $8 for every $1 spent on its investigations and returns more than $4 billion dollars to the US Treasury every year.[10]

As these statistics show, prevention of fraud and abuse should be a top priority for healthcare administration, and a basic understanding of the major criminal and civil fraud statutes is therefore essential. The following are some of the most obvious types of healthcare fraud and abuse:

- Filing claims for services not rendered or not medically necessary
- Misrepresenting the time, location, frequency, duration, or provider of services
- Assigning a higher payment than the procedure or diagnosis warrants (upcoding)
- Billing a battery of services (e.g., laboratory tests) separately (unbundling)
- Violating the "three-day rule," which states that outpatient diagnostic procedures performed on any of the three days before hospitalization are deemed part of the Medicare diagnosis-related group payment and are not to be billed separately
- Paying kickbacks to induce referrals or the purchase of goods or services
- Billing for services said to have been "incident to" a physician's services but that were not provided under the physician's direct supervision
- Referring patients to entities in which the physician has a financial interest (self-referral)

The major statutes that these kinds of activities may violate include the civil and criminal False Claims Act, the antikickback law, and the physician self-referral statute (known as the Stark law). Depending on the facts of the case, other statutes that may be implicated include mail fraud and wire fraud statutes; the Racketeer Influenced and Corrupt Organizations Act; money-laundering statutes; the FCPA; and various criminal statutes relating to theft, embezzlement, bribery, conspiracy, and obstruction of justice. Whereas this chapter focuses on the major healthcare fraud statutes and does not address violations of the other laws mentioned, myriad legal standards (both state and federal) apply to healthcare organizations, and the importance of competent legal counsel and a process for preventing criminal activity cannot be overemphasized.

False Claims Act

The federal government's main weapon in the so-called war on fraud and abuse is the False Claims Act (FCA), which provides that a person is liable for penalties if he

- "knowingly presents, or causes to be presented, to an officer or employee of the United States . . . a false or fraudulent claim for payment or approval";
- "knowingly makes, uses, or causes to be made or used, a false record or statement to get a false or fraudulent claim paid or approved by the Government";
- "conspires to defraud the Government by getting a false or fraudulent claim allowed or paid"; or
- "knowingly makes, uses, or causes to be made or used, a false record or statement to conceal, avoid, or decrease an obligation to pay or transmit money or property to the government." (This provision was added in 1986 to deal with *reverse false claims*—attempts to avoid paying money owed to the government.)[11]

Most states have similar laws. Penalties for the civil type of FCA violations can be as much as $11,000 per claim plus three times the amount of damages sustained by the government. In addition, the costs of the prosecution are charged to the defendant. If the claim is found to be false, penalties and costs may be assessed even if the claim was not paid and the government suffered no damages.[12]

Interestingly, the FCA was enacted during the Civil War to stem the practice of overcharging the Union Army for goods and services. Apparently the term *claim* was better understood then than it is now because it is not defined in the statute. In healthcare, the definition of claim has been a matter of some dispute. For example, each procedure code on a billing form could be considered a separate claim. Therefore, up to $11,000 in penalties could be assessed for each false code. By this line of reasoning, more than $200,000 plus damages and court costs could be assessed for 20 false codes. The definition of claim was addressed in the appeal of *Krizek*, in which the court of appeals held that each billing form was one claim, irrespective of the number of false codes it contained. The court asserted that the form was merely one request for payment of the total sum it represented.[13] This definition seems logical and is consistent with other cases defining a claim as "a demand for money or for some transfer of public property."[14]

scienter
knowledge by a defendant that his acts were illegal or his statements were fraudulent

Another interesting question is that of **scienter**: Did the defendant deliberately and willfully break the law? Or, in the words of the FCA, did the defendant do so "knowingly"? First-year law students are painfully aware of the question-and-answer exchange that could attend the definition of *knowingly*. The following dialogue is an example:

PROFESSOR KINGSFIELD. Mr. Showalter, what if I sign a claim form, put it in a stamped envelope, and mail it to Medicare? Have I knowingly submitted that claim?

STUDENT SHOWALTER. I guess so. Unless you were drunk or mentally incompetent, you knew what you were doing. You were mailing a claim form and expecting to get paid.

KINGSFIELD. How much did I expect to get paid?

SHOWALTER. Whatever amount is on the form.

KINGSFIELD. What if I didn't look at the amount but just signed a bunch of forms my staff gave me at the end of the day and those forms had errors on them?

SHOWALTER. Well . . .

KINGSFIELD. Well, what? Are the forms that have errors on them false claims?

SHOWALTER. Well, they're erroneous. But if you didn't know they had errors and just assumed that your staff were doing their jobs correctly . . .

KINGSFIELD. Assumed? Never assume anything in this class or in any legal matter!

SHOWALTER. Sorry.

KINGSFIELD. Let's consider another case. Suppose that I know my claims contain the occasional error—some are over, some are under—but I think they will all balance out in the end, sort of the "no harm, no foul" approach to billing. And suppose I think that the False Claims Act applies only to overbilling the government on purpose, which I haven't done. What say you now?

SHOWALTER. Hmm. You knew you were submitting a bill, but you didn't know that the particular bill was wrong, and you didn't know that submitting incorrect bills is illegal when you should have had a system in place to check them for errors. Good question!

So goes this Socratic dialogue for a few more uncomfortable minutes. In 1986, Congress addressed the issue of scienter by amending the FCA to say that "no proof of specific intent to defraud" is required. Instead, the person must either (1) have actual knowledge that the information is false, (2) act in deliberate ignorance of the truth or falsity of the information, or (3) act with reckless disregard of whether it is true or false.[15] As stated in the committee report accompanying the 1986 amendments,

> the Committee is firm in its intentions that the act not punish honest mistakes or incorrect claims submitted through mere negligence. But the Committee does believe the civil False Claims Act should recognize that those doing business with the Government have an obligation to make a limited inquiry to ensure the claims they submit are accurate.[16]

The *Krizek* case (discussed earlier) shows how this standard is used. Although Dr. Krizek was not personally involved in the billing process, the court found that he and the other defendants had submitted the claims knowingly: "These were not 'mistakes' [or] merely negligent conduct. Under the statutory definition of 'knowing' conduct, the court is compelled to conclude that the defendants acted with *reckless disregard as to the truth or falsity of the submissions*" [italics added].[17]

This standard requires healthcare providers—and their top management and governing board members—to have mechanisms in place to verify the accuracy of their organization's claims. A further incentive to comply is the threat of exclusion from participation in Medicare and Medicaid: The government may exclude from participation any individual who (1) has a direct or indirect ownership or control interest in a sanctioned entity and has acted in "deliberate ignorance" of the information or (2) is an officer or a managing employee of a convicted or excluded entity, irrespective of whether the individual participated in the offense.[18] Any excluded person who retains ownership or control or who continues to serve as an officer or a managing employee in such entity may be fined $10,000 per day.[19] This threat and the potential for criminal convictions and massive fines have been the major forces motivating healthcare organizations to adopt corporate compliance programs (discussed later in this chapter).

FCA cases are usually investigated by the Office of Inspector General and brought by a US attorney or the DOJ. An unusual feature of the statute, however, allows private citizens to sue on their own behalf and, as stated earlier, on behalf of the government to recover damages and penalties. These *qui tam* (whistle-blower) lawsuits have become an important factor in FCA enforcement because, if successful, the plaintiff (a *relator* in legal parlance) can share in the amount of the award (see exhibit 15.3 on p. 550 and Legal Brief on p. 556).

Any person with information about healthcare fraud can be a qui tam plaintiff (relator). *Person* is defined as "any natural person, partnership, corporation, association, or other legal entity, including any State or political subdivision of a State."[20] The relator must file the complaint, which is

Legal Brief

Qui tam is shorthand for a Latin phrase that means "he who sues for the king as well as for himself." In such a case, the relator files suit as a kind of private attorney general on behalf of the government. The government can choose to take over the prosecution, but if it declines to do so the relator can proceed alone.

Qui tam cases are cited as *United States ex rel.* [name] *v.* [name of defendant]. *Ex rel.* means "by the relation of" (or, more loosely, "at the request of") and indicates the name of the relator.

immediately sealed and thus not made public pending an investigation, and file a copy with the US attorney general and the appropriate US attorney. The government then has 60 days, plus extensions for good cause, to determine whether to pursue the case. If the government decides to take over the case, the relator will receive 15–25 percent of the amount recovered. If the government declines, the relator may still pursue the matter and, if successful, will receive up to 30 percent of the recovery.

To file suit, the potential qui tam plaintiff and the allegations must meet certain conditions. Substantially, the same allegations or transactions must not have been disclosed publicly at an earlier date—unless the qui tam plaintiff is the original source of the previously disclosed information. *Original source* means someone who gave the government the information in the first place or who has information additional to that previously disclosed.[21] If the jurisdictional barriers are met and the facts of the case warrant recovery, the qui tam plaintiff can proceed to assist the government or pursue the case individually, often to significant financial advantage.

Federal law provides a remedy for whistle-blowers who are discharged, demoted, harassed, or otherwise discriminated against because they filed a qui tam case.[22] Given the financial incentives and the protection against employment-related retaliation, the qui tam lawsuit has become a popular and effective means of combating fraud and abuse.

Occasionally, qui tam plaintiffs in healthcare cases argue that a claim involving a kickback or an illegal physician self-referral (described in more detail in the following sections) violates the FCA, even though the claim is otherwise legitimate.[23] For example, in *United States ex rel. Woodard v. Country View Care Center, Inc.*,[24] the defendants had submitted Medicare cost reports that included among their expenses some payments to "consultants" that were actually kickbacks for referrals. Because the defendants' reimbursement was based on the cost reports, the court held that the FCA applied. *United States v. Kensington Hospital*,[25] filed after the advent of the prospective payment system, brought a new twist to the argument. The defendants asserted that because their Medicaid reimbursement was a set amount, the government could not have suffered a loss and the cost of the kickbacks did not make the claims false. Citing *United States ex rel. Marcus v. Hess* and other cases, the court disagreed, holding that the government was not required to show actual damages to prove an FCA violation.

In neither *Country View* nor *Kensington Hospital* did the plaintiffs specifically base their claim of FCA liability on the antikickback or self-referral statutes. Some subsequent cases did so, however, and they have survived scrutiny by the courts. For example, in *United States ex rel. Pogue v. American Healthcorp*,[26] a trial court refused to dismiss an FCA case based on violations of the antikickback and the Stark self-referral laws. The court agreed with the relator's contention that "participation in any federal program involves an *implied certification* [emphasis added] that the participant will abide by and adhere to all statutes, rules, and regulations governing that program."[27] It held, in effect, that Stark violations create prohibited financial relationships that taint the Medicare claims and that the FCA therefore applies.

In 2016, the US Supreme Court held the implied certification rationale to be valid in certain circumstances, and the theory has been followed in some cases and questioned in others.[28] Thus, though the concept that an FCA case can be based on violation of the antikickback or self-referral laws appears to be consistent with the 1986 amendments, it remains to be seen in what fact situations it will be applied.

In addition, the ACA codifies the implied certification rationale, at least insofar as the antikickback statute is concerned. The ACA states that "a claim that includes items or services resulting from a violation of the [antikickback statute] constitutes a false or fraudulent claim for purposes of [the civil False Claims Act]."[29] Thus, compliance with the antikickback statute is a precondition for payment, and non-compliance with the antikickback statute will support an FCA claim. The Medicare claim form adds weight to this position (see Legal Brief).

A separate provision of federal law makes filing false claims a criminal offense.[30] If convicted, an organization may be fined $500,000 or twice the amount of the false claim, whichever is greater. An individual may be fined the greater of $250,000 or twice the amount of the false claim and may be sentenced to up to five years in prison. Of course the standards of proof are higher in criminal prosecutions than in civil cases. In a civil FCA action, the

> **Legal Brief**
>
> When the government wants to make regulatory compliance a precondition for payment, it clearly knows how to do so. The Medicare claim form (CMS-1500) states in boldface: **"Any person who knowingly files a statement of claim containing any misrepresentation or any false, incomplete or misleading information may be guilty of a criminal act punishable under law and may be subject to civil penalties."**
>
> It also includes the following language:
>
> NOTICE: This is to certify that the foregoing information is true, accurate and complete. I understand that payment and satisfaction of this claim will be from Federal and State funds, and that any false claims, statements, or documents, or concealment of a material fact, may be prosecuted under applicable Federal or State laws.
>
> This notice appears to turn what would otherwise be an implied certification into an express condition for payment.

standard is merely "a preponderance of the evidence"—in other words, it is more likely than not that the defendant did what is alleged. In criminal FCA cases, the government must prove beyond a reasonable doubt that the defendant knew the claim was false. For this reason, and because the penalties in civil actions are already severe, fewer criminal false claims cases are brought than civil cases.

Antikickback Statute

Federal law that has come to be known as the "antikickback statute" (AKS) imposes severe criminal penalties for fraudulent acts involving federal healthcare programs. Except for certain state plans and the health plan of federal employees, both of which are dealt with separately, the AKS applies to "any plan or program that provides health benefits, whether directly, through insurance, or otherwise, which is funded directly, in whole or in part, by the United States Government."[31]

The law prohibits making false statements to receive reimbursement for claims and sets the standard of care as follows:

> (1) Whoever knowingly and willfully solicits or receives any remuneration (including any kickback, bribe, or rebate) directly or indirectly, overtly or covertly, in cash or in kind—
>> (A) in return for referring an individual to a person for the furnishing or arranging for the furnishing of any item or service for which payment may be made in whole or in part under a Federal health care program, or
>> (B) in return for purchasing, leasing, ordering, or arranging for or recommending purchasing, leasing, or ordering any good, facility, service, or item for which payment may be made in whole or in part under a Federal health care program,
>
> shall be guilty of a felony and upon conviction thereof, shall be fined not more than $25,000 or imprisoned for not more than five years, or both.
>
> (2) Whoever knowingly and willfully offers or pays any remuneration (including any kickback, bribe, or rebate) directly or indirectly, overtly or covertly, in cash or in kind to any person to induce such person—
>> (A) to refer an individual to a person for the furnishing or arranging for the furnishing of any item or service for which payment may be made in whole or in part under a Federal health care program, or
>> (B) to purchase, lease, order, or arrange for or recommend purchasing, leasing, or ordering any good, facility, service, or item for which payment may be made in whole or in part under a Federal health care program,
>
> shall be guilty of a felony and upon conviction thereof, shall be fined not more than $25,000 or imprisoned for not more than five years, or both.[32]

Thus, both sides of such a transaction—the one who offers or provides the remuneration and the one who solicits or receives it—are potentially liable for kickback violations. In addition to fines and prison time, offenders may be excluded from participation in the Medicare and Medicaid programs[33] and may be assessed civil money penalties of up to $50,000 per violation plus three times the amount of the remuneration involved.[34]

Certain types of remuneration are exempt from the statute, such as the following:

- Discounts reflected in Medicare cost reports
- Amounts paid by an employer to an employee to provide healthcare services
- Certain amounts paid by a vendor to agents of a group purchasing entity
- Waivers of coinsurance for Public Health Service beneficiaries
- Certain remuneration through risk-sharing arrangements (e.g., under capitation)[35]

Pursuant to authority granted to the secretary of HHS, detailed regulations provide for the following *safe harbors*—categories of activities in which providers may lawfully engage:

- Fair market value leases for rental of space or equipment
- Commercially reasonable personal services (e.g., consulting, peer review) and management contracts
- Purchase of physician practices by hospitals
- Payments to referral services for patients, so long as the payment is not related to the number of referrals made
- Properly disclosed warranties
- Properly disclosed discounts contemporaneous with the original sale
- Bona fide employment relationships
- Discounts available to members of a group purchasing organization
- Waivers of coinsurance and deductibles for indigent persons
- Marketing incentives offered by health plans to enrollees
- Price reductions offered by providers to health plans

The point of these exceptions and safe harbors is to decriminalize legitimate activities that might otherwise seem to induce referrals or purchases. For example, the very purpose of a manufacturer's warranty is to induce purchase of the product. If that product is a medical device that will be paid for by "a federal health care program," it would seem to offend the literal language of the AKS; a safe harbor for legitimate warranties is thus eminently reasonable.

These regulations are quite technical, and an in-depth analysis of their provisions is beyond the scope of this chapter. Suffice to say that although the AKS is one of the most important laws affecting healthcare today, it is also one of the most complicated and ambiguous. Congress recognized the statute's complexity when it wrote in 1987 that "the breadth of the statutory language has created uncertainty among health care providers as to which commercial arrangements are legitimate, and which are proscribed."[36] Although the 1987 amendments specifying safe harbors were intended to provide guidance and clarity, much uncertainty remains.

What Is a "Referral"?

One point of uncertainty in the AKS is the meaning of *referral*, one of the law's key terms. For example, when one member of a multispecialty group practice sends a patient to another member of the same group, has she made a referral? If the referring physician's compensation depends in part on the volume of services she orders from other group members, a literal reading of the statute would call the practice into question. A group practice safe harbor under the Stark self-referral law (discussed in the next section) seems to suggest that regulators believe a referral has been made in those circumstances. If such action is not a referral, why have a safe harbor for it? Because intragroup referrals are not Stark violations, the government is unlikely to take enforcement action under the AKS for such referrals, but the uncertainty remains.

Ownership of a hospital by a medical group presents a similar situation. Under traditional indemnity insurance plans, the physicians benefit financially if they admit patients to their own hospital, yet distribution of the hospital's profits to the physician owners appears to violate the statute. A proposed regulatory safe harbor for such situations was abandoned in 1993. The ACA bars physician groups from opening new hospitals after December 31, 2010, and prevents expansion of existing ones except under limited circumstances.[37]

What Is "Remuneration"?

Another uncertainty lies in the meaning of *remuneration*. The AKS merely hints at a definition. The passage quoted earlier indicates that remuneration includes kickbacks, bribes, and rebates. A later paragraph states that remuneration "includes the waiver of coinsurance and deductible amounts . . . and transfers of items or services for free or for other than fair market value."[38] The same section (as amended by the ACA) then lists a number of arrangements that are *not* considered remuneration:

- The statutory exceptions described earlier
- Certain waivers and differentials of coinsurance and deductibles
- Incentives for preventive care

- Retailers' coupons available to the general public
- Certain items or services provided to persons in financial need
- Waivers of first copayments under a Medicare prescription drug plan
- "Other remuneration which promotes access to care and poses a low risk of harm to patients"

Lacking a precise definition from which to work, the courts are left to divine the AKS's import and apply this indistinct concept to real-life situations. *Hanlester Network v. Shalala* provides an example.[39]

In *Hanlester*, certain physicians were limited partners in a network of clinical laboratories to which they referred their patients. The network contracted with Smith Kline Bio-Science Laboratories (SKBL) to manage the laboratory facilities for a fee of $15,000 per month or 80 percent of the laboratories' collections, whichever was greater. (The 80 percent figure was usually higher than the fixed monthly fee.) Because performing the tests at SKBL's own laboratories was more economical, 85 to 90 percent of the Hanlester labs' testing was done at the main SKBL lab rather than at the network's satellite facilities (see Legal Decision Point).

The Ninth Circuit held that even though the cash payments under the arrangement flowed from the Hanlester Network labs to SKBL, the arrangement was a scheme by which SKBL offered a 20 percent discount—the prohibited kickback/remuneration—for the physicians' referrals. In other words, but for the

Legal Decision Point

Before reading further, refer to exhibit 15.4 and try to determine where the kickbacks and referrals are located in the *Hanlester* scenario.

EXHIBIT 15.4
Hanlester Network Structure

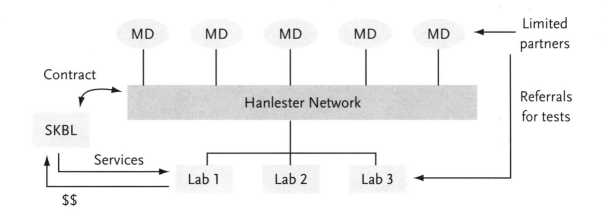

existence of the Hanlester Network, SKBL would have received 100 percent of the lab fees and the physicians would not have earned their 20 percent share. (Today, the arrangement would also violate the physician self-referral law, discussed later in this chapter.)

Although the AKS and regulations do not define *remuneration*, the law clearly applies to the provision of anything that has a value. The 20 percent "discount" in *Hanlester* is one example. Likewise, the provision of free goods or services has an economic value and is prohibited.[40] Remuneration of minimal amounts is not an exception; in one case, a physician was excluded from the Medicare program for receiving a kickback of $30.[41]

Consider provision (1)(B) of the AKS quoted earlier. The AKS prohibits payments "in return for purchasing, leasing, ordering, or arranging for or recommending purchasing, leasing, or ordering any good, facility, service, or item for which payment is made in whole or in part by a Federal healthcare program."[42] For example, a company that provides patient transportation would clearly be acting illegally if it bribed a hospital employee to choose the company's services. The cases are seldom that obvious, however. For example, the question might arise whether a hospital or clinic violates the AKS if it provides free transportation for patients as an encouragement for them to select the provider.

That was the situation in *United States v. Recovery Management Corp. III*. A psychiatric hospital pleaded guilty to an antikickback violation after it gave patients free airfares to induce them to choose the facility.[43] Thus we learn that the AKS applies even in the absence of a literal referral—the "referral" in this case being the patient's own choice of the facility.

The AKS also applies to the provision of anything of value that induces patients or providers to purchase or order services. Waiver of coinsurance and deductibles is such an inducement and is prohibited, except in limited circumstances (such as in documented cases of financial need). Civil money penalties can be assessed against any person who

> offers to or transfers remuneration to any individual eligible for benefits under [Medicare] or a State health care program . . . that such person knows or should know is likely to influence such individual to order or to receive [goods or services] from a particular provider, practitioner or supplier.[44]

Thus, routine waiver of coinsurance and deductibles (especially if advertised in the hope of stimulating business) is considered a violation of the AKS.

mens rea
the mental element of a crime; one's awareness that one's conduct is criminal

A Question of Intent

What kind of **mens rea**—guilty mind—must a defendant have to violate the AKS? This question is another classic, first-year law school issue and is closely related to the concept of *scienter*, discussed earlier. The *Hanlester* court answered the question this way: "We construe 'knowingly and willfully'. . . of the anti-kickback statute as requiring appellants to (1) know that Sec. 1128B prohibits offering or paying remuneration to induce referrals, and (2) engage in prohibited conduct with the specific intent to disobey the law."[45]

Three years after *Hanletser*, the Supreme Court decided *Bryan v. United States*, in which it stated:

> The word "willfully" is sometimes said to be "a word of many meanings" whose construction is often dependent on the context in which it appears. Most obviously it differentiates between deliberate and unwitting conduct, but in the criminal law it also typically refers to a culpable state of mind. As we explained [in a 1933 case], a variety of phrases have been used to describe that concept. As a general matter, when used in the criminal context, a "willful" act is one undertaken with a "bad purpose." In other words, in order to establish a "willful" violation of a statute, "the Government must prove that the defendant acted with knowledge that his conduct was unlawful."[46]

The *Bryan* decision quotes favorably the following statement from a standard jury instruction:

> A person acts willfully if he acts intentionally and purposely and with the intent to do something the law forbids, that is, with the bad purpose to disobey or to disregard the law. Now, the person need not be aware of the specific law or rule that his conduct may be violating. But he must act with the intent to do something that the law forbids.[47]

Following *Bryan*, the Eleventh Circuit decided *United States v. Starks*. Mindful of the preceding language from the Supreme Court, the *Starks* court phrased the willfulness standard as follows: "The word willfully . . . means the act was committed voluntarily and purposely, with the specific intent to do something the law forbids, that is with a bad purpose, either to disobey or disregard the law."[48] It reminded the parties that ignorance of the law is no excuse and stated that the AKS is no exception:

malum in se
an act that is evil in itself because it violates basic moral principles of society (e.g., murder, rape, burglary)

> [The AKS] is not a highly technical tax or financial regulation that poses a danger of ensnaring persons engaged in apparently innocent conduct. Indeed, the giving or taking of kickbacks for medical referrals *is hardly the sort of activity a person might expect to be legal*; compared to the licensing provisions that the *Bryan* Court considered, such kickbacks are more clearly **malum in se**, rather than **malum prohibitum**.[49] [Emphasis added.]

malum prohibitum
an act that is not inherently wrong but is illegal because it is prohibited by statute (e.g., tax avoidance or violation of traffic laws)

As this discussion shows, "criminal intent" is difficult to define precisely; its meaning depends on the statute and circumstances involved. Congress tried to clarify the concept in a provision of the ACA, which states that "no proof of specific intent to defraud is required" to violate the AKS. Therefore, willfulness under the AKS is established by showing that the defendant (1) consciously committed an illegal act (offered/paid or solicited/received remuneration) and (2) had a nefarious purpose in mind (medical referrals or purchases) even if he was unaware of the exact law he was violating.

The issue of intent raises another question: Assuming remuneration has been solicited or received, must its *sole* purpose be to induce referrals or purchases? Or is it sufficient for the government to show that such an inducement was one of multiple reasons for offering the remuneration?

These questions were at the heart of *United States v. Greber* and *United States v. McClatchey* (see the first two The Court Decides features at the end of this chapter). In both cases, payments made for legitimate purposes also appeared to have been intended to induce referrals. In both cases, the court held that even if the remuneration was given for legitimate reasons, the statute was violated if another purpose was to induce referrals.

Stark Self-Referral Law

The Ethics in Patient Referrals Act[50] was championed by former California Representative Fortney "Pete" Stark. The act's purpose, like that of the AKS, was to remove conflicts of interest from physician decision making and to discourage overuse of healthcare services. In summary, the law and its regulations prohibit physicians (i.e., those with MD, DO, DDS, DPM, OD, or DC degrees) from referring Medicare patients for *designated health services* to entities with which the physician or an immediate family member has a financial relationship, unless an exception applies. The statute also prohibits the entity to which the referral was made from billing for the requested services. The Stark law is a strict liability statute for the physician, which means that if a prohibited referral was made, liability is automatic regardless of whether the physician intended to break the law (see Legal Brief).

Financial relationship means a compensation arrangement or an ownership or investment interest. Unless an exception applies (see list of exceptions on p. 568), if a physician or an immediate family member has a financial relationship with an entity, the physician may not refer patients to the entity for any of the following "designated health services":

- Clinical laboratory services
- Physical, occupational, and speech therapy

Legal Brief

The Stark law applies only to physician referrals. Intent is irrelevant; thus, violations are automatic if the physician has a financial interest in the entity to which she is referring patients.

The relevant regulations can be found at 42 C.F.R. §§ 411.350 et seq.

- Radiology and certain other imaging services (e.g., MRIs, CT scans, ultrasound)
- Radiation therapy services and supplies
- Durable medical equipment and supplies
- Parenteral and enteral nutrients, equipment, and supplies
- Prosthetics, orthotics, and prosthetic devices and supplies
- Home health services
- Outpatient prescription drugs
- Inpatient and outpatient hospital services
- Outpatient speech-language pathology services

With regard to the penultimate item on that list, physicians originally were permitted to refer to hospitals in which they had an ownership interest (so-called doctors' hospitals) if that ownership interest was "in the hospital itself (and not merely in a subdivision of the hospital)."[51] This exception to the Stark law was eliminated by the ACA, which "grandfathered" physician-owned hospitals that existed on December 31, 2010, but prevented their further expansion; it also barred physicians from opening new doctors' hospitals after that date.

The penalties for Stark violations are severe. They include denial of payment for the services, an obligation to refund any payments made, civil money penalties of up to $15,000 for each illegal referral, and exclusion from the Medicare and Medicaid programs. In addition, a physician or an entity that enters into a scheme to bypass the Stark law may be fined up to $100,000 for each such arrangement and excluded from the programs.

Tuomey and Halifax

The draconian nature of the law is exemplified by two well-publicized recent cases. The first involved Tuomey Healthcare System, a nonprofit hospital located in a small, rural community in South Carolina. When many of its physicians began performing outpatient surgery in their offices, Tuomey sought to prevent the loss of hospital revenue by offering them part-time employment contracts. The contracts guaranteed an annual salary plus "productivity bonuses" based in part on the "facility fees" that the hospital billed when the physicians performed procedures in the hospital. The more procedures performed at the hospital, the more facility fees Tuomey was able to bill for, and the more compensation the physicians received in the form of bonuses.

Legal counsel, a national consulting firm, and a former inspector general of HHS advised Tuomey about the terms of the proposed employment relationship, and 19 physicians accepted it. One balked, however, citing the Stark law and False Claims Act concerns. He believed the compensation package did not meet Stark's exception for "bona fide employment relationships" and did not reflect fair market value.

Given those concerns, Tuomey and the reluctant physician jointly consulted Kevin McAnaney, an attorney and former government official who had written a "substantial portion" of the Stark law regulations. McAnaney advised that the proposed contracts raised significant "red flags" and would not pass the "straight-face test." He also warned that the contracts presented "an easy case to prosecute" for the government.

The physician declined to enter into the agreement and sued under the *qui tam* provisions of the False Claims Act, alleging that Tuomey had submitted false claims because the contracts with the 19 other physicians were illegal. The government intervened in the case, and a verdict of more than $237 million was the result.

A significant factor in the final outcome on appeal was "evidence indicating that Tuomey shopped for legal opinions approving of the employment contracts, while ignoring negative assessments." The court continued,

> The district court noted—and we agree—that a reasonable jury could have concluded that Tuomey was . . . no longer acting in good faith reliance on the advice of its counsel when it refused to give full consideration to McAnaney's negative assessment of the part-time employment contracts and terminated his representation. . . . Thus, a reasonable jury could conclude that Tuomey ignored McAnaney because it simply did not like what he had to say.[52]

The *Tuomey* drama evolved coincident with a saga involving Halifax Hospital Medical Center in Daytona Beach, Florida. That case was brought by one of the hospital's own compliance officials, who had suggested that the bonuses being paid to certain oncologists might be illegal. As in the Tuomey case, the hospital–physician contracts in Halifax were based on an opinion of validity by competent legal counsel. Notwithstanding that opinion, the employee filed suit as a *qui tam* relator and a settlement in the amount of $85 million resulted.[53] (See The Court Decides at the end of this chapter for excerpts from the *Halifax* case.)

Both *Tuomey* and *Halifax* involved huge verdicts and serious consequences for the defendant hospitals. Halifax is run by a special taxing district (a government entity), so the taxpaying residents of that part of Florida will foot the bill. Tuomey was so beleaguered by the verdict that it had to merge with a larger healthcare system or face bankruptcy. Questions remain about how the verdict against Tuomey will be paid.

Perhaps the most distressing aspect of these cases is the inability of attorneys, consultants, and even the courts to make sense out of the complexities and implications of the Stark law. The concurring judge in the *Tuomey* case states the conundrum well:

> I write separately to emphasize the troubling picture this case paints: An impenetrably complex set of laws and regulations that will result in a likely death sentence for a community hospital in an already medically underserved area.

> . . . It seems as if, even for well-intentioned health care providers, the Stark
> Law has become a booby trap rigged with strict liability and potentially ruinous
> exposure—especially when coupled with the False Claims Act.[54]

Even the author of the original Stark law, former congressman Pete Stark, seems to agree. He has been quoted in a leading health administration journal as saying the law should be repealed.[55]

Stark's Applicability to Medicaid

On its face, the Stark law applies only to Medicare, and for years, healthcare providers and their attorneys failed to consider its possible effect on Medicaid claims and the FCA. However, the DOJ now takes the position that the Stark law affects Medicaid-reimbursable services too. The theory is based on a 1993 amendment that prohibits Medicaid payments for services furnished "on the basis of a physician referral that would result in the denial of payment under the Medicare program if Medicare covered the service to the same extent."[56] Thus one of the government's arguments in the Halifax case was that the alleged false claims in question were not those that the hospital submitted to Medicaid but were the claims that Florida Medicaid submitted to the federal government for Florida's Medicaid money.

No definitive ruling was issued in *Halifax*, the issue has been disputed elsewhere, and it will need to be decided eventually by the appellate courts. The point is that the DOJ and plaintiffs' attorneys may try to bootstrap the Stark law onto Medicaid and thus stretch the FCA even further. This issue may be purely academic—because compliance with Stark for Medicare purposes should prevent Medicaid problems as well—but it will remain a legal and regulatory quagmire until it is resolved.

Statutory Exceptions

Congress provided for certain exceptions to the self-referral ban because, without the exceptions, the Stark law's sweeping language would have made illegal many legitimate, laudable, and even necessary arrangements. For example, the law excepts referrals for services provided by other physicians in the same group practice and also most in-office ancillary services furnished "personally by the referring physician, personally by a physician who is a member of the same group practice . . . or personally by individuals who are directly supervised by the physician or by another physician in the group practice."[57] Likewise, because the financial incentive for self-referral does not exist in prepaid health plans (e.g., health maintenance organizations), the statute does not apply when a physician refers beneficiaries of those plans for designated health services.

In addition to exceptions for certain referrals, the following financial relationships do not trigger the Stark law:

- Owning stocks or bonds in a large, publicly traded company or mutual fund
- Owning or investing in certain rural providers or hospitals in Puerto Rico
- Reasonable rent for office space or equipment
- Amounts paid under bona fide (fair and legitimate) employment relationships
- Reasonable payments for services provided unrelated to designated health services
- Compensation under a legitimate incentive plan (such as by withholds, capitation, or bonuses in managed care)
- Reasonable payments to induce a physician to relocate to the hospital's service area
- Isolated transactions, such as a onetime sale of property or a practice
- An arrangement that began before December 19, 1989, in which services are provided by a physician group but are billed on its behalf by a hospital with which it is affiliated
- Reasonable payments by a physician for clinical laboratory services or for other items or services

The exceptions to Stark are much more complicated than this list implies. What publicly traded companies qualify? What is a rural provider? How does one determine reasonable rent or salaries? What is an isolated transaction? This last question is an especially good example of the ambiguities generated by the exceptions. Does the isolated transactions exception apply to the purchase of a physician's practice made in installment payments rather than in a lump sum? CMS originally took the position that the exception did not apply and that installment payments were prohibited, but eventually the exception was redefined and the regulations now permit "a transaction that involves integrally related installment payments" if certain additional provisos are met.[58] Those conditions, however, create other ambiguities.

Each attempt at guidance and clarification—although helpful in some respects—adds new uncertainties, increases healthcare providers' unease, and makes the practice of law in this area extremely difficult (or profitable, depending on your point of view). Because of the ambiguities and complexities involved, the importance of expert legal counsel cannot be overemphasized.

Foreign Corrupt Practices Act

In addition to domestic concerns, healthcare is becoming a global sector. Devices, drugs, and other items are increasingly available from the world market, and individuals engage in medical tourism to seek care that is unavailable or too expensive in the United States. These developments bring into play the possibility of international fraud.

The FCPA[59] prohibits making payments to foreign government officials to assist in obtaining or retaining business, and it specifically prohibits paying bribes (or anything of value) if all or a portion of the payment will be used to influence a foreign official. These provisions apply to all US persons and to foreign firms and individuals doing business in this country. The DOJ and the Securities and Exchange Commission share enforcement authority.[60]

Although few cases to date have involved healthcare providers directly, improper payments to foreign officials can clearly be prosecuted under the FCPA. Healthcare executives should ensure that their practices do not expose them to FCPA liability.

Corporate Compliance Programs

Violations of law can occur in any company, and given the amount of money at stake, healthcare organizations are especially fertile soil for white-collar crime and its resultant criminal convictions and financial penalties. Punishments for fraud and abuse of the payment system can be levied against both the perpetrators and the corporation itself, even if the offense occurred at the lowest levels and was contrary to express company policy. Even though they may never have authorized the act or had knowledge of it, officers and managers may be held personally accountable if they deliberately or recklessly disregarded the possibility that illegal conduct might occur. Therefore, executives who believe that "what I don't know can't hurt me" are mistaken.

One of the most effective tools for minimizing the exposure of an organization and its board and management is a corporate compliance program (CCP; see Legal Brief). CCPs help healthcare organizations develop internal controls that promote adherence to federal and state laws and the program requirements of federal, state, and private health plans. For many years, adoption and implementation of CCPs was strongly recommended but remained voluntary. Now the ACA makes a CCP mandatory for "providers of services and suppliers" under Medicare, Medicaid, and the Children's Health Insurance Program.[61] All hospitals, nursing homes, rehabilitation facilities, hospice programs,

Legal Brief

The term *corporate compliance program* is used in this book because it has gained purchase in the field and has made its way into statutory language. However, *compliance* has a reactive connotation, as if saying, "Fine, we will comply if we have to." A more positive, good-citizen, "we are on the side of the angels" term might be preferable—perhaps one that includes words such as *integrity*, *ethics*, and *responsibility*.

The CCP concept gained prominence after the publication of the *Federal Sentencing Guidelines for Organizations* in 1991. Federal judges use the *Guidelines* to promote uniform, predictable sentencing.[62]

home health agencies, and other healthcare facilities; drug and device manufacturers; and physicians and other practitioners must have a CCP in place if they wish to participate in federally funded health insurance programs.

Whether voluntary or mandatory, CCPs help significantly in the effort to prevent fraud, abuse, and waste. They promote legal compliance and corporate integrity, they guide the governing body and top management in the efficient management and operation of the entity, and they help healthcare practitioners and all employees achieve and document quality patient care. CCPs are especially critical for regulating reimbursements and payments, because claims and billing operations often are sources of fraud and abuse and subject to governmental scrutiny. Elements essential to an effective CCP are identified in exhibit 15.5.

Healthcare organizations, including their governing boards and senior management, must take seriously the possibility that criminal violations (including fraud and abuse) may occur and that civil liability may arise in the course of their business. Although the cost of developing a CCP is significant, substantial benefits may accrue in the form of reduced exposure to whistleblower lawsuits or criminal prosecution. Furthermore, the consequences of having an ineffective CCP—especially one that is considered a sham—can be dire if illegal or unethical activity occurs because in that case the civil or criminal penalties would be increased.

CCPs are an important part of most healthcare organizations' operations. Initially, they emphasized the detection and prevention of fraud and abuse as well as compliance with regulations. As they matured, many became more proactive, focusing on the ethical integrity of the corporation through education and information sharing. The compliance officer should be seen as a valuable resource for questions relating to corporate ethics, conflicts of interest, human subject research, privacy and security of healthcare information, and other subjects—from antitrust to zoning.

CCPs typically benefit organizations by doing the following:

- Demonstrating the organization's commitment to honest, ethical, and responsible corporate conduct
- Improving billing practices and thus increasing revenue
- Creating a centralized source of information related to healthcare statutes and regulations
- Identifying and preventing criminal and unethical conduct
- Identifying weaknesses in internal systems and management
- Exposing possible fraud and abuse by employees or contractors
- Enabling employees to report potential problems
- Facilitating prompt, thorough investigation of alleged misconduct and appropriate corrective action

EXHIBIT 15.5
Elements of a Corporate Compliance Program

Item	The CCP Must:	Comment
(A)	Contain established compliance standards and procedures	Management must publish standards of conduct outlining legal and ethical requirements in all areas of the organization's operations, including antitrust, document retention, employment and employee benefits, environmental compliance, Medicare/Medicaid fraud and abuse, occupational safety, patient protection, and taxation.
(B)	Be overseen by high-level personnel	Most organizations assign the CCP function to an individual who reports to the chief executive officer and has a relationship with the governing board and general counsel.
(C)	Provide that no discretionary authority in the organization may be vested in persons who are known (or should be known) to be likely to engage in criminal conduct	The organization must have a mechanism (e.g., routine criminal background checks) that prevents it from hiring persons who, for example, have previously been convicted of healthcare offenses or who have been excluded from federal healthcare programs.
(D)	Effectively communicate its procedures and standards of conduct to employees and agents of the organization	The organization must educate all employees and agents about CCP standards and procedures and must continually publicize the topic in employee newsletters and similar media. Everyone in the organization—the board and senior management and lower-level employees alike—must understand and be committed to a culture of compliance.
(E)	Contain reasonable methods for achieving compliance with the standards of conduct	These methods should include ongoing monitoring activities, periodic audits of various operational departments, and anonymous reporting of suspicious activities (e.g., through hotlines or written reports).
(F)	Provide for, and the organization must carry out, appropriate and consistent discipline	Discipline includes possible termination of employment for those who violate the standards of conduct or fail to report violations.
(G)	Appropriately and consistently respond to violations that are detected	Corrective action must be established to prevent recurrence of violations.
(H)	Periodically reassess and revise the program as necessary	The CCP must keep pace with regulatory changes and changes within the organization.

Source: Data from ACA § 6102 (relating to skilled nursing facilities). ACA § 6401 (which applies to Medicare, Medicaid, and CHIP providers generally) does not list specific CCP program elements but only directs the Secretary of HHS to establish "core elements" for such programs. These elements will undoubtedly match those listed in this table because they are the same as the CCP elements contained in the Office of Inspector General program guidance documents.

- Minimizing loss to the government from false claims and thus reducing the hospital's exposure to civil damages and penalties, criminal sanctions, and administrative remedies such as program exclusion
- Helping document improvements in the quality of patient care

Summary

This chapter addresses one of the most salient issues in healthcare today: the prevention of fraud and abuse in governmental healthcare programs. The major fraud laws—the False Claims Act, the antikickback statute, and the Stark self-referral law—are reviewed. The aggressive enforcement activities of federal and state regulators and the severe monetary and criminal penalties that can be imposed for violations of these laws are emphasized. The chapter also discusses some of the changes to the fraud laws occasioned by the passage of the ACA, and it reviews the basics of a corporate compliance program (CCP)—one of the most effective programs a healthcare organization can establish to prevent fraud, promote integrity, and improve billing accuracy. A CCP is both an important preventive measure and a valuable resource for a wide range of legal and ethical issues.

Discussion Questions

1. What factors motivate healthcare organizations to maintain programs aimed at compliance and corporate ethics?
2. What kinds of fraudulent or abusive behavior related to federal healthcare payment programs can occur in hospital operations?
3. What are the most significant statutes related to healthcare fraud, and how have they been affected by the ACA?
4. What do the terms *kickback* and *self-referral* describe in the healthcare setting?
5. Explain the essential provisions of the Stark law, including to whom it applies and what types of transactions it prohibits.

The Court Decides

United States v. Greber
760 F.2d 68 (3rd Cir. 1985)

WEIS, Circuit Judge

[The defendant was convicted of fraud related to his durable medical equipment company's billing practices. The company supplied Holter monitors—portable devices worn by patients to record their heartbeats for later interpretation. For this service, Dr. Greber's company, Cardio-Med, billed Medicare and remitted a portion of each payment to the referring physician. For this practice, he was found guilty of having violated the AKS even though the payments were made for consultative services rendered. Dr. Greber was also convicted of submitting false statements concerning the length of time the monitors were operated (Medicare requires at least eight hours of operation to qualify for payment) and mail fraud (by using the mail to bill for services that were medically unnecessary or were never provided). Only the kickback issue is addressed in the following excerpt.]

On appeal, defendant raises several alleged trial errors. He presses more strongly, however, his contentions that the evidence was insufficient to support the guilty verdict on the Medicare fraud counts, and that the charge to the jury on that issue was not correct. . . .

I. Medicare Fraud

The Medicare fraud statute was amended [in 1977]. Congress, concerned with the growing problem of fraud and abuse in the system, wished to strengthen the penalties to enhance the deterrent effect of the statute. To achieve this purpose, the crime was upgraded from a misdemeanor to a felony.

Another aim of the amendments was to address the complaints of the United States

Attorneys who were responsible for prosecuting fraud cases. They informed Congress that the language of the predecessor statute was "unclear and needed clarification."

A particular concern was the practice of giving "kickbacks" to encourage the referral of work. Testimony before the Congressional committee was that "physicians often determine which laboratories would do the test work for their Medicaid patients by the amount of the kickbacks and rebates offered by the laboratory. . . . Kickbacks take a number of forms including cash, long-term credit arrangements, gifts, supplies and equipment, and the furnishing of business machines."

To remedy the deficiencies in the statute and achieve more certainty, the present version of 42 U.S.C. § 1395nn(b)(2) was enacted. It provides:

> whoever knowingly and willfully offers or pays any remuneration (including any kickback, bribe or rebate) directly or indirectly, overtly or covertly in cash or in kind to induce such person . . . (B) to purchase, lease, order, or arrange for or recommend purchasing . . . or ordering any . . . service or item for which payment may be made . . . under this title, shall be guilty of a felony.

[The evidence showed that the defendant had paid physicians "interpretation fees" for the doctors' consultation services and for explaining the test results to the patients. Some evidence existed that physicians received interpretation fees even though Dr. Greber had actually evaluated the monitoring

(continued)

(continued from previous page)

data. Moreover, the fixed percentage paid to the referring physician was more than Medicare allowed for such services.]

The district judge instructed the jury that the government was required to prove that Cardio-Med paid . . . some part of the amount received from Medicare; that defendant caused Cardio-Med to make the payment; and did so knowingly and willfully as well as with the intent to induce Dr. Avallone to use Cardio-Med's services for patients covered by Medicare. The judge further charged that even if the physician interpreting the test did so as a consultant to Cardio-Med, that fact was immaterial if a purpose of the fee was to induce the ordering of services from Cardio-Med.

Defendant contends that the [instruction to the jury] was erroneous. He insists that absent a showing that the only purpose behind the fee was to improperly induce future services, compensating a physician for services actually rendered could not be a violation of the statute. The government argues that Congress intended to combat financial incentives to physicians for ordering particular services patients did not require.

The language and purpose of the statute support the government's view. Even if the physician performs some service for the money received, the potential for unnecessary drain on the Medicare system remains. The statute is aimed at the inducement factor.

The text refers to "any remuneration." That includes not only sums for which no actual service was performed but also those amounts for which some professional time was expended. "Remunerates" is defined as "to pay an equivalent for service." Webster Third New International Dictionary (1966). By including such items as kickbacks and bribes, the statute expands "remuneration" to cover situations where no service is performed. That a particular payment was a remuneration (which implies that a service was rendered) rather than a kickback, does not foreclose the possibility that a violation nevertheless could exist.

In United States v. Hancock the court applied the term "kickback" found in the predecessor statute to payments made to chiropractors by laboratories which performed blood tests. The chiropractors contended that the amounts they received were legitimate handling fees for their services in obtaining, packaging, and delivering the specimens to the laboratories and then interpreting the results. The court rejected that contention and noted, "The potential for increased costs to the Medicare-Medicaid system and misapplication of federal funds is plain, where payments for the exercise of such judgments are added to the legitimate cost of the transaction. . . . [T]hese are among the evils Congress sought to prevent by enacting the kick-back statutes. . . ."

Hancock strongly supports the government's position here, because the statute in that case did not contain the word "remuneration." The court nevertheless held that "kickback" sufficiently described the defendants' criminal activity. By adding "remuneration" to the statute in the 1977 amendment, Congress sought to make it clear that even if the transaction was not considered to be a "kickback" for which no service had been rendered, payment nevertheless violated the Act.

We are aware that in United States v. Porter the Court of Appeals for the Fifth Circuit took a more narrow view of "kickback" than did the court in Hancock. Porter's interpretation of the predecessor statute[,] which did not include "remuneration[,]" is neither binding nor persuasive. . . . We conclude that the more expansive reading is consistent with the impetus for the 1977 amendments and therefore hold that the district court correctly instructed the jury. If the payments were intended to induce the physician to use Cardio-Med's services, the statute was violated, even if the payments were also intended to compensate for professional services.

Discussion Questions

1. How, if at all, can you distinguish *Greber* from other instances of payments for professional services? Suppose the percentage Dr. Greber paid to the physicians had not exceeded Medicare's guidelines. Would that payment still amount to prohibited remuneration in this court's eyes?
2. Suppose you are a lawyer or a compliance officer advising a hospital cardiology department. The department has a contract under whose terms it will pay a certain cardiology group a fixed dollar amount for every electrocardiogram (ECG) it interprets, and the hospital will bill Medicare accordingly. The dollar amount is equal to Medicare's allowable charge for a basic ECG and report (less than $10 at this writing), and all readings are medically necessary. You ask why the hospital does not just let the doctors bill Medicare themselves, and the reply is, "Oh, it's such a hassle for them. We already have a billing department, and we can do it for them easily." What is your response, and why?

The Court Decides

United States v. McClatchey
217 F.3d 823 (10th Cir. 2000)

MURPHY, Circuit Judge

[Fifteen years after Greber, *the type of intent required to violate the AKS was still an open question.* Greber *determined that if any purpose of the remuneration was to induce referrals, the act was violated even if other purposes were legitimate. The following case excerpt illustrates some of the difficulties of this interpretation.*

The case involved two physicians who were the principals in a group practice (BVMG) that provided care to nursing home patients. In 1984, the physicians approached Baptist Medical Center in Kansas City, Missouri, and proposed that they would move their patients from other hospitals to Baptist

if the hospital would buy BVMG. Baptist rejected the proposal, but after much negotiation the parties agreed that the physicians would provide various services to the hospital in return for $75,000 each per year. (Among other findings, testimony indicated that the fee was determined before the physicians had agreed on the services.) The physicians then began admitting their patients to Baptist.

The contractual arrangement continued until 1993, even though as early as 1986 attorneys for Baptist's new owner, the Health Midwest system, were concerned that it did not comply with the safe harbor regulations that had since been issued by the US

(continued)

(continued from previous page)

government. Additionally, in late 1991 or early 1992, Baptist learned that the physicians were not performing some of the contractual services, but the fees continued to be paid and the contract was renewed.

The jury convicted the hospital chief executive officer, the two physicians, and McClatchey (Baptist's chief operating officer) of violating the AKS. Two attorneys for Health Midwest who were involved in the negotiations to renew the contract were charged with conspiracy but were found not guilty by the judge on motions for acquittal. The judge also granted McClatchey's motion for acquittal on the ground that no reasonable jury could find that he deliberately intended to violate the law. Thus, the issue on appeal concerned the type of criminal intent necessary to violate the AKS.]

. . .

In Instruction 32, the district court charged the jury as follows:

In order to sustain its burden of proof against the hospital executives for the crime of violating the Anti-Kickback statute, the government must prove beyond a reasonable doubt that the defendant under consideration offered or paid remuneration with the specific criminal intent "to induce" referrals. To offer or pay remuneration to induce referrals means to offer or pay remuneration with the intent to gain influence over the reason or judgment of a person making referral decisions. The intent to gain such influence must, at least in part, have been the reason the remuneration was offered or paid.

On the other hand, defendants Anderson, Keel, and McClatchey cannot be convicted merely because they hoped or expected or believed that referrals may ensue from remuneration that was designed wholly for other purposes.

Likewise, mere oral encouragement to refer patients or the mere creation of an attractive place to which patients can be referred does not violate the law. There must be an offer or payment of remuneration to induce, as I have just defined it.

McClatchey contends this instruction was incorrect and warrants a new trial, because a defendant should not be convicted under the Act when his offer or payment of remuneration was motivated merely in part to induce referrals, but rather the motivation to induce referrals must be the defendant's primary purpose. . . .

Whether the "at least in part" or "one purpose" standard applied in the instant case constitutes a correct interpretation of the Act is an issue of first impression in this Circuit. McClatchey urges this court to reject the test set out in Instruction 32 as too broad, because "[e]very business relationship between a hospital and a physician is based 'at least in part' on the hospital's expectation that the physician will choose to refer patients." This argument, however, ignores the actual instruction given in the instant case, in which the district court specifically informed the jury that "McClatchey cannot be convicted merely because [he] hoped or expected or believed that referrals may ensue from remuneration that was designed wholly for other purposes." According to this instruction, therefore, a hospital or individual may lawfully enter into a business relationship with a doctor and even hope for or expect referrals from that doctor, so long as the hospital is motivated to enter into the relationship for legal reasons entirely distinct from its collateral hope for referrals.

The only three Circuits to have decided this issue have all adopted the "one purpose" test. *[One of these was* Greber, *which is set forth earlier.]* In Greber, a doctor who owned a diagnostic laboratory was convicted of violating the Act because he paid "interpretation fees" to other physicians to induce them to refer Medicare patients to use his laboratory's services. Defendant Greber asserted that these interpretation fees compensated the physicians both for providing initial consultation services and for explaining the test results to the patients. On appeal, Greber argued that a jury instruction much like Instruction 32 was erroneous, because the Act requires the government to prove that the only purpose for the interpretation fees was to induce referrals and that compensation for services actually rendered could not constitute a violation of the Act. Carefully examining the language and purpose of the Act, the Third Circuit rejected Greber's proposed interpretation and instead held that "if one purpose of the payment was to induce referrals, the [Act] has been violated." . . . The Greber court thus concluded that the "one purpose" test is consistent with the legislative intent behind the amended Act.

This court agrees with the sound reasoning in Greber and thus holds that a person who offers or pays remuneration to another person violates the Act so long as one purpose of the offer or payment is to induce Medicare or Medicaid patient referrals. Because the district court accurately informed the jury of the applicable law, McClatchey is not entitled to a new trial based on the jury instructions.

. . .

This court concludes that the government presented sufficient evidence from which a reasonable jury could infer McClatchey knowingly, voluntarily, and purposefully entered into an agreement with the specific intent to violate the Act. . . . We therefore REVERSE the judgment of acquittal and the alternative order for a new trial entered by the District Court for the District of Kansas and REMAND to that court with instructions to reinstate the verdict rendered by the jury. ∎

Discussion Questions

1. Determining difficult questions of fact is the jury's job. If you had been a juror in this case and had heard "Instruction 32," where would you have drawn the line between an intent to induce referrals and a mere hope that referrals might ensue?
2. The summary given here leaves out many important facts. What other facts might have been important to you as a juror?
3. Recognizing that physicians are their lifeblood, hospitals have long provided certain amenities to keep them happy. Among these perks are preferred parking, free meals, and "professional courtesy" (discounted care for themselves and their family members). Because the one-purpose test now appears to be the accepted standard under the FCA, and because a purpose of "keeping the docs happy" is to encourage them to refer patients to the facility, are these types of benefits illegal?

~ ▥ ~

The Court Decides

United States ex rel. Baklid-Kunz v. Halifax Hospital Med. Ctr.
U.S. Dist. Ct., M.D. Fla., No: 6:09-cv-1002-Orl-31TBS

Nov. 13, 2013
ORDER

This matter comes before the Court without a hearing on the Motion for Partial Summary Judgment filed by the United States of America, the response in opposition filed by the Defendants, and the reply filed by the Government.

I. Background
Halifax Hospital Medical Center ("Halifax Hospital") is a special taxing district that operates a community hospital of the same name in Volusia County, Florida. Halifax Staffing, Inc. is an instrumentality of Halifax Hospital. Halifax Staffing employs the individuals who work for Halifax Hospital. Halifax Hospital pays all of the expenses and obligations of Halifax Staffing, including payroll, either directly or by transfer of funds into Halifax Staffing's payroll account.

Halifax Staffing entered into employment agreements with six medical oncologists. . . . The employment agreements provided that the Medical Oncologists would receive a salary and bonuses.

The Medical Oncologists treated patients at Halifax Hospital on both an inpatient and outpatient basis and, *inter alia,* ordered or requested outpatient prescription drugs for their patients. Whenever one of the Medical Oncologists personally performed a Medicare-reimbursable procedure, Halifax Hospital would submit two claims for payment to Medicare—one for the physician's services and a second for the facility fee, which would include items such as providing space and equipment. . . .

In fiscal year 2005, the Medical Oncologists became eligible to receive a bonus (henceforth, the "Incentive Bonus" pursuant to the following provision of their employment agreements:

> Compensation [Halifax Staffing] shall pay to Employee as compensation for services the following:
>
> . . .
>
> c. Beginning with the fiscal year ending September 30, 2005, an equitable portion of an Incentive Compensation pool which is equal to 15% of the operating margin for the Medical Oncology program as defined by the financial statements produced by the Finance Department on a quarterly basis. The amount of the incentive compensation distributed to the Employee shall be determined by the Medical Oncology Practice Management Group. This compensation shall be paid annually according to the operating margin for the fiscal year.

. . . In response to an interrogatory from the Government, the Defendants stated that the operating margin for the Medical Oncology program was made up of "revenue and direct expenses from outpatient medical oncology services" and that "[r]evenue consisted of outpatient medical oncology services, physician services, and related outpatient oncology pharmacy charges." The Defendants admit that the revenue at issue included fees for services that were not personally performed by the Medical Oncologists, such as fees for services related to the administration of chemotherapy.

The Incentive Compensation pool was divided between the six Medical Oncologists based on each individual oncologist's personally performed services. Halifax Staffing paid the Incentive Bonuses to the Medical Oncologists for fiscal years 2005–2008. During this time frame, Halifax Hospital submitted thousands of claim forms to Medicare in which one or more of the Medical Oncologists was identified as an attending physician or an operating physician.

The Relator, Elin Baklid-Kunz . . . filed this *qui tam* action on June 16, 2009, alleging that the Defendants, *inter alia,* violated the Stark Law by billing Medicare for items provided as a result of referrals from physicians with whom the Defendants had improper financial relationships. On October 4, 2011, the Government announced that it had elected to intervene as to certain of the Relator's claims, including her Stark Act claim involving the Medical Oncologists. By way of the instant motion, the Government seeks summary judgment as to the alleged Stark Act violation; as well as related claims under the False Claims Act, for unjust enrichment and for payment by mistake; plus a number of affirmative defenses asserted by the Defendants.

. . . .

[After reviewing the applicable laws and regulations in considerable detail, the court proceeds with the following.]

III. Analysis
A. Stark Law Compliance
The Government contends that during the period when the Medical Oncologists were eligible to receive the Incentive Bonus, the Defendants violated the Stark Law by submitting Medicare claims resulting from referrals made by the Medical Oncologists for designated health services. The Defendants dispute this contention on two grounds. The Defendants argue that the compensation arrangement with the Medical Oncologists fit within the Stark Law exception for bona fide employment relationships and therefore referrals by the Medical Oncologists were not

prohibited by the Stark Law. The Defendants also argue that the Government has failed to produce any evidence that the Medical Oncologists actually made referrals of DHS during the pertinent time frame.

1. Bona Fide Employment Relationship
It is undisputed that the Medical Oncologists had a financial relationship with Halifax Hospital. Because of this, the burden shifts to Halifax Hospital to show that the compensation arrangement with the Medical Oncologists fit within one of the Stark Law's exceptions. Halifax contends that the Medical Oncologists' compensation arrangement satisfied the exception for bona fide employment relationships, which requires a showing that:

(A) the employment is for identifiable services,
(B) the amount of remuneration under the employment—
(i) is consistent with the fair market value of the services, and
(ii) is not determined in a manner that takes into account (directly or indirectly) the volume or value of any referrals by the referring physician,
(C) the remuneration is provided pursuant to an agreement which would be commercially reasonable even if no referrals were made to the employer, and
(D) the employment meets such other requirements as the Secretary may impose by regulation as needed to protect against program or patient abuse. 42 U.S.C. § 1395nn(e)(2).

The Government contends that the requirements of this exception were not satisfied because the Incentive Bonus, and therefore the Medical Oncologists' remuneration, varied based on referrals for designated health services. More particularly, the Government

(continued)

(continued from previous page)

points out that the pool from which the Incentive Bonus was drawn was equal to 15 percent of the operating margin of the Medical Oncology program, and the program's revenue included fees for designated health services such as outpatient prescription drugs and outpatient services not personally performed by the Medical Oncologists. Thus, revenue from referrals made by the Medical Oncologists would flow into the Incentive Bonus pool, and additional referrals would be expected to increase the size of the pool. All other things being equal, this would in turn increase the size of the Incentive Bonus received by the referring Medical Oncologist.

Halifax points out that the requirement in the bona fide employment exception that the remuneration not be "determined in a manner that takes into account (directly or indirectly) the volume or value of any referrals by the referring physician," is itself subject to an exception. The final sentence of 42 U.S.C. § 1395(e)(2) provides that "[s]ubparagraph (B)(ii) shall not prohibit the payment of remuneration in the form of a productivity bonus based on services performed personally by the physician (or an immediate family member of such physician)". The Incentive Bonus, the Defendants argue, was just such a bonus, because "it is undisputed the bonus pool was divided up based on [each] oncologist's personally performed services." (Emphasis in original).

This is not enough to bring the Incentive Bonus within the bona fide employment exception. The Incentive Bonus was not a "bonus based on services personally performed" by the Medical Oncologists, as the exception requires. Rather, as described by the Defendants themselves, this was a bonus that was divided up based on services personally performed by the Medical Oncologists. The bonus itself was based on factors in addition to personally performed services—including revenue from referrals made by the Medical Oncologists for DHS. The fact that each oncologist could increase his or her share of the bonus pool by personally performing more services cannot alter the fact that the size of the pool (and thus the size of each oncologist's bonus) could be increased by making more referrals.

During the time period when the Incentive Bonus was being paid, the compensation arrangement between Halifax Staffing and the Medical Oncologists did not satisfy the requirements for the bona fide employment exception. As a result, the Medical Oncologists were prohibited from making referrals to Halifax Hospital for DHS, and Halifax Hospital was prohibited from submitting Medicare claims for services furnished pursuant to such referrals.

[The court thus held that a violation of the Stark Law had been proven but that the extent of the violation—in other words, the amount of damages—was still in question. For these reasons, complete summary judgment was denied and further proceedings were ordered to determine the amount of damages that should be awarded. Reading the handwriting on the wall, Halifax proceeded to negotiate a settlement of $86 million about a year after this decision was announced.] ■

Discussion Questions

1. What does the judge mean by the "instant motion"?
2. Can you explain the terms of the compensation agreement between Halifax and the oncologists?
3. Why does the incentive bonus fail to meet the "bona fide employment relationship" exception?
4. What changes to the agreement should Halifax have made to avoid Stark Law liability?

~ 🏛 ~

Notes

1. US Department of Justice, *Foreign Corrupt Practices Act* (updated July 20, 2016), at https://www.justice.gov/criminal-fraud/foreign-corrupt-practices-act.

2. Centers for Medicare & Medicaid Services, *National Health Expenditure Data: Historical* (last modified December 3, 2015), at https://www.cms.gov/Research-Statistics-Data-and-Systems/Statistics-Trends-and-Reports/NationalHealthExpendData/NationalHealthAccounts Historical.html.

3. Statistics are from Centers for Medicare & Medicaid Services, http://www.cms.gov. For the latest historical information and projections, drill down to: Research, Statistics, Data and Systems > National Health Expenditure Data.

4. In the mid-1990s, healthcare fraud was considered the Department of Justice's (DOJ's) number two priority, second only to violent crime. US Department of Justice, Department of Justice Healthcare Fraud Report, Fiscal Year 1994 (March 2, 1995). Healthcare fraud is now perhaps number three because the "war on terror" has ascended on the DOJ's priority list.

5. 768 F. Supp. 1127 (E.D. Pa. 1991).

6. United States v. Krizek, 859 F. Supp. 5, 8 (1994).

7. *Id.* at 11.

8. *Id.* at 14.

9. United States v. Krizek, 7 F. Supp. 2d 56, 60 (D.D.C. 1998). The *Krizek* case appears numerous times in the law reports. In addition to the final decision are these other opinions: 859 F. Supp. 5 (D.D.C. 1994), the original trial court decision; 909 F. Supp. 32 (D.D.C. 1995), a memorandum opinion assessing damages; and 111 F.3d 934 (D.C. Cir. 1997), the appellate decision remanding the case for additional hearings.

10. *See, e.g.,* US Department of Health and Human Services and US Department of Justice, *Health Care Fraud and Abuse Control Program: Annual Report for Fiscal Year 2013* (published February 2014), at http://oig.hhs.gov/publications/docs/hcfac/FY2013-hcfac.pdf.

11. 31 U.S.C. §§ 3729–3732.

12. *See, e.g.,* Rex Trailer Co. v. United States, 350 U.S. 148 (1952), *and* Fleming v. United States, 336 F.2d 475 (10th Cir. 1964).

13. United States v. Krizek, 111 F.3d 394 (D.C. Cir. 1997).

14. *See, e.g.,* United States v. McNinch, 356 U.S. 595 (1958).

15. 31 U.S.C. § 3729(b).

16. S. Rep. No. 345, 99th Cong., 2d Sess. 7.

17. 859 F. Supp. at 13. *But see* United States v. Nazon, 1993 WL 410150 (N.D. Ill. 1993).

18. 42 U.S.C. § 1320a–7(b)(15) (permissive exclusions).

19. 42 U.S.C. § 1320a–7a (civil money penalties).

20. 31 U.S.C. § 3733(k)(4).

21. These conditions were loosened somewhat by § 10104 of the ACA, thus making it easier for a qui tam plaintiff to sustain a lawsuit. *See* 31 U.S.C. § 3730(3)(4).

22. 31 U.S.C. § 3730(h).

23. *See* United States ex rel. Marcus v. Hess, 317 U.S. 537 (1943), in which a government contractor's claims were based on a contract obtained through collusion. The opinion held, "The government's money would never have been [paid] had its agents known the bids were collusive." *See also* United States v. Forster Wheeler Corp., 447 F.2d 100 (2d Cir. 1971) (invoices submitted on contract that was based on inflated cost estimates are false claims) *and* United States v. Veneziale, 268 F.2d 504 (3d Cir. 1959) (fraudulently induced contract may create liability when the contract later results in payment by the government).

24. 797 F.2d 888 (10th Cir. 1986).

25. 760 F. Supp. 1120 (E.D. Pa. 1991).

26. 914 F. Supp. 1507 (M.D. Tenn. 1996).

27. *Id.* at 1509.

28. The Supreme Court case was *Universal Health Services, Inc. v. United States ex rel. Escobar,* __ U.S. __ (2016). In earlier cases the rationale was followed in *U.S. ex rel. Thompson v. Columbia/HCA Healthcare Corp.*, 20 F. Supp. 2d 1017 (S.D. Tex. 1998), but it was rejected in *U.S. ex rel. Conner v. Salina Regional Health*, 543 F.3d 1211 (10th Cir. 2008). In a footnote, the *Conner* opinion recognizes that "several other courts have followed Thompson's reasoning," but it declined to follow it for other reasons. See also *U.S. ex rel Spicer v. Westbrook*, 751 F.3d 354 (5th Cir. 2004): "[A] false certification of compliance, without more, does not give rise to a false claim for payment unless payment is conditioned on compliance."

29. ACA § 6402(f); 42 U.S.C. § 1320a–7b(g).

30. 18 U.S.C. § 287.

31. *See* 42 U.S.C. § 1320a–7b.

32. 42 U.S.C. § 1320a–7b(b).

33. 42 U.S.C. § 1320a–7.

34. 42 U.S.C. § 1320a–7a(a)(7).

35. 42 U.S.C. § 1320a–7b(b)(3).

36. S. Rep. No. 109, 100th Cong., 1st Sess. 27.

37. ACA § 6001 et seq., *amending* 42 U.S.C. § 1395nn *and* § 1301 et seq.

38. 42 U.S.C. § 1320a–7a(i)(6).

39. 51 F.3d 1390 (9th Cir. 1995).

40. Office of Inspector Gen., US Dept. of Health and Human Servs., Advisory Op. No. 97-6 (October 8, 1997).

41. Levin v. Inspector General, CR No. 343 (HHS Dept. App. Bd. November 10, 1994).

42. *See* 42 U.S.C. §§ 1320a–7b(b)(1)(B) *and* (2)(B).

43. Unreported decision cited in *Psychiatric Hospital Firm Pleads Guilty to Violating Anti-Kickback Statute*, 4 HEALTH L. REP. (BNA) 687 (1995).

44. 42 U.S.C. § 1320a–7a(a)(5).

45. Hanlester v. Shalala, *supra* note 39 at 1400.

46. 524 U.S. 184 (1998).

47. *Id.* at 185.

48. United States v. Starks, 157 F.3d 833, 837-38 (11th Cir. 1998).

49. *Id.* at 838.

50. 42 U.S.C. § 1395nn.

51. 42 U.S.C. § 1395nn(d)(3)(C).

52. United States ex rel. Drakeford v. Tuomey, 792 F.3d 364, 375 (4th Cir. 2015).

53. United States ex rel. Baklid-Kunz v. Halifax Hospital Medical Center, No. 6:09-cv-1002-ORL-31TBS (M.D. Fla.) available at http://bit.ly/1GbEk5U.

54. *Supra* note 52 at 391, 395.

55. Joe Carlson, *Pete Stark: Repeal the Stark Law*, MODERN HEALTHCARE (August 2, 2013), at http://www.modernhealthcare.com/article/20130802/blog/308029995.

56. *Medicare and Medicaid Programs: Physicians' Referrals to Health Care Entities with Which They Have Financial Relationships, Proposed Rule*, 63 Fed. Reg. 1659, 1672 (January 9, 1998). This proposed rule was later withdrawn and, as of this writing, has not been replaced.

57. 42 U.S.C. § 1395nn(b).

58. 42 C.F.R. § 411.351.

59. 15 U.S.C. §§ 78dd–1, et seq.

60. The DOJ maintains a website dedicated to the FCPA and its enforcement. *See* US Department of Justice, *Foreign Corrupt Practices Act* (updated July 20, 2016), at https://www.justice.gov/criminal-fraud/foreign-corrupt-practices-act.

61. *See* ACA §§ 6102 *and* 6401, *amending* 42 U.S.C. §§ 1301 et seq. *and* § 1395cc(j), respectively.

62. 56 Fed. Reg., No. 95, May 16, 1991. *See generally* US Sentencing Commission, http://www.ussc.gov.

GLOSSARY

accountable care organizations (ACOs): organizations of hospitals, physicians, and other providers who—under a shared governance structure—coordinate patient care, are accountable for the quality and cost of that care, and receive bonuses when they deliver care more efficiently

admiralty: the system of law that applies to accidents and injuries at sea, maritime commerce, alleged violations of rules of the sea over shipping lanes and rights of way, and crimes aboard a ship

ad valorem tax: tax imposed in proportion to the value of the property being assessed

Affordable Care Act (ACA): the health reform law enacted by Congress in 2010; full name: Patient Protection and Affordable Care Act, Pub. L. No. 111-148

apparent agency or **agency by estoppel:** closely related doctrines that can be used to counter the independent contractor defense

arbitration: an extrajudicial hearing sometimes used in medical liability cases to avoid a court trial and conducted by a person or a panel of people who are not necessarily judges

assumption of risk: a situation that is so obviously dangerous that the individual knows he could be injured but might (or did) take the chance anyway

business associates: outside persons or organizations that use protected health information while providing services on behalf of a "covered entity" (a healthcare organization); business associate functions include billing, claims processing, utilization review, and so on.

cause of action: the basis of a lawsuit; sufficient legal grounds and alleged facts that, if proven, would constitute all the requirements for the plaintiff to prevail

charitable immunity: the venerable principle (now discredited) that a charitable organization is not to be held liable for the tortious actions of its agents

charity: an organization that exists to help those in need or to provide religious, educational, scientific, or similar aid to the public

common law: the body of law based on custom and judicial precedents, as distinct from statutory law; its historical roots are the traditional laws of England that developed over many centuries and were carried over to the American colonies and thus the United States.

concierge medicine: a relationship between a patient and a primary care physician in which the patient pays an annual fee in return for direct, personalized care; also known as *boutique medicine*

consideration: essentially, payment; something of value (not necessarily money) that is given (or promised) in return for what is received (or promised)

consolidation: a transaction in which two or more organizations combine to form a new corporation, thereby dissolving the predecessor companies; sometimes used as a general term inclusive of *merger* and *acquisition*

contributory negligence and **comparative negligence:** common-law doctrines relating to allocation of responsibility when the plaintiff was partially at fault

corporate charter: the fundamental document (usually articles of incorporation) of a corporation's legal authority

corporation: an organization formed with governmental approval to act as an artificial person to carry on business (or other activities), which can sue or be sued and (unless not-for-profit) can issue shares of stock to raise capital

covered entity: a health plan, healthcare clearinghouse, or healthcare provider that transmits any health information in electronic form

credentialing: a process for establishing the qualifications and competence of medical staff applicants through review of their training, licensure, and practice history

defamation: the act of making untrue statements about another that damage the person's reputation

de minimis: inconsequential or of minor importance; a reference to the legal maxim *de minimis non curat lex* (Latin meaning "the law does not concern itself with trifles")

dictum plural, **dicta**): Latin meaning "remark"—a comment in a legal opinion that is not binding because it is not required to reach the decision but that states a related legal principle

due process of law: a fundamental principle of fairness in legal matters, both civil and criminal; the requirement that all legal procedures set by statute and court practice be followed so that no unjust treatment results

exculpatory: absolving or clearing of blame

ex parte hearing: a hearing in which only one party is present

fiduciary: an individual or entity (e.g., a bank or a trust company) that has the power and duty to act for another (the beneficiary) under circumstances that require trust, good faith, and honesty

Good Samaritan statutes: provisions of law that provide immunity from liability for persons who provide emergency care at the scene of an accident

guardian ad litem: a guardian appointed by a court to represent the interests of a minor or an incompetent person

hearsay: an out-of-court statement offered into evidence to prove the truth of the matter asserted in the statement

in camera: in secret; privately (from Latin: *room, chamber*)

informed consent: agreement to permit a medical procedure after disclosure of all relevant facts needed to make an intelligent decision

intentional tort: a category of torts that describes a civil wrong resulting from an intentional act on the part of the tortfeasor

inure: a term used but not defined in IRC section 501(c)(3); in context, it means a charity's income or assets may not benefit, accrue to, or be distributed to private interests.

joint venture: a mutual endeavor by two or more organizations for a specific purpose or for a limited duration

judgment NOV (non obstante veredicto): a verdict "notwithstanding the verdict" entered by the court when a jury's verdict is clearly unsupported by the evidence

justiciable: capable of being settled by a court of law

law: a system of standards to govern the conduct of people in an organization, a community, a society, or a nation

liability: legal responsibility for one's acts or omissions

lobbying: activity intended to influence the outcome of pending legislation

malum in se: an act that is evil in itself because it violates basic moral principles of society (e.g., murder, rape, burglary)

malum prohibitum: an act that is not inherently wrong but is illegal because it is prohibited by statute (e.g., tax avoidance or violation of traffic laws)

medical tourism: travel of people to another country to obtain medical treatment, usually because of cost considerations or the treatment's unavailability in their home country

mens rea: the mental element of a crime; one's awareness that one's conduct is criminal

merger or acquisition: the joining of two or more corporations, whereby one or more of the organizations transfers assets to another (the survivor) and then is dissolved

negligence: failure to comply with established standards for the protection of others; departure from the conduct expected of a reasonably prudent person acting under the same or similar circumstances

not-for-profit (or nonprofit): a type of organization in which legal and ethical restrictions prohibit distribution of profits to owners or shareholders

parens patriae: the doctrine that the government is the ultimate guardian of all people who have a legal disability, such as minors and the mentally ill

peradventure: chance or uncertainty; doubt; question

per curiam: literally, "by the court"; a decision issued by all or a majority of the judges deciding a case and for which individual authorship is not given

physician: for purposes of federal healthcare programs (42 U.S.C. § 1395x(r)), doctors of medicine (MD), doctors of osteopathy (DO), doctors of dental surgery or dental medicine (DDS or DMD), doctors of podiatric medicine (DPM), doctors of optometry (OD), and chiropractors (DC)

positive predictive value: the probability that subjects with a positive screening test truly have the disease

pretermit: to disregard, overlook, or intentionally omit

prima facie: containing enough evidence to win unless the defendant presents contradictory evidence

privileging: the process whereby the specific scope and content of patient care (clinical) services are authorized for a healthcare practitioner by a healthcare organization on the basis of evaluation of the individual's credentials and performance

protected health information (PHI): any health-related information that identifies or can be used to identify the individual to whom it pertains

proximate cause: the act or omission from which an injury results as a natural, direct, uninterrupted consequence and without which the injury would not have occurred; the legal cause of the damages to the plaintiff; the cause that immediately precedes and produces the effect (as contrasted with a remote or an intermediate cause)

public policy: the common sense and common conscience of the citizenry as a whole that is applied to matters of public health, safety, and welfare; the general, well-settled (and usually unwritten) sense of public opinion relating to the duties of citizens to one another

remittitur: a judge's order reducing an excessive jury award

res ipsa loquitur: a rule of law that one is presumed to be negligent if one had exclusive control of the cause of the accident or injury, even though there is no specific evidence of negligence

respondeat superior: a doctrine in the law of agency that provides that a principal—the employer (superior)—is responsible for the actions of her agent done in the course of employment

school rule: the principle that healthcare practitioners are judged by the standards of their own branch of medicine

scienter: knowledge by a defendant that his acts were illegal or his statements were fraudulent

sovereign immunity: an ancient legal doctrine exempting the sovereign (monarch or state) from liability for wrongs

standard of care: the caution and prudence that a reasonable person would exercise under the circumstances or that are required by appropriate authority for such situations

stare decisis: the principle that a court must respect decisions of higher courts (precedents) on a settled legal issue applicable to the instant case

statute of limitation: a law setting the maximum period one can wait before filing a lawsuit, depending on the type of case or claim

strict liability: automatic responsibility (without having to prove negligence) for damages as a result of possession or use of inherently dangerous equipment, such as explosives, wild and poisonous animals, or assault weapons

subpoena duces tecum: a court order, issued at the request of one of the parties to a suit, that asks a witness to bring to court or to a deposition any relevant documents under the witness's control

suspect class: a group of people often subjected to discrimination because of stereotyping; criteria for suspect classification and thus careful judicial review include race, religion, national origin, gender, and so on.

third-party payers: managed care organizations, government programs, employee benefit plans, private insurance plans, and similar entities responsible for paying for health services

tort: a civil offense not founded on contract; a failure to conduct oneself in a manner considered proper under the given circumstances

tortfeasor: a wrongdoer; a person who commits a tort

utilization management (UM): proactive techniques to improve the efficiency and to control the cost of health services by influencing providers' medical decision making; UM typically includes concurrent peer review processes.

utilization review (UR): systematic (usually retrospective) review of the efficiency and medical necessity of healthcare services on the basis of established guidelines

vicarious liability: attachment of responsibility to a person whose agent caused the plaintiff's injuries

writ of certiorari: an order from a higher court to a lower court, requesting that the record of a case be sent up for review

CASE INDEX

Note: Italicized page locators refer to cases in exhibits.

Abbott Laboratories v. Portland Retail Druggists Association, Inc., 474

Addington v. Texas, 104n35

Ad Hoc Executive Comm. of the Medical Staff of Memorial Hosp. v. Runyan, 289n6

Adler v. Montefiore Hospital Association of Western Pennsylvania, 275–76, 292n62

Aetna Health, Inc. v. Davila, 236

Alexandridis v. Jewett, 124–25

Allen v. Sisters of St. Joseph, 532

Am. College of Obstetricians v. Thornburgh, 543n76

Am. Hosp. Ass'n v. Hansbarger, 214n12

Anderson v. Moore, 105n53

Andrews-Clarke v. Travelers Ins. Co., 252n69

Ardoin v. Hartford Accident & Indem. Co., 250n31

Arizona v. Maricopa County Medical Society, 479

Arrington v. Wong, 359, 360

Atlanta Oculopic Surgery, P.C. v. Nestlehutt, 179n86

Aultman Hosp. Ass'n v. Evatt, 466n30

Ayotte v. Planned Parenthood of Northern New England, 530

Azzolino v. Dingfelder, 539n14, 541n43

Baber v. Hospital Corporation of America, 357–59, 378n66

Bader v. United Orthodox Synagogue, 250n30

Bailie v. Miami Valley Hosp., 106n62

Baird v. Sickler, 164

Baldetta v. Harborview Medical Center, 257

Baldor v. Rogers, 175n2

Bang v. Charles T. Miller Hospital, 386

Baptist Health v. Murphy, 277–78, 292n72

Baptist Memorial Hosp. System v. Sampson, 223, 249n20

Barcia v. Society of N. Y. Hosp., 377n53

Barefoot v. Estelle, 80

Barnes Hosp. v. Leggett, 466–67n36, 467n37

Barnes Hospital v. Collector of Revenue, 452, 458

Barnett v. Bachrach, 128

Barrett v. United Hosp., 289n9, 289n10

Bartling v. Superior Court, 426n41

Bauer v. Bowen, 179n76

Baxter v. State, 429n85

Beal v. Ann Doe, 545n98

Becker v. Schwartz, 539n13, 540n27, 541n35, 541n36

Bedard v. Notre Dame, 106n62

Bellah v. Greenson, 341n34

Beller v. Health and Hospital Corp. of Marion County, 360, 372–74

Berkey Photo, Inc. v. Eastman Kodak Co., 503n55

Berlin v. Nathan, 179n85

Berman v. Allan, 539n14, 540n26, 540n33, 541n35

INDEX

Note: Italicized page locators refer to figures or tables in exhibits.

Hill-Burton Act and mandated free care, *77–79*; nation's health dollar 2014: where it came from, *548*; nation's health dollar 2014: where it went, *549*; patient registration and admission, 71–77; private law and, 9; "right" to, 61–62, 71; rising costs of, factors contributing to, 548–50; Sherman Act and applications to, 484–86; top five fraud settlements of 2014, *550*; traditional principles on access to, 70–79

Health Care and Education Reconciliation Act of 2010, 63

Healthcare Financial Management Association, 58

Health Care Fraud and Abuse Control Program, 552

Healthcare institutions. *See also* Hospitals; Taxation of healthcare institutions: consent cases and role of, 384–85; duty of, 219

Healthcare Integrity and Protection Data Bank, 275

Health Care Quality Improvement Act of 1986, 263, *471,* 480, *481*; definitions and reports, 297–99; Kadlec Medical Center v. Lakeview Anesthesia Associates and peer review under, 271–72; National Practitioner Data Bank, 266, 267, 274–75; Patrick v. Burget and peer review under, 266–67; peer review under, 265–73; Poliner v. Texas Health System and peer review under, 267–71, 272; professional review action defined by, 270; promotion of professional review activities, 294–96; reporting of information, 296–97

Healthcare reform. *See also* Affordable Care Act: advertising and, 48; charitable hospitals and, 444; Clinton administration and, 48–49; history of efforts for, 108–9; tax code and, 446–47

Healthcare systems: multi-institutional, 198, *199*

Healthcare workforce: ACA definition of, 281

Health information: access to, 309–27; covered entity and, 302; HIPAA definition of, 302; liability for unauthorized disclosure of, 314–19; protected, 302–3; storage media for, 302

Health Information and Management Systems Society, 59

Health information management, 301–45; access to health information, 309–27; covered entity, protected health information, and de-identification, 302–3; federal government's access to personal health information, 328–30; form and content of records, 303–4, 306–8; health records used in legal proceedings, 327–28; overview, 301–2; state open meeting and public records laws, 330–31

Health Information Technology for Economic and Clinical Health Act, 304, 325; privacy breaches and, 323–24

Health insurance: Blue Cross and Blue Shield plans, 41–42; history of, 40

Health insurance exchanges, 64

Health Insurance Portability and Accountability Act (HIPAA), 130, 312, 318, 319, 325; duty to warn third parties, health information, and, 312; health information defined by, 302; law enforcement and, 329–30; legacy of, 301; patient's right to access under, 309–11; privacy regulations, 316–17; state and federal confidentiality laws and, 320; telemedicine services and, 326; uses and disclosures of personal health information, 321–23

Health Maintenance Organization Act (1973), 45, 59

ABOUT THE AUTHOR

J. Stuart Showalter, JD, MFS, has spent most of his career dealing with health law issues. He has a law degree from Washington University in St. Louis, Missouri, and a master's degree in forensic science from George Washington University in Washington, DC. He served in the US Navy from 1972 to 1980 in various positions, including in-house counsel to a large Navy medical center, malpractice claims defense attorney, and counsel to the US Navy Surgeon General.

From 1980 to 1996, Mr. Showalter was vice president of the Catholic Health Association of the United States, headquartered in St. Louis. Thereafter, he was a partner in a St. Louis law firm, where he specialized in health law and corporate compliance until joining the Orlando Regional Health System as director of compliance in March 1998. He later served as compliance officer for a health system in Baton Rouge, Louisiana.

While in St. Louis, Mr. Showalter taught health law and public policy in the health administration program at Washington University School of Medicine, where he was twice named teacher of the year. He has also held teaching positions at St. Louis University, the University of Central Florida, San Diego State University, and, most recently, La Sierra University.

Mr. Showalter is now semiretired and lives in San Diego, California. He is a contributing editor to the Healthcare Financial Management Association's *Legal and Regulatory Forum*.